Development and Manufacture of Yogurt and Other Functional Dairy Products

Edited by

Fatih Yildiz

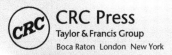

CRC Press
Taylor & Francis Group
Boca Raton London New York

CRC Press is an imprint of the
Taylor & Francis Group, an **informa** business

CRC Press
Taylor & Francis Group
6000 Broken Sound Parkway NW, Suite 300
Boca Raton, FL 33487-2742

First issued in paperback 2019

© 2010 by Taylor and Francis Group, LLC
CRC Press is an imprint of Taylor & Francis Group, an Informa business

No claim to original U.S. Government works

ISBN-13: 978-1-4200-8207-4 (hbk)
ISBN-13: 978-0-367-38483-8 (pbk)

Library of Congress Cataloging-in-Publication Data

Development and manufacture of yogurt and other functional dairy products / editor, Fatih Yildiz.
    p. ; cm.
Includes bibliographical references and index.
ISBN 978-1-4200-8207-4 (hardcover : alk. paper)
  1. Yogurt--Microbiology. 2. Dairy microbiology. 3. Fermentation. I. Yildiz, Fatih.
  [DNLM: 1. Yogurt--microbiology. 2. Dairy Products--microbiology. 3. Fermentation.
4. Foods, Specialized. 5. Nutritional Physiological Phenomena. QW 85 D489 2010]

QR121.D48 2010
641.3'7--dc22

2009031466

Visit the Taylor & Francis Web site at
http://www.taylorandfrancis.com

and the CRC Press Web site at
http://www.crcpress.com

Contents

Preface

Yogurt and related yogurt-like dairy beverages (ayran, kefir, and koumiss) are unique in taste and nutrition and are probably the first functional foods to be researched by the scientific community. They have a very long history of being in the homemade foods category and have many nutritional attributes. Yogurt holds the secrets behind good health and nutrition, which have not been completely understood even after 5000 years of consuming it. It is a perfect alternative to the junk and snack foods and beverages consumed today.

The Russian bacteriologist Ilya Metchnikoff was the first scientist to perform research on yogurt, yogurt beverages, and human longevity, which he did when he was the director of the Louis Pasteur Institute in Paris, France, from 1889 until his death in 1916. Mechnikoff received the Nobel Prize in 1908 for his work on phagocytosis in relation to wounds, diseases, immunity, and normal healthy life.

Yogurt products include plain yogurt, fruit yogurts, pasteurized and sterilized yogurts, dried yogurts, yogurt mixes and instant yogurt, acidophilus yogurt, liquid yogurt, frozen yogurts, and many others. Yogurt can be consumed as a complete lunch, breakfast, dinner, between-meal snack, as a beverage, or with many vegetable dishes, at any time of the day. Yogurt-related beverages include cacık and several other probiotic beverages.

During the past two decades, there has been renewed interest in the study and understanding of the nutritional and therapeutic aspects of dairy products; this book will enlarge our knowledge of these less-known aspects of fermented dairy products.

Beneficial effects attributed to yogurt and fermented dairy beverages include the anticarcinogenic and immunological properties of lactic acid bacteria (LAB), bone and gastrointestinal health, and many others.

The health benefits of cultured milk products with viable and nonviable bacteria are now well recognized, but there is still much confusion that needs to be solved.

This book will definitely be of great help to all those involved in the manufacture or study of milk and dairy products.

Fatih Yıldız

Acknowledgments

I would like to acknowledge and extend my heartfelt thanks to the following people who have made the completion of this book possible:

My friends and colleagues:

Prof. Dr. Celalettin Koçak of Ankara University
Prof. Dr. Barbaros Özer of Abant Izzet Baysal University
Prof. Dr. Candan Gürakan of Middle East Technical University
Prof. Dr. Theodoros H. Varzakas of the Technological Educational Institute
   of Kalamata

Thanks are due to the contributors of this book, that is, 20 scientists from 12 different universities, whose names and affiliations are given in this book.

Special thanks to Edmund Zottola, Professor Emeritus at the University of Minnesota, who helped me to understand the dairy industry.

Special thanks to my family and friends for their patience during the preparation of this book.

And finally, many thanks to Stephen Zollo, Kari Budyk and Rachael Panthier of Taylor & Francis for producing this book.

Editor

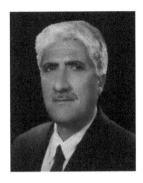

Fatih Yıldız received his BS degree from Atatürk University, Erzurum, Turkey, as an agricultural engineer. He also received a BS degree in biochemistry from the University of Wisconsin. Later he received his MS and PhD degrees in food biochemistry from the University of Maryland. He worked as a faculty member at the University of Maryland for five years. In 1980, Dr. Yıldız joined the Middle East Technical University (METU) Department of Chemical Engineering and was actively involved in the establishment of the food engineering, biochemistry, and biotechnology departments at that university. Dr. Yıldız also worked as a professor at the University of Minnesota, Department of Food Science and Nutrition. He has done research at the French National Institute for Agricultural Research (INRA), France, as a visiting professor in 1997. Additionally he has done research projects with FAO, UNIDO, UNICEF, and NATO as a project director.

Currently he is teaching and doing research at the Middle East Technical University, Food Engineering and Biotechnology Departments, Ankara, Turkey.

Dr. Yıldız has published more than 130 research and review papers in international and national journals as the major author. His papers have been cited by *Science Citation Index* many times. He has coauthored a book entitled *Minimally Processed and Refrigerated Fruits and Vegetables*, published by Chapman & Hall in 1994, which was then a new concept in the food industry.

His current research interests include health nutrition, and the safety attributes of the Mediterranean Diet. He is the editor of the first book on phytoestrogens, entitled *Phytoestrogens in Functional Foods* published by CRC Press.

Professor Yıldız is listed in *Who's Who in Turkey and Europe* and serves on numerous advisory committees of the Ministry of Health and Agriculture in Turkey. He is a member of 10 scientific and academic organizations in the United States, France, and Turkey.

Contributors

Neslihan Altay
Department of Food Engineering
Middle East Technical University
Ankara, Turkey

Ioannas S. Arvanitoyannis
School of Agricultural Sciences
University of Thessaly
Volos, Greece

Yahya Kemal Avşar
Department of Food Engineering
Mustafa Kemal University
Antakya-Hatay, Turkey

Bilkay Baştürk
Department of Immunology
Gazi University
Besevler, Ankara, Turkey

Eugenia Bezirtzoglou
Department of Food Science
    and Technology
Democritus University of Thrace
Orestiada, Greece

Aysun Cebeci
Department of Food Engineering
Middle East Technical University
Ankara, Turkey

Costas Chryssanthopoulos
Department of Physical Education and
    Sports Science
University of Athens
Athens, Greece

Meltem Yalinay Cirak
Department of Microbiology
    and Clinical Microbiology
Gazi University
Besevler, Ankara, Turkey

Annel K. Greene
Department of Animal and Veterinary
    Sciences
Clemson University
Clemson, South Carolina

G. Candan Gürakan
Department of Food Engineering
Middle East Technical University
Ankara, Turkey

Zeynep Guzel-Seydim
Department of Food Engineering
Suleyman Demirel University
Isparta, Turkey

Yonca Karagül-Yüceer
Department of Food Engineering
Çanakkale Onsekiz Mart University
Çanakkale, Turkey

Tarkan Karakan
Department of Gastroenterology
Gazi University
Ankara, Turkey

Hüseyin Avni Kırmacı
Department of Food Engineering
Harran University
Sanlııurfa, Turkey

Celalettin Koçak
Department of Dairy Technology
Ankara University
Ankara, Turkey

Tuğba Kök-Taş
Department of Food
    Engineering
Süleyman Demirel University
Isparta, Turkey

Maria Maridaki
Department of Physical Education and
    Sports Science
University of Athens
Athens, Greece

Barbaros Özer
Department of Food Engineering
Abant Izzet Baysal University
Golkoy, Bolu, Turkey

Theodoros H. Varzakas
Department of Food Technology
Technological Educational Institute
    of Kalamata
Kalamata, Greece

Fatih Yıldız
Department of Food Engineering and
    Biotechnology
Middle East Technical University
Ankara, Turkey

1 Overview of Yogurt and Other Fermented Dairy Products

Fatih Yıldız

CONTENTS

1.1 HISTORICAL PERSPECTIVES

Humans have evolved in close contact with Nature, and the first food that Nature provided for man was milk. Throughout most of the evolution of the human history, from 200,000 years BP (before present) up to 15,000 BP, the sole source of milk was from mother to newborn baby. In early times, when Nature failed to give milk to the child with a lactating mother, the baby either suckled another mother or died [1].

1

Then, as man domesticated animals, at first goat and sheep (about 13,000 BP) and later cow (9000 BP), milk from other mammals became available to provide essential nutrients. Since that time (13,000 BP), young and old, men and women, and all humans have been using milk as food [2].

The importance of milk to humans as food:

a. Domestication of animals has made it possible for humanity to have a secure source of milk all year round (Figure 1.1) [2]
b. Milk has contributed for the nutrition of humans of all ages, decreasing infant mortality and increasing well-being of mammalian infants [1]
c. Fermented milk consumption has increased adult human height, bone density, adult body mass, longevity, and adult brain volume (cm^3) over the last 13,000 years [3]

There is evidence of cultured milk products being produced as food for at least 8000 years. The earliest yogurts were probably spontaneously fermented by wild bacteria living on the goat skin bags carried by nomadic people. Today, many different countries claim yogurt as their own invention, yet there is no clear evidence as to where it was first discovered, and it may have been independently discovered several times [4].

The use of yogurt by mediaeval Turks is recorded in the books *Diwan Lughat al-Turk* by Mahmud Kashgari [5] and *Kutadgu Bilig* by Yusuf Has Hajib [6] written in the eleventh (1070 AD) century. In both texts the word "yogurt" is mentioned in different sections and its use by nomadic Turks is described. These two books are the earliest recorded information about yogurt. The first account of a European encounter with yogurt occurs in French clinical history: Francis I suffered from a severe diarrhea that no French doctor could cure. His ally Suleiman the Magnificent, an Ottoman sultan, sent a doctor, who allegedly cured the patient with yogurt [7].

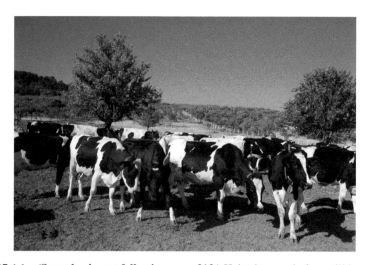

FIGURE 1.1   (See color insert following page 212.) Holstein cows before milking.

In 1908, Elie Metchnikov, Nobel Laureate for the discovery of phagocytic (cell-eating) cells, proposed in his book "The Prolongation of Life" [8] that the secret to longevity lies in maintaining healthy colon bacteria. He even named the bacteria responsible, *Lactobacillus bulgaricus* (LB), after the Bulgarians, whose health and longevity he attributed to the large quantities of yogurt they typically ate. While his conclusions were met with skepticism for many years, healthy gut bacteria are now decidedly back as probiotics.

1.2 YOGURT ETYMOLOGY AND SPELLING

The word is derived from the Turkish word *yoğurt* [9] and is related to *yoğurmak* "to knead" and *yoğun* "dense" or "thick" [10]. The letter ğ was traditionally rendered as "gh" in transliterations of Turkish, which used to be written in a variant of the Arabic alphabet until the introduction of the Latin alphabet in 1928. In older Turkish the letter denoted a voiced velar fricative |γ|, but this sound is elided between back vowels in modern Turkish, in which the word is pronounced (yoğurt, jogurt). Some eastern dialects retain the consonant in this position, and Turks in the Balkans pronounce the word with a hard /g/ [11].

1.3 YOGURT

Yogurt is made by introducing specific bacteria strains into milk, which is subsequently fermented under controlled temperatures (42–43°C) and environmental conditions (in fermentation tank), especially in industrial production (Figure 1.2). The bacteria ingest natural milk sugars and release lactic acid as a waste product. The increased acidity causes milk proteins to coagulate into a solid mass (curd) in a process called denaturation [12]. The increased acidity (pH = 4–5) also prevents the proliferation of potentially pathogenic bacteria. In most countries, to be named

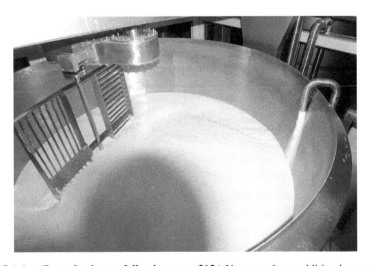

FIGURE 1.2   **(See color insert following page 212.)** Yogurt culture addition in a tank.

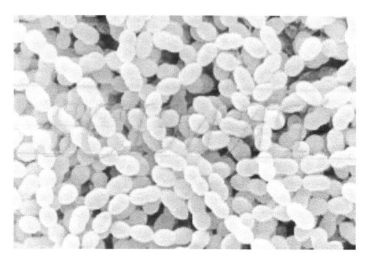

FIGURE 1.3   (See color insert following page 212.) *Streptococcus salivarius* subsp. *thermophilus.*

yogurt, the product must be made with the bacterial species *Streptococcus salivarius* subsp. *thermophilus* (ST) and *Lactobacillus delbrueckii* subsp. *bulgaricus* (Figures 1.3 through 1.5). Often these two are cocultured with other lactic acid bacteria for taste or health effects (see Chapter 6). These include *Lactobacillus acidophilus* (LA), *Lactobacillus casei*, and *Bifidobacterium* species. In the United States and in the European Union countries, a product may be called yogurt only if live bacteria are present in the final product. In the United States, nonpasteurized yogurt can be marketed as "live" or containing "live active culture." A small amount of live yogurt can be used to inoculate a new batch of yogurt, as the bacteria reproduce and multiply

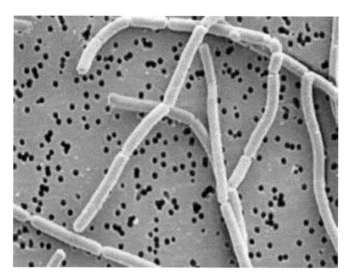

FIGURE 1.4   (See color insert following page 212.) *Lactobacillus delbrueckii* subsp. *bulgaricus.*

FIGURE 1.5 (See color insert following page 212.) *Lactobacillus delbrueckii* subsp. *bulgaricus* in coagulated milk.

during fermentation [13]. Pasteurized products, which have no living bacteria, may be called fermented milk product. When yogurt is pasteurized, even though its main aim is to kill harmful bacteria, it kills large amounts of essential bacteria too, such as *Acidophilus*, *Bifidus*, and *Lactobacillus rhamnosus*. Yogurt is a semisolid fermented milk product. Its popularity has grown and is now consumed in most parts of the world. Although the consistency, flavor, and aroma may vary from one region to another, the basic ingredients and manufacturing are essentially consistent [14]. Important parameters in yogurt manufacturing include ingredients, starter culture, and manufacturing methods (see Chapters 2 and 3).

1.3.1 YOGURT TYPES

a. *Set yogurt*: A solid set where the yogurt forms in a consumer container and is not disturbed (Figure 1.6).

b. *Stirred yogurt*: Yogurt is first made in a large container and then spooned or otherwise dispensed into secondary serving containers. The consistency of the "set" is broken and the texture is less firm than set yogurt. This is the most popular form of commercial yogurt.

c. *Drinking sweet yogurt*: Stirred yogurt to which additional milk and flavors are mixed in. Fruit or fruit syrups are added to taste. Milk is added and mixed to achieve the desired thickness. The shelf life of this product is 4–10 days, since the pH is raised by fresh milk addition. Some whey separation will occur and is natural [13].

d. *Fruit yogurt*: Fruit, fruit syrups, or pie filling can be added to the yogurt. They are placed on top, on bottom, or stirred into the yogurt (Figure 1.7) [12].

e. *Yogurt cheese*: It is a fresh cheese made by draining overnight by separating the whey. The flavor is similar to that of a sour cream with the texture of a soft cream cheese. A liter of yogurt will yield approximately 500 mL of

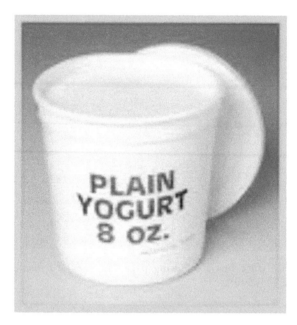

FIGURE 1.6   **(See color insert following page 212.)** Plain yogurt in consumer container.

cheese. Yogurt cheese has a shelf life of approximately 7–14 days when wrapped and placed in the refrigerator and kept at less than 4°C [15].
   f. *Frozen yogurt*: After manufacturing yougurt, it is frozen by batch or continuous freezers.
   g. *Dried yogurt* (Kurut in Turkey): Yogurt is sun dried for longer preservation.

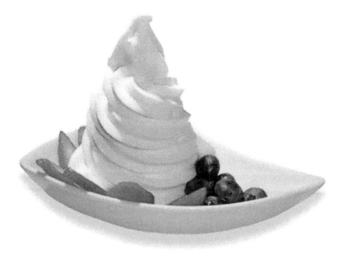

FIGURE 1.7   **(See color insert following page 212.)** Low fat frozen yogurt with fruits.

1.3.2 OTHER VARIANTS

Strained yogurts are types of yogurts that are strained through a cloth or paper filter, traditionally made of muslin, to remove the whey, giving a much thicker consistency, and a distinctive, slightly tangy taste. Some types are boiled in open vats first, so that the liquid content is reduced. The popular East Indian dessert, Mishti Dahi, is a variation of traditional Dahi, offers a thicker, more custard-like consistency, and is usually sweeter than Western yogurts [16].

Dadiah, or Dadih, is a traditional West Sumatran yogurt made from water buffalo milk. It is fermented in bamboo tubes [16].

Labneh is a strained yogurt used for sandwiches popular in Arab countries. Olive oil, cucumber slices, olives, and various green herbs may be added. It can be thickened further and rolled into balls, preserved in olive oil, and fermented for a few more weeks. It is sometimes used with onions, meat, and nuts as a stuffing for a variety of pies or kebabs [16].

Tarator and *Cacık* are popular cold soups made from yogurt, popular during summertime in Bulgaria, Republic of Macedonia, and Turkey. They are made with ayran, cucumbers, dill, salt, olive oil, and optionally garlic and ground walnuts [17].

Rahmjoghurt, a creamy yogurt with much higher milk fat content (10%) than most yogurts offered in English-speaking countries (Rahm is German for cream), is available in Germany and other countries [18].

Jameed is a yogurt that is salted and dried to preserve it. It is popular in Jordan.

Raita is a yogurt-based South Asian/Indian condiment, used as a sauce or dip. The yogurt is seasoned with cilantro (coriander), cumin, mint, cayenne pepper, and other herbs and spices. Vegetables such as cucumber and onions are mixed in. The mixture is served chilled. Raita has a cooling effect on the palate, which makes it a good foil for spicy Indian dishes [15].

Zabady is the yogurt made in Egypt. It is essentially famous in Ramadan fasting as it is thought to prevent feeling thirsty during fasting all day long [15].

Bihidasu, of the thicker variety of plain yogurt in Japan sold in 500 g containers, comes with a package of powdered sugar [15].

Sour cream is cultured cream and usually has a fat content of between 12% and 30%, depending on the required properties. The starter is similar to that used for cultured buttermilk. The cream after standardization is usually heated to 75–80°C and is homogenized at >13 MPa to improve the texture. Inoculation and fermentation conditions are also similar to those for cultured buttermilk, but the fermentation is stopped at an acidity of 0.6% [19].

Low-fat probiotic yogurt (commercial name Activia): Activia is a low-fat probiotic yogurt-like drink produced by a company, either a semisolid yogurt or a yogurt drink, and is sold in small and larger packages in more than 30 countries worldwide. Activia contains the probiotic bacterium *Bifidobacterium animalis*. Activia is available in plain, strawberry, raspberry, peach, mango, oatmeal, pear, walnut, coconut, vanilla, blueberry, prune, fig, pineapple, aloe vera, fibers, fruit of the forest, kiwi cereals, and rhubarb varieties, but not all varieties are available in every country [20].

Manufacturers claim that the "Bifidus Regularis" or "Bifidus Actiregularis" (both are brand names of *B. animalis*) helps digestive discomfort and irregularity [21].

Activia is in the category of functional foods designed to address digestive health. Such products typically contain a proprietary strain of probiotics and may also contain prebiotics.

1.3.3 INGREDIENTS

Although milk of various animals has been used for yogurt production in various parts of the world, most of the industrialized yogurt production uses cow's milk. Whole milk, partially skimmed milk, skim milk, or cream may be used. To ensure the development of the yogurt culture, the following criteria for the raw milk must be met:

- Low bacteria count
- Free from antibiotics, sanitizing chemicals, mastitis milk, colostrum, and rancid milk
- No contamination by bacteriophages

Other yogurt ingredients may include some or all of the following:

Other dairy products: Concentrated skim milk, nonfat dry milk, whey, and lactose. These products are often used to increase the nonfat solids content
Sweeteners: Glucose or sucrose, and high-intensity sweeteners (e.g., aspartame)
Stabilizers: Gelatin, carboxymethyl cellulose, locust bean guar, alginates, carrageenans, and whey protein concentrate
Flavors: Fruit preparations, including natural and artificial flavoring, and color [22]

1.3.4 STARTER CULTURE

The starter culture for most yogurt production is a symbiotic blend of *Str. salivarius* subsp. *thermophilus* and *L. delbrueckii* subsp. *bulgaricus*. Although they can grow independently, the rate of acid production is much higher when used together than either of the two organisms grown individually. ST grows faster and produces both acid and carbon dioxide. The formate and carbon dioxide produced stimulates LB growth. On the other hand, the proteolytic activity of LB produces stimulatory peptides and amino acids for use by ST. These microorganisms are ultimately responsible for the formation of typical yogurt flavor and texture. The yogurt mixture coagulates during fermentation due to the drop in pH. The streptococci are responsible for the initial pH drop of the yogurt mix to approximately 5. The lactobacilli are responsible for a further decrease to pH 4. The following fermentation products contribute to flavor [22]: lactic acid, acetaldehyde, acetic acid, and diacetyl (see Chapters 2 and 3 for details).

1.3.5 MANUFACTURING METHOD

Yogurt can be made from any source of milk of any fat content, but mostly fat-free milk yogurt, skim milk yogurt, and full-fat yogurt is made with cow's milk.

The milk is clarified and separated into cream and skim milk and then standardized to achieve the desired fat content. The various ingredients are then blended together in a mix tank equipped with a powder funnel and an agitation system. The mixture is then pasteurized using a continuous plate heat exchanger for 30 min at 85°C or 10 min at 95°C. These heat treatments, which are much more severe than fluid milk pasteurization, are necessary to achieve the following:

• Produce a relatively sterile and conducive environment for the starter culture
• Denature and coagulate whey proteins to enhance the viscosity and texture

The mix is then homogenized using high pressures of 2000–2500 psi. Besides thoroughly mixing the stabilizers and other ingredients, homogenization also prevents creaming and wheying off during incubation and storage. Stability, consistency, and body are enhanced by homogenization. Once the homogenized mix has cooled to an optimum growth temperature, the yogurt starter culture is added [23].

A ratio of 1:1, ST to LB, inoculation is added to the jacketed fermentation tank. A temperature of 43°C is maintained for 4–6 h under quiescent (no agitation) conditions (Figure 1.8). This temperature is a compromise between the optimums for the two microorganisms (ST 39°C; LB 45°C). The titratable acidity (TA) is carefully monitored until the TA is 0.85–0.90%. At this time the jacket is replaced with cool water and agitation begins, both of which stop the fermentation. The coagulated product is cooled to 5–22°C, depending on the product (Figure 1.9). Fruit and flavor may be incorporated at this time and then packaged. The product is now cooled and stored at refrigeration temperatures (5°C) to slow down the physical, chemical, and microbiological degradation (see Chapter 2). There are two types of plain yogurt manufacturing methods: stirred style yogurt and set style yogurt.

The above description is essentially the manufacturing procedures for stirred style. In set style, the yogurt is packaged immediately after inoculation with the

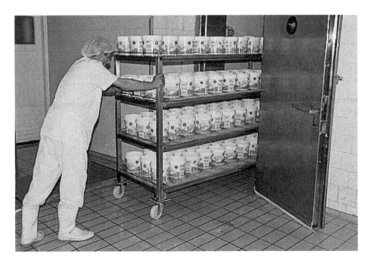

FIGURE 1.8   (See color insert following page 212.) Yogurt containers on the shelves of an incubation room at 42–43°C.

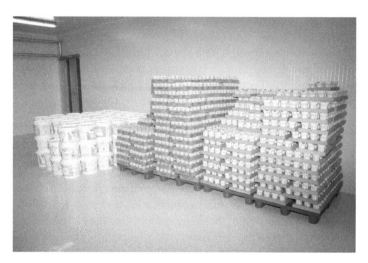

FIGURE 1.9   (See color insert following page 212.) Yogurt in cold storage room after incubation at 5–22°C.

starter and is incubated in the packages. Other yogurt products include fruit-on-the-bottom style: the fruit mixture is layered at the bottom followed by inoculated yogurt and incubation occurs in the sealed cups.

Soft-serve and hard pack frozen yogurt (Continental, French, and Swiss): stirred style yogurt with fruit preparation [24].

1.4   FERMENTED MILK DRINKS

Ayran is a yogurt-based, salty drink, popular in Turkey, Azerbaijan, Iranian Azerbaijan, Bulgaria, Republic of Macedonia, Kazakhstan, and Kyrgyzstan (Figure 1.10). It is made by mixing yogurt with water and adding salt. The same drink is known as "Dough" in Iran, "Tan" in Armenia, "Laban Ayran" in Syria and Lebanon, "Shenina" in Jordan, "Moru" in South India, and "Laban Arbil" in Iraq. A similar drink, doogh, is popular in the Middle East between Lebanon and Afghanistan; it differs from ayran by the addition of herbs, usually mint, and is carbonated, usually with mineral, water. *Ayran* or *airan* (from Turkish *ayran*) is a drink made of yogurt and water, popular in Turkey, Armenia, Azerbaijan, Iran, Lebanon, Bulgaria, and other parts of the Balkans, the Middle East, and Central Asia. It is similar to Armenian *tahn* and Iranian *doogh*, although doogh can be naturally carbonated. In Cyprus, it is referred to as *ayrani*. Ayran is a mixture of yogurt, water, and salt. It is thought to have originated as a way of preserving yogurt by adding salt. It can also be made with cucumber juice in place of some or all of the water, or flavored with garlic. It may be seasoned with black pepper, although this is uncommon in Bulgaria, where ayran is also often served without salt. Another recipe popular in some regions includes finely chopped mint leaves mixed into the ayran. In countries such as Bosnia and Herzegovina, extra salt is added to give the drink the flavor of salt water and is often consumed in large quantities at Turkish eateries (see Chapter 4) [25].

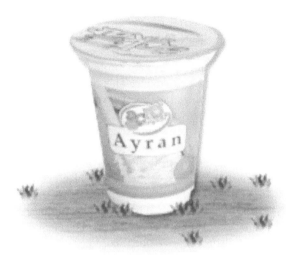

FIGURE 1.10   **(See color insert following page 212.)** Single serve ayran package.

Lassi is a yogurt-based beverage originally from the Indian subcontinent that is usually slightly salty or sweet. Lassi is a staple of Punjab; in some parts of the subcontinent, the sweet version may be commercially flavored with rosewater, mango, or other fruit juice to create a totally different drink. Salty lassi is usually flavored with ground, roasted cumin, and red chillies; this salty variation may also use buttermilk, and is interchangeably called Ghol (Bangladesh), Mattha (North India), Tak (Maharashtra), or Chaas (Gujarat). Lassi is also very widely drunk in Pakistan [15].

Kefir is a fermented milk drink that originated in the Caucasus. A related Central Asian Turco-Mongolian drink made from mare's milk is called kumis, or airag in Mongolia. Some American dairies have offered a drink called "kefir" for many years with fruit flavors but without carbonation or alcohol (see Chapter 5).

Sweetened yogurt drinks are the usual forms in the United States and United Kingdom containing fruit and added sweeteners, such as honey. These are typically called "drinking/drinkable yogurt" [26].

Cacık (IPA pronunciation: dʒɑːdʒik/) is a Turkish dish of seasoned, diluted yogurt, eaten throughout the former Ottoman world. In Greece it is called tzatziki. It is served cold in very small bowls, usually as a side dish or with ice cubes. Cacık is made of yogurt, salt, olive oil, crushed garlic, chopped cucumber, dill, mint, and lime juice, diluted with water to a low consistency, and garnished with sumac. Among these ingredients, olive oil, lime juice, and sumac are optional. Dill and mint (fresh or dried) may be used alternately. Cacık, when consumed as a meze, is prepared without water but follows the same recipe. Ground paprika may also be added when it is prepared as a meze. As a rarer recipe, when prepared with lettuce or carrots instead of cucumber, it is named *kış cacığı* (winter cacık). A similar side dish prepared in India is known as raita. Particularly popular in the state of Maharashtra, it is prepared with cucumbers, onions, tomatoes, and quite often, grated carrots. Unlike other versions, lime juice is not used in raita. Further differences in the Indian dish include heated oil, mustard seeds, or the other vegetables are given to the consistency of yogurt [25].

Acidophilus milk *Lactobacillus acidophilus* (LA) is one species in the genus *Lactobacillus*. It is sometimes used commercially together with *Str. salivarius* and *Lactobacillus delbrueckii* ssp. *bulgaricus* in the production of acidophilus-type yogurt. LA gets its name from *lacto-*, meaning milk, *-bacillus*, meaning rod-like in shape, and *acidophilus*, meaning acid-loving. This bacterium thrives in more acidic environments than most of the related microorganisms (pH 4–5 or lower) and grows best at 30°C. LA occurs naturally in the human and animal gastrointestinal (GI) tract, mouth, and vagina. LA ferments lactose into lactic acid, like many (but not all) lactic acid bacteria. Certain related species (known as heterofermentive) also produce ethanol, carbon dioxide, and acetic acid this way. LA itself (a homofermentative microorganism) produces only lactic acid. Like many bacteria, LA can be killed by excess heat, moisture, or direct sunlight. Some strains of LA may be considered probiotic or "friendly" bacteria. These types of healthy bacteria inhabit the intestines and vagina and protect against some unhealthy organisms. The breakdown of nutrients by LA produces lactic acid, hydrogen peroxide, and other by-products that make the environment hostile for undesired organisms. LA also tends to consume the nutrients many other microorganisms depend on, thus outcompeting possibly harmful bacteria in the digestive tract. During digestion, LA also assists in the production of niacin, folic acid, and pyridoxine. LA can assist in bile deconjugation, separating amino acids from bile acids, which can then be recycled by the body [27].

Some research has indicated that LA may provide additional health benefits, including improved GI function, a boosted immune system, and a decrease in the frequency of vaginal yeast infections. Some people report that LA provides relief from indigestion and diarrhea. A study found that feed supplemented with LA and fed to cattle resulted in a 61% reduction of *Escherichia coli* 0157:H7. Research has also indicated that LA may be helpful in reducing serum cholesterol levels [28].

Acidophilus milk is a traditional milk fermented with LA, which has been thought to have therapeutic benefits in the GI tract. Skim or whole milk may be used. The milk is heated to high temperature, for example, 95°C for 1 h, to reduce the microbial load and favor the slow-growing LA culture. Milk is inoculated at a level of 2–5% and incubated at 37°C until coagulated. Some acidophilus milk has an acidity as high as 1% lactic acid, but for therapeutic purposes 0.6–0.7% is more common [27].

Another variation has been the introduction of a sweet acidophilus milk, one in which the LA culture has been added but there has been no incubation. It is thought that the culture will reach the GI tract where its therapeutic effects will be realized, but the milk has no fermented qualities, thus delivering the benefits without the high acidity and flavour, considered undesirable by some people [29].

1.4.1 YOGURT BEVERAGES

Drinking yogurt is essentially stirred yogurt, which has a total solids content not exceeding 11% and which has undergone homogenization to further reduce the viscosity; flavoring and coloring are invariably added. Heat treatment may be applied to extend the storage life. High temperature short time (HTST) pasteurization with aseptic processing will give a shelf life of several weeks at 2–4°C, which ultra high temperature (UHT) processes with aseptic packaging will give a shelf life of several weeks at room temperature [26].

1.4.2 OTHER FERMENTED MILK BEVERAGES

Cultured buttermilk: This product was originally the fermented by-product of butter manufacture, but today it is more common to produce cultured buttermilks from skim or whole milk. The culture most frequently used is *Streptococcus lactis*, perhaps also spp. *cremoris*. Milk is usually heated to 95°C and cooled to 20–25°C before the addition of the starter culture. Starter is added at 1–2% and the fermentation is allowed to proceed for 16–20 h, to an acidity of 0.9% lactic acid. This product is frequently used as an ingredient in the baking industry, in addition to being packaged for sale in the retail trade [30].

Buttermilk is a fermented dairy product produced from cow's milk with a characteristically sour taste. The product is made in one of two ways. Originally, buttermilk was the liquid left over from churning butter from cream. In India, buttermilk (chaas) is known to be the liquid leftover after extracting butter from churned curd (dei). Today, this is called *traditional buttermilk*. On the other hand, artificially made buttermilk, also known as *cultured buttermilk*, is a product where lactic acid bacteria called *Str. lactis* have been added to milk. Whether traditional or cultured, the tartness of buttermilk is due to the presence of acid in the milk. The increased acidity is primarily due to lactic acid, a by-product, naturally produced by lactic acid bacteria while fermenting lactose, the primary sugar found in milk. As lactic acid is produced by the bacteria, the pH of the milk decreases and casein, the primary protein in milk, precipitates, causing the curdling or clabbering of milk (Figures 1.11 and 1.12). This process makes buttermilk thicker than plain milk. While both traditional and cultured buttermilk contain lactic acid, traditional buttermilk tends to be thinner, whereas cultured buttermilk is much thicker [31].

Koumiss (*Kumis*) (Turkish:kımız) is a fermented dairy product traditionally made from mare's milk. The drink remains important to the people of the Central Asian steppes, including the Turks, Bashkirs, Kazakhs, Kyrgyz, Mongols, Yakuts, and Uzbeks (see Chapter 5).

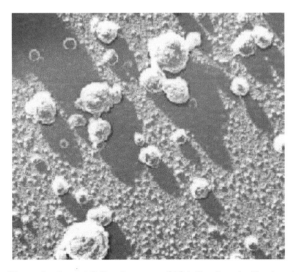

FIGURE 1.11 **(See color insert following page 212.)** Casein micelles in milk.

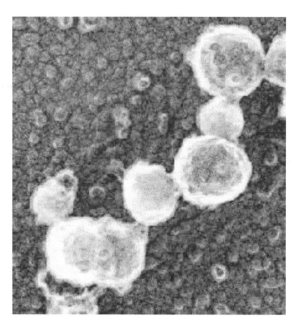

FIGURE 1.12 (**See color insert following page 212.**) Casein micelles form chains in yogurt before coagulation.

Koumiss is a dairy product similar to kefir, but is produced from a liquid starter culture, in contrast to the solid kefir "grains." Because mare's milk contains more sugars than the cow's or goat's milk fermented into kefir, koumiss has a higher, though still mild, alcohol content.

Even in the areas of the world where koumiss is popular today, mare's milk remains a very limited commodity. Industrial-scale production of koumiss therefore generally uses cow's milk, which is richer in fat and protein but lower in lactose than the milk from a horse. Before fermentation, the cow's milk is fortified in one of several ways. Sucrose may be added, to allow a comparable fermentation. Another technique adds modified whey in order to better approximate the composition of mare's milk (see Chapter 5).

Many of these have developed in regional areas and, depending on the starter organisms used, have various flavors, textures, and components from the fermentation process, such as gas or ethanol.

1.5 NUTRIENT CONTRIBUTION OF FERMENTED MILK IN HUMAN DIET

Milk is a natural source of 15 essential nutrients. These nutrients include proteins; vitamins: A, B_6, B_{12}, thiamine, riboflavin, niacin, folic acid, and pantothenic acid; and minerals: calcium, potassium, zinc, selenium, phosphorus, and magnesium. In addition, vitamin D if it is fortified should be mentioned. Milk is also an effective thirst quencher [32] (Table 1.1).

TABLE 1.1

Basic Nutritional Contribution of Fermented Dairy Products to Human Diet

a. Source of Ca, B_{12}, and riboflavin

b. Live and active cultures facilitate the digestion of milk

c. Milk proteins and minerals help children and babies to grow

d. Bone density and strength increase, which build and maintain strong bones

e. Good bacteria keep the bad bacteria away from the human digestive system

f. High-quality proteins maintain muscles

g. Flavor, texture, and taste are satisfying and give fullness

It is common knowledge that milk, yogurt, and cheese are great sources of calcium, but they also have many other nutrients. The contribution of their nutrients to the overall quality of the average diet is substantial. The various nutrients provided by milk products are given in Table 1.2 [33].

An American study [35] (n = 18,000) evaluated the impact of milk products on nutrient intakes in the United States. Intakes of all micronutrients examined, with the exception of vitamin C (of which milk products are not a source), were higher with increasing quartiles of total intakes of milk and milk products. Those who met or surpassed the "adequate intake" for calcium consumed 1.8 more servings of total milk products, 1.4 more servings of milk, and 0.4 more servings of cheese than those who did not. Individuals who got their calcium from sources other than milk products failed to meet the nutrient profile of those who consumed milk products. In addition to more calcium, higher intakes of milk and milk products were associated with

TABLE 1.2

Percentage Nutrient Contribution of Dairy Products to U.S. and Canada Populations

- 72% of the calcium
- 60% of the vitamin D (if the milk is fortified with vitamin D)
- 29% of the phosphorus
- 30% of the riboflavin
- 23% of the vitamin A
- 31% of the vitamin B_{12}
- 20% of the protein
- 17% of the potassium
- 18% of the zinc
- 15% of the magnesium
- 18% of the fat
- But a mere 13% of the calories [34]

Sources: Adapted from Refs. [33–36].

significantly higher intakes of magnesium, potassium, zinc, iron, vitamin A, riboflavin, and folate, suggesting that individuals who choose milk products make better food choices in general [36].

Choosing a variety of milk products also contributes significantly to the nutrient profile. Women who consumed an additional daily serving of milk products improved the nutrient quality of their diet, and those who also consumed an additional type of fermented milk products improved it even more [37].

1.5.1 FERMENTED MILK PRODUCTS FOR BABIES AND CHILDREN

Since babies are not supposed to have cow's milk before the age of one, is it okay to feed them dairy products, such as yogurt or cheese? After 6–9 months of age, dairy products such as yogurt and cheese can make an important contribution to a baby's diet. Dairy products contain protein and calcium, as well as several important vitamins.

Yogurt is a perfect baby food due to its smooth texture and rich tangy flavor. Small cubes of soft cheese are a great finger food for older babies.

If you have a family history of allergies and/or asthma it would be wise to wait until your baby is older to introduce cow's milk in hopes of avoiding an allergic response.

Note: Babies are not supposed to be given cow's milk until at least the age of one. Cow's milk is higher in protein than mothers' milk or formula, and can stress their kidneys and cause intestinal bleeding. This is because a baby's digestive system is still immature and has not yet totally developed. By the age of one, a baby's system has matured enough that cow's milk can now become the primary source of milk.

The Institute of Medicine released a report listing the requirements for daily calcium intake. How much calcium a person needs to maintain good health varies by age group. Recommendations from the report are shown in Table 1.3 [38].

TABLE 1.3

Daily Calcium Requirements and Dairy Products in the Human Life Cycle

Age Group	Amount of Calcium to Consume Daily (mg)	Fluid Milk (mL) to be Consumed/Day to Meet 100% Ca Requirement	Yogurt (g) to be Consumed/Day to Meet 100% Ca Requirement	Soft Cheese (g) to be Consumed/Day to Meet 100% Ca Requirement
0–6 months	400			
6–12 months	600	530	490	120
1–5 years	800	700	650	160
6–10 years	1200	1060	990	250
11–24 years	1200–1500	1060–1330 g/day	990–1240	250–305
19–50 years	1000	885	820	200
51–70+ years	1500	1330	1240	305

Source: Virginia, A. Stallings and Christine, L. Taylor (Eds), Nutrition standards and meal requirements for National School Lunch and Breakfast Programs: Phase I. Proposed Approach for Recommending Revisions, Report, Food and Nutrition Board (FNB) Institute of Medicine (IOM), p. 192, 2008.

In addition, pregnant and nursing women need between 1200 and 1500 mg of calcium daily [38].

1.5.2 FUNCTIONAL DAIRY INGREDIENTS

Milk is a very complex food system. Its physiological bioactivity is essential for neonatal growth and development, providing protection against disease and infection. Cow's milk is composed of 3.6% protein, 4.1% fat, 5.0% sugar, 0.7% ash, and 86.6% water. To be more specific, milk consists of approximately nine major protein types and eight different types of lipids and lactose, plus nine vitamins and five minerals. These components perform specific functions in the body, both individually and in combination, resulting in real health benefits throughout life. Table 1.4 lists some of the functional dairy components [39].

TABLE 1.4
List of Functional Milk Components (Ingredients)

1. α-Lactalbumin
2. β-Lactoglobulin [40]
3. Bovine serum albumin [41]
4. Immunoglobulins and immune system components [42]
   - Cytokines
   - Neutrophils
   - T-lymphocytes
   - Nucleotides
5. Lactoferrin [42]
6. Lactoferricin [42]
7. Lactoperoxidase [43]
8. Lysozyme [43]
9. Biotin-binding protein
10. Epidermal growth factor
11. Fibroblast growth factor
12. Riboflavin-binding protein
13. Vitamin B_{12}-binding protein
14. Whey protein peptides include
    - Casein macropeptide [44]
    - α-Lactorphin [44]
    - β-Lactorphin [44]
15. Lipids include
    - Conjugated linoleic acid (CLA) [45]
    - Sphingomyelin [45]
    - Milk fat globule membrane
    - Butyric acid
    - Arachidonic acid

---

continued

TABLE 1.4   (continued)

16. Hormones
    - Pituitary hormones
    - Steroid hormones
    - Leptin
    - Thyroid hormones
17. Carbohydrates
    - Oligosaccharides
    - Mucins
    - Lactose

1.6   HEALTH BENEFITS OF FERMENTED DAIRY PRODUCTS

Milk is a complex physiological liquid that simultaneously provides nutrients and bioactive components that facilitate the successful postnatal adaptation of the newborn infant by stimulating cellular growth and digestive maturation, the establishment of symbiotic microflora, and the development of gut-associated lymphoid tissues. The number, the potency, and the importance of bioactive compounds in milk and especially in fermented milk products are probably greater than previously thought. They include certain vitamins, specific proteins, bioactive peptides, oligosaccharides, and organic (including fatty) acids. Some of them are normal milk components, and others emerge during digestive or fermentation processes (Table 1.4). Fermented dairy products and probiotic bacteria decrease the absorption of cholesterol [28]. Whey proteins, medium-chain fatty acids, and in particular calcium and other minerals may contribute to the beneficial effect of dairy food on body fat and body mass. There has been growing evidence of the role that dairy proteins play in the regulation of satiety, food intake, and obesity-related metabolic disorders. Milk proteins, peptides, probiotic lactic acid bacteria, calcium, and other minerals can significantly reduce blood pressure. Milk fat contains a number of components having functional properties. Sphingolipids and their active metabolites may exert antimicrobial effects either directly or upon digestion. A large body of scientific research indicated that the consumption of the recommended level of milk and fermented dairy products, as part of a healthy diet, can contribute and reduce the risk of many diseases [46]. Table 1.5 summarizes some of these diseases on which research has been done.

Fermented dairy products include probiotics that contain sufficient levels of certain live and active cultures, which can help to improve the balance of "beneficial" versus "undesirable" bacteria in the intestinal tract. In addition to promoting intestinal health, research on fermented dairy products suggests that these products may have an impact on the modulation of the immune system. "Scientific researchers are investigating the use of fermented dairy products to help improve immune function in the body while simultaneously providing a defense system against harmful toxins and carcinogens" (see Chapter 11).

TABLE 1.5

List of Diseases that have been Clinically Investigated Regarding Whether Risk of them is Reduced by Intake of Milk and Dairy Products

1. GI system diseases
2. Cardiovascular system diseases
3. Musculoskeletal system diseases
4. Urogenital system diseases
5. Dermatology
6. Immune system diseases
7. Allergy
8. Nervous system diseases
9. Cognitive system diseases
10. Weight control, obesity
11. Aging
12. Nutrigenomics of fermented dairy foods
13. Dental health

While the past several years have seen a growing awareness of the health-promoting actions of fermented dairy products, their potential role in helping to prevent chronic diseases and intestinal disorders is now being studied more frequently by scientists. According to a recent study, "Research suggests that several nonnutrient yogurt properties, such as sphingolipids, conjugated linoleic acid and butyric acid may play a role as anti-cancer agents" [47].

Another emerging area of probiotics is their positive effect on food allergies in children. "Recent studies in infants have shown that probiotics can modify the response to potentially harmful antigens (substances that induce allergies), as well as reduce their allergenic potential" [48].

A good example of functional foods is fermented dairy products. "Many organized Symposiums are particularly encouraging because the scientific research supports the role of yogurt and other fermented dairy products as functional foods and suggests an emerging role for their future, in enhancing the immune system and in disease prevention." "It is a good, and in some cases an excellent, source of nutrients such as calcium, protein and potassium" [49].

1. *Dental (oral) health*: It is known that calcium in milk helps build strong teeth, but few know that cheese is an important ally against tooth decay, helping to prevent both coronal and root cavities [50]. Plaque bacteria that stick to the teeth use sugary foods to produce organic acids that attack the teeth, causing tooth-mineral loss. Calcium from milk products (particularly in cheese) and milk protein help restore lost tooth minerals. The calcium and phosphate in cheese are absorbed into the plaque, helping to prevent cavities. Cheese also increases the secretion of saliva, not just while eating it but for a good 5 minutes thereafter and alters its composition, neutralizing both plaque pH and acids, and increasing the clearance of food from the mouth [51]. For maximum protection, cheese should be eaten by itself, at the end of

a meal. In addition, milk protein prevents bacteria from collecting in the mouth and modifies dental plaque, thereby reducing cavities [52]. Finally, milk fat coats the teeth, decreasing the amount of fermentable carbohydrates retained in the mouth and preventing acid from penetrating the teeth [52]. One study conducted with children aged 3–6 years in day care centers evaluated the ability of milk containing *L. rhamnosus* GG to reduce the incidence of dental caries. Only a subset of the study group, children aged 3–4 years, showed any statistically significant reduction in dental caries incidence. Other studies have documented that other probiotics, for example, *Lactobacillus reuteri* or *B. animalis* DN173 010, can reduce salivary levels of cariogenic *Streptococcus mutans* in young adults [50,52].

2. *Hypertension*: About 50–60 million (~22%) people in the United States are estimated to have hypertension, or elevated blood pressure, and are therefore at greater risk of heart disease and stroke [53]. Antihypertensive effects have been documented in animal models and in mildly hypertensive adults for three compounds derived from the growth of certain lactobacilli: (1) fermented milk containing two tripeptides derived from the proteolytic action of *Lactobacillus helveticus* on casein in milk; (2) bacterial cell wall components from cell extracts of lactobacilli; and (3) fermented milk containing fermentation-derived γ-amino butyric acid. Systolic blood pressure was decreased in the order of 10–20 mm Hg. These results suggest that consumption of certain lactobacilli, or products made from them, may reduce blood pressure in mildly hypertensive people. Viability of the *Lactobacillus* is not required for the effect. Such fermentation-derived, but nonprobiotic, products have been developed in Japan [a peptide, Lactotripeptide (Ameal S®)] and in Europe (Evolus®), but these products have not been approved by FOSHU or EFSA [54]. The Panel notes that Evolus products, which provide daily doses of 5 mg tripeptides as recommended by the applicant for the claimed effect, have not been tested with regard to their effect on arterial stiffness. On the basis of the data presented, the Panel concluded that a cause-and-effect relationship has not been established between the consumption of *L. helveticus* fermented Evolus low-fat milk products and the reduction of arterial stiffness in mildly hypertensive subjects [54]. The fermented milk drink Evolus helps to control blood pressure and the effect is based on peptides from milk protein. These bioactive peptides are produced by fermenting milk casein with certain lactic acid bacteria. *L. helveticus* bacterium splits casein to the ile–pro–pro and val–pro–pro tripeptides that help to control blood pressure. Fermentation is a normal dairy process, and the *L. helveticus* bacterium is generally used in cheese-making. The effect of Evolus in helping to control blood pressure has been documented in several clinical trials [55].

The Dietary Approaches to Stop Hypertension (DASH) study assessed the effects of dietary patterns on blood pressure and found that adults who consumed a diet high in fruits and vegetables (8–10 servings/day) had lower blood pressure than those who did not [56]. However, the addition of three servings of milk products to a diet rich in fruits and vegetables doubled the blood pressure-lowering effect—enough to treat mild hypertension and prevent it in those with normal blood pressure. The DASH diet—rich in milk products, fruits, and vegetables and low in fat—lowers blood pressure in men and women, regardless of age. Reductions in blood pressure of the magnitude achieved by the DASH diet could translate into a 15% reduction in coronary heart disease and a 27% reduction in stroke [53]. The diet also lowers serum homocysteine levels, an independent risk factor for heart disease [57], as well as total and low-density lipoproteins (LDL) cholesterol [56]. In their guidelines for the year 2000, the American Heart Association recommended the DASH diet for heart health [57].

3. *Cancer:* In general, cancer is caused by mutation or activation of abnormal genes that control cell growth and division. (A substance that causes a mistake in genes is known as a mutagen.) Most of these abnormal cells do not result in cancer since normal cells usually out-compete abnormal ones. Also, the immune system recognizes and destroys most abnormal cells [58]. Many processes or exposures can increase the occurrence of abnormal cells. Precautions that minimize these exposures decrease the risk of cancer. Among the many potentially risky exposures are chemical exposures. Cancer-causing chemicals (carcinogens) can be ingested or generated by metabolic activity of microbes that live in the GI tract. It has been hypothesized [59] that probiotic cultures might decrease the exposure to chemical carcinogens by (a) detoxifying ingested carcinogens, (b) altering the environment of the intestine and thereby decreasing populations or metabolic activities of bacteria that may generate carcinogenic compounds, (c) producing metabolic products (e.g., butyrate), which improve a cell's ability to die when it should die (a process known as apoptosis or programmed cell death), (d) producing compounds that inhibit the growth of tumor cells, or (f) stimulating the immune system to better defend against cancer cell proliferation.

Research suggests [60] that the consumption of probiotic cultures may decrease cancer risk. Researchers testing the effect of the consumption of fermented milks, probiotic bacteria, components of bacteria, or extracts of bacteria have found

- A reduction in the incidence of chemically induced tumors in rats
- A reduction of the activity of fecal enzymes (β-glucuronidase, azoreductase, nitroreductase, and 7-α-dehydrogenase) postulated to play a role in colon cancer in human and animal subjects
- Degradation of nitrosamines
- A weakening of mutagenic activity of substances tested in the laboratory
- Prevention of damage to DNA in certain colonic cells
- *In vitro* binding of mutagens by cell wall components of probiotic bacteria
- Enhancement of immune system functioning

Taken together, these results suggest that probiotic cultures may positively influence the GI environment to decrease the risk of cancer. However, cancer reduction must be demonstrated in humans to confirm the significance of these observations. The impact of consumption of milk fermented by *L. casei* strain Shirota on recurrence of superficial bladder cancer was tested [61]. The recurrence-free period for the *Lactobacillus*-consuming group was found to be almost twice as long as the control group. In another study, this same strain was found to decrease atypical recurrent polyps in subjects with previous history of colonic polyp [62]. The EU-sponsored Synbiotics and Cancer Prevention in Humans project tested a synbiotic (oligofructose plus *L. rhamnosus* GG and *Bifidobacterium lactis* Bb12) in patients at risk for colonic polyps and looked at intermediate end points that can be used as biomarkers of colon cancer risk. This study found that the synbiotic decreased uncontrolled growth of intestinal cells. These results must still be considered preliminary, but are encouraging that impacting the colonic environment may improve cancer occurrence [63].

Breast cancer: Finnish researchers were among the first to suggest that milk drinkers have a significantly lower risk of developing breast cancer [64]. More recently, the Norwegian Women and Cancer Study of 48,844 premenopausal women found that those who drank milk during both childhood and adulthood had a substantially reduced risk of breast cancer [65]. And the more milk, the better. Compared to those who drank little or no milk, moderate milk drinkers were shown to have one quarter the risk of breast cancer, while heavy milk drinkers had half [66]. These findings may be due in part to the conjugated linoleic acid (CLA) content of milk. CLA, a class of fatty acids found mainly in milk fat, slows the development and growth of mammary tumors in animals [66], and it appears to have similar effects in women. Postmenopausal women with the highest intake of CLA-rich foods, particularly cheese, had higher levels of CLA in their blood, and more importantly, at least a 70% lower risk of breast cancer [67]. Questions about the impact of milk products on breast cancer risk remain, in part because the assessment of dietary factors in relation to cancer risk is notoriously difficult and subject to bias [68].

Colon cancer: The third most common cause of cancer death in United States, colon cancer owes more to environmental and lifestyle factors than to genetics. A pooled analysis of 10 prospective cohort studies in five countries has shown that higher consumption of milk and calcium is associated with a lower risk of colorectal cancer [69]. And it does not take that much milk. These studies followed the milk product consumption habits of 534,536 individuals, among whom 4992 new cases of colorectal cancer were diagnosed between 6 and 16 years of follow-up. The data showed that those who drank at least one glass of milk (250 mL) per day were 15% less likely to develop colorectal cancer than those who drank little or no (<70 mL/day) milk (P_{trend} < 0.001) [69]. Moreover, each 500 mL per day increase in milk intake (about two glasses) was associated with a 12% reduced rate of colorectal cancer risk. The inverse association between milk intake and colorectal cancer risk was limited to cancers of the distal colon and rectum [69]. On the other hand, cheese and yogurt consumption had little impact, possibly because people ate much less of them [69]. The authors also measured the independent effects of calcium and vitamin D intake and found that the relative risk was lowest (RR = 0.74) for persons in the highest category of both total calcium and total vitamin D intake compared with the lowest category of intake for both nutrients [69]. A randomized trial of 803 individuals has shown that calcium supplementation and vitamin D status appear to act in synergy to reduce the risk of colorectal adenoma recurrence [70].

Furthermore, a recent study of the overall relationship between diet and colorectal cancer on 60,000 women found that consumption of high-fat milk products was linked to a reduced risk of colon cancer, even after adjusting for calcium intake [71].

Protection against cancer: Dairy foods (and/or calcium) appear to be protective against colonic polyps and the risk of colorectal cancer. CLA found in milk fat, identified as a potent cancer inhibitor, reduces breast cancer risk in adult women [72,67].

4. *The role of fermented milk products in weight management*: Increased intake of milk products can help one lose weight where it counts—around the middle. Epidemiological studies suggest that, over time, adults [73–75] and children [76,77] who consume a low-calcium or low-milk-product diet gain more weight and more body fat than those with higher intakes. Dietary calcium markedly accelerates the burning of fat for energy (lipolysis) and helps prevent the conversion of excess carbohydrates to fat (lipogenesis), resulting in less fat storage [78].

In research studies [79,80] of both mice and human subjects, calcium from milk and milk products was substantially more effective (from 50% to 100%) than calcium supplements in reducing both body fat and body weight, particularly for those on a calorie-reduced diet [81]. In a 24-week trial, 32 obese but otherwise healthy adults were randomized to diets different in milk product intake and designed to promote a 0.5 kg weight loss per week [75]. Only those in the high-milk-product group (1200 mg of calcium, including three servings of milk products/day) had significant decreases in total body fat, trunk fat, and blood pressure, and an increase in lean muscle mass [77]. In another similarly designed trial, researchers followed 105 overweight/obese adults on calorie-restricted diets over a 12-week period.

Individuals on the high-milk-product diet (three servings of milk products, ~1400 mg of calcium/day) [79] experienced an almost two-fold greater decrease in fat loss, trunk fat loss, and waist circumference than those on the low-calcium (~600 mg/day) or high-calcium (~1400 mg/day) diets [79]. The high-milk-product diet was associated with the greatest weight loss and the greatest increase in percentage of lean tissue [82]. Other researchers [83] had similar findings with their 16-week, randomized, controlled trial of three weight-reduction diets. Outpatients on the 800-calorie milk and yogurt-only diet lost 11.2 kg. Those on a standard 800-calorie control diet lost less than 3 kg, whereas those on a 1300-calorie diet, consisting of milk and yogurt plus one other food daily, lost almost three times more: 8.2 kg [83].

5. *Osteoporosis*: Osteoporosis affects one in every four women and one in eight men over the age of 50, that is, approximately 200 million people worldwide; an estimated 75 million people in Europe, United States, and Japan have osteoporosis. That number could be cut in half if adequate intakes of calcium and vitamin D were assured [84]. Adequate calcium maximizes peak bone mass achieved by the time we reach our twenties and minimizes age-related bone loss later in life [84]. Children who do not drink milk may fail to reach their genetic potential for peak bone mass, making them more vulnerable to osteoporotic fractures as adults [85].

Unlike the short-term benefits of calcium supplements [86], dairy intake during childhood has demonstrated persistent, long-term benefits to bone [87,88]. In fact, data from the National Health and Nutrition Examination Survey (NHANES) III Study ($n = 3251$ women) indicate that among women aged 20–49 years, bone mineral content was significantly lower in those with low milk intake in childhood and adolescence. Women aged 50+ years who drank less than one serving of milk per week during childhood doubled their risk of hip fracture compared to those who drank at least one serving of milk per day [89]. Studies have also shown that along with adequate calcium and vitamin D, higher intakes of protein are associated with significant gains in bone mineral density in elderly men and women [90,91]. In addition to calcium, milk provides protein, phosphorus, vitamins A and D, zinc, and magnesium—bone-building nutrients that are important for long-term bone health [92].

Protection against osteoporosis: Avoidance of dairy foods is most likely an important factor in the increased osteoporosis risk observed in individuals who are, or simply believe themselves to be, lactose intolerant [85].

6. *Insulin resistance syndrome*: Insulin resistance syndrome (IRS) is a combination of at least two interrelated conditions, including obesity, impaired glucose metabolism, hypertension, low high-density lipoproteins (HDL) cholesterol, and high triglyceride concentrations. Estimated to affect approximately 25% of the adult population, IRS interferes with the body's ability to control blood sugar, thereby increasing the risk of type 2 diabetes and cardiovascular disease. Overweight individuals are most vulnerable to IRS. The *Coronary Artery Risk Development in Young Adults* (CARDIA) Study followed 3157 adults aged 18–30 years over a 10-year period [93]. Overweight subjects (i.e., body mass index ≥25) who consumed less than 1.5 servings of milk products per day tripled their risk of developing IRS, compared with those who consumed at least five servings per day [93]. Each daily serving of milk or a milk product (regular or low fat) was associated with a 21% lower risk of IRS or one of its related components [93]. This was independent of other lifestyle factors, dietary variables, sex, age, and race. Moreover, contrary to established belief, consuming more milk products did not increase LDL cholesterol, a major risk factor in heart disease, but not a component of IRS [93]. In the *Bogalusa Heart Study*, young adults (18–38 years) with no risk factors for IRS were found to consume significantly more low-fat milk products than did those with three or more risk factors [94]. It is important to note that milk (GI = 33), yogurt (GI = 27), and cheese (GI = 0) are foods with a very low glycemic index, compared to the reference standard glucose (GI = 100) [95].

7. *Kidney stones*: Contrary to popular opinion, high calcium intake does not increase the risk of developing kidney stones. In fact, evidence to the contrary is compelling. While most stones are composed of calcium oxalate, it is the oxalate—not the calcium—that is chiefly responsible for stone formation. Since dietary calcium binds with oxalate in the intestine, thereby inhibiting its absorption, low calcium diets could actually increase the risk of stones. Studies have shown that increased consumption of calcium-rich milk products reduces the risk of kidney stones in both men [96] and women [97]. Calcium supplements have not demonstrated the same protection, perhaps because they are usually taken without food. Food is necessary if calcium is to bind with oxalate and prevent the formation of kidney stones.

High levels of oxalate in the urine are a risk factor for the development of kidney stones. Utilization of oxalate by intestinal microbes limits its absorption. A probiotic preparation that contained bacteria that were able to degrade oxalate *in vitro* was shown to reduce oxalate fecal excretion in six patients. These results suggest that manipulation of the gut flora with the right probiotic bacteria may have a positive impact on GI tract oxalate levels and may decrease oxalate absorption. These results are intriguing, but preliminary [98].

8. *Premenstrual syndrome (PMS)*: Calcium-rich milk products are the most effective dietary approach for alleviating the majority of mood and physical symptoms

associated with PMS. Women with PMS appear to suffer from abnormalities of calcium metabolism, suggesting that PMS is actually a manifestation of calcium deficiency that occurs following increases in estrogen during the menstrual cycle. In intervention studies, women with PMS in the high-calcium groups (1000– 1300 mg), either from supplements or from milk products, experienced significant improvements in mood, behavior, pain, and bloating during the menstrual cycle [99,100]. What's more, at least two studies indicate that women with PMS are prone to lower bone mass or increased risk of fractures, confirming the link between PMS and low calcium intake [99,100].

9. *Milk allergies*: Milk allergies are rare in adults and should not be confused with lactose intolerance. People who have a confirmed milk allergy and need to eliminate milk products from their diets should be careful to ensure that they obtain all the nutrients they need.

Less than 1% of adults and 3% of children have a clinically proven milk allergy, and children tend to outgrow a milk allergy by the age of 3 [101]. Because most children outgrow a milk allergy by the age of 3 and since milk is an important source of more than 15 essential nutrients, the sooner it can be reintroduced into your child's diet the better. There are a wide range of milk allergy symptoms that can involve the GI tract, respiratory tract, and skin complaints [102,103]. GI tract symptoms may present as abdominal pain, vomiting, or diarrhea and account for about half of presenting milk allergy symptoms. Respiratory tract symptoms can include nasal congestion, coughing, and wheezing, and typically account for about one-fifth to one-third of presenting symptoms. Skin complaints, such as rash, eczema, and hives, are present in about one-third to two-third of suffering individuals. Other symptoms such as mucus formation, colic, inner ear infections, migraines, and behavioral problems, sometimes associated with milk allergy, have not been substantiated. Infantile colic—prolonged episodes of irritability, fussiness, and crying—is often attributed to an allergy to cow's milk protein [104]. However, evidence fails to support that an allergy to cow's milk is the cause of colic. The exact cause of colic remains unknown. Lactose intolerance, also known as "lactose maldigestion," and milk allergy are not the same and should be distinguished since they require different treatments [105].

10. *Lactose intolerance*: Individuals with idiopathic gastric complaints often assume, inappropriately, that they are lactose intolerant. Most people—even those who consider themselves to be severely lactose intolerant—can comfortably consume at least 250 mL of milk (12 g lactose/day) [106–108]. The best defence against lactose intolerance is the consumption of milk products. The human colon adapts to continue exposure to lactose, thereby reducing symptoms [109–111].

1.6.1 THE FACTS ABOUT LACTOSE INTOLERANCE

Lactose is the principal carbohydrate in milk. Barring a rare congenital deficiency, virtually all mammals are born with high levels of lactase, a unique intestinal enzyme that breaks down lactose, enabling its absorption [107,111]. In individuals with lactose maldigestion, the lactose that is not completely digested in the small intestine passes into the large intestine, where it is fermented by colonic microflora, producing short-chain fatty acids and gases, principally hydrogen [111].

Testing: GI symptoms are often misdiagnosed as lactose intolerance by consumers and health professionals. The diagnosis can be confirmed by breath hydrogen analysis—an objective, noninvasive, inexpensive, and easily performed test, appropriate for both adults and children [108]. Symptoms of lactose intolerance are highly subjective and may or may not accompany lactose maldigestion [108].

Primary lactase deficiency: This deficiency can begin to develop after weaning. More common in certain racial or ethnic groups, including Africans, Asians, and Native Americans, it is relatively rare in Caucasians [108]. Offspring of Caucasians and African-Americans, however, have reduced prevalence of lactose maldigestion. The degree of lactose intolerance depends on a balance between the level of remaining lactase activity, the amount of lactose consumed, the adaptation of intestinal flora, and the irritability of the colon [108].

Secondary lactase deficiency: This deficiency is temporary. It is a response to GI factors that harm the intestinal mucosa (e.g., certain medical conditions, some medications, etc.). It can occur at any age and is reversible upon correction of the causative factor [112]. Testing for other underlying conditions (such as Crohn's disease, infectious diarrheal disease, and celiac disease) may be in order.

Colonic adaptation: According to breath hydrogen tests, newborns are unable to completely hydrolyze the lactose in mothers' milk. Nevertheless, infants thrive on lactose-containing breast milk and formula, perhaps due to colonic absorption of the fermentation by-products of undigested lactose [113]. Blinded, controlled, crossover studies have been conducted in adult lactose maldigesters to determine whether continuous lactose challenges could cause bacteria in the colon to metabolize lactose and reduce symptom severity.

Gradually increasing lactose intake significantly increased the ability of colonic bacteria to break it down [110]. Subjects experienced a decrease in breath hydrogen (suggesting that the lactose was being digested) and, concomitantly, a significant reduction in flatulence, one of the principal symptoms of lactose intolerance. Often, despite a continued inability to digest lactose, confirmed by breath hydrogen testing, subjects can still tolerate more and more lactose with minimal symptoms [111,112].

A recent 21-day intervention study assessed the effects of a dairy-rich diet in 14 African-American girls (11–15 years old). Confirmed lactose maldigesters, all were self-proclaimed nondrinkers of milk. The diet contained four servings of dairy products (primarily milk, some cheese, and yogurt), providing about 33 g of lactose and 1200 mg of calcium throughout the day. In addition to a significant decrease in breath hydrogen [113], GI symptoms were negligible during the milk challenges and throughout the study period, likely due to colonic adaptation [113]. The message is clear: Even individuals who are lactose intolerant can consume milk and milk products.

The amount of daily milk intake is important. Double-blind, controlled studies have demonstrated time and again that primary lactase deficiency should not be an obstacle to meeting calcium needs with milk and milk products [106,107,113,114]. Lactose intolerance is dose dependent. Most individuals with primary lactase deficiency—even adolescents and adults who perceive themselves to be severely lactose intolerant—can easily tolerate one cup (250 mL) of milk with a meal or two cups (500 mL) consumed in divided doses, for example with breakfast and dinner [115].

Women with limited lactose digestion can comfortably consume enough milk, yogurt, and cheese to provide up to 1500 mg of calcium/day [116]. Interestingly, increased tolerance to lactose appears to be a by-product of pregnancy [117,118], possibly because intestinal transit time slows down [119,120]. According to a research in lactose intolerance, people can recondition their digestive systems to accept dairy foods without discomfort [121]. Smaller quantities, taken with meals or other foods and spread throughout the day, increase lactose tolerance [121].

A significant portion of the population avoids milk products unnecessarily. Although the consequences may be similar, that is, avoidance of milk products, there is a difference between lactose intolerance and milk protein intolerance. It is not unusual for individuals with milk intolerance to experience placebo-induced symptoms in double-blind studies. Sometimes intolerance to milk has absolutely nothing to do with lactase deficiency or the inability to digest lactose [118,122]. Rather, it is affected by psychological factors or cultural attitudes. This phenomenon not only distorts clinical trial results, it exaggerates the prevalence of lactose intolerance and prevents too many people from the nutritional benefits and enjoyment that milk and milk products provide.

Reconditioning the gut [123]: Lactose-intolerant patients find their own unique levels of tolerance. The following tips will help the digestive process of these patients:

- **Start small**
  Start with less than 125 mL of milk, 2–3 times a day, and slowly increase the amount over a few weeks
- **Enjoy with other foods**
  Drink milk with fermented milk products or with other foods, not by itself
- **Watch the quantity**
  Avoid too much at one time. For some people, two glasses of milk could be a lactose overdose
- **Consume other dairy foods**
  Try firm cheeses that contain small amounts of lactose
  Try yogurt with active cultures
- **If all else fails**
  Try only fermented and active culture-containing dairy products

Its prevalence is grossly overestimated. Self-diagnosis is frequently inaccurate. Most lactose-intolerant individuals can consume milk products with minimal symptoms [108,109]. Lactose-intolerant individuals who consume fermented dairy milk products have fewer symptoms than those who consume regular dairy products. The colon adapts to regular exposure, increasing tolerance [124]. It has been documented scientifically that many lactose-intolerant individuals are better able to consume fermented dairy products, such as yogurt, with fewer symptoms than the same amount of unfermented milk. Yogurt was found to aid digestion of lactose because the lactic acid bacteria used to make yogurt deliver lactase to the small intestine, where it breaks down the lactose before it reaches the colon. In addition to yogurt starter bacteria, LA and bifidobacteria have been shown by several studies to improve digestion of lactose, although generally to a lesser extent than the yogurt starter cultures, LB and ST [125].

11. *Milk as brain food*: All people, especially pregnant women, children, and older adults, should be encouraged to consume recommended daily intakes of milk and milk products, the most bioavailable source of naturally occurring B_{12} in the diet [34].

The only natural source of vitamin B_{12} is food of animal origin. Foods rich in B_{12} include dairy, fish, meat, poultry, eggs, and shellfish. Inadequate intakes have been shown to be an important contributor to low vitamin B_{12} serum concentrations. Recent studies show that the vitamin B_{12} in meat, the major source of vitamin B_{12} for most individuals, may be less available than the vitamin B_{12} in dairy products [126]. Nutritional B_{12} deficiency can develop easily in strict vegetarians and those who follow macrobiotic diets (whole grain, soya-based diet) since they typically avoid the foods that are rich in B_{12}. There is little information on the prevalence of B_{12} deficiency in many countries. But a recent cross-sectional study of 1424 pregnant women in Canada (Newfoundland) found that 43.6% of women were B_{12} deficient or had marginal B_{12} levels [127]. We know that specific nutrient deficiencies can cause low birth weight and spina bifida, so it is also possible to envisage nutrient deficiencies affecting brain development in infants causing adverse effects. Reports of B_{12}-deficient infants (several of strict vegetarian mothers) showed anemia, irritability, anorexia, and failure to thrive, as well as marked developmental regression and poor brain growth [128,129]. The age of onset of symptoms may be important, as may be the duration of symptoms. Although the response to treatment in the short term is encouraging, complete neurologic recovery may never be complete [128]. In a review, only two of six reported cases had normal intellectual outcome at 9–11 years. Another study reporting on older children discovered that B_{12} deficiency early in life, due to macrobiotic diet consumption to the age of 6 years, may not be overcome in adolescence following moderate consumption of B_{12} after the age of 6 years [130]. Children on macrobiotic diets until the age of 6 with marginal vitamin B_{12} status were not able to overcome cognitive problems, due to the deficiency, regardless of moderate B_{12} intakes in later years [131]. In fact, previously "macrobiotic" subjects with low or normal vitamin B_{12} status scored significantly lower in intelligence tests measuring reasoning, capacity to solve complex problems, abstract thinking ability, and ability to learn [128]. These studies demonstrate the potential long-term risk in cognitive function that can occur in children who persistently avoid animal products due to medical reasons, beliefs, poverty, or eating habits during the formative years.

Vitamin B_{12} deficiency is estimated to affect 10–15% of people over age 60 [132]. Prevalence of B_{12} deficiency increases with age, especially over 65, and is frequently associated with Alzheimer's disease [133]. Neurologic complications are found in 75–90% of individuals with clinically apparent vitamin B_{12} deficiency. While low serum cobalamin levels are often found in apparently normal older subjects, a major worry of leaving vitamin B_{12} deficiency untreated is that it may lead to subtle deterioration in cognitive function [132].

Cognitive syndromes such as dementia, hallucination, frank psychosis, paranoia, depression, violent behavior, and changes in personality are not frequent, but vitamin

B_{12} deficiency should be considered as a possible cause of these symptoms [134]. In fact, vitamin B_{12} assay is part of the routine investigation of dementia in the United Kingdom. A study [135] of 1432 patients found a positive treatment effect of B_{12} among patients presenting with cognitive impairment. However, in the same study, none of the B_{12} deficiency-related dementia was reversed with the treatment of B_{12}.

12. *Milk and mucus*: Scientific evidence indicates that milk does not cause excess mucus production [136]. It has been suggested that milk and dairy products increase mucus production, and that avoiding milk will therefore alleviate respiratory symptoms, especially those commonly associated with colds. However, there is no scientific evidence to support this belief.

Studies have been conducted to investigate this hypothesis [137,138], but these have found no statistically significant association between milk intake and the symptoms of mucus production. Those subjects who believed that milk caused increased mucus production perceived themselves to have more respiratory symptoms after drinking milk [139], although they did not produce higher levels of mucus than non-believers. The symptoms experienced were related to difficulty in swallowing and the perceived thickness of the mucus and salivary secretions, rather than excessive mucus production. Furthermore, in a randomized, double-blind study using a milk drink and a soy placebo, a research [138] has demonstrated that the "milk–mucus effect" is not specific to cow's milk, but can be duplicated by a soy drink with similar sensory characteristics, for example, "mouthfeel." Milk does tend to leave a slightly filmy coating in the mouth or throat, but this is the result of milk's creamy texture and perhaps a little saliva production, not mucus. It has also been reported [140] that there is no basis for believing that, in the absence of an allergic response to milk, the intake of milk increases mucus production during upper respiratory tract infections. It has been common in folk medicine to advise asthmatics to avoid milk in the belief that its stimulation of mucus production can exacerbate asthma symptoms. However, it was [141] found no evidence that milk intake increased mucus congestion in adults with asthma. A more recent study by researchers [142] supports this assertion, demonstrating no association between the intake of dairy products and either the inducement of bronchoconstriction or changes in asthma symptoms in patients with asthma. Woods et al. actually warn against the unnecessary avoidance of dairy products in the diet of asthmatics, pointing out that asthmatics who use corticosteroids regularly require a good intake of calcium since they are particularly vulnerable to osteoporosis [142].

13. *Allergy*: Allergy is on the rise in industrialized nations. It is estimated that the incidence of asthma in the United States doubled between 1980 and 2000. Scientists have proposed a hypothesis known as the "hygiene hypothesis" to explain the rise in allergic conditions such as asthma and eczema [143]. This hypothesis is based on observations that lower allergy incidence is associated with environments that have greater numbers of microbes, such as day care centers, farms, or in homes with siblings or pets. Sanitary living environments and the consumption of processed foods have limited the number of microbes in the diet. The hypothesis suggests that the exposure of infants to microbes before the age of 6 months helps the immune system mature to be more tolerant of exposure to allergens later in life. Certainly, microbial colonization of the gut in early life is important to the development of a properly functioning immune system [144].

Of course, increasing exposure to microbes must be done safely. This hypothesis led researchers in Finland to conduct a study evaluating the effects of a *Lactobacillus* strain on incidence of atopic eczema in 132 infants at high risk of developing eczema [145]. The study was double-blinded and placebo-controlled. Pregnant mothers 2–4 weeks before delivery and newborn babies through 6 months of age were given *L. rhamnosus* GG. Infants were followed through 2 years of age and incidence of recurring atopic eczema was recorded. The study reported a 50% drop in incidence of recurring atopic eczema in the group receiving the probiotic supplement. A follow-up study of these same children indicated that these same trends were still present at 4 years of age. However, no impact on other allergic conditions was observed through seven years of age [146]. These results suggest that exposure to the right types of microbes early in life may decrease the risk of atopic dermatitis. However, a different research group using a very similar protocol and the same probiotic microbe as the Finnish group recently reported that no impact on incidence of atopic eczema was observed with supplementation with *L. rhamnosus* [147].

14. *Diarrhea*: Many types of diarrheal illnesses, with many different causes, disrupt intestinal function. The ability of probiotics to decrease the incidence or duration of certain diarrheal illnesses is perhaps the most substantiated health effects of probiotics. A paper published in 2001 reviewed nine studies on the effect of *Lactobacillus* as therapy for diarrhea in children [148]. This paper concluded that "*Lactobacillus* is safe and effective as a treatment for children with acute infectious diarrhea." Although this meta-analysis can be criticized for combining data from different species and strains of *Lactobacillus* into one analysis, the positive nature of the conclusion suggests that at least for this indication and for these strains, positive results have been obtained [149].

One common form of diarrhea is that associated with the consumption of antibiotics. The purpose of antibiotics is to kill harmful bacteria. Unfortunately, they can kill normal bacteria as well, and consequently disturb normal intestinal function. (Note that it is certainly NOT true that antibiotics "wipe out" all normal flora, but they can act broadly and exact a toll on normal, nonpathogenic bacteria.) It is important to realize that the microbiota of the healthy person is quite resilient and will return to a preantibiotic status with no intervention [150]. But it is hypothesized that supplementing the intestine with probiotics might help stabilize the antibiotic-induced dysbiosis and minimize disruptive effects [151]. One recent study documented that a probiotic containing four *Lactobacillus* and *Bifidobacterium* strains did lead to a quicker return to normal microbiota in antibiotic-consuming adults [152]. A paper published in 2006 reviewed seven studies (881 total patients) on the impact of probiotics (*L. rhamnosus* GG or *Saccharomyces boulardii*) on antibiotic-associated diarrhea [153]. The paper concluded that probiotics can be used to prevent antibiotic-associated diarrhea, but that no strong effect on the ability of probiotics to treat such diarrhea exists. How these probiotics accomplish this task is not known. Not all studies have shown positive results in the prevention of antibiotic-associated diarrhea or other symptoms associated with antibiotic therapy.

A serious complication of antibiotic therapy can be the onset of colitis due to *Clostridium difficile* [154]. This condition can be refractory to subsequent antibiotic treatment, resulting in ongoing recurrences. A few small studies have suggested that certain probiotics can prevent relapses of *Cl. difficile* colitis. A recent meta-analysis concluded that the probiotic yeast, *Sac. boulardii*, was the most effective probiotic treatment [154].

Another common form of diarrhea is experienced by travelers. Studies evaluating the effect of probiotics on travelers' diarrhea are equivocal. There is a need for further research in this area for more convincing findings. One meta-analysis of 12 studies on travelers' diarrhea concluded that certain probiotic products may offer a safe and effective method to prevent travellers' diarrhea with no indication of serious adverse events [150].

15. *Lowering of blood cholesterol level:* Cholesterol is essential for many functions in the human body. It acts as a precursor to certain hormones and vitamins and it is a component of cell membranes and nerve cells. However, elevated levels of total blood cholesterol or other blood lipids are considered risk factors for developing coronary heart disease. Although humans synthesize cholesterol to maintain minimum levels for biological functioning, diet is also known to play a role in serum cholesterol levels. The extent of influence varies significantly from person to person. Probiotic cultures have been evaluated for their effect on serum cholesterol levels. Clinical studies on the effect of lowering cholesterol or low-density lipid levels in humans have not been conclusive. There have been some human studies that suggest that blood cholesterol levels can be reduced by consumption of probiotic-containing dairy foods by people with elevated blood cholesterol, but in general the evidence is not overwhelming. It is likely that some strains may demonstrate this property while others do not, or that only subsets of people with elevated cholesterol respond [155].

16. *Helicobacter pylori:* It is a bacterium that colonizes the stomach and can cause gastric ulcers and gastric cancer. The effect of probiotics on *H. pylori* has been studied. Mechanistic studies in laboratory assays or in animal models have shown that antibacterial substances including (but not limited to) organic acids produced by some lactobacilli inhibit the growth and survival of this pathogen. When tested in humans, results are mixed. Results in humans suggest that some probiotic strains or milk fermented with a probiotic strain can reduce metabolic activity or colonization by *H. pylori*, but eradication has not been achieved. Probiotics have also been used to manage side effects of triple antibiotic therapy used to treat *H. pylori* infections. In these studies, the use of probiotics decreases the side effects of antibiotics, improves patient compliance with taking the prescribed therapy, and increases the rate at which *H. pylori* is eradicated [156].

17. *Irritable bowel syndrome (IBS):* This is a functional bowel disorder that can be characterized by symptoms of abdominal pain, cramps, gas, bloating, diarrhea, and constipation. Surveys estimate the prevalence rate ranging from 10% to 20% of the adult population and the condition is diagnosed three times more often in women than men. Only a few controlled studies have been conducted evaluating probiotics and IBS [157]. Some symptom relief (primarily from diarrhea or abdominal pain or bloating) has been reported in studies published to date (see Chapter 13).

18. *Inflammatory bowel disease (IBD):* IBDs, such as ulcerative colitis and Crohn's disease, are serious intestinal diseases that can lead to the surgical removal of the colon. The cause of these diseases is not known but it has been hypothesized that an intolerance to the normal microbiota in the gut leads to inflammation and resulting pathology. Efforts to identify a single microbe associated with the disease

have failed, leading some to suggest that it is a pathogenic microbial community, not a single microbe, that is responsible for IBD. The role of gut flora in the progression of these diseases has led some researchers to study the impact certain probiotic bacteria might have on maintaining the state of reduced inflammation that occurs during remission stages of the diseases. Several controlled, clinical trials have shown that high levels of certain probiotic strains can extend the disease-free remission period. Studies also have documented this effect on remission of pouchitis. But not all studies have shown benefits. Additional research in this area is progressing in Europe and in the United States (see Chapter 13) [158].

19. *Immune system modulation*: The immune system defends against microbial pathogens that have entered our bodies. The immune system is extremely complex, involving both cell-based and antibody-based responses to potential infectious agents. Immunodeficiency can result from certain diseases (e.g., cancer, AIDS, and leukemia) or, to a lesser extent, from more normal conditions such as old age, pregnancy, or stress. Autoimmune diseases (e.g., allergies, rheumatoid arthritis, and IBD) can also occur due to misdirected immune system activity (see Chapter 12).

Probiotic cultures have been shown in a variety of test systems to stimulate certain cellular, biochemical, and antibody functions of the immune system. Animal and some human studies have shown an effect of yogurt or lactic acid bacteria on enhancing levels of certain immunoreactive cells (e.g., macrophages and lymphocytes) or on regulation of immune factors (cytokines, immunoglobulins, and interferon). In addition, some studies have shown improved survival of pathogen-infected laboratory animals consuming probiotic cultures as compared to animals consuming a control diet. Results accumulated so far suggest that probiotics may provide an additional tool to help body protect itself [159].

An exciting area of research has been documenting the ability of certain probiotic bacteria to modulate immune dysregulation. Studies have shown that probiotics are effective in decreasing the development of allergy and relapse of IBD [160].

20. *Necrotizing enterocolitis (NEC)*: NEC is a GI disease that mostly affects premature infants. It is characterized by infection and inflammation leading to death of tissue of the large intestine. Probiotic supplementation may reduce the risk of NEC in preterm infants. A recent review of studies targeting efficacy and safety of probiotics for infants at risk for developing NEC was conducted. Taken together, studies suggest that probiotics lower the risk of mortality in preterm infants, but additional studies on best strains for this application, short- and long-term safety, and required dose must be conducted [161].

21. *Small bowel bacterial overgrowth*: Under certain conditions (production of low stomach acid, kidney dialysis, and others), microbial populations in the small intestine can increase beyond normal levels. This is termed small bowel bacterial overgrowth. The misplaced microbes can produce by-products from their growth that can be toxic. Researchers have found that feeding high levels of certain probiotic strains can control the toxic effects of these microbes. This is another example of the ability of probiotic strains fed in high numbers to modulate the activity of other intestinal bacteria [162].

22. *Vaginosis*: The vagina and its microbiota form a finely balanced ecosystem. Disruption of this ecosystem can lead to a microbiological imbalance and symptoms

of vaginosis. Vaginosis used to be considered a mere annoyance, but now is being examined for a role in serious conditions including pelvic inflammatory disease, pregnancy-related complications (such as low-birth-weight babies), and increased susceptibility to AIDS infection [163]. Vaginosis can be caused by several different organisms, and in many cases, the causative agent may not be identified. What is known is that lactobacilli predominate in the healthy vagina, and a lack of lactobacilli is a risk factor for vaginosis. The lactobacilli are thought to maintain a favorable vaginal pH in the acidic range and to inhibit pathogens, possibly through the production of hydrogen peroxide and other antimicrobial factors. The most conclusive human studies to date on the impact of lactobacilli on bacterial vaginosis showed that *L. rhamnosus* GR-1 and *L. reuteri* RC-14 administered in milk could pass through the intestine, ascend to the vagina, and restore a normal lactobacilli microbiota in women prone to infections [164]. These strains were delivered in yogurt to African women with bacterial vaginosis and shown to improve therapeutic outcomes. These studies have provided the best evidence to date for successful probiotic intervention to improve vaginal health. Some other recent studies have not shown positive results, highlighting the importance of use of effective strains and delivery systems [165].

1.7 PROBIOTICS AND FERMENTED DAIRY PRODUCTS

Staying healthy: The value of probiotics to reduce the risk of, rather than treat, disease has recently become appreciated more fully. Studies have been conducted in healthy populations, with end points such as decreasing the incidence of colds [166], winter infections, or even absences from work or day care. These controlled human studies provide support that certain probiotic strains consumed as part of a daily diet will increase the number of illness-free days or, in the case of younger population, improved growth for undernourished children [167]. This effect is likely mediated by immune enhancement functions or more direct inhibition of pathogens, but mechanistic studies have not always accompanied positive clinical indications. Probiotic bacteria are frequently, but not always, chosen from bacteria that normally inhabit the GI system of humans. Sometimes the term "probiotic" is used as a synonym to "commensal, beneficial bacteria," but this is an incorrect usage. Commensal flora may be beneficial, but until they are isolated, characterized, and shown in human studies to impart a health benefit, they cannot be accurately called "probiotic." Also, probiotics must be safe [168].

Once destined for commercial use, these bacteria are purified, grown to large numbers, concentrated to high doses, and preserved. They are provided in products in one of three basic ways:

- As a culture concentrate added to a food at medium levels, with little or no opportunity for culture growth
- Inoculated into a milk-based food (or dietary supplement) and allowed to grow to achieve high levels in a fermented food
- As concentrated and dried cells packaged as dietary supplements such as powders, capsules, or tablets, and delivered at a range of doses

Probiotic bacteria have a long history of association with dairy products [169]. This is because some of the same bacteria that are associated with fermented dairy products also make their homes in different sites on the human body, including the mouth, the GI tract, and the vagina. Some of these microbes, therefore, can play a dual role in transforming milk into a diverse array of fermented dairy products (yogurt, cheese, kefir, etc.), and contributing to the important role of colonizing bacteria.

Dairy products may provide a desirable "probiotic delivery vehicle" for several reasons. To date, however, there is little research on the impact of delivery vehicle and probiotic efficacy for any of the possible formats. This is an important area for future research.

Dairy foods can protect the probiotic bacteria: Traveling through the human digestive tract can be a challenge for bacteria. High acid levels in the stomach and exposure to pancreatic secretions such as digestive enzymes and bile in the small intestine can lead to the injury and death of a percentage of orally administered probiotics. Although some bacteria are more resistant than others to this stress, consumption of probiotics with food, including milk, yogurt, and other dairy products, buffers stomach acid and can increase the chance that the bacteria will survive in the intestine.

Refrigerated storage of dairy products helps promote probiotic stability: Although the lactic acid content of yogurt can be a barrier to culture stability, short-term refrigeration generally promotes stability.

Live cultures in dairy foods carry a positive image: The consuming public may have a generally negative image of bacteria in foods, but they are aware of "live, active cultures" in fermented dairy foods, and these cultures convey a positive, healthful image. Probiotic bacteria in dairy foods can be an extension of the comfortable association of cultures in dairy products, and make it easier to communicate health messages to the public (see Chapter 6).

The healthful properties of probiotic bacteria blend with the healthful properties of milk products: A dairy product containing probiotics makes a healthy, "functional food package." In addition to the vitamins, calcium, other minerals, and protein obtained from milk products, modern research has suggested healthful properties of fermentation-derived peptides and butyric acid found in some dairy products. Dairy products have recently been shown to be important components of a healthy diet, for more than the prevention of osteoporosis. Consumption of three or more servings of dairy products each day has been associated with lower levels of obesity among Americans. Obesity is associated with diabetes, hypertension, and heart disease. The DASH diet also recommends three servings of low-fat dairy products [53].

Choosing a probiotic: Over 400 bacterial species are living in the human intestinal digestive system. There are three main classifications of probiotics: genus, species, and strain. Table 1.6 lists the classification and functions of probiotic bacteria [170].

The potential benefits of probiotic cultures seem vast. The applications range from helping to treat acute intestinal infections to aiding in the digestion of lactose and contributing, over the longer term, to improved health and possibly reduced risk of disease. Since the beginning of the first microbiological health claims [171], about yogurt intake with active bacteria, its importance increased with time.

What should be considered when choosing a probiotic [172]? Microbiologists agree that it cannot be assumed that research published on one strain of probiotic

TABLE 1.6
Classification and Functions of Probiotic Bacteria

A. *Genus*: The two most common probiotic genera found in the digestive system are *Lactobacillus* and *Bifidobacterium* [173].

    a. The *Lactobacillus* genus is a group of lactic acid-producing bacteria that play a important role in the digestive tract, most specifically in the small intestine.

    b. Bifidobacteria are the major inhabitants of the large intestine. When sufficient numbers of bifidobacteria are present, they make it extremely difficult for pathogenic invaders such as the yeast *Candida albicans* to exist in the gut. Bifidobacteria produce acetic and lactic acids; they also assist in the absorption of B complex vitamins.

B. *Species*: Some species belonging to the *Lactobacillus* genus include [174] the following:

LA is a colonizing bacterium that establishes itself primarily in the small intestine, and prevents invaders. LA is also part of the normal vaginal flora and helps control the growth of fungus, thus preventing yeast infections. There are over 200 species of acidophilus with approximately 13 of those capable of producing antimicrobial and antibacterial substances.

LB is a transient species of bacteria that is used in the production of yogurt. This species works synergistically with LA to break down lactose and aid digestion. It has been know to alleviate many digestive problems such as acid reflux.

L. casei is another transient species of bacteria found both in the intestine and in the mouth. This species has been found to assist in the propagation of other desirable bacteria such as LA.

L. rhamnosus is another lactic acid-producing species that inhibits the growth of harmful bacteria in the gut and it is used as a natural preservative in yogurt and other dairy products. There is some debate as to whether *L. rhamnosus* is a colonizing or transient bacteria.

Lactobacillus plantarum is a very versatile species found in many fermented foods such as pickles.

Some species belonging to the *Bifidobacterium* genus include the following [175]:

Bifidobacterium infantis is the primary inhabitant of the digestive tract of newborn infants. It is also found in the vagina along with LA. This anaerobic species does not require oxygen and produces lactic and acetic acids, both of which prevent the colonization of harmful pathogens.

Bifidobacterium longum assists in the production and absorption of B complex vitamins and inhibits harmful pathogens by lowering pH in the intestine with production of acetic and lactic acids.

Bifidobacterium breve assists in the production and absorption of B complex vitamins and inhibits harmful pathogens by lowering pH in the intestine with production of acetic and lactic acids.

B. lactis and *B. animalis* are the same species; these lactic acid-producing microbes compete for nutrients and intestinal wall space, thus forcing invaders out of the digestive tract.

C. *Strains*

The strain is the most specific classification of bacteria and is based on individual characteristics such as how strong and aggressive the microorganism is. For example, some strains of LA, such as the DDS-1 Super Strain, are much more effective in producing antibiotic substances and inhibiting harmful pathogens. While other strains of LA may not be as strong to survive the acidic stomach environment or have the capacity to produce antimicrobial substances.

Following is a list of strains by species that have been researched and proven effective in treating disorders such as the IBS and viral diarrhea as well as improving digestive and overall health.

Lactobacillus strains [173]

    L. acidophilus DDS-1

    L. acidophilus NCFM

    L. acidophilus LA02

continued

TABLE 1.6   (continued)

L. acidophilus R0052

L. acidophilus T20

L. bulgaricus LB-51 (supreme strain)

L. casei DN-114 001

L. casei Shirota

L. plantarum 299v

L. plantarum LP01

L. rhamnosus GG, LGG

L. rhamnosus GR-1

L. rhamnosus HN001, DR20

L. rhamnosus 19070-2

L. rhamnosus R0011, Rosell-11

Bifidobacterium strains [176]

B. animalis DN-173 010

Bifidobacterium bifidum Malyoth Super Strain

B. breve BR03

B. breve C50

B. breve Yakult, BBG

B. breve YIT4064

B. infantis 35624

B. infantis NLS Super Strain

B. lactis Bb-12

B. lactis HN019, DR10

B. longum BB536, BB356

applies to another strain, even of the same species. (Remember that, for the strain "*L. rhamnosus* GG," the genus is *Lactobacillus*, the species is *rhamnosus* and the strain designation is GG. Another strain of *L. rhamnosus*, for example strain GR-1, has different probiotic properties.) Therefore, documentation of type of bacteria (genus, species, and strain), potency (number of viable bacteria per dose), purity (presence of contaminating or ineffective bacteria), and the extent of research that has been published on health effects, must be provided for any strain being used in a product. Interactions of species and strains are also important aspect of use and selection of cultures [177]. Usually the culture or product manufacturer can provide this information.

REFERENCES

1. Campbell, J.R. and Marshall, R.T., *The Science of Providing Milk for Man*, McGraw-Hill, New York, pp, 1–24, 1975.
2. Bogart, R., *Scientific Farm Animal Production*, Burgess Publishing Company, Minneapolis, Minnesota, pp. 1–19, 1977.

3. de Beer, H., Observations on the history of Dutch physical stature from the late-Middle Ages to the present. *Econ. Hum. Biol.* 2 (1), 45–55, 2004.
4. Reay Tannahill., *Food in History*, Three Rivers Press, New York, pp. 27–29, 1988.
5. Kaşgarlı and Mahmud., *Divanü Lügati't-Türk*, First published in Bagdat, 1074 A.D., 725 pages, ISBN: 9759970130, Translated by Serap Tuğba Yurtsever. Kabalcı Publishing Company, İstanbul, 2005.
6. Yusuf Has hacip., *Kutadgu Bilig*, First published in Balasagun, Central Asia in 1070 A.D., 1285pp., ISBN: 9759970651, Translated by Reşit Rahmeti Arat. Kabalcı Publishing Company, İstanbul, April 2006.
7. Maguelonne Toussaint-Samat, *History of Food*, translated by Anthea Bell. Barnes & Noble Books, New York, pp. 119–20, 1992.
8. Ilya Ilyich Metchnikoff; *The Prolongation of Life: Optimistic Studies*, Springer, New York, NY, p. 360, 2004.
9. Bruce Moore (Ed.), Yoghurt n, *The Australian Oxford Dictionary*, 2nd edition, Oxford University Press, Oxford, 2004. Oxford Reference Online. Accessed on January 14, 2009.
10. Peters, Pam, *The Cambridge Guide to English Usage*, Cambridge University Press, Cambridge, pp. 587–588, 2004.
11. Yogurt., In *Merriam-Webster Online Dictionary*, Retrieved January 14, 2009, from http://www.merriam-webster.com/dictionary/yogurt.
12. Robinson, R.K. and Tamime, A.Y., Recent developments in yoghurt manufacture, in *Modern Dairy Technology*, B.J.F. Hudson, Ed., Elsevier Applied Science Publishers, London, pp. 1–36, 1986.
13. Ramesh C. Chandan (Ed.), Charles H. White (Associate Ed.), Arun Kilara (Associate Ed.), Hui, Y.H. (Associate Ed.), *Manufacturing Yogurt and Fermented Milks*, Wiley-Blackwell Publishers, New York, p. 364, 2006.
14. Robinson, R.K., Manufacturing yogurt and fermented milks, *Int. J. Dairy Technol.* (Blackwell Publishing), 60 (3), 237–237, 2007,
15. Keçeli, T., Robinson, R.K., and Gordon, M.H. The role of olive oil in the preservation of yogurt cheese (labneh anbaris), *Int. J. Dairy Technol.*, 52 (2), 68–72, 1999.
16. Crawford, R.J.M. (Ed.), The technology of traditional milk products in developing countries, FAO Animal Production and Health Papers No. 85, T0251/E, 333pp., FAO Publication, 1990.
17. Prakash, S. and Urbanska, A.M., Fermented milk products and use thereof, World Intellectual Property Organization, WO/2007/140613. Publication date: 13712/2007.
18. Sieber, R., Collomb, M., Aeschlimann, A., Jelen, P., and Eyer, H., Impact of microbial cultures on conjugated linoleic acid in dairy products—a review, *Int. Dairy J.*, 14, 1–15, 2004.
19. Tamime, A.Y., *Yoghurt Science and Technology*, 3rd edition, CRC Press/Taylor & Francis, London, UK, 791pp., 2007.
20. Coudeyras, S., Marchandin, H., Fajon, C., and Forestier, C., Taxonomic and strain-specific identification of the probiotic strain lactobacillus rhamnosus 35 within the lactobacillus casei group, *Appl. Environ. Microbiol.*, 74, 2679–2689, 2008.
21. Agrawal, A., Houghton, L.A., Morris, J., Reilly, B., Guyonnet, D.N., Schlumberger, A., Jakob, S., and Whorwell, P.J., Clinical trial: The effects of a fermented milk product containing *Bifidobacterium lactis* DN-173 010 on abdominal distension and gastrointestinal transit in irritable bowel syndrome with constipation, *Alimen. Pharmacol. Ther.*, 29 (1), 104–114, 2009.
22. Vinderola, C.G., Mocchiutti, P., and Reinheimer, J.A., Interactions among lactic acid starter and probiotic bacteria used for fermented dairy products, *J. Dairy Sci.* (American Dairy Science Association), 85 (4), 721–729, 2002.

23. Walstra, P., Wouters, J.T.M., and Geurts, T.J., *Dairy Science and Technology*, 2nd edition, CRC Press, USA, 2005.
24. Gregory, D.M., Jarvis, J.K., and Mcbean, L.D., *Handbook of Dairy Foods and Nutrition*, 3rd edition, National Dairy Council, USA, 432pp., 2006.
25. Kucukoner, E., Tarakci, Z., and Sagdic, O., Physicochemical and microbiological characteristics and mineral content of herby cacik, a traditional Turkish dairy product, *J. Sci. Food Agri.*, 86 (2), 333–338, 2006.
26. Choi, H.S. and Kosikowski, F.V., Sweetened plain and flavored carbonated yogurt beverages, *J. Dairy Sci.*, 68 (3), 613–619, 1985.
27. Gıllıland, S.E. and Speck, M.L., Instability of lactobacillus acidophilus in yogurt, *J. Dairy Sci.*, 9, 1394–1398, 1977.
28. Anderson, J.W. and Gilliland, S.E., Effect of fermented milk (yogurt) containing *Lactobacillus Acidophilus* L1 on serum cholesterol in hypercholesterolemic humans, *J. Am. College Nutr.*, 18 (1), 43–50, 1999.
29. Onwulata, C.I., Rao, D.R., and Vankineni, P., Relative efficiency of yogurt, sweet acidophilus milk, hydrolyzed-lactose milk, and a commercial lactase tablet in alleviating lactose maldigestion, *Am. J. Clin. Nutr.*, 49, 1233–1237, 1989.
30. Fankhause, D.B., *Making Buttermilk*, University of Cincinnati, Clermont College. http://biology.clc.uc.edu/Fankhauser/Cheese/buttermilk.htm. Retrieved on 01/25/2009.
31. Mistry, V.V., Metzger, L.E., and Maubois, J.L., Use of ultrafiltered sweet buttermilk in the manufacture of reduced fat cheddar cheese, *J. Dairy Sci.*, 79 (7), 1137–1145, 1996.
32. Bishpo-McDonald, H., Dairy food consumption and health: State of the science on current topics, *J. Am. College Nutr.*, 24 (6), 525S, 2005.
33. Statistics Canada: www.statcan.gc.ca, Accessed 25/01/, 2009.
34. Huth, P.J., Dirienzo, D.B., and Miller, G.D., Major scientific advances with dairy foods innutrition and health, *J. Dairy Sci.*, 89, 1207–1221, 2006.
35. Hiza, H.A.B., Bente, L., and Fungwe, T., Nutrient content of the U.S. food supply, 2005 Home Economics Research Report No. 58, Center for Nutrition Policy and Promotion U.S. Department of Agriculture, 2008. http://www.cnpp.usda.gov/USFoodSupply htm.
36. Weinberg, L.G., Berner, L.A., and Groves, J.E., Nutrient contributions of dairy foods in the United States, continuing survey of food intakes by individuals, 1994–1996, 1998, *J. Am. Diet. Assoc.*, 104 (6), 895–902. 2004.
37. Foote, J.A., Suzanne, P., Murphy, L. R. Wilkens, P., Peter, B., and Carlson, A., Dietary variety increases the probability of nutrient adequacy among adults, *J. Nutr.* 134, 1779–1785, 2004.
38. Virginia, A. Stallings and Christine, L. Taylor (Eds), Nutrition standards and meal requirements for National School Lunch and Breakfast Programs: Phase I. Proposed Approach for Recommending Revisions, Report, Food and Nutrition Board (FNB) Institute of Medicine (IOM), p. 192, 2008.
39. Shortt, C. and O'Brien, J. (Eds), *Handbook of Dairy Products*. CRC, Taylor & Francis, London, UK, 312pp., 2003.
40. Kontopidis, G., Holt, C., and Sawyer, L., Invited review: Beta-lactoglobulin: Binding properties, structure, and function, *J. Dairy Sci.*, 87, 785–796, 2004.
41. Marincic, P.Z., Mccune, R.W., and Hendricks, D.G., Cow's-milk-based infant formula heterogeneity of bovine serum albumin content, *J. Am. Diet. Assoc.*, 99 (12), 1575–1578, 1999.
42. Peyrouset, A. and Spring, F., Process of extraction of lactoferrine and immunoglobulins of milk. US Patent no. 4436658, Issue date: 13 March 1984.
43. Elagamy, E.I., Ruppanner, R., Ismail, A., Champagne C.P., and Assaf R., Purification and characterization of lactoferrin, lactoperoxidase, lysozyme and immunoglobulins from camel's milk, *Int. Dairy J. (Elsevier)*, 6 (2), 129–145, 1996.

44. Eskin, M. and Snait, T., *Dictionary of Nutraceuticals and Functional Foods*, CRC Press, Taylor & Francis, New York, NY, London, p. 520, 2005.
45. Ebringer, L., Ferencik, M., and Krajcovic, J., Beneficial health effects of milk and fermented dairy products—review, *Folia Microbiol.*, 53 (5), 378–394, 2008.
46. Mattila-Sandholm, T. and Saarela, M., *Functional Dairy Products*, CRC Press, Taylor & Francis, 395pp., 2003.
47. Sanders, M.E., Hamilton-Miller, J., Reid, G., and Gibson, G., A non-viable preparation of *L. acidophilus* is not a probiotic, *Clin. Infect. Dis.*, 44, 886, 2007.
48. Isolauri, E. and Allan Walker, W. (Eds), Allergic diseases and the environment: 53rd Nestle Nutrition Workshop, Pediatric Program, Lausanne, April 6–10, 2003, Vol. 53, Karger, S., 2004.
49. Carla, R., Victor, L.F., Douglas, D., Huth, P.J., Kurilich, A.C., and Gregory, D.M., Contribution of dairy products to dietary potassium intake in the United States population, *J. Am. College Nutr.*, 27 (1), 44–50, 2008.
50. Kashket, S. and DePaola, D.P., Cheese consumption and the development and progression of dental caries, Nutr. Rev., 60, 97–103, 2002.
51. Papas, A.S., Joshi, A., Belanger, A.J., Kent, R.L., Palmer, C.A., and DePaola, P.F., Dietary models for root caries, *Am. J. Clin. Nutr.*, 61 (Suppl), 417S–422S, 1995.
52. Jenkins, G.N. and Hargreaves, J.A., Effect of eating cheese on Ca. and P concentrations of whole mouth saliva and plaque, *Caries. Res.*, 23, 159–64, 1989.
53. Appel, L.J., Moore, T.J., and Obarzanek, E., A clinical trial of the effects of dietary patterns on blood pressure (DASH Collaborative Research Group), *N. Eng. J. Med.*, 336, 1117–1124, 1997.
54. European Food Safety Authority (EFSA), Scientific Opinion of the Panel on Dietetic Products, Nutrition and Allergies on a request from Valio Ltd. on the scientific substantiation of a health claim related to *Lactobacillus helveticus* fermented Evolus® low-fat milk products and reduction of arterial stiffness. *EFSA J.*, 824, 1–2, 2008.
55. Jauhiainen, T., Rönnback, M., Vapaatalo, H., Wuolle, K., Kautiainen, H., and Korpela R., *Lactobacillus helveticus* fermented milk reduces arterial stiffness in hypertensive subjects, *Int. Dairy J.*, 17, 1209–11, 2007.
56. Obarzanek, E.,Velletri, P.A., and Cutler, J.A., Dietary protein and blood pressure, *JAMA*, 275 (20), 1996.
57. Krause, R.M., et al., AHA Dietary Guidelines (2000): A statement for healthcare professionals from the Nutrition Committee of the American Heart Association, Circulation, 102, 2284–2299, 2000.
58. Ingrid Wollowski, I., Rechkemmer, G., and Pool-Zobel, B., Protective role of probiotics and prebiotics in colon cancer, *Am. J. Clin. Nutr.*, 73 (2), 451S–455S, 2001.
59. Hirayama, K. and Rafter, J., The role of probiotic bacteria in cancer prevention, *Microbes Infect.* (Elsevier B.V.), 2 (6), 681–686, 2000.
60. Rafter, J., Lactic acid bacteria and cancer: Mechanistic perspective, *British J. Nutr.* (Cambridge University Press), 88, S89–S94, 2002.
61. Kıkuchı-Hayakawa, H., Shıbahara-Sone, H., Osada, K., Onodera-Masuoka, N., Ishikawa, F., and Watanuki, M., Lower plasma triglyceride level in Syrian hamsters fed on skim milk fermented with *Lactobacillus casei* strain Shirota, *Biosci. Biotechnol. Biochem.*, 64, 466–475, 2000.
62. Ishikawa, H., Akedo, I. Otani Suzuki, T., Miyo Nakamura, T., Takeyama, I., Miyaoka, E., and Kakizoe, T., Randomized trial of dietary fiber and *Lactobacillus* casei administration for prevention of colorectal tumors, *International J. Cancer* (UICC International Union Against Cancer), 116 (5), 762–767, 2005.
63. Kampman, E., Goldbohm, A., van den Brandt, A., and van 't Veer, P., Fermented dairy products, calcium, and colorectal cancer in the Netherlands cohort study, Cancer Res., 54, 3186–3190, 1994.

64. Knekt, P., Jarvinen, R., Seppanen, R., Pukkala, E., and Aromaa, A., Intake of dairy products and the risk of breast cancer, *Br. J. Cancer*, 73, 687–691, 1996.
65. Hjartaker, A., Laake, P., and Lund, E., Childhood and adult milk consumption and risk of premenopausal breast cancer in a cohort of 48,844 women–The Norwegian women and cancer study, *Int. J. Cancer*, 93, 888–893, 2001.
66. Ip, C., et al., Conjugated linoleic acid-enriched butter fat alters mammary gland morphogenesis and reduces cancer risk in rats, *J. Nutr.*, 129, 2135–2142, 1999.
67. Aro, A., et al., Inverse association between dietary and serum conjugated linoleic acid and risk of breast cancer in postmenopausal women, *Nutr. Cancer*, 38, 151–157, 2000.
68. Moorman, P.G. and Terry, P.D., Consumption of dairy products and the risk of breast cancer: A review of the literature, *Am. J. Clin. Nutr.*, 80, 5–14, 2004.
69. Cho, E., et al., Dairy foods, calcium, and colorectal cancer: A pooled analysis of 10 cohort studies, *JNCI J. Nat. Cancer Inst.*, 96, 1015–1022, 2004.
70. Grau, M.V., et al., Prolonged effect of calcium supplementation on risk of colorectal adenomas in a randomized trial, *JNCI J. Nat. Cancer Inst.*, 99, 129–136, 2007.
71. Larsson, S.C., Bergkvist, L., and Alicja Wolk, A., Calcium and dairy food intakes are inversely associated with colorectal cancer risk in the cohort of Swedish men, *Am. J. Clin. Nutr.*, 83, 667–673, 2006.
72. Parodi, P.W., Conjugated linoleic acid and other anticarcinogenic agents of bovine milk fat, *J. Dairy Sci.*, 82 (6), 1339–1349, 1999.
73. Pereira, M.A., Jacobs, Jr., D.R., Horn, L.V., Slattery, M.L., Kartashov, A.I., and Ludwig, D.S., Dairy consumption, obesity, and the insulin resistance syndrome in young adults: The CARDIA study, *JAMA*, 287, 2081–2089, 2002.
74. Jacqmain, M., Doucet, E., Després, J.-P., Bouchard, C., and Tremblay, A., Calcium intake, body composition, and lipoprotein–lipid concentrations in adults, *Am. J. Clin. Nutr.*, 77 (6), 1448–1452, 2003.
75. Yi-Chin, L., Roseann, M.L., McCabe, L.D., McCabe, G.M., Connie, M.P., and Teegarden, D., Dairy calcium is related to changes in body composition during a two-year exercise intervention in young women, *J. Am. College Nutr.*, 19 (6), 754–760, 2000.
76. Lovejoy, J.C., Champagne, C.M., Smith, S.R., de Jonge, L., and Xie, H., Ethnic differences in dietary intakes, physical activity, and energy expenditure in middle-aged, premenopausal women: The healthy transitions study, *Am. J. Clin. Nutr.*, 74, 90–95, 2001.
77. Zemel, M.B., Richards, J., Mathis, S., Milstead, A., Gebhardt, L., and Silva, E., Dairy augmentation of total and central fat loss in obese subjects, *Int. J. Obesity*, 29, 391–397, 2005.
78. Sun, X. and Zemel, M.B., Leucine and calcium regulate fat metabolism and energy partitioning in murine adipocytes and muscle cells, *Lipids*, 42 (4), 297–305, 2007.
79. Zemel, M.B., The role of dairy foods in weight management, *J. Am. College Nutr.*, 24 (6 Suppl), 537S–46S, 2005.
80. Loos, R.J.F., Rankinen, T., Leon, A.S., Skinner, J.S., Wilmore, J.H., Rao, D.C., and Bouchard, C., Calcium intake is associated with adiposity in black and white men and white women of the Heritage Family Study, *J. Nutr.*, 134, 1772–1778, 2004.
81. Moore, L.L., Bradlee, M.L., Di Gao, and Singer, M.R., Low dairy intake in early childhood predicts excess body fat gain, *Obesity*, 14, 1010–1018, doi:10.1038/oby.2006.
82. Novotny, R., Daida, Y.G., Acharya, S., Grove, J.S., and Vogt, T.M., Dairy intake is associated with lower body fat and soda intake with greater weight in adolescent girls, *J. Nutr.*, 134, 1905–1909, 2004.
83. Summerbell, C.D., Watts, C., Higgins, J.P.T., and Garrow, J.S., Randomised controlled trial of novel, simple, and well supervised weight reducing diets in outpatients, *BMJ*, 317, 1487–1489, 1998.
84. International Osteoporosis Foundation, Facts and statistics about osteoporosis and its impact. I. Available at http://www.iofbonehealth.org/facts-and-statistics.html. Accessed January 29, 2009.

85. Heaney, R.P., Calcium, dairy products and osteoporosis, *J. Am. College Nutr.*, 19 (90002), 83S–99S, 2000.
86. Cadogan, J., Eastell, R., Jones, N., and Barker, M.E., Milk intake and bone mineral acquisition in adolescent girls: Randomised, controlled intervention trial, *BMJ*, 315 (7118), 1255–1260, 1997.
87. Ruth, E.B., Sheila, M.W., Ianthe, E.J., and Ailsa, G., Children who avoid drinking cow milk have low dietary calcium intakes and poor bone health, *Am. J. Clin. Nutr.*, 76, 675–680, 2002.
88. Lee, W.T.K., Leung, S.S.F., Leung, D.M.Y., Wang, S.-H., Xu, Y.-C., Zeng, W.-P., and Cheng, J.C.Y., Bone mineral acquisition in low calcium intake children following the withdrawal of calcium supplement, *Acta Paediatr.*, 86, 570–576, 1997.
89. Bonjour, J.-P., Chevalley, T., Ammann, P., Slosman, D., and Rizzoli, R., Gain in bone mineral mass in prepubertal girls 3–5 years after discontinuation of calcium supplementation: A follow-up study, *Lancet*, 358 (9289), 1208–1212, 2001.
90. Heidi, J., Kalkwarf, H., Khoury, J.C., Bean, J., and Elliot, J.G., and Vitamin, K., bone turnover, and bone mass in girls, *Am. J. Clin. Nut.*, 80 (4), 1075–1080, 2004.
91. Dawson-Hughes, B., Harris, S., Palermo, N.J., Castaneda-Sceppa, C., Rasmussen, H.M., and Dallal, G.E., Treatment with potassium bicarbonate lowers calcium excretion and bone resorption in older men and women, *J. Clin. Endocrinol. Metab.*, 94 (1), 96–102, 2009.
92. Promislow, J.H.E., Gladen, B.C., and Sandler, D.P., Maternal recall of breastfeeding duration by elderly women, *Am. J. Epidemiol.*, 161 (3), 289–296, 2005.
93. Pereira, M.A., Jacobs, D.R., Horn, L.V., Slattery, M.L., Kartashov, A.I., and Ludwig, D.S., Dairy consumption, obesity, and the insulin resistance syndrome in young adults, *JAMA*, 287, (16), 2081–2089, 2002.
94. Yoo, S., et al., Comparison of dietary intakes associated with metabolic syndrome risk factors in young adults: The Bogalusa heart study, *Am. J. Clin. Nutr.*, 80, 841–848, 2004.
95. Kaye Foster-Powell, K., Holt, S.H.A., and Brand-Miller, J.C., International table of glycemic index and glycemic load values: 2002, *Am. J. Clin. Nutr.*, 76 (1), 5–56, 2002.
96. Curhan, G.C., et al., Calcium and kidney stones, *N. Engl. J. Med.*, 328, 833–838, 1993.
97. Curhan, G.C., Willett, W.C., Speizer, F.E., Spiegelman, D., and Stampfer, M.J., Comparison of dietary calcium with supplemental calcium and other nutrients as factors affecting the risk for kidney stones in women, *Ann. Intern. Med.*, 126 (7), 497–504, 1997.
98. Lieske, J.C., Goldfarb, D.S., De Simone, C., and Regnier, C., Use of a probiotic to decrease enteric hyperoxaluria, *Kidney Int.*, 68 (3), 1244–1249, 2005.
99. Bendich, A., The potential for dietary Supplements to reduce premenstrual syndrome (PMS) symptoms, *J. Am. Coll. Nutr.*, 19, 3–12, 2000.
100. Thys-Jacobs, S., Micronutrients and the premenstrual syndrome: The case for calcium, *J. Am. Coll. Nutr.*, 19, 220–227, 2000.
101. Sicherer, S.H., Food allergy, *The Lancet*, 360 (9334), 701–710, 2002.
102. Brigino, E. and Bahna, S.L., Clinical features of food allergy in Infants, *Clin. Rev. Allergy Immunol.*, 13, 329–345, 1995.
103. Schrander, J.J.P., et al., Cow's milk protein intolerance in infants under 1 year of age: A prospective study, *Eur. J. Pediatr.*, 152, 640–644, 1993.
104. Zeiger Robert, S., Dietary aspects of food allergy prevention in infants and children-supplement contents, *J. Pediatr. Gastroentero. Nutr.*, 30 (1), S77–S86, 2000.
105. Johnson, A.O., Semenya, J.G., Buchowski, M.S., Enwonwu, C.O., and Scrimshaw, N.S., Correlation of lactose maldigestion, lactose intolerance, and milk intolerance, *Am. J. Clin. Nutr.*, 57, 399–401, 1993.
106. Suarez, F.L., et al., Tolerance to the daily ingestion of two cups of milk by individuals claiming lactose intolerance, *Am. J. Clin. Nutr.*, 65, 1502–1506, 1997.

107. Suarez, F.L., et al., A comparison of symptoms after the consumption of milk or lactose-hydrolysed milk by people with self-reported severe lactose intolerance, *N. Engl. J. Med.*, 333, 1–4, 1995.

108. Miller, G.D., et al., *Lactose Intolerance. Dans: Handbook of Dairy Foods and Nutrition*, 2e éd., Chap. 8, pp. 311–354, CRC Press, Boca Raton, FL, 2000.

109. Hertzler, S.R., et al., Fecal hydrogen production and consumption measurements, Response to daily lactose ingestion by lactose maldigesters. *Dig. Dis. Sci.*, 42, 348–353, 1997.

110. Hertzler, S.R., and Savaiano, D.A., Colonic adaptation to the daily lactose feeding in lactose maldigesters reduces lactose intolerance, *Am. J. Clin. Nutr.*, 64, 1232–1236, 1996.

111. Johnson, A.O., et al., Adaptation of lactose maldigesters to continued milk intakes, *Am. J. Clin. Nutr.*, 58, 879–881, 1993.

112. Briet, R., et al., Improved clinical tolerance to chronic lactose ingestion in subjects with lactose intolerance: A placebo effect? *Gut*, 41, 632–635, 1997.

113. Pribila, B.A., et al., Improved lactose digestion and intolerance among African-American adolescent girls fed a dairy-rich diet, *Am. J. Diet. Assoc.*, 100, 524–528, 2000.

114. Suarez, F.L. and Savaiano, D.A., Lactose digestion and tolerance in adult and elderly Asian-Americans, *Am. J. Clin. Nutr.*, 59, 1021–1024, 1994.

115. Sampson, H.A. and Metcalfe, D.D., Food allergies, *JAMA*, 268, 2840–2844, 1992.

116. Suarez, F.L., et al., Lactose maldigestion is not an impediment to the intake of 1500 mg calcium daily as dairy products, *Am. J. Clin. Nutr.*, 68, 1118–1122, 1998.

117. Johnson, A.O., et al., Correlation of maldigestion, lactose intolerance and milk intolerance, *Am. J. Clin. Nutr.*, 57, 399–401, 1993.

118. Villar, J., et al., Improved lactose digestion during pregnancy: A case of physiologic adaptation? *Obstet Gynecol*, 71, 697, 1988.

119. Szilagyi, A., et al., Lactose handling by women with lactose malabsorption is improved during pregnancy, *Clin. Invest. Med.*, 19, 416, 1996.

120. Paige, D., et al., Lactose intolerance in pregnant African-American women, *J. Am. Coll. Nutr.*, 16 (Abstract 69), 488, 1997.

121. Savaiano, D., Managing lactose intolerance: A food lover's guide. Presentation. The Smart Gourmet. Dairy Foods for Health and Pleasure. Montréal, Québec (19 février 2001), 2001.

122. Iacono, G., et al., The "red umbilicus": A diagnostic sign of cow's milk protein intolerance, *J. Pediatr. Gastroenterol Nutr.*, 42 (5), 531–534, 2006.

123. McBean, L.D. and Miller, G.D., Allaying fears and fallacies about lactose intolerance, *J. Am. Diet. Assoc.*, 98 (6), 671–676, 1998.

124. Antonio Tursi, Factors influencing lactose intolerance, *Eur. J. Clin. Invest.*, 34 (4), 314–315, 2004.

125. Vesa, T.H., Marteau, P., and Riitta Korpela, R., Lactose intolerance, *J. Am. College Nutr.*, 19 (90002), 165S–175S, 2000.

126. Tucker, K.L., et al., Plasma vitamin B12 concentrations relate to intake source in the Framingham Offspring Study, *Am. J. Clin. Nutr.*, 71, 514–522, 2000.

127. House, J.D., et al., Folate and vitamin B12 status of women in Newfoundland at their first prenatal visit, *Can. Med. Assoc. J.*, 162 (11), 1557–1559, 2000.

128. Graham, S.M., et al., Long-term neurologic consequences of nutritional vitamin B12 deficiency in infants, *J. Pediatr.*, 121 (5, part 1), 710–714. 1992.

129. Stollhoff, K. and Schulte, F.J., Vitamin B12 and brain development, *Eur. J. Pediatr.*, 146 (2), 201–205, 1987.

130. Van Dusseldorp, M., et al., Risk of persistent cobalamin deficiency in adolescents fed a macrobiotic diet in early life, *Am. J. Clin. Nutr.*, 60, 661–667, 1999.

131. Louwman, M.W.J., et al., Signs of impaired cognitive function in adolescents with marginal cobalamin status, *Am. J. Clin. Nutr.*, 72, 762–769, 2000.

132. Baik, H.W. and Russell, R.M., Vitamin B12 deficiency in the elderly, *Annu. Rev. Nutr.*, 19, 357–377, 1999.

133. Wynn, M., et al., The danger of B_{12} deficiency in the elderly, *Nutr. Health*, 12 (4), 215–226, 1998.

134. Zucker, D.K., et al., B_{12} deficiency and psychiatric disorders: Case report and literature review, *Biol. Psychiatry*, 16 (2), 197–205. 1981.

135. Eastley, R., et al., Vitamin B12 deficiency in dementia and cognitive impairment: The effects of treatment on neuropsychological function, *Int. J. Geriatr. Psychiatry*, 15 (3), 226–233, 2000.

136. Brunello Wüthrich, B., Schmid, A.,Walther, B., and Sieber, R., Milk consumption does not lead to mucus production or occurrence of asthma, *J. Am. College Nutr.*, 24 (90006), 547S–555S, 2005.

137. Pinnock, C.B., et al., Relationship between milk intake and mucus production in adult volunteers challenged with rhinovirus-2, *Am. Rev. Resp. Dis.*, 141 (2), 352–356, 1990.

138. Pinnock, C.B. and Arney, W.K., The milk-mucus belief: Sensory analysis comparing cows milk and a soy placebo, *Appetite*, 20, 61–70, 1993.

139. Arney, W.K. and Pinnock, C.B., The milk-mucus belief: Sensations associated with the belief and characteristics of believers, *Appetite*, 20, 53–60. 1993.

140. Finberg, L., Milk effect on mucus production during upper respiratory tract infection, *JAMA*, 266 (9), 1289, 1991.

141. Haas, F., et al., Effect of milk ingestion on pulmonary function in healthy and asthmatic subjects, *J. Asthma*, 28 (5), 349–355, 1991.

142. Woods, R.K., et al., Do dairy products induce bronchoconstriction in adults with asthma? *J. Allergy Clin. Immunol.*, 101, 45–50, 1998.

143. Yazdanbakhsh, M., Kremsner, P.G., and Ree, R.V., Allergy, parasites, and the hygiene hypothesis, *Science*, 296 (5567), 490–494, 2002.

144. Romagnani, S., The increased prevalence of allergy and the hygiene hypothesis: Missing immune deviation, reduced immune suppression, or both? *Immunology*, 112 (3), 352–363, 2004.

145. Kalliomäki, M., Salminen, S., Poussa, T., Arvilommi, H., Isolauri, E., Probiotics and prevention of atopic disease: 4-year follow-up of a randomised placebo-controlled trial, *Lancet*, 361 (9372), 1869–1871, 2003.

146. Rosenfeldt, V., Benfeldt, E., Nielsen, S.D., Michaelsen, K.F., Jeppesen, D.L., Valerius, N.H., and Paerregard, A., Effect of probiotic **Lactobacillus** strains in children with atopic dermatitis, *The J. Allergy Clin. Immunol.* (Elsevier), 111 (2), 2003.

147. Pessi, T., Sütas, Y., Hurme, M., and Isolauri, E., Interleukin-10 generation in atopic children following oral Lactobacillus rhamnosus GG, *Clin. Exp. Allergy* (Wiley Interscience), 30 (12), 1804–1808, 2000.

148. Hania, S., and Mrukowicz, J.Z., Probiotics in the treatment and prevention of acute infectious diarrhea in infants and children: A systematic review of published randomized, double-blind, placebo-controlled trials, *J. Pediatr. Gastroenterol. Nutr.*, 33 (Suppl. 2), S17–S25, 2001.

149. Hania, S., Marek, R., and Andrzej, R., Probiotics in the prevention of antibiotic-associated diarrhea in children: A meta-analysis of randomized controlled trials, *J. Pediatr.*, 149 (3), 367, 2006.

150. Lynne V. McFarland, Meta-analysis of probiotics for the prevention of traveler's diarrhea, *Travel Med. Infect. Dis.*, 5 (2), 97–105, 2007.

151. Sartor, R.B., Therapeutic manipulation of the enteric microflora in inflammatory bowel diseases: Antibiotics, probiotics, and prebiotics, *Gastroenterology*, 126 (6), 1620–1633, 2004.

152. Bartlett, J.G., Antibiotic-associated diarrhea, *New Engl. J. Med.*, 346 (5), 334–339, 2002.

153. Lynne V. McFarland, Meta-analysis of probiotics for the prevention of antibiotic associated diarrhea and the treatment of *Clostridium difficile* disease, *The Am. J. Gastroenterol.*, 101 (4), 812–822, 2006.
154. Kelly, C.P. and LaMont, J.T., Clostridium difficile infection. *Ann. Rev. Med.*, 49, 375–390, 1998.
155. Kiessling, G., Schneider, J., and Jahreis G., Long-term consumption of fermented dairy products over 6 months increases HDL cholesterol, *Eur. J. Clin. Nutr.*, 56 (9), 843–849, 2000.
156. Hamilton-Miller, J.M.T., The role of probiotics in the treatment and prevention of Helicobacter pylori infection, *Int. J. Antimicrobial Agents*, 22, (4), 360–366, 2003.
157. Saito, Y.A., Schoenfeld, P., and Richard Locke III, R., The epidemiology of irritable bowel syndrome in North America: A systematic review, *The Am. J. Gastroenterol.*, 97 (8), 1910–1915, 2004.
158. Bouma, G. and Strober, W., The immunological and genetic basis of inflammatory bowel disease, *Nat. Rev. Immunol.*, 3 (7), 521–533, 2003.
159. De simone, C., Vesely, R., Bianchi Salvadori, B., and Jirillo, E., The role of probiotics in modulation of the immune system in man and in animals, 9 (1), 23–28, 1993.
160. Takeshi, M. and Ames, C., Modulating immune responses with probiotic bacteria, *Immunol. Cell Biol.*, 78 (1), 67–73, 2000.
161. Kliegman, R.M. and Willoughby, R.E., Prevention of necrotizing enterocolitis with probiotics, *Pediatrics*, 115 (1), 171–172, 2005.
162. Rial, D. and Rolfe, R.D., The role of probiotic cultures in the control of gastrointestinal health, *J. Nutr.*, 130, 396S–402S, 2000.
163. Gregor, R. and Alan, B., The potential for probiotics to prevent bacterial vaginosis and preterm labor, *Am. J. Obstetr. Gynecol.*,189 (4), 1202–1208, 2003.
164. Gregor, R., Burton, J., Hammond, J.-A., and Bruce, A.W., Nucleic acid-based diagnosis of bacterial vaginosis and improved management using probiotic lactobacilli, *J. Med. Food*, 7 (2), 223–228, 2004.
165. Falagas, M.E., Betsi, G.I., and Athanasiou, S., Probiotics for the treatment of women with bacterial vaginosis, *Clin. Microbiol. Infect.*, 13 (7), 657–664, 2007.
166. de Vrese, M., et al., Probiotic bacteria reduced duration and severity but not the incidence of common cold episodes in a double blind, randomized, controlled trial, *Vaccine*, 24, (44–46), 6670–667410, 2006.
167. Saran, S., Gopalan, S., and Krishna, T.P., Use of fermented foods to combat stunting and failure to thrive, *Nutrition*, 18 (5), 393–396, 2002.
168. Schrezenmeir, J. and de Vrese, M., Probiotics, prebiotics, and synbiotics—approaching a definition, *Am. J. Clin. Nutr.*, 73 (2), 361S–364S, 2001.
169. Heller, K.J., Probiotic bacteria in fermented foods: Product characteristics and starter. organisms, *Am. J. Clin. Nutr.*, 73 (2), 374S–379S, 2001.
170. Axelsson, L., Lactic acid bacteria: Classification and physiology, in *Lactic Acid Bacteria: Microbiology and Functional Aspects*; S. Salminen and A. van Wright (Eds), Marcel Dekker Inc., New York, pp. 1–66, 2004.
171. Metchnikoff, E., *The Prolongation of Life*, G.P. Putnam's Sons, New York, 1908.
172. Klaenhammer, T.R. and Kullen, M.J., Selection and design of probiotics, *Int. J. Food Microbiol.*, 50 (1–2), 45–57, 1999.
173. Coeuret, V., Gueguen, M., and Vernoux, J.P., Numbers and strains of lactobacilli in some probiotic products, *Int. J. Food Microbiol.* (Elsevier B.V.), 97 (2), 147–156, 2004.
174. Jacobsen, C.N.V., Nielsen, R., Hayford, A.E., Møller, P.L., Michaelsen, K.F., Pærregaard, A., Sandström, B., Tvede, M., and Jakobsen, M., Screening of probiotic activities of forty-seven strains of lactobacillus spp. by *in vitro* techniques and evaluation of the colonization ability of five selected strains in humans, *Appl. Environ. Microbiol.*, 65 (11), 4949–4956, 1999.

175. Prasad, J., Gill, H., Smart, J., and Gopal, P.K., Selection and characterisation of lactobacillus and bifidobacterium strains for use as probiotics, *Int. Dairy J.*, 8 (12), 993–1002, 1998.
176. Zavaglia, A.G., Guillermo, K., Pablo, P., and Graciela, De. A., Isolation and characterization of bifidobacterium strains for probiotic formulation, *J. Food Protect.*, 61 (7), 865–873, 1998.
177. Yıldız, F. and Westhoff, D., Associative growth of lactic acid bacteria in cabbage juice, *J. Food Sci.*, 46, 962–963, 1981.

2 Strategies for Yogurt Manufacturing

Barbaros Özer

CONTENTS

2.1   INTRODUCTION

Although there are no records available regarding the origin of yogurt, it is thought that it was first found as early as 2000 BC in mid-Eastern civilizations as a way to preserve milk. The word yogurt is Turkish in origin. The ancient Assyrian word for yogurt, "lebeny" meant life. Surprisingly, the word "probiotic" can literally be translated to "for life." There has been a longstanding belief that eating yogurt or the consumption of some types of cultured milk products is associated with longevity due to the friendly bacteria's ability to fight disease. According to the legends, Abraham owned his fruitfulness and longevity to yogurt. This legend was later turned into a theory by Elie Metchnikoff (1845–1916) who devoted the last decade of his life to investigating the means of increasing human longevity and advocating the consumption of lactic acid-producing bacteria. His works toward understanding the role of lactic acid bacteria in the improvement of the immune system wheeled the scientific researches on yogurt and fermented milks. In parallel to the development in human history, yogurt production evolved as well. This evolution can be summarized as follows:

- The use of the same utensils in the manufacture
- The addition of fresh milk onto fermented milk to provide sustainability in production
- Boiling of milk in open vats to obtain a more viscous product with extended shelf life
- The use of the previous day's soured milk to ferment the fresh milk
- Improvement of the aroma/flavor of yogurt by incorporating acid-resistant lactic acid bacteria in the manufacture

Since the mid-19th century, a rapid evolution in yogurt science and technology was noted. The developments in the field of yogurt science, technology, and microbiology are chronologically presented below:

1910–1925   The longevity theory developed by Metchnikoff stimulated the researches on the relationship between yogurt consumption and healthy life.

1925–1935   *Lactobacillus delbrueckii* subsp. *bulgaricus* was found not to withstand gastric acid. This triggered new studies in yogurt microbiology and *Lactobacillus acidophilus* was demonstrated to be able to keep its viability in the gastrointestinal tract.

1945–1950	Yogurt was still consumed by a limited group of consumers in Europe.
1950–1960	Aromatized yogurt was introduced into the European market and yogurt consumption in Europe increased slightly.
1970s	Evaporation and membrane techniques were introduced into yogurt industry and continuous yogurt production became common.
1980s	The scientific studies on the therapeutic effects of probiotic bacteria were intensified and commercial probiotic yogurts were introduced into yogurt market.
1990s	Depending on the improvements in genetic engineering, yogurt starters with improved phage-resistance and aroma/texture formation capabilities were developed, and automation and mechanization in industrial yogurt production became common.
2000s	Studies have been carried out to improve the genetic traits of yogurt starters. In addition, studies on the development of novel yogurt-derived products such as $\omega - 3$ enriched oil yogurt, transglutaminase (TGase) yogurt, fat-substitute yogurt, chemically acidified yogurt, vegetable oil yogurt, and health-promoting yogurt have been conducted.

2.2 PRETREATMENTS OF YOGURT MILK

2.2.1 MILK RECEPTION

The quality of raw milk is of critical importance for the sensory, chemical, and microbiological quality of the final product. Milk may be supplied to the dairy in milk churns or by a tanker after it has been cold stored at the farm. During transport, milk in churns usually has a temperature of >10°C, up to 20–30°C according to the climate. Bacterial growth likely occurs between milking and milk arrival at the dairy, as this interval may take as long as a day. The level of bacterial contamination is determined by the quality of the hygiene during milking, temperature, and the storage period [1]. In order to prevent postmilking contamination, all the measures must be taken between milking and processing. Overall, raw yogurt milk should

- Have low acidity
- Be clean
- Be milked from a healthy animal
- Have a good microbiological quality
- Have a normal taste and odor
- Not include residues of antibiotics, neutralizers, detergents, bacteriophages, and so on
- Have normal chemical composition

2.2.1.1 Acidity Control

After milking, the fresh milk has a pH of 6.6–6.7 (0.16–0.17% lactic acid). Following milking, milk is rapidly contaminated with microorganisms originating mainly from milking environments, utensils, and staff. While mesophilic bacterial contamination may spoil milk through lactic acid fermentation, heavy contamination with polluted water (e.g., pseudomonads) may cause a nonsouring spoilage. Development of acidity of raw milk during cold storage partly causes destabilization of casein micelles, which may end up with coagulation during heat treatment of yogurt milk base. Therefore, the acidity of raw milk should be between 0.17% and 0.19% lactic acid. Lower levels of lactic acid may indicate that milk contains residues of neutralizing agents (e.g., hydrogen peroxide and alkaline residues) or is obtained from cows with mastitis.

2.2.1.2 Mastitis Control

Milk drawn aseptically from the healthy udder is not sterile but contains low numbers of microorganisms, the so-called udder commensals [2]. Udder commensals are predominantly micrococci and streptococci. Also, coryneform bacteria (mainly *Corynebacterium bovis*) are common in fresh milk. None of these bacteria have any adverse effect on milk yield or quality. Mastitis is the inflammation of the mammary gland. This disease and resulting infection can significantly reduce milk production. The bacterial content of freshly drawn milk is significantly increased by mastitis. The mastitis-causing organisms enter the udder through the duct at the teat tip. The milk obtained from cows with mastitis contains lower levels of protein, lactose, and milk fat than the milk of healthy animals. Mastitis causes increase in serum protein, potassium, and chloride levels in milk and decrease in heat-stabilization of milk proteins, which may lead to coagulation during heat treatment. Yogurt processing requires intense heat treatment (i.e., 85–90°C for 10–30 min) and the bacteria causing mastitis are largely destroyed during heating. However, in the case that the somatic cell count in yogurt milk is higher than 4×10^5 mL^{-1}, the metabolic activities of yogurt starter bacteria may be reduced. At higher somatic cell counts (>10^6 mL^{-1} of milk), the yogurt starter bacteria are completely inhibited [3]. To obtain a good sensory quality yogurt, the somatic cell count should be lower than 2.5×10^5 mL^{-1} of milk [4].

2.2.1.3 Control of Antibiotic Residues

Antibiotics and other antimicrobial drugs are widely used in the treatment of mastitis. Penicillin G, ampicillin, tetracyclines, chloramphenicol, bacitracin, neomycin, polymyxin, and sulfa drugs, such as sulfamethazine, are the most common antibiotics used in mastitis treatment. These antibiotics have negative effects on the growth and metabolic activities of yogurt starter bacteria [5,6]. Some antibiotics can remain in milk up to 4 days. In the case of use of penicillin, the residual penicillin should be inactivated by adding penicillinase or penicillinase-synthesizing bacteria (e.g., *Micrococcus* spp.) into raw milk. High heat treatment causes inactivation of the majority of residual antibiotics; however, some antibiotics such as tetramycin and chloramphenicol cannot be influenced by heat treatment at 85°C for 20 min [7]. *Streptococcus thermophilus* was reported to be sensitive to very low concentrations of penicillin (<0.003 unit mL^{-1}). Similarly, the resistance of *Streptococcus thermophilus* against chloramphenicol and tetracyclines is fairly low [8]. Table 2.1 shows the antibiotic resistance levels of yogurt starter bacteria.

TABLE 2.1

Antibiotic Resistance of *Streptococcus thermophilus* and *L. delbrueckii* subsp. *bulgaricus* (mL^{-1})

Antibiotic	*Streptococcus thermophilus*	*L. delbrueckii* subsp. *bulgaricus*	Mixed Culture (IU)
Penicillin	0.004–0.01 IU	0.02–0.1 IU	0.01
Streptomycin	0.38 IU	0.38 IU	1.0
Tetracycline	0.13–0.5 µg	0.3–2.0 µg	1.0
Chlorotetracycline	0.06–1.0 µg	0.06–1.0 µg	0.1
Oxytetracycline	0.4 IU	0.7 IU	0.4
Bacitracin	0.04–0.12 IU	0.04–0.1 IU	0.04
Erythromycin	0.3–1.3 mg	0.7–1.3 mg	0.1
Chloramphenicol	0.8–13.0 mg	0.8–13.0 mg	0.5

Source: After Tamime, A.Y. and Robinson, R.K., *Yoghurt Science and Technology*, 3rd edition, Woodhead Publishing, Cambridge, p. 808, 2007.

IU, international unit.

2.2.1.4 Control of Bacteriological Quality of Milk

The ideal aim in producing high-quality milk is that it should be produced in an esthetic environment using suitable sanitary practices permitting only minimal bacterial contamination of milk. However, milk is always prone to contamination of microorganisms from the milking environment. Since the initial bacteriological quality of raw milk directly affects the quality of the final product, implementation of quality milk production programs is of critical importance. Total counts of bacteria in raw milk should be less than 100,000 cfu mL^{-1} (in special cases, up to 250,000 cfu mL^{-1} is permitted) [5]. Since the early 1990s, a monitoring program for total colony counts and somatic cell counts in raw milk has been conducted by the European Union. Similar programs have been in effect in many developed countries for more than two decades. The major strategy to extend shelf life of raw milk is to provide rapid refrigeration. However, in some cases, alternative methods other than refrigeration would be employed as well. Carbonation of raw milk or activation of lactoperoxidase (LP) system in raw milk is among the practical alternatives to farm cooling, if farm cooling is impractible.

2.2.1.4.1 Carbon Dioxide (CO$_2$) Application

Decreasing the storage temperature from 6°C to 2°C increases the time for the psychrotrophic count to reach 10^6 cfu mL^{-1} from 2.9 to 5 days [9]. However, cooling does not prevent the growth of psychrotrophs that are present as normal contaminants in raw milk [10]. Several authors have reported on the use of CO$_2$ as an antimicrobial agent in foods including dairy products [11–13]. King and Mabbitt [14] demonstrated an extension in storage life of both poor and good quality milks by the addition of 30 mM CO_2. The incorporation of carbon dioxide can be achieved by several ways, for example, addition of carbonated water into raw milk, injection of CO_2, or addition of metal carbonates. Vinderola et al. [15] demonstrated that injection of CO_2 into yogurt milk reduced the fermentation time significantly without adversely affecting the growth and metabolic activities of the yogurt starter bacteria. The level of CO_2 added is of critical importance since excess CO_2 reduces milk pH and causes partly destabilization of casein micelles, which makes raw milk sensitive to coagulation during heat treatment. CO_2 shows antimicrobial effect over a wide range of pH in raw milk [16,17].

2.2.1.4.2   LP System Activation

The activation of the LP system is currently the only approved method for raw milk preservation, apart from refrigeration, in Codex Alimentarius. The LP system operates by the reactivation of the enzyme LP, which is naturally present in raw milk, by the addition of thiocyanate and a source of peroxide. This results in the blocking of bacterial metabolism thereby preventing the multiplication of bacteria present in milk. The LP system is promoted by Food and Agriculture Organization of the United Nations (FAO) as an effective means of extending the shelf life of raw milk in developing countries where technical, economical, and/or practical reasons do not allow the use of cooling facilities for maintaining the quality of raw milk [18].

The LP system strongly inhibits the growth of Gram(−) microorganisms in raw milk. The efficiency of the LP system depends on the storage temperature of raw milk [19]. Özer et al. [20] demonstrated that the fermentation period was extended in yogurt made from milk in which the LP system was activated. Residual peroxide may also cause partial inhibition of thermophilic yogurt starter bacteria [21]. Additionally, the physical properties of the final product made from the LP system activated milk was weakened due to H_2O_2-induced oxidation of protein thiol groups [20,22,23]. Therefore, parameters required for the activation of the LP system should be selected carefully. Özer [7] reports the ideal concentrations of H_2O_2 and thiocyanate as 20–40 mg kg^{-1}.

2.2.2   FAT STANDARDIZATION

The fat content of yogurt can vary from 0.1% to over 10% in order to meet existing regulations. Also, milk fat content may show seasonal variation during a lactation period, which makes standardization of the final product difficult. Therefore, standardization of milk fat prior to yogurt manufacturing is essential. To adjust the level of milk fat, a number of practical ways are employed:

- Removal of part of the fat from milk through mechanical separation
- Addition of cream onto fresh skimmed, semiskimmed, or full-fat milk
- Mixing full cream milk with skimmed milk
- Combination of some of the methods given above

During the last two decades, automatic systems have been designed for continuous standardization of the fat content in the milk and surplus cream. *CompoMaster type KCC*, developed by APV Nordic, Denmark, is one of the well-designed automatic fat standardization systems. This system operates together with a milk separator. The fat content of milk is automatically determined using a density transmitter. The capacity of the system varies between 7.000 and 60.000 L h^{-1} and operates in the temperature range of 55–65°C. Calibration of the equipment is done only once every second year. Another automatic fat standardization system, called *Automatic Direct Standardization (ADS) System*, was developed by Tetra Pak A/B, Sweden. The system consists of a number of flow and density transmitters, modulating and other valves, and a control panel (Figure 2.1). The control panel contains the control system and an operator interface. The operator interface may be incorporated into a central control panel. The milk and cream fat content set-points as well as the required total production quantities of milk and cream are preset on the operator interface. The transmitters are integrated with the computer in a Cascade Control System, which ensures fast process response and accurate standardization of both cream and milk [5,24].

Another automatic fat standardization system, OL 7000F, was developed by On-Line Instrumentation Inc., USA. This system relies on measuring the density of the skimmed milk and cream phase after separation, and therefore on controlling the flow of each component to standardize the milk to the desired fat content. The principles of operating the OL-7000 standardization system are illustrated in Figure 2.2.

2.2.3 STANDARDIZATION OF SOLIDS NONFAT (SNF) CONTENT OF YOGURT MILK BASE

It is well known that raising the level of SNF in bovine milk above the typical value of 8.5–9.0% improves the gel strength of set yogurt and viscosity of the stirred yogurt. The values for these physical parameters tend to increase with levels of SNF

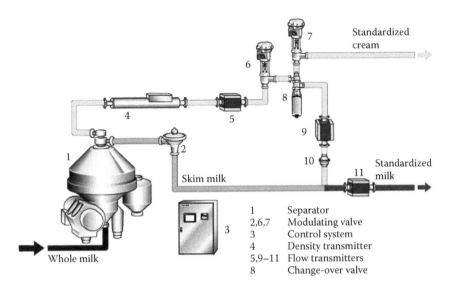

1	Separator
2,6,7	Modulating valve
3	Control system
4	Density transmitter
5,9–11	Flow transmitters
8	Change-over valve

FIGURE 2.1 Illustration of a Tetra Alfast Plus separator for standardization of fat content in milk and cream. (Courtesy of On-Line Instrumentation Inc., New York, USA; Tetra Pak A/B, Lund, Sweden.)

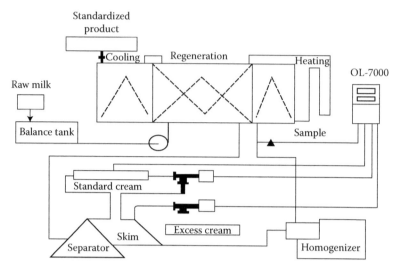

FIGURE 2.2   Schematic illustration of the OL-7000 automatic fat standardization system. (Courtesy of On-Line Instrumentation Inc., New York, USA.)

up to a maximum of 16% [25], but the benefits of exceeding this figure are usually marginal—at least as measured by the penetrometer or viscometer. As a result of increasing the level of SNF in the mix, the titratable acidity of the milk is raised owing to the buffering action of the additional proteins, phosphates, citrates, lactates, and other miscellaneous milk compounds [5]. This function can lead to a reduced gel formation time. Different levels of SNF can affect the growth kinetics of the yogurt starter bacteria and optimum SNF levels for the growth of *Streptococcus thermophilus* and *L. delbrueckii* subsp. *bulgaricus* were 14% and 12%, respectively. There are a number of different methods for the fortification of SNF levels in the yogurt milk base. These methods are as follows:

- Boiling
- Addition of milk powder (MP)
- Addition of buttermilk powder (BP)
- Addition of whey powder (WP) or whey concentrate (WC), whey protein powder (WPP), or whey protein concentrate (WPC)
- Addition of caseinate
- Evaporation
- Membrane techniques [ultrafiltration (UF) or reverse osmosis (RO)]

In Table 2.2, the effects of SNF fortification methods on the gross composition of milk are presented.

2.2.3.1 Boiling

Boiling is the oldest way of increasing the SNF of the yogurt mix. Apart from home scale productions, this method is completely deserted by the yogurt manufacturers.

TABLE 2.2

Effects of Different SNF Methods on the Milk Constituents

Method	Fat	Protein	Lactose	Ash
Boiling	+	+	+	+
Addition of SMP	−	+	+	+
Addition of BP	−[a]	+	−	+
Addition of WPP or WPC	−	+	−	−
Addition of WP or WC	−[b]	+[c]	+	+
Addition of caseinate	−	+	−	−[d]
Evaporation	+	+	+	+
UF	+	+	−	−[d]
RO	+	+	+	+

[a] Fat content is slightly increased due to the trace amount of phospholipids.

[b] Fat content is increased since the additives contain low level of milk fat (0.5–0.6%).

[c] Contains mainly WP fractions.

[d] Mineral contents of yogurt is increased due to casein micelle-bound minerals.

2.2.3.2 Addition of MP

Fortification of milk SNF level by adding skimmed MP (SMP) or whole MP is a common practice in the small-scale yogurt production plants. Whole MP has a shorter shelf life and may lead to the formation of oxidized aroma in the yogurt; therefore, SMP is more widely used for this purpose [26]. In practice, the level of SMP added into the yogurt mix varies between 1% and 6%, but exceeding the critical level of 3–4% may cause lumpy texture and powdery taste in the yogurt [27]. Although in some countries, yogurt is produced totally using SMP (12% SNF) and anhydrous milk fat (99.9% fat), in some other countries including Italy and Denmark, addition of MP to the yogurt mix is prohibited.

Seasonal variations in milk components are the major handicap of the yogurt industry in ensuring product standardization. This handicap can be overcome by adjusting the protein content of the milk using SMP [28].

In line with the latest development in membrane technology, high-protein MPs have gained popularity in the yogurt market [29,30]. The use of ultrafiltered MPs offers advantages in preventing after-acidification in yogurt due to the reduced level of lactose in the MP [7]. Such powders have been commercialized by New Zealand Milk Products (ALACO) and DMV International (Excellion, with 51–85% protein level). Both special powders have been reported to increase the texture, viscosity, and mouthfeel and reduce the whey separation in the yogurt [31]. Fortification of yogurt mix by SMP is more suitable for the set-type yogurts rather than the stirred-type yogurts [32]. Specifications of the MP are determinative for the quality of the final product. Medium heat-treated SMPs (120–125°C/30 s), with a whey protein nitrogen index (WPNI) of 4.00–5.99 mg g^{-1}, are more suitable for yogurt production. Additionally, the cysteine, thiol, and heat numbers of the powders should be 38–48, 7.5–9.4, and 80–83, respectively.

2.2.3.3   Addition of BP

Although it is not a common practice at industrial level, fortification of yogurt mix with BP may result in a yogurt with desired sensory and physical properties [33]. Guinee et al. [34] reported that the whey separation was reduced in yogurts made from milk fortified with BP compared to the yogurt with added SMP. The level of BP should not exceed 4.5–5.0% for an acceptable yogurt [35]. Fortification of unconcentrated fresh buttermilk with SMP or by UF or nanofiltration (NF) is another alternative to obtain good textural and sensory quality yogurt [36].

2.2.3.4   Addition of Whey-Derived Powders

Since the early 1990s, the use of whey products and blended dairy powders in the manufacture of yogurt has been widely investigated [34,37]. The most common forms of whey are as follows:

- WC [38–40]
- WP [41,42]
- WPC [5,32]
- WPP [5]
- Hydrolyzed whey concentrate (WCH) [43,44]
- Whey isolate (WI) [5].

The level of WP and WPP added into milk may vary between 0.6% and 4.0%. However, in order to minimize the risk of development of unacceptable aroma/flavor in the yogurt, the level of fortification should be about 2–3% [45,46]. In order to improve the characteristic aroma/flavor in yogurt, preincubation of whey with yogurt starter bacteria is recommended. The prefermented whey is then spray dried and the powder is used in the manufacture of yogurt [47]. In the case of use of WC or WPC (with 28–30% total solids), the level of fortification should not exceed 20–25%; otherwise the color of the yogurt turns greenish and the texture of the product is weakened [48]. Since yogurt milk is heated at relatively high temperatures (e.g., 85–90°C for 10–30 min), the WPs present in WPC are flocculated and the water-holding capacity of the curd is reduced. To overcome this handicap, milk and WPC should be heated separately or heating temperature should be lower than 82°C, which is the critical temperature for WP flocculation [7]. WP or WPC may result in development of salty taste in the yogurt. This can be overcome by demineralizing the WP or WPC via UF/microfiltration (MF). Demineralization was reported to prolong the incubation period of the yogurt as well as adversely affecting the textural properties. Therefore, the incorporation of demineralized WP/WPC is recommended for the stirred-type yogurts rather than the set-type product [49]. The effects of WP or WPC fortification on the properties of yogurt are summarized in Table 2.3.

2.2.3.5   Addition of Caseinates

Although it is not a common practice, various forms of caseinates may be used for the fortification of SNF of yogurt base. Addition of casein powders to yogurt mix

TABLE 2.3

Summary of the Results of Recent Studies on the Application of WP and/or WPC in Yogurt Manufacturing

Application	Effect on Yogurt	Reference
Increased substitution of milk solids with WPC	Low viscosity and weak gel development	[32,61,62]
Excessive level of WPs	Development of a grainy texture in the yogurt	[63]
Fortification of milk base with demineralized whey and heating at 90°C	Improvement in the viscosity of the 14-day-old yogurts	[49]
Blending WPC (25% or 80% protein) with SMP at various levels	Change in the casein-to-fat (C:N) ratio in milk base; the physical properties of the yogurt were improved with a reduced C:N ratio	[64,65]
Fortification of milk base with acetylated WPC (made by heat precipitation of salted whey or UF of sweet whey)	The best sensory quality yogurt was obtained from milk fortified with 2% UF-WPC	[40]
Adding WPC into yogurt mix along with cysteine	Improved firmness in the final product, stimulation of health-promoting bacteria in yogurt	[38,66–68]
Treatment of WPI with microbial TGase	Increase in the intrinsic viscosity, decrease in gelation temperature, stronger gel structure	[69]
Addition of milk protein hydrolysate	Reduced fermentation time, decreased viscosity and graininess of yogurt	[53]
Addition of casein hydrolysate to yogurt base	Enhancement of the cell counts of probiotics in yogurt	[70]
Incorporation of caseinolytic enzymes into yogurt base to hydrolyze κ-CN	Improved gelation capacity of fermenting milk	[71]
Addition of WPC to the milk base	No influence on the viability of yogurt starters	[72]

leads to improvement in the physical properties of the resulting product without impairing the sensory properties. On the other hand, excessive use of casein powders causes a very dense protein matrix leading eventually to whey separation during storage [50]. It is important that the ratio between milk serum proteins and caseins (20:80 in cow's milk) should be maintained to have a product with desired rheological properties. Therefore, in the case of adding casein powder to increase SNF of yogurt mix, WPP or WPC should also be included to restore the casein to serum protein balance [51]. Small- or medium-size free amino acids derived from hydrolyzed caseins were demonstrated to stimulate the growth of *Streptococcus thermophilus* [52]. Sodini et al. [53] used casein and WP hydrolysates in yogurt, and concluded that the addition of hydrolysates reduced fermentation time, decreased viscosity and graininess, and the structure of the gel was more open and less branched. It was reported that the viscosity of yogurt with added 1% of protein hydrolysate was improved by 30% [54].

2.2.3.6 Vacuum Evaporation

Small factories with a low throughput of product tend to rely on the addition of powder, whereas large factories may find that the financial investment in process plant is more than offset by the economies offered by vacuum evaporation (EV). EV operates on the basis of removal of vaporized water by lowering the boiling point of milk under low pressure (~−0.5 bar). The vast majority of the large-scale yogurt manufacturers use multiple effect evaporators equipped with either thermal or mechanical vapor recompression unit (Figure 2.3).

During evaporation, the concentrations of all the milk constituents increase with the concentration factor, with the exception of minor losses of volatile compounds in the concentrate. To reach the target protein level in yogurt mix (5.5–6.0%) for obtaining a better textural quality yogurt, the concentration factor should be high. This eventually leads to prolonging the processing time. On the other hand, vacuum evaporators are very common in medium and/or large-scale yogurt plants since they are relatively cheap and easy to operate. For a good-quality yogurt, the TS level of yogurt mix concentrated by EV should be 16–18%, as recommended by Baltadzhieva et al. [55]. Removal of entrapped air during evaporation under vacuum contributes to the stability of the coagulum and reduces syneresis during storage [56]. EV is also widely employed in the manufacture of WP, WC, WPP, WPC, and SMP.

2.2.3.7 Membrane Techniques

Membrane techniques (especially UF) have been successfully used in the yogurt industry for more than two decades. The usual membrane processes are RO, UF, MF, and NF. The basic differences of these techniques are summarized in Tables 2.4 and 2.5. MF separates particles and suspended materials of sizes in the order of 0.1–10 μm. Therefore, it is widely used in the separation of bacteria and milk fat

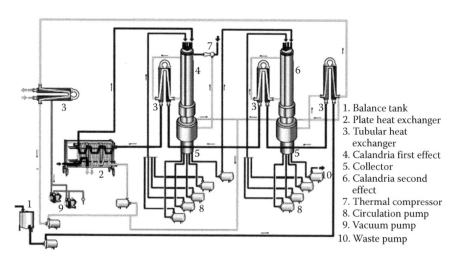

1. Balance tank
2. Plate heat exchanger
3. Tubular heat exchanger
4. Calandria first effect
5. Collector
6. Calandria second effect
7. Thermal compressor
8. Circulation pump
9. Vacuum pump
10. Waste pump

FIGURE 2.3 Multieffect falling film evaporator. (Courtesy of Tetra Pak A/B, Lund, Sweden.)

TABLE 2.4

Efficiency of Different Membrane Processes in Separation of Milk Components

Milk Compounds	RO	NF	UF	MF
Water	–	–	–	–
Minerals	+ / –	–	–	–
Lactose, amino acids, and nonprotein nitrogen	+	+	–	–
Proteins	+	+	+	–
Fat and bacteria	+	+	+	+

Source: After Tamime, A.Y. and Robinson, R.K., *Yoghurt Science and Technology*, 3rd edition, Woodhead Publishing, Cambridge, p. 808, 2007.

+, retained in the retentate; –, passes through the membrane into the permeate.

globules from the milk [57]. This system is also effective in defatting of whey, which is then processed to WPC or WPI. RO allows separation of small molecules and ions (molecular weight <1.000; molecular size <0.001 μm) from the milk or whey. RO is widely employed for concentrating whey and UF permeate. Application of RO in concentrating yogurt milk is far less common. NF separates selectively low-molecular-weight solutes from aqueous solution. The permeability of NF is higher than RO but less than UF and operates at pressures of 2–3 MPa. NF is a common technology in partial demineralization/desalination of whey, UF permeate, or retentate [5].

Several reports on the use of UF-treated milk for the manufacture of high-quality yogurt have been published. In general, yogurt made from UF-concentrated milk

TABLE 2.5

Specifications of RO, UF, and MF Systems

Parameters	MF	UF	RO
Size of solutes retained	>10^6 Da (0.01–10 μm)	10^3–10^6 Da (0.001–0.02 μm)	<1000 Da (<0.001 μm)
Operating pressure (bar)	<2	1–15	>20
Operating temperature (°C)	45–50	35–45	30–50
Mechanism of membrane retention	Molecular screening	Molecular screening	Diffusive transport, possibly molecular screening
Typical flux (L m^{-2} h^{-1})	>300	30–300	3–30

Source: After Renner, E. and Abd-El Salam, M.H., *Application of Ultrafiltration in the Dairy Industry*, Elsevier Applied Science, London, p. 132, 1991.

1 bar = 0.1 MPa = 1 kg cm^{-2} = 14.5 psi = 10^5 N m^{-2} (1 N = 10^5 dyne).

had a firmer body than the samples produced from RO milk, milk with added MP, or unconcentrated milk [58]. Ferguson [59] urged the use of UF milk in the manufacture of yogurt, as it eliminates the homogenization stage and gives rise to a smooth and creamy texture. Similarly, Becker and Puhan [60] demonstrated that UF resulted in a yogurt rated as superior to yogurt made from milk concentrated by EV or adding SMP.

Yogurt has a weak viscoelastic gel structure formed from a three-dimensional network, which immobilizes the liquid phase [25]. The physical quality of gel network is largely determined by the protein concentration of the yogurt mix, since protein–protein bonds triggered by heat treatment and acidity development are essential for the formation of gel network in which fat globules are also entrapped. Therefore, increasing the protein and fat content of milk is the prime target of SNF fortification systems in the yogurt industry. During UF, lactose, a major component of milk total solids, is effectively removed through the permeate and the increase in the levels of protein and fat is relatively higher compared with the other SNF fortification methods. The utilization of UF-concentrated milk for the manufacture of yogurt strengthens the yogurt coagulum, increases viscosity, and prevents whey separation and syneresis [73]. For a good-quality yogurt, a high ratio of casein to noncasein protein is required. Although, during UF, the casein to noncasein protein ratio in milk is not largely changed, somewhat increased formation of lactic acid in UF yogurt results in firmer coagulum compared with other fortification systems. A protein to lactose ratio of 1.2 was reported to be ideal for yogurt with improved textural properties [74].

The growth of yogurt starter bacteria is enhanced in UF concentrated milk because of the presence of greater amounts of nutrients available. On the other hand, proteolytic capacity of yogurt starters is to some extent weakened by UF [75]. The increased buffer capacity due to the high protein concentration protects starter organisms against the low pH value [76–78]. This effect has been confirmed by calculations of maximum generation times (G_{max}) for the mixed yogurt cultures [79]. If the ultrafiltered milk is heated to 85–90°C, the acidification time of yogurt is reduced, which is explained by the decreased oxygen content that exhibits an inhibitory effect on *Streptococcus thermophilus* in the yogurt culture [80].

UF is applied to the manufacture of concentrated yogurt as well. Two different systems of UF have been developed for the manufacture of concentrated yogurt. First, the fermentation of UF retentate (Figure 2.4a) that has the solids content desired in concentrated yogurt, about 24% [81–90], and second, the UF of yogurt at 40–50°C until the targeted level of total solids in the product is reached [83,86,88,91–94] (Figure 2.4b). Although the final chemical compositions of both products are similar to each other, the physical and organoleptic properties are considerably different [95]. The concentration of milk by UF prior to concentrated yogurt-making carries the risk of bitterness in the final product since the calcium content will be higher. The main advantages of the UF technique as compared with other conventional methods are higher yield (i.e., increases by 10%), shorter processing time (e.g., by 25%), and lower wheying-off [81,83,86,88,93]. In addition, the volumes of milk, starter cultures, and salt (optional) are reduced by about 10%, 80%, and 50%, respectively. It was reported that the concentrated yogurt produced using the

(a)   (b)

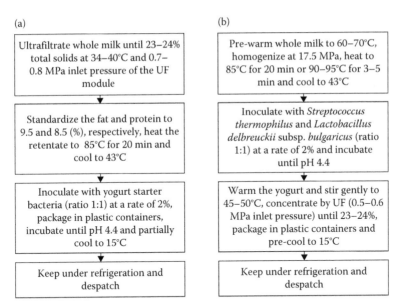

Ultrafiltrate whole milk until 23–24% total solids at 34–40°C and 0.7–0.8 MPa inlet pressure of the UF module	Pre-warm whole milk to 60–70°C, homogenize at 17.5 MPa, heat to 85°C for 20 min or 90–95°C for 3–5 min and cool to 43°C
Standardize the fat and protein to 9.5 and 8.5 (%), respectively, heat the retentate to 85°C for 20 min and cool to 43°C	Inoculate with *Streptococcus thermophilus* and *Lactobacillus delbrueckii* subsp. *bulgaricus* (ratio 1:1) at a rate of 2% and incubate until pH 4.4
Inoculate with yogurt starter bacteria (ratio 1:1) at a rate of 2%, package in plastic containers, incubate until pH 4.4 and partially cool to 15°C	Warm the yogurt and stir gently to 45–50°C, concentrate by UF (0.5–0.6 MPa inlet pressure) until 23–24%, package in plastic containers and pre-cool to 15°C
Keep under refrigeration and despatch	Keep under refrigeration and despatch

FIGURE 2.4 Production of concentrated yogurt from (a) UF whole milk retentate and (b) UF warm yogurt. (After Özer, B.H., *Yogurt Bilimi ve Teknolojisi*, Sidas Yayincilik, Izmir, p. 496, 2006.)

UF method had a smoother body and texture, and more palatable in taste than those manufactured by the traditional method [7].

Milk can be concentrated by UF to the desired total solids level without any difficulty, but the efficiency of the UF plant in concentrating warm yogurt is largely dependent on the operational temperature and operational pressures [96]. At low processing temperatures (i.e., 30–35°C), the permeability of the aqueous phase across the membrane is rather slow. Temperatures above 50°C cause an increase in the fouling rate of the UF membrane, which may affect the processing conditions in large-scale operations [97]. In general, with the increase in processing temperature, the flux rate and the firmness of the yogurt increase, but at >50°C, the total viable counts of the yogurt starter organisms decline. The ideal operational temperature for UF yogurt is 35–45°C. The inlet pressure of the UF plant should not exceed 0.7–0.8 MPa, and the difference between the inlet and outlet pressures should be about 0.25–0.30 MPa [95,96]. In order to prevent membrane fouling and increase the membrane efficiency, UF of skimmed milk is a practical option. After the desired total solids level has been reached, the skimmed milk is mixed with pasteurized cream (Figure 2.5).

2.2.4 Additives

The popularity of low-calorie yogurts has increased dramatically during the last 10–15 years. The production of low-calorie products can be achieved by using any one or combinations of the following methods: (i) replacement of the carbohydrate

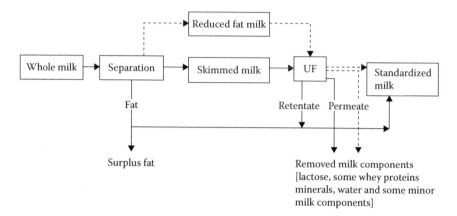

FIGURE 2.5 Continuous membrane filtration of yogurt milk. Dotted lines indicate the UF model for the fat content of preadjusted milk. (Courtesy of APV Nordic A/S, Aarhus, Denmark.)

with artificial sweeteners, (ii) reducing the carbohydrate content using fiber or bulking ingredients (i.e., hydrocolloids such as carrageenan or guar gum), (iii) lowering the fat content in traditional food products, and (iv) using fat substitutes to replace fat in food while keeping the same functional and organoleptic properties as fats without the calories [98].

2.2.4.1   Fat Substitutes

Fat substitutes used in the yogurt production are given in Table 2.6. Some scientific data are available on the use of different types of milk fat replacement during the

TABLE 2.6

Origin and Specifications of Fat Substitutes Potentially Used in Yogurt Production

Commercial Name	Origin	Reference
I. Hydrocolloid and carbohydrates		
Guar		
Carrageenan	Natural gums	[104]
Xanthan		
N-Oil®2	Tapioca (3.75 kcal g^{-1})	[105]
Litesse™	Polydextrose (1 kcal g^{-1})	[106]
Lycadex®100 and 200	Potatoes	[107]
Avicel®	Cellulose (0 kcal g^{-1})	[108]
II. Microparticulated proteins		
Simplesse®	Milk/egg white	[105,109]
Miprodan®	Milk	[110]
Dairy-Lo™	WPs	[111]

manufacture of yogurt. The number of fat-substitute products is far beyond the ones listed in Table 2.6. However, not all the fat substitutes are available for scientific investigations either because they are not fully developed or because they are awaiting establishment of their safety status. As a consequence, the availability of fat substitutes is somewhat restricted. Some of the commercially available fat substitutes are Litesse™, Paselli®SA2, N-Oil®2, Simplesse®, Lycadex®100 and 200, Maltodextrin, Dairy-Lo™, and P-fibre 150C and 285F [7].

It was demonstrated that the metabolic activities of yogurt starter bacteria including lactose metabolism, acidity development, and organic acid production were not affected by fat substitutes [99]. On the other hand, fat substitutes caused a decrease in the casein micelle size and casein micelles became shorter, which eventually led to improvement of rheological properties in yogurt [100,101]. Similarly, sensory properties of the yogurt were improved greatly when fat substitutes were used in the manufacture of set-type fat-free yogurt [102,103].

However, incorporation of fat substitutes at high concentrations (>1.5%) weakened the physical and sensory properties of the yogurt [111,112]. Recently, it has been shown that the use of β-cyclodextrin as partial fat replacer has improved the characteristic aroma of the yogurt [113].

Since fat substitutes are used in placement of milk fat, the uptake of oil-soluble vitamins is restricted. Therefore, in the case of use of fat substitutes in the manufacture of yogurt, A, D, E, and K vitamins should be added into yogurt mix to keep the balance of healthy diet.

2.2.4.2   Stabilizers

Although many consumers prefer yogurts to be "additive-free," stabilizers are widely added into stirred yogurts to improve viscosity and texture, and reduce susceptibility to syneresis. Stabilizers also improve mouthfeel and permit reduction in calories while maintaining the organoleptic quality [2]. Stabilizers are hydrocolloids including gelatin and carbohydrates such as pregelatinized starch, agar, guar gum, pectin, and carrageenan. Stabilizers are divided into three groups based on their origin [5]:

1. Natural stabilizers
2. Modified natural or semisynthetic stabilizers
3. Synthetic stabilizers.

The stabilizers permitted by FAO/WHO [114] are listed in Table 2.7.

Stabilizers have two main functions: (i) water binding and (ii) increasing viscosity [115]. Stabilizers can form a three-dimensional gel network and this network can limit movement of free water by binding it [116] and increasing the water-binding capacity of milk components (mainly proteins) by interacting with these compounds [117], and increasing the stabilization of protein molecules in the gel network [117]. The suggested levels of some stabilizers used in yogurt production are presented in Table 2.8.

The level of stabilizers added into yogurt mix is determined by their effects on the physical and chemical properties of the final product and by total solids level of

TABLE 2.7
Some Stabilizers Permitted by FAO/WHO

Natural	Function in Yogurt	Modified, Natural, or Semisynthetic	Function in Yogurt
Arabic gum	Thickener, stabilizer	Cellulose derivatives	Thickener
Targacanth	Thickener	i. Carboxymethylcellulose	
Karaya		ii. Methylcellulose	
Pectins	Stabilizer, gelling agent	iii. Hydroxymethylcellulose	
Carob	Thickener	iv. Hydroxypropylcellulose	
Guar	Thickener	v. Hydroxypropylmethylcellulose	
Agar	Stabilizer, gelling agent	vi. Microcrystallinecellulose	
Alginates	Thickener, stabilizer, gelling agent	Xanthan (by microbial fermentation)	Thickener, stabilizer
Carrageenan	Stabilizer, gelling agent	Miscellaneous derivatives	
Furcelleran	Thickener, stabilizer, gelling agent	i. Low-methoxy pectin	
Gelatin	Stabilizer	ii. Propylene glycole alginate	
		iii. Pregelatinized starches	
		iv. Modified starches	

Source: Adapted from Tamime, A.Y. and Robinson, R.K., *Yoghurt Science and Technology*, 3rd edition, Woodhead Publishing, Cambridge, p. 808, 2007.

the yogurt. In general, the higher the total solids level of yogurt mix, the lesser the amount of stabilizer added. It was reported, for example, that with the increase in the total solids level of yogurt mix from 12.5% to 22%, the level of gelatin/plant origin gums mixture was reduced to 0.25% from 0.5% [5]. The type of stabilizer is one of the parameters determining the incubation temperature. For instance, in the case of

TABLE 2.8
The Suggested Concentrations of Some Stabilizers Used in the Manufacture of Yogurt

Stabilizers	Concentrations (%)	Reference
Pectin or modified starch	0.02–0.70	[124,125]
Pectin	0.05	[126]
Agar–agar, guar gum, alginate, gelatin, Carrageenan or carboxymethylcellulose	0.05–0.60	[127]
Starch preparations	1.00–2.00	[128]
Guar gum	0.10–0.50	[129]
Sugar beet fiber	0.50–2.00	[130]
Gelodan	0.35	[131]
Na-alginate	0.30	[132]
Na-alginate + β-cyclodextrin	0.20 + 0.10	[133]

use of modified starch (≤1% conc.), incubation temperature should be decreased from 43°C to 35–36°C [62,119]. The level and/or type of stabilizers used in the production of yogurt are determined by the production model of the yogurt. For example, for long life or ultra high temperature (UHT) yogurts, locust bean gum, the mixture of agar–agar and xanthan [120], or starch derivatives [121] were recommended. Similarly, the use of modified starch was reported to cause textural defects in frozen yogurt or yogurt-ice [122]. Protein-based stabilizers are more suitable for improvement of viscosity in the stirred yogurts [123].

The majority of the stabilizers are solidified at <10°C, except agar–agar and gelatin that are solidified at 25°C and 42–45°C, respectively. Therefore, in the case of use of gelatin or agar–agar in the manufacture of the stirred yogurt, the yogurt should be passed through a fine metal sieve to avoid lumpiness in the final product. The effects of some stabilizers on the physical and sensory properties of yogurt are summarized in Table 2.9.

2.2.4.3 Sweeteners

2.2.4.3.1 Nutritive Sweeteners

In the manufacture of flavored yogurt, it is usually desirable to add a sweetening agent to the yogurt base. For this purpose, sucrose is widely used in either liquid (60–67% total solids) or granulated form [134]. In the case of use of liquid sucrose, the total solids content of the resulting product should be taken into consideration to avoid the dilution of the total solids of the yogurt mix. Due to the inhibitory effect of sugar on the yogurt starter bacteria, the level of added sugar should not exceed the level of 10–11%. It has been reported that on the addition of sucrose at 8% or higher, the production of acetaldehyde (major carbonyl compound of yogurt) is suppressed [135]. For safety reasons, the sweeteners that are added after fermentation must be pasteurized prior to use. Using liquid sugar is more widely preferred by the yogurt manufacturers, because of efficiency of its handling. Although liquid sugar may seem to be more economical, conversion from dry sugar to liquid sugar set-up requires capital cost for sugar storage tanks, appropriate pumps, heaters, strainers, and meters [134]. All measures have to be taken to avoid microbial growth in sugar storage tanks. These measures include attachment of a UV light source to the storage tanks and proper ventilation of the tanks to avoid moisture condensation and resulting microbial growth. Other nutritive sweeteners such as corn sweeteners, maltodextrins, high fructose corn syrup, crystalline fructose, and invert sugar are far less commonly used in the manufacture of yogurt, but they are mostly preferred for the manufacture of low/nonfat frozen yogurt or frozen desserts. Crystalline fructose is widely used to effect flavor improvement in light yogurt by rounding off the sweet flavor of aspartame and other nonnutritive sweeteners [134].

2.2.4.3.2 Artificial Sweeteners

Artificial sweeteners are chemicals that offer the sweetness of sugar without the calories. Because the substitutes are much sweeter than sugar, it takes a much smaller quantity of them to create the same sweetness. Therefore, products made with artificial sweeteners have a much lower calorie count than do those made with sugar. During the last two decades, consumer demand over low-calorie fruit yogurts has

TABLE 2.9

Effect of Various Stabilizers on the Physical and Sensory Properties of Yogurt

Stabilizers	Effect on Yogurt	Reference
Xanthan (≤0.01%)	Viscosity was increased without impairing organoleptic properties in stirred yogurt	[136]
Gelatin and starch	More effective on the physical properties of the stirred yogurt than synthetic or modified synthetic stabilizers	[137,138]
Gellan gum (microbial origin)	Viscosity was improved and whey separation was reduced significantly in the stirred yogurt	[139]
Gelatin	At concentrations of ≥0.8%, sensory defects were noted and viscosity was decreased	[140,141]
Arabic gum and carboxymethylcellulose	Development of atypical aroma/flavor in the yogurt	[142]
Locust bean gum	At ≥0.02% concentrations, the syneresis was stimulated in the yogurt	[143]
Modified starch	Replacing nonfat dry milk with up to 40% modified starch did not significantly affect the flavor, body and texture, and appearance	[140]
Pectin and starch	Negatively affected the formation of carbonyl compounds in yogurt	[144]
Locust bean gum	Positively affected the formation of aroma/flavor compounds	[144]
Starch and pectin	Interaction of starch or pectin with esters (e.g., pentyl acetate or ethyl pentoate), aldehydes [hexanal (E)-2-hexenal] and lactones (γ-octalactone) increased the concentrations of aroma compounds	[145]
Tapioca-based starch	0.6% Tapioca-based starch was able to replace 2% SNF without affecting the properties of yogurt	[146]
Low-methoxy pectin, λ-carrageenan, guar gum, locust bean gum, xanthan	Stabilization of casein aggregates improved with the increase in the level of low-methoxy pectin and λ-carrageenan	[147]
λ-Carrageenan	No adverse affect on the properties of the yogurt up to the level of 0.03%	[148]

increased tremendously. Therefore, replacement of natural sugar with artificial sweeteners, such as aspartame, saccharin, acesulfame, and sucrose, has been studied in detail and commercialized. The level of artificial sweeteners added into the yogurt mix depends on the acidity and relative sweetness of the sugar of fruit. The effect of sweeteners on the aroma/flavor of fruit yogurt is determined by pH and temperature [149]. The natural or modified sweeteners are readily degraded at high temperatures. One method of manufacturing set-type flavored yogurt involves the addition of sweeteners to the base mix before fermentation. In stirred-type fruit yogurts, the sweeteners are added just before the packaging.

The fruit preparations used by the yogurt industry may be prepared in two different ways: (i) fruit preserves that do not contain any added sweetening agent and (ii) fruits with added sweeteners. Addition of sweeteners with fruit is more common and the level of added sweeteners in processed fruits for yogurt manufacture ranges from 25% to 65%, with the most popular level being 30–35% [5].

The sweeteners added into yogurt mix may affect the metabolic activity of yogurt starter bacteria. Overall, with the increase in the level of sweeteners, the metabolic activity of the starter bacteria is weakened, leading to low viscosity and acidity development in the final product [150]. The levels of inhibitory effect of various sweeteners on yogurt starters are shown in Table 2.10.

The inhibitory effect of sweeteners is directly related with the water activity (a_w) and osmotic pressure of the environment [151]. With the increase in the total solids level of yogurt mix, the a_w decreases. In normal circumstances, the metabolic activities of the starter bacteria are fairly slowed down at a_w levels of 0.65–0.70. In addition, due to the hygroscopic effect of sugar, the level of water available for the metabolic activities of starter bacteria decreases. The origins and technical specifications of some sweeteners are given in Table 2.11.

The function of artificial sweeteners is not limited to the contribution to the aroma/flavor of the yogurt. They also play active roles in modifications and size of casein micelle during acidification of the milk [152]. The stability of sweeteners throughout the storage period is one of the prime criteria in the selection of the sweeteners for yogurt manufacturing [153]. The current trend in the use of high-intensity (artificial) sweeteners in yogurt is blending two or more sweeteners to optimize the flavor profile of yogurt.

2.2.4.4 Addition of Preservatives

In the yogurt industry, preservatives are commonly used in the preparation of fruit yogurts and concentrated yogurts. The basic function of the preservatives is to prevent the growth of undesired microorganisms contaminating yogurt during or

TABLE 2.10
Inhibitory Levels of Different Sweeteners on the Yogurt Starter Bacteria

Sweeteners	Level of Inhibitory Effect (%)
Sucrose	>4.00
Fructose	>2.70
Aspartame	>0.02
Fructo-oligosaccharides	>7.30
Isomalto-oligosaccharides	>7.70

Source: After Song, T.B., et al., *Dairy Sci. Abstr.*, 58, 243, 1996.

TABLE 2.11

Origins and Technical Specifications of Some Sweeteners Used in the Manufacture of Fruit Yogurt

Sweeteners	Specifications	Origin	Reference
Xylitol, fructose, cyclamate, saccharin	Xylitol inhibits the growth of bacteria and it is recommended to be used with sucrose	Carbohydrate	[160]
Thaumatin	Optimum level of thaumatin is 0.0002–0.0003%	Protein	[161]
Aspartame	It is suggested to be used with stabilizers such as methoxy pectin and Na-hexametaphosphate. Aspartame causes slow development of aroma in yogurt. There is a direct relationship between the fat level of yogurt and perception of sweetness of aspartame. Optimum level of addition of aspartame is 0.1–0.75	Protein	[162]
Sorbitol	No adverse effect on the aroma/flavor properties of yogurt is noted when sorbitol is used together with polydextrose	Carbohydrate	[163]
Corn syrup with high level of fructose	This is preferred when a highly sweet yogurt-type product is desired. It does not have any effect on the basic carbonyl compounds of yogurt	Carbohydrate	[164]
Neohesperidine	Stability of this sweetener is maintained during cold storage. It is suggested for use together with aspartame	Carbohydrate	[165]
Actilight®	It stimulates the growth of *Lactobacillus* spp. and *Bifidobacterium* spp.	Carbohydrate	[166]
Sucrose	It is being used in light and low carbohydrate yogurt, drinks and smoothies, with no problem. It is poorly absorbed (11–27%) in the gastrointestinal tract. No negative effect of sucrose on the growth of yogurt starters has been reported	Carbohydrate	[134,167,168]
Neotame™	It is stable at yogurt processing temperatures and fermentation conditions. It enhances the flavor of yogurt	Protein	[134]
Acesulfame-K	Degree of sweetness is dependent on the stabilizers used. The optimum effect is obtained when Acesulfame-K is used with locust bean gum	Acetoacetic acid derivatives	[169]

Source: Rajmohan, S. and Prasad, V., *Cheiron*, 23, 26–31, 1994.

after fermentation [154]. Particularly, the risk of contamination of yeasts and molds in fruit yogurt is high; therefore, preparation of fruit pulps and/or syrups should be handled with care. The count of yeasts and moulds in fruit yogurt should be <1 g^{-1} of yogurt [155]. Some yeasts including *Candida famata* and *Kluyweromyces marxianus* can grow at low temperatures in fruit yogurt [156]. The basic principle of manufacturing traditional concentrated yogurt is to extract water from plain yogurt until the desired total solids level (22–25%) has been reached [7]. During the extraction of water through gravity drainage, which takes about 12–18 h, undesired microorganisms likely contaminate the concentrating yogurt. The major contaminants of concentrated yogurt are yeasts [157]. In addition to the hygienic measures taken in the production of fruit and concentrated yogurts, in some countries, the use of preservatives to prevent the growth of undesirable microorganisms is permitted [158]. FAO/WHO [114] permits the use of sorbic acid (including Na, K, and Ca salts), benzoic acid, and sulfur dioxide in yogurt. The maximum permitted level in the final product is 50 mg kg^{-1} (singly or in combination) [5].

Mycostatic effect of sorbic acid salts is more pronounced at pH ≤ 6.5. Sorbic acid and/or sorbic acid salts prevent the growth of yeasts by blocking their dehydrogenase system. Potassium sorbate not only prevents the growth of yeasts and molds, but also the metabolic activity of the yogurt starter bacteria is partly decelerated by this preservative agent, leading to prolonged fermentation. K-sorbate and Na-benzoate (≤ 400 mg kg^{-1}) are very effective against *Saccharomyces* spp., *Debaryomyces* spp., *Candida* spp., and *Geothricum candidum* in concentrated yogurt [157,170]. Both K-sorbate and Na-benzoate have no adverse effect on the texture and aroma/flavor of yogurt [171].

In recent years, synthetic and semisynthetic preservatives have been replaced by the natural bacteriocins [158]. Among the natural bacteriocins, nisin, which is a polycyclic peptide antibacterial with 34 amino acid residues, is the most commonly used food preservative. Nisin has a relatively limited effect against yeasts and Gram(−) bacteria. On the contrary, Gram(+) bacteria such as *Clostridium* spp. and *Bacillus* spp. are strongly affected by nisin [7]. The use of nisin in yogurt is limited by the sensitivity of the starter culture to nisin, which may impair the fermentation depending on the concentration of nisin and the strains used [172]. It was reported that yogurt starter bacteria are largely inhibited in the presence of nisin at levels of 100–200 RU mL^{-1}, thereby preventing subsequent overacidification of the yogurt [173]. In general, *Streptococcus thermophilus* shows more resistance to nisin than *L. delbrueckii* subsp. *bulgaricus* [174]. Typical application levels of nisin are in the range of 0.50–1.25 mg kg^{-1}. The action of nisin is pH-dependent; it is more effective in low-pH food systems.

Natamycin, also known as pimaricin, is a naturally occurring antimicrobial agent produced by *Streptomyces natalensis*. It is a polyene antibiotic, especially effective against yeasts and molds. On the contrary, natamycin does not have any effect on yogurt starters [175]. Since natamycin can withstand high-temperature and low-pH conditions, it may be added into yogurt mix prior to pasteurization and can maintain its activity up to 2–3 weeks of storage. Although it is not legally permitted for use in yogurt in many countries, natamycin is successfully used in the manufacture of plain or fruit yogurt without affecting the chemical and/or physical properties of the final product [176]. One example of the common commercial mycostatic preservatives in which natamycin is the major active component is Delvocid® (Gist-Brocades Delft, the Netherlands). Other mycostatic preservatives used in the yogurt-making are listed in Table 2.12.

TABLE 2.12
Preservatives Used in the Yogurt-Making and Their Inhibitory Effect on Yogurt Starters

Preservatives	Yeasts	Molds	Streptococcus thermophilus	L. delbrueckii subsp. bulgaricus
Benzoic acid and benzoates	+	+	±[a]	±[a]
Sulfur dioxide	+	+	−	−
Sorbic acid and sorbates	+	+	±[a]	±[a]
Nisin	+	+	−[b]	+
Natamycin	+	+	−	−
Nitrate/nitrite[c]	+	+	+	+
Lysozyme	+	+	−[d]	+[d]
Microgard™				
Ethyl carbamate	+	+	−	−

Source: Baranova, M., et al., Dairy Sci. Abstr., 59, 58, 1997; Kontova, M. and Prekoppova, J., Proc. XXIII Int. Dairy Congr., Vol. II, p. 352, 1990; and Salih, M.A. and Sandine, W.E., J. Dairy Sci., 73, 887–893, 1990.

[a] It is ineffective on yogurt starters up to 0.06 g/100 g.
[b] Resistant up to 25 RU mL^{-1}.
[c] Causes low acidity and viscosity development.
[d] Ineffective against yogurt starters up to 0.5–10 mg/100 g.
[e] Addition at lower concentrations is allowed. At higher concentrations, a carcinogenic risk occurs.

2.2.5 HOMOGENIZATION

Milk is an oil-in-water emulsion, with the fat globules dispersed in a continuous SM phase. If raw milk is left to stand, however, the fat would rise and form a cream layer.

Homogenization is a mechanical treatment of the fat globules in milk brought about by passing milk under high pressure through a tiny orifice, which results in a decrease in the average diameter and an increase in the number and surface area of the fat globules. The net result, from a practical view, is a much reduced tendency for creaming of fat globules.

As a result of homogenization, a number of physical and/or chemical changes occur in yogurt. The adsorption capacity of the newly formed fat globules, for example, onto the casein micelle increases, which leads to an increase in the effective total volume of suspended matter and, therefore, viscosity. There is also an improvement in the consistency of the yogurt and greater stability against whey separation due to the increased hydrophilicity (Table 2.13) [134,180]. Changes in protein–protein interaction as a result of some denaturation and shift in salt balance occur during homogenization. Homogenization triggers some undesirable changes in yogurt as well. For example, total fat surface area available to lipase is increased (up to 4–6 folds), causing extended lipolysis [181]. Depending on the increase in the level of phospholipids in the

TABLE 2.13
Physical Properties of Yogurts Homogenized under
Different Pressures

Pressure[a]	Consistency[b]	Viscosity[c]
0	338.6	868.7
50	338.3	870.0
100	319.5	1050.0
150	315.7	1130.0
200	303.5	1258.3
250	285.7	1385.7
300	278.3	1556.7

Source: Atamer, M., Yildirim, Z., and Sezgin, E., *Gida*, 17, 255–258, 1992.
[a] kg cm^{-2}.
[b] 1/10 mm.
[c] cP.

skimmed milk phase, pumping of yogurt milk can cause foaming in the incubation tanks [5]. Development of oxidized flavor is also likely in the homogenized yogurts.

Homogenization is usually achieved at temperatures ranging between 55°C and 80°C with homogenization pressures between 100 and 250 bar [182]. In yogurt-making, single-stage homogenizers are usually preferred since reclustering of fat globules in yogurt milk is unlikely. The optimum operating temperature for homogenization is 65–70°C where the milk fat is in liquid form. Homogenization is usually applied prior to heat treatment; however, some researchers claim that homogenization after heat treatment improves the physical properties of yogurt [5]. In this case, establishment of aseptic working conditions is essential. However, in a model system developed by APV Nordic A/S (Aarhus, Denmark), milk is subject to heat treatment before and after homogenization, which exempts the necessity of aseptic working conditions (Figure 2.6). Some yogurt manufacturers employ two-stage homogenization. In the two-stage system, homogenization takes place in the first stage. The second stage helps improving the homogenization efficiency through serving as a constant and controlled back-pressure supplier to the first stage. The second stage also prevents the clumping of fat globules that can occur immediately following the first-stage homogenization [134].

2.2.6 HEAT TREATMENT

The milk for the manufacture of yogurt has to be heat treated in such a way that the entire pathogenic flora, most vegetative cells of all microorganisms, and indigenous enzymes contained therein are destroyed. From microbiological point of view, heat-induced destruction of competitive microorganisms creates an environment conducive to the growth of desirable yogurt bacteria. When the milk used in the manufacture of yogurt is kept in cold store for a long period (i.e., 2–3 days), heat-stable lipases from psychrotrophic bacteria such as *Pseudomonas* spp., *Acinetobacter* spp., *Serratia*

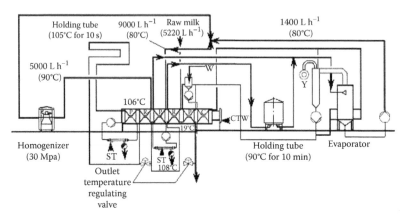

FIGURE 2.6   APV Nordic A/S homogenizing–heating–evaporating system flow diagram. ST, steam; W, water; CW, chilled water. (Courtesy of APV Nordic A/S, Aarhus, Denmark.)

spp., *Aerobacter* spp., *Alcaligenes* spp., and *Moraxella* spp. can act on milk fat that results in increases in free fatty acid concentration, leading to bitterness in the end product [183].

During heat treatment, some substances formed can stimulate or inhibit the growth of yogurt starter bacteria [5]. These substances are listed in Table 2.14. Cold stored milk is usually saturated with oxygen, and during heat treatment (especially in open systems), oxygen is expelled, which produces conditions favorable to yogurt starter bacteria. Using conventional closed heating systems this oxygen cannot escape from the milk. The content of oxygen of yogurt milk will be higher than 4 mg kg^{-1}, which results in a stagnation of growth of the yogurt starter bacteria

TABLE 2.14
Stimulatory/Inhibitory Compounds Formed During Heat Treatment of Yogurt Mix

Effect	Reaction	Heating Norm
Stimulation	Release of cysteine, glutathione or thiogluconate	62°C/30 min
		72°C/40 min
	Degradation of toxic sulfide groups	90°C/60–180 min
		120°C/15–30 min
Inhibition	Increase in the level of toxic sulfide groups depending on the excess cysteine accumulation	72°C/45 min
		82°C/10–120 min
		90°C/1–45 min
	Unknown	120°C/>30 min

Source: Adapted from Tamime, A.Y. and Robinson, R.K., *Yoghurt Science and Technology*, 3rd edition, Woodhead Publishing, Cambridge, p. 808, 2007.

after some time [184]. This stagnation period depends on the incubation temperature and the oxygen content.

2.2.6.1 Effect of Heat Treatment on Milk Protein Interactions and Gel Formation Characteristics of Yogurt

Proteins are the determinant components for the physical quality of yogurt. Therefore, much attention has been paid to the relationships between heat treatment and changes in the functional properties of milk proteins. Milk proteins are composed of caseins and WPs, and WPs are very sensitive to heat treatment, with the exception of proteose-peptone (PP). However, caseins precipitate with decrease in pH, but they are heat stable at pasteurization temperature [95]. Unlike caseins, WPs have three-dimensional structures or configurations. Each configuration is stabilized by hydrogen and hydrophobic bonds, and other forces. Secondary and tertiary structures of WPs tend to be broken down by heat treatment because hydrogen and hydrophobic bonds are weakened by heating [185]. The reactivity of thiol (-SH) groups, which are mainly present in β-lactoglobulin, is increased by heat treatment. Milk WPs, which contain cysteine and cystine, are able to undergo sulfhydryl oxidation and/or disulfide interchange reactions, which lead to the formation of aggregates, as shown below [186]:

$$\text{Protein-S-S-protein}' + \text{R-S}^- \longrightarrow \text{protein}'\text{-S}^- + \text{R-S-S-protein}'.$$

It has long been recognized that heat treatment of milk above 70°C causes denaturation of WPs, some of which complex with the casein micelles and this determines many characteristics of milk and milk products [187]. Below 65°C, at least in theory, denaturation or functional changes of WPs—mainly β-lactoglobulin—are reversible, but above 70°C irreversible functional changes in WPs occur [188]. Heat-induced aggregation of milk WPs is a multistage process. The first step of aggregation involves thiol–disulfide groups interactions. However, the second stage includes not only these bonds, but also calcium bridges, hydrogen, and hydrophobic bonds. After the aggregation is completed, the aggregated β-lactoglobulin interacts with κ-casein, and the rate of aggregation depends on the β-lactoglobulin variants present. Calcium ions promote the association of β-lactoglobulin with casein micelles [95], perhaps due to the ability of ions to influence the degree of electrostatic attraction or repulsion between β-lactoglobulin and κ-casein by providing an ionic environment around the interacting molecules. Additionally, salts could be affecting the reactivity of thiol groups. The level of WP denaturation is largely affected by milk pH. At lower pH values, the denaturation rate is increased [189]. Lactose concentration is a limiting factor for the WP denaturation. The glucosyl residues are bound to β-lactoglobulin via gluconic acid or melibionic acid, making this WP fraction stable against heat treatment [190]. Lactose concentrations of milk with normal chemical composition do not have any negative effect on the rate of WP denaturation. However, if the lactose level of yogurt milk is increased during SNF fortification by adding SMP or by RO, rate of WP denaturation is likely reduced. In order to overcome this handicap, milk should be heat-treated at >90°C for 10–15 min [7].

As stated above, the β-lactoglobulin and κ-casein interaction plays a determinative role in the formation of the yogurt gel. In addition to this interaction, the existence of the interactions between other WPs and casein fractions has also been proved [191].

Mottar et al. [191] pointed out that the ratio between β-lactoglobulin and α-lactalbumin associated with casein micelles seemed to affect their reactivity and texture formation in yogurt, and that this ratio is directly related to the time–temperature combination used. It was demonstrated that heat treatment at 90°C for 10 min is the optimum heat treatment norm to obtain yogurt with a good textural quality. With this combination, α-lactalbumin associates with the casein micelle and, subsequently, the water-holding capacity and hydrophilic properties of proteins increase.

2.2.6.2   Effect of Heat Treatment on the Textural Properties of Yogurt

Heat treatment is one of the most effective technological steps affecting the rheology of yogurt. Dannenberg and Kessler [192] revealed that the holding time of milk at a given temperature, which causes 99% denaturation of β-lactoglobulin, determines the characteristics of the yogurt gel. In general, firmness improves with an increase in heat intensity but when the holding time was increased to 2.5 times that necessary for 99% denaturation of β-lactoglobulin, the firmness of the yogurt gel was reduced; similar adverse effects were noted at temperatures >120°C. Labropoulous et al. [193] suggested that the method of heat treatment affects the level of WP denaturation. According to their findings, Vat processed milks (82°C for 15 min or 65°C for 30 min) had considerably higher gel firmness than those prepared from indirect-UHT-treated milk (at 149°C for 0–12 s). In a further study, it was demonstrated that yogurt from UHT milk showed lower gel firmness and apparent viscosity and higher spreadability than yogurt made from milk to which the 82°C for 30 min temperature–time combination had been applied [194]. Krasaekoopt et al. [195,196] found that yogurt made from UHT milk had lower gel firmness and viscosity but showed less tendency to whey separation. In general, high-temperature–short-time (HTST) combinations, such as HTST at 98°C for 0.5–1.8 min [197], and direct or indirect UHT [191] give low gel firmness and poor textural quality compared with the conventional Vat system. On the contrary, yogurt made from milk subjected to the HTST process had higher water-holding capacity followed by yogurt made from UHT-treated milk [196]. Overall, heat treatment at 85°C for 30 min represents the best process and is recommended for industrial productions, as long as the yogurt starter activity is concerned.

In yogurt production, a plate heat exchanger, a scrapped/swept surface heat exchanger, or a tubular heat exchanger is used to pasteurize the milk. The plate heat exchanger and tubular heat exchanger are more common in the pasteurization of yogurt milk base. The swept surface heat exchanger is more widely used for the heat treatment of fruit preparations. There are some factors considered in the selection of size and configuration of any type of heat exchanger [198]. These are as follows:

1. Production flow rate
2. Physical properties of liquids to be processed
3. Temperature programme
4. Permission pressure drops
5. Heat exchanger design
6. Cleaning requirements
7. Required running or operation time

The equipment for continuous heat processing is made up from the following sections:

1. Regeneration section
2. Heating/cooling section
3. Holding unit

Rising energy costs and an increased sense of environmental awareness mean that reduced energy consumption is critical to dairy operations. HTST pasteurizers typically have a regeneration section to optimize the heat recovery between a cold raw product and the same hot pasteurized product. Below is the typical regeneration protocol developed by Anonymous [198] and analyzed in detail by Tamime and Robinson [5].

Step 1. Prewarming yogurt milk base from 5°C to 60°C by regeneration (utilizing the energy available in the concentrate from the evaporator)

Step 2. Heating milk to 85–90°C with hot water before vacuum evaporating

Step 3. Heating the concentrated milk (at ~70°C) to 82°C by regeneration (utilizing the energy available from already heated milk)

Step 4. Heating the concentrated milk from 82°C to 85–90°C with hot water

Step 5. Cooling the heated milk from 85–90°C to 78°C by regeneration (transfer of energy to the concentrated milk at 70°C)

Step 6. Cooling the milk base from 78°C to 42–43°C by cold water

For further information on the design of heating equipment and regeneration efficiency, readers are recommended to refer to Tamime and Robinson [5] and Anonymous [198].

2.2.7 FERMENTATION

Following the heat treatment stage, the milk is cooled to 42–43°C and inoculated with the starter culture consisting of a 1:1 mixture of *L. delbrueckii* subsp. *bulgaricus* and *Streptococcus thermophilus*. Inoculation may be achieved either by growing cultures on-site to the volume needed to inoculate the process milk (bulk culture) or by incorporating concentrated freeze-dried or frozen cultures. In the former case, the milk is more prone to problems of infection and liable to lead to changes in culture with respect to the balance between strains of given species. Additionally, it may be possible that during replication the variant may lose a plasmid-controlled characteristic [199]. Therefore, today, most manufacturers prefer either deep-frozen or freeze-dried cultures with specified properties. In the case of use of bulk culture, the optimum rate of culture inoculation is 2 g/100 mL. The addition rate for concentrated freeze-dried or frozen culture is usually set by the suppliers [200]. The rate of inoculation is determinative for the final textural and sensory characteristics of yogurt. Lower levels of inoculation can cause slow acidity development during fermentation, extending the fermentation period and weak coagulum leading to whey separation. On the contrary, excessive levels of inoculation may lead to fast acidity development, decrease in protein hydration capacity, and stimulated wheying off during storage. Once the milk has been inoculated with starter culture, it will be filled into cups for fermentation (set yogurt) or it will be fermented in a bulk tank (stirred yogurt). In the small-scale productions, the cartons of yogurt are stacked into cardboard trays holding 9 or 12 units and then placed on a shelf in the incubator. Alternatively, in the large-scale productions, the yogurt trays can be placed on a conveyor belt that slowly runs through a tunnel operated at the same temperature (stage 1) and followed by forced air cooling (stage 2) [5200] (Figure 2.7). Heating and cooling are achieved by circulating warm and chilled air. The speed of the conveyor belt is adjusted considering the rate of acid development in the yogurt milk. When the yogurt cups enter into the cooling stage (stage 2), the pH of the fermenting milk should be about 4.5–4.6.

In the production of stirred yogurt, fermentation is achieved in a bulk tank fitted with temperature and pH recorders, and once the preset pH has been reached, the coagulum is stirred gently and pumped to the filling machine. The fermentation tanks are generally designed conically to discharge to yogurt from the base more easily. This type of tank is water jacketed and warm water at 40–45°C is circulated during the incubation period, followed by cold or chilled water for partial cooling of the coagulum [5]. In order to provide a hygienic environment, the fermentation tanks are usually fitted with air filters, preventing entrance of particles larger than 0.3 μm.

The typical fermentation temperature for yogurt is 42°C. However, some yogurt manufacturers may prefer lower incubation temperatures (i.e., 40°C). At lower fermentation temperature, the gelation time will be prolonged and the size of the casein particles will be increased due to a reduction in hydrophobic interactions, which, in turn, leads to a coagulum with firmer body and lower whey separation [201,202]. On the other hand, at lower incubation temperatures, the formation of aroma compounds is weakened [7].

Determination of incubation end point is of critical importance with regard to the textural characteristics of the final product. Since the water holding and hydration capacity of yogurt is optimum at pH 4.2–4.6, the fermentation stage usually ends at pH 4.5–4.6. During fermentation, depending on the metabolic activities of lactic acid bacteria, the concentrations of lactate and ammonium increase, which, in turn, lead to increase in the electrical conductivity (EC) of the milk. On-line measurements of pH and EC data have made it possible to access time and rate feature points of

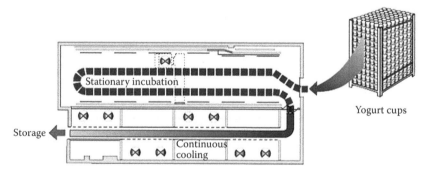

FIGURE 2.7   Combined incubation room and cooling tunnel. (Courtesy of Tetra Pak A/B, Lund, Sweden.)

thermophilic lactic acid fermentations. The EC-meters designed for the yogurt production are gaining popularity in the yogurt industry.

2.2.7.1 Microbiology of Fermentation

For a satisfactory flavor to develop, approximately equal numbers of *Streptococcus thermophilus* and *L. delbrueckii* subsp. *bulgaricus* should be present. The essential flora of yogurt show obligate symbiotic relationship during fermentation. The rates of acid and flavor production by mixed yogurt culture are considerably higher than by either of the two organisms grown separately [134]. Energy and nitrogen are required by yogurt starter bacteria to maintain their life cycle. The cell-bound proteases of *L. delbrueckii* subsp. *bulgaricus* (especially *prtB*) are capable of forming small peptides and amino acids, the main amino acid being valine [203]. The peptides and amino acids formed by the lactobacilli are utilized by *Streptococcus thermophilus* for their growth. Proteinase activity of *Streptococcus thermophilus* is much weaker than *L. delbrueckii* subsp. *bulgaricus*; however, peptidases of *Streptococcus thermophilus* can hydrolyze the intermediate products of casein proteolysis from *L. delbrueckii* subsp. *bulgaricus*, which is an important aspect of the synergistic relationship between the two organisms in yogurt [204]. *Streptococcus thermophilus* produces purine, pyrimidine, CO_2, formic acid, oxaloacetic acid, and fumaric acids that stimulate the growth of *L. delbrueckii* subsp. *bulgaricus*. Formic acid and CO_2 are the prime growth factors for *L. delbrueckii* subsp. *bulgaricus*. Formic acid production can only be possible when the oxygen concentration of the milk is <4 mg O_2 L^{-1}. During the growth in milk, *L. delbrueckii* subsp. *bulgaricus* apparently exhibits a preference for utilizing β-casein over other proteins as a nitrogen source, indicating that the type of protein is also an important factor influencing the growth of this culture [204].

The practical result of the synergy is that both species grow rapidly and actively metabolize sufficient lactose to lactic acid to complete the fermentation of milk to yogurt within 3.5–4.0 h. In addition, metabolites liberated by the two species give yogurt flavor that is distinctly different from any other fermented milk [200]. The concentration of acetaldehyde, a major component of the flavor profile, may go up to 40 mg kg^{-1} during fermentation by the mixed culture.

2.2.7.2 Mechanism of Gel Formation

Yogurt gel, which primarily comprises macromolecules, mainly caseins and fat globules, has a particulate structure [205,206]. As compared with literature data on model casein gels and microstructural findings on yogurt, the results imply that a permanent network that is composed by covalent (–SH/S–S) and noncovalent protein interactions (hydrophobic, electrostatic, etc.) exists in yogurt [207]. Yogurt is a typical weak viscoelastic gel [208]. The formation of yogurt gel relies on the interaction between acid-destabilized κ-casein and heat-denatured WPs (mainly β-lactoglobulin) [86,88]. Depending on the environmental conditions of the gelation, yogurt gels with different physical properties can be obtained. Formation of yogurt gel is summarized below [5]:

1. Lactose (milk sugar) is utilized by yogurt starter bacteria for their energy requirements. As a result of the metabolic activities of the starters, lactose is converted mainly to lactic acid.

2. The increase in the concentration of lactic acid causes destabilization of the casein micelle/denatured WP complex produced by heat treatment. Colloidal calcium phosphate in micelle plays a key role in this mechanism.

3. When the pH reaches 5.2–5.1 (isoelectric point of β-casein) aggregation starts, and at about pH 4.6–4.7 aggregation of the micelles is extensively completed.

4. The interaction of α-lactalbumin and β-lactoglobulin with κ-casein via thiol–disulfide bridges prevents the formation of coarse aggregations and gives rise to a fine gel network, which entraps within it water and other milk compounds.

Gel formation solely depends on destabilization of the casein micelle, and the characteristics of the destabilizing forces define the structure; the forces contributing to its integrity help us to understand the gel formation of yogurt. During acidification of yogurt milk, calcium phosphate is completely released from the micelle at pH 5.0–5.1. Therefore, its cementing role in keeping the individual casein molecules together in the form of a micelle is reduced, and κ-casein and β-casein begin to dissociate from the micelle [209]. In this dissociation, the zeta potential of the micelles plays an important role. The zeta potential of the micelles in normal milk (pH 6.7) is about −13 mV, and hydration, steric repulsion, and a negative surface charge protect the micelle against aggregation [95].

When the pH drops to 5.2, the zeta potential is minimal but, at lower pH values, the zeta potential begins to increase again. The main reason for this fluctuation of the zeta potential is the anomalous behavior of β-casein. At pH 5.2, β-casein entirely passes into the serum phase; at this point, the zeta potential is minimal. Between 4.8 and 5.2, the β-casein, which is positively charged in this pH range, reacts with α_s-casein, which is negatively charged in this pH range, by electrostatic bonds [209].

Another important factor related to micelle stability is heat treatment. The importance of heat treatment is reviewed in depth in Section 2.2.6. After heat treatment, an interaction occurs between κ-casein and serum proteins (mainly β-lactoglobulin) at pH 6.4. This interaction leads to an increase in hydrophobicity as the hydration barrier preventing the aggregation of casein micelles is reduced [209]. Consequently, micellar aggregation and gelation start at pH 5.2. A second possible reason for the onset of gelation at pH 5.2 could be a change in micellar composition at this pH. Thus, at higher pHs, the concentration of heat-treated micellar α-casein is increased and, because of the higher sensitivity of α_s-casein than the other caseins to calcium, the sensitivity of the micelles to calcium increases.

As briefly described above, development of acidity and heat treatment are the key components of the gel formation during fermentation. Homogenization is also a key step in the manufacture of yogurt. Homogenization of milk disrupts fat globules and increases their fat surface area by a factor of 5–6. The reformed fat globules become coated with a protein layer consisting of casein micelles, submicelles, and to a lesser extent WP [210]. The recombined fat globule membrane can become an integral part of the gel network during acid gelation in the manufacture of yogurt. This results in a gel with improved physical properties (e.g., increase in viscosity and firmness and reduction in whey separation).

In physical terms, the formation of yogurt gel can be described as a multistage process as follows:

1. Initial lag period of low viscosity
2. A stage of rapid viscosity change depending on the rapid bacterial multiplication, and start of gelation
3. A stage of high constant viscosity (almost completion of gelation)
4. Syneresis stage (the death phase of starter bacteria).

The period of fermentation is largely affected by a number of factors including incubation temperature, total solids level of milk, starter bacteria strain, and mechanical handling of fermenting milk. Especially, acid-producing capacity and inoculation rate of starter bacteria are of critical importance in gelation kinetics [211,212]. Gel onset point and gel development rate (k) are the two parameters that are widely used in determining incubation conditions.

Gel development rate (k): $2.303/t \log(G^*_\infty - G^*_{t1}/G^*_\infty - G^*_{t2})$

G^* : Gel firmness (complex modulus)
G^*_∞ : Gel firmness at the end of incubation
G^*_{t1} : Gel firmness at the beginning of incubation
G^*_{t2} : Gel firmness at the stage of high viscosity
t : Time (s)

Complex modulus
$|G^*| = |G'^2 + iG''^2|^{1/2}$
G': storage modulus (elastic character of the gel) (m Nm)
G'': loss modulus (viscous character of the gel) (m Nm)

2.2.8 COOLING

The metabolic activities of the yogurt starter bacteria are largely hindered at <10°C. Therefore, development of postfermentation acidity can be controlled by rapidly cooling the fermenting milk after the desired pH level (pH 4.6–4.7) is attained. In practice, two cooling systems are available: single-phase cooling and two-phase cooling. In single-phase cooling, the temperature of fermenting milk is directly reduced from 43°C to <10°C. This model is more appropriate for plain set-type yogurt production. Two-phase cooling is more widely employed in the yogurt industry. In the first phase, fermenting milk is stirred gently in a tank to obtain a homogeneous body, and cooled to 20–24°C. Addition of fruit to yogurt and filling up the yogurt cups are achieved at this stage, and the filled cups are then cooled to <10°C over a period of 10–12 h. In general, the temperature of the yogurt cups is subjected to an air temperature of 7–10°C for 5–6 h, and then the air temperature is reduced to 1–2°C for the rest of cooling. The rate of cooling is of critical importance in obtaining a product with desired textural quality. Too fast cooling can cause a weak body and stimulates whey separation during cold storage. The construction of a cold room and materials used for the packaging are the key elements of cooling efficiency. In large-scale yogurt installations, intermediate cooling is achieved in a chill tunnel before final cooling to 2–4°C [24,94,198]. White [213] proposed an alternative model for cooling yogurt as follows:

shock cooling → intermediate cooling → lact-less cooling → holding phase
(43–30°C)   (30–20°C)   (20–14°C)   (2–4°C)

2.2.9 ADDITION OF FRUIT PREPARATIONS

Although there is a market in some countries for flavored set yogurts, stirred fruit yogurt remains the most popular type in Western societies. In the manufacture of fruit yogurt, the use of fresh fruit is limited due to high risk of spoilage. Instead, the use of processed fruit preparations is found to be a more attractive option by the yogurt manufacturers. Frozen fruits are also available to manufacturers who demand to use only natural fruits in yogurt-making. According to Robinson and Tamime [199], the advantages of the use of processed fruits in fruit yogurt production are as follows:

- They are entirely free from yeasts and molds
- The level of color can be adjusted to ensure a uniform appearance in the final product
- The degree of sweetness in the final product can be adjusted by adding sucrose

Major fruit processing techniques available in the market include canning, freezing, drying, preservation with sugar syrups, concentrating by moisture removal, and preservation with chemicals [134]. These techniques can be used alone or in combination of two or more of them.

The basic steps of processing of fruit preparations are summarized by O'Rell and Chandan [134] as follows:

- Mixing fruit, 75% of the sugar, 50% of the water, and preservatives (most commonly potassium sorbate and sodium benzoate) in a stainless steel jacketed tank
- In a second tank, mixing the remaining 50% of the water and starch
- Adding the preparation of the second tank into the first tank and preheating the mixture at 37–38°C for 3 min
- Addition of flavor and color ingredients to the pasteurized preparation and checking the quality control (pH, °Brix and color)
- Heating the mixture by using a scrapped surface heat exchanger (88–93°C for 3 min) and cooling the pasteurized mixture to 27–32°C through a scrapped surface heat exchanger
- Aseptic filling and dispatch

Various types of fruit or flavored yogurts are available in the market. These are as follows:

- Stirred-type fruit yogurts
  - Yogurt with mixed fruit before packaging

- – Fruit corner yogurt (yogurt and fruit preparation is mixed at the time of consumption)
- – Fruit-flavored stirred yogurt
- Set-type fruit yogurts
  - – Fruit-on-the-bottom yogurt
  - – Fruit-on-the-top yogurt
  - – Aromatized set-type yogurt
- Drinking yogurt with added fruit syrup

There are two possible options to blend the yogurt base with the fruit preparation automatically (Figure 2.8). In the first option, correct amounts of fruit and yogurt base dosed by metering devices are mixed through a static in-line mixer to ensure a uniform distribution of fruit throughout the coagulum (bold lines). In the second option, yogurt base and fruit preparations are drawn by separate feeding pumps into a mixing chamber and the mixture is sent to the filling machine directly. The mixing chamber is fitted with a dynamic agitator.

Blending temperature of fruit preparations and yogurt base is of critical importance for the textural quality of the final product. In general, fruit preparation is added after cooling the yogurt base. Mixing of fruit with yogurt base at high temperature may cause a weak body and a sandy texture in the end product. The optimum temperature for fruit addition is <10°C. The speed of the mixer should be adjusted appropriately to avoid mechanical damage in the yogurt. In the production of fruit-on-the-bottom-type set yogurt, the pH and the osmotic pressure generated by the fruit preparation at the interface of fruit and yogurt base should be taken into consideration to assure compatibility of the two layers during incubation of the cup. Low pH and osmotic pressure difference between the fruit and yogurt base may cause a lumpy or gritty texture in the final product. Set- (fruit-on-the-bottom-type) and stirred-type fruit yogurt production flow charts are illustrated in Figure 29a–c.

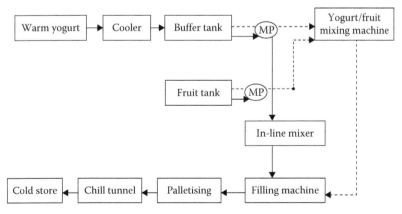

FIGURE 2.8 Flow diagram of stirred fruit yogurt. MP, metering pump. (Courtesy of Sheffield Academic Press.)

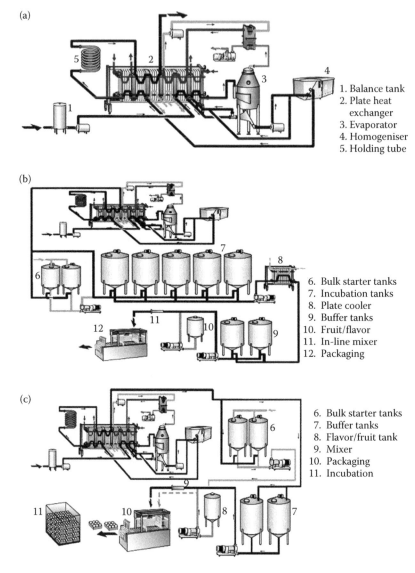

(a)

5   2

3

4

1. Balance tank
2. Plate heat
   exchanger
3. Evaporator
4. Homogeniser
5. Holding tube

(b)

7

8

6

11

12   10

9

6. Bulk starter tanks
7. Incubation tanks
8. Plate cooler
9. Buffer tanks
10. Fruit/flavor
11. In-line mixer
12. Packaging

(c)

6

9

11   10   8   7

6. Bulk starter tanks
7. Buffer tanks
8. Flavor/fruit tank
9. Mixer
10. Packaging
11. Incubation

FIGURE 2.9   Flow chart of (a) pretreatment of yogurt milk, (b) fruit/flavored stirred yogurt, and (c) fruit/flavored set yogurt. (Courtesy of Tetra Pak A/B, Lund, Sweden.)

2.2.10   PACKAGING

The selection of packaging material in the yogurt industry is important in protecting the natural properties of the product as efficiently as possible during the storage and marketing and in conforming to food safety standards at the highest level. The packaging material should conform to the below specifications:

- It should resist environmental and mechanical effects
- It should be suitable for serial filling in packaging machines

- It should prevent migration of light, odor, and so on
- It should not contain any toxic material(s) and not react with the product
- It should be environmentally friendly

There are two packaging models widely used in the yogurt industry. These are (i) preformed polypropylene (PP) cups and (ii) thermoformed cups. The first option is more attracted by the small-scale yogurt manufacturers. The second option (form-fill-seal) is more suitable for the large-scale productions as it offers flexibility to the manufacturers. The yogurt manufacturers can fill up to four different products (e.g., yogurts added with four different fruits) at the same time. Additionally, the cartons suitable for thermoforming are thinner than the conventional preformed cartons, offering an economical benefit to the yogurt manufacturers. The most common packaging materials in the yogurt industry are PP, polystyrene (PS), and polyethylene (PE) [214,215]. Recently, biopackaging materials (i.e., polylactate) are gaining popularity in the yogurt industry [216]. The polylactate packaging materials were first used in Germany (Danone) and Finland (Valio Ltd) [217]. The polylactates offer certain advantages in preventing (i) color changes, (ii) formation of hydroperoxides, and (iii) decrease in β-carotene and riboflavin concentrations in the final product [216]. On the other hand, polylactates show slightly poorer resistance against migration from outside compared with the PS materials. Some properties of the common packaging materials are given in Table 2.15.

Migration level of monomers from the materials to the product is the major limiting factor in the selection of packaging materials. Ideally, migration from the packaging materials to the product should be prevented efficiently. The level of migration is related to the acidity and fat level of the product, relative humidity of the environment, and filling temperature of the inoculated milk [219]. Styrene and ethylbenzene are commonly present in industrial yogurts, ranging from 0.08 to 200 μg kg^{-1}. Styrene may trigger flavor defects in the end product (with a threshold level of >0.2 μg g^{-1}) [7]. Cumin and o-xylene are other monomers having the potential to migrate from the packaging materials to the yogurt.

TABLE 2.15

Some Properties of PS, PP, and PVC Materials Used in Yogurt Packaging

Properties	PS	PP	PVC
Density[a]	1.05	0.9	1.35
Form stability (°C)	95	140	80
Oxygen permeability[b]	10	6	0.3
Vapor permeability[c]	10	0.5	2
Light permeability[d]	~90	~60	~90

Source: After Ucuncu, M., *Gidalarin Ambalajlanmasi*, Ege Universitesi Basimevi, Izmir, p. 689, 2000.

[a] g cm^{-3}.

[b] cm^3 100 μm m^{-2} day atm × 10^{-3}.

[c] g 100 μm m^{-2} day.

[d] %.

In large-scale installations, filling and packaging are achieved by employing fully automated systems. The capacity of the filling machines can vary between 5.000 and 70.000 pots h^{-1}. The internal design of an aseptic filling machine developed by Erca-Formseal Inc. (France) and the external design of a Pure Pack P-S50 filling machine are illustrated in Figures 2.10 and 2.11, respectively. The filled yogurt containers are nested in cardboard trays before being palletized.

2.3   FUTURE PERSPECTIVES

The future of yogurt manufacturing will focus on the novel or emerging technologies such as high hydrostatic pressure (HHP) application or improvement of the textural properties of the end product by the enzymatic way (e.g., by TGase). The preliminary works have revealed that HHP reduces the fermentation time of yogurt milk. Additionally, the stability of the product during the storage period is improved by HHP [220,221]. HHP may also be applied to cold yogurt after fermentation to increase the viscosity and stability of the final product [222]. More study needs to be carried out before the HHP application is commercialized by the yogurt industry. The incorporation of TGase into yogurt production to improve the textural properties of yogurt is also a promising approach. Özer et al. [223] showed that TGase-treated yogurts had higher viscosity and gel firmness and lower whey separation compared with the untreated control sample. However, the TGase-treated samples had remarkably lower concentrations of carbonyl compounds and sensory scores. Therefore, the reason(s) for the adverse effect of TGase on typical yogurt flavor should be investigated further in detail. The development of new flavors and longer lasting yogurts will continue to be the prime targets of researches on yogurt. The nutritional aspects of yogurt will be more thoroughly investigated in the near future as well. In this respect, more studies will be expected to be carried out before commercializing the yogurt-derived nutritive products such as $\omega - 3$ enriched yogurt, vegetable oil yogurt, health-promoting yogurt, fat-substitute yogurts, cholesterol-free yogurt, vitamin-enriched yogurt, or bifidogenic yogurt.

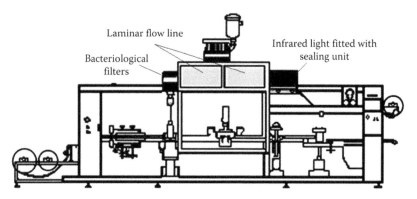

FIGURE 2.10   Internal design of an aseptic fruit yogurt filling machine. (Courtesy of Erca-Formseal Inc., France.)

(a)

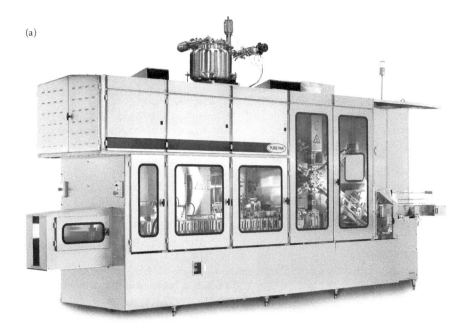

(b)

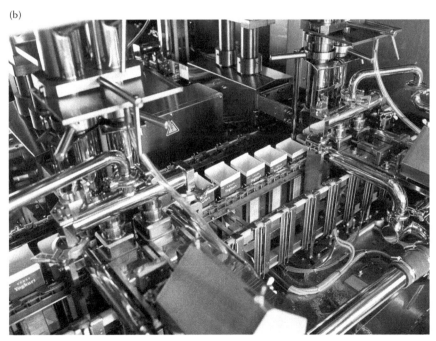

FIGURE 2.11 (a) External and (b) internal appearance of Pure-Pak P-S50S-med filling machine. (Reproduced with permission from Elopak AS, Skippestad.)

REFERENCES

1. Walstra, P., Geurts, T.J., Nooman, A., Jellema, A., and van Boekel, M.A.J.S., *Dairy Technology: Principles of Milk Properties and Processes*, Marcel Dekker, New York, pp. 181–185, 1999.
2. Varnam, A.H. and Sutherland, J.P., *Milk and Milk Products: Technology, Chemistry and Microbiology*, Chapman & Hall, London, p. 451, 1994.
3. Mitic, S., Jakimov, N., Otenhajmer, I., Milenkovic, D., Bubanja, N., Grubac, D., and Markovic, D., Influence of somatic cell count on growth of *Streptococcus thermophilus* and *Lactobacillus bulgaricus* strains used in yoghurt manufacture, in *Proc. XXI Int. Dairy Congr.*, Vol. 1, pp. 275–276, 1982.
4. Oliveira, C.A.F., Fernandes, A.M., Cunha Neto, O.C., Fonseca, L.F.L., Silva, E.O.T., and Balian, S.C., Composition and sensory evaluation of whole yoghurt produced from milk with different somatic cell counts, *Aus. J. Dairy Technol.*, 57, 192–196, 2002.
5. Tamime, A.Y. and Robinson, R.K., *Yoghurt Science and Technology*, 3rd edition, Woodhead Publishing, Cambridge, p. 808, 2007.
6. Metin, M., *Sut Teknolojisi*, 1st edition, E.U. Muhendislik Fakultesi Yayinlari, Izmir, p. 786, 1999.
7. Özer, B.H., *Yogurt Bilimi ve Teknolojisi*, Sidas Yayincilik, Izmir, p. 496, 2006.
8. Aslim, B., Yücel, N., and Beyatli, Y., Effect of a bacteriocin-like substances (BLS) produced by *Streptococcus thermophilus* strains on *Listeria* spp., *J. Food Procces. Preserv.*, 28, 241–250, 2004.
9. Griffiths, M.W., Phillips, J.D., and Muir, D.D., Effect of low temperature storage on the bacteriological quality of raw milk, *Food Microbiol.*, 4, 285–291, 1987.
10. Gueimonde, M., Alonso, L., Delgado, T., Bada-Gancedo, J.C., and Reyes-Gavilan, C.G., Quality of plain yogurt made from refrigerated and CO_2-treated milk, *Food Res. Int.*, 36, 43–48, 2003.
11. Dixon, N.M. and Kell, D.B., The inhibition by carbon dioxide of the growth and metabolism of microorganisms, *J. Appl. Bacteriol.*, 67, 109–136, 1989.
12. Haas, G.J., Prescott, H.E., Dudley, E., Jr., Dik, R., Hintlian, C., and Keane, L., Inactivation of microorganisms by carbon dioxide under pressure, *J. Food Saf.*, 9, 253–265, 1989.
13. Calvo, M.M., Montilla, A., and Cobos, A., Lactic acid production and rheological properties of yogurt made from milk acidified with carbon dioxide, *J. Sci. Food Agric.*, 79, 1208–1212, 1999.
14. King, J.S. and Mabbitt, L.A., Preservation of raw milk by the addition of carbon dioxide, *J. Dairy Res.*, 49, 439–447, 1982.
15. Vinderola, C.G., Gueimonde, M., Delgado, T., Reinheimer, J.A., and Reyes-Gavilan, C.G., Characteristics of carbonated fermented milk and survival of probiotic bacteria, *Int. Dairy J.*, 10, 213–220, 2000.
16. Ma, Y., Barbarno, D.M., Hotchkiss, J.H., Murphy, S., and Lynch, J.M., Impact of CO_2 addition to milk on selected analytical testing methods, *J. Dairy Sci.*, 84, 1959–1968, 2001.
17. Ma, Y. and Barbarno, D.M., Impact of temperature of CO_2 addition on the pH and FP of milks and creams, *J. Dairy Sci.*, 86, 1578–1589, 2003.
18. Özer, B.H., Kırım, B., and Atamer, M., Effect of hydrogen peroxide treatment on the quality of raw cream, *Int. J. Dairy Technol.*, 53, 83–86, 2000.
19. Kamau, D.V., Doores, S., and Pruitti, K.M., Antibacterial activity of the lactoperoxidase system against *Listeria monocytogenes* and *Staphylococcus aureus* in milk, *J. Food Protect.*, 53, 1010–1014, 1990.
20. Özer, B.H., Grandison, A.S., Robinson, R.K., and Atamer, M., Effects of lactoperoxidase and hydrogen peroxide on the rheological properties of yoghurt, *J. Dairy Res.*, 70, 227–232, 2003.

21. Nakada, M., Dosako, S., Hirano, R., Ooka, M., and Nakajima, I., Lactoperoxidase suppresses acid production in yoghurt during storage under refrigeration, *Int. Dairy J.*, 6, 33–42, 1996.
22. Hirano, R., Hirano, M., Ooka, M., and Hatanaka, K., Effects of lactoperoxidase on gelation properties of yoghurt, *Food Res. Int.*, 31, 1–6, 1998.
23. Hirano, R., Hirano, M., Oooka, M., Dosako, S., Nakajima, I., and Igoshi, K., Lactoperoxidase effects on rheological properties of yoghurt, *J. Food Sci.*, 63, 35–38, 1998.
24. Bylund, G., *Dairy Processing Handbook*, Tetra Pak Processing Systems A/B, Lund, Sweden, 1995.
25. Lankes, H., Özer, B.H., and Robinson, R.K., The effect of elevated milk solids and incubation temperature on the physical properties of natural yoghurt, *Milchwissenschaft*, 53, 510–513, 1998.
26. McKenna, A.B., Examination of whole milk powder by confocal laser scanning microscopy, *J. Dairy Res.*, 64, 423–432, 1997.
27. Thomopoulous, C., Tzia, C., and Milkas, D., Influence of processing of solids-fortified milk on coagulation time and quality properties of yogurt, *Milchwissenschaft*, 48, 426–430, 1993.
28. Kieseker, F.G. and Healey, D., Protein-adjusted non-fat milk powders, *Aus. J. Dairy Technol.*, 51, 101–126, 1996.
29. Mistry, V.V., Hassan, H.N., and Robinson, D.J., Effect of lactose and protein on the microstructure of dried milk, *Food Struct.*, 11, 73–82, 1992.
30. Aguilar, C.A. and Ziegler, G.R., Physical and microscopic characterization of dry whole milk with altered lactose content. 1. Effect of lactose concentration, *J. Dairy Sci.*, 77, 1198–1204, 1994.
31. Harnett, M. and Mueller, B., Ingredients made from milk for yoghurt products, *Deutsche Milchwirt.*, 45, 841–842, 1994.
32. Augustin, M.A., Cheng, L.J., Glagovskaia, O., Clarke, P.T., and Lawrence, A., Use of blends of skim milk and sweet whey protein concentrates in reconstituted yoghurt, *Aus. J. Dairy Technol.*, 58, 30–35, 2003.
33. Guler, Z., Sezgin, M., and Atamer, M., Yayikalti tozunun yogurt uretiminde kullanim olanaklarinin arastirilmasi, *Gida*, 21, 317–322, 1996.
34. Guinee, T.P., Mullins, C.G., and Cotter, M.P., Physical properties of stirred-curd unsweetened yoghurts stabilised with different dairy ingredients, *Milchwissenschaft*, 50, 196–200, 1995.
35. Trachoo, N. and Mistry, V.V., Application of ultrafiltered sweet buttermilk and sweet buttermilk powder in the manufacture of nonfat and low fat yoghurts, *J. Dairy Sci.*, 81, 3163–3171, 1998.
36. Corredig, M., Roesch, R.R., and Dalgleish, D.G., Production of a novel ingredient from buttermilk, *J. Dairy Sci.*, 86, 2744–2750, 2003.
37. Rohm, H. and Schmidt, W., Influence of dry matter fortification on flow properties of yoghurt. I. Evaluation of flow curves, *Milchwissenschaft*, 48, 556–560, 1993.
38. Dave R.I. and Shah, N.P., The influence of ingredient supplementation on the textural characteristics of yoghurt, *Aus. J. Dairy Technol.*, 53, 180–184, 1998.
39. Bozanic, R., Tratnik, L., and Maric, O., The influence of whey protein concentrate addition on the viscosity and microbiological quality of yoghurt during storage, *Mljekarstvo*, 50, 15–24, 2000.
40. Zedan, M.A., Zedan, A.N., Kebary, K.M.K., and Mahmoud, S.F., Effects of fortification of cows milk with acetylated whey protein concentrates on the quality of set yoghurt, *Egypt. J. Dairy Sci.*, 29, 285–297, 2001.
41. Kailasapathy, K., Supriadi, D., and Hourigan, J.A., Effect of partially replacing skim milk powder with whey protein concentrate on buffering capacity of yoghurt, *Aus. J. Dairy Technol.*, 51, 89–93, 1996.

42. Penna, A.L.B., Baruffaldi, R., and Oliviera, M.N., Use of demineralized whey powder in yoghurt production. II. Sensory evaluation, in *Proc. IFT Annual Meeting*, IFT, New Orleans, p. 216, 1996.
43. Atamer, M., Aydin, G., and Sezgin, E., Hidrolize peyriraltı suyu konsantresinin yogurt uretiminde kullanim olanaklarinin arastirilmasi, *Gida*, 18, 83–88, 1993.
44. Shah, N.P., Spurgeon, K.R., and Gilmore, T.M., Use of dry whey and lactose hydrolysis in yoghurt basis, *Milchwissenschaft*, 48, 494–498, 1993.
45. González-Martínez, C., Becerra, M., Chafer, M., Albors, A., Carot, J.M., and Chiralt, A., Influence of substituting milk powder for whey powder on yoghurt quality, *Trend Food Sci. Technol.*, 13, 334–340, 2002.
46. Kailasapathy, K. and Supriadi, D., Effect of whey protein concentrate on the survival of *Lactobacillus acidophilus* in lactose hydrolysed yoghurt during refrigerated storage, *Milchwissenschaft*, 51, 565–569, 1996.
47. van der Schaft, P.H., European Patent Application, EP 0426210 A2, 1995.
48. Kailasapathy, K., Nyugen, M., Khan, N.M., and Hourigan, J.A., Effect of membrane concentrated cottage cheese whey on yoghurt production, *Food Aus.*, 48, 281–284, 1996.
49. Djurdjevic, D.J., Macej, O., and Jovanovic, S., The influence of investigated factors on viscosity of stirred yoghurt, *J. Agric. Sci.*, 47, 219–231, 2002.
50. Guzman-Gonzalez, M., Morais, F., Ramos, M., and Amigo, L., Influence of skimmed milk concentrate replacement by dry dairy products in a low fat set-type yoghurt model systems: I: Use of whey protein concentrates, milk protein concentrates and skimmed milk powder, *J. Sci. Food Agric.*, 79, 1117–1122, 1999.
51. Gonc, S. and Uysal, H.R., Degisik oranlarda yogum katilarak yapilan yogurtlarin ozellikleri uzerine arastirmalar, *Ege Univ. Ziraat Fak. Der.*, 28, 137–150, 1991.
52. Nakamura, T., Syukunobe, Y., Doki, R., Shimoda, K., Yoshida, T., and Kuwazuru, M., Stimulating effect of milk casein hydrolysates on the growth of *Streptococcus thermophilus*, *J. Japan. Soc. Food Sci. Technol.*, 38, 858–863, 1991.
53. Sodini, I., Lucas, A., Tissier, J.P., and Corrieu, G., Physical properties and microstructure of yoghurts supplemented with milk protein hydrolysates, *Int. Dairy J.*, 15, 29–35, 2005.
54. Kim, Y.J. and Hwang, I.H., Culture condition on viscosity of lactic acid bacteria isolated from market yoghurt, *Dairy Sci. Abst.*, 58, 799, 1996.
55. Baltadzhieva, B.G., European Patent Application, BG 19850071321, 1987.
56. Mangashetti, L., Balasubramanyam B.V., Jayaraj Rao K., Ghosh Bikash C., and Kulkarni, S., Suitability of concentrated milk for dahi preparation, *Ind. J. Dairy Sci.*, 56, 359–362, 2003.
57. International Dairy Federation (IDF), Implications of microfiltration on hygiene and identity of dairy products, *Bull. Int. Dairy Fed.*, 320, 8–40, 1997.
58. Abrahamsen, R.K. and Holmen, T.B., Yoghurt from hyperfiltrated, ultrafiltrated and evaporated milk and from milk with added milk powder, *Milchwissenschaft*, 35, 399–401, 1980.
59. Ferguson, P.H., Membrane processing in food and dairy industry, in *Process Engineering in the Food Industry-Developments and Opportunities*, R.W. Field and J.A., Howell, Eds, Elsevier Applied Sciences, London, p. 237, 1989.
60. Becker, T. and Puhan, Z., Effect of different processes to increase the milk solids non-fat content on the rheological properties of yoghurt, *Milchwissenschaft*, 44, 626–629, 1989.
61. Onwulata, C.I., Konstance, R.P., and Tomasula, P.M., Minimizing variations in functionality of whey protein concentrates from different sources, *J. Dairy Sci.*, 87, 749–756, 2004.
62. Williams, R.P.W., Glakovskaia, O., and Augustin, M.A., Properties of stirred yoghurts with added starch: Effects of blends of skim milk powder and whey protein concentrate on yoghurt texture, *Aus. J. Dairy Technol.*, 59, 214–220, 2004.

63. Lucey, J.A. and Singh, H., Formation and physical properties of acid milk gels: A review, *Food Res. Int.*, 30, 529–542, 1997.
64. Puvanenthiran, A., Williams, R.P.W., and Augustin, M.A., Structure and viscoelastic properties of set yoghurt with altered casein to whey protein ratio, *Int. Dairy J.*, 12, 383–391, 2005.
65. Antunes, A.E.C., Antunes, A.J., and Cardello, M.A.B., Chemical, physical, microstructural and sensory properties of set fat-free yogurts stabilized with whey protein concentrate, *Milchwissenschaft*, 59, 161–165, 2004.
66. Tamime, A.Y., Saarela, M., Korslund Sondergaard, A., Mistry, V.V., and Shah, N.P., Production and maintenance of viability of probiotic microorganisms in dairy products, in *Probiotic Dairy Products*, A.Y. Tamime, Ed., Blackwell Publishing, Oxford, pp. 39–72, 2005.
67. Amatayakul, T., Zisu, B., Sherkat, F., and Shah, N.P., Physical characteristics of set yogurts as affected by co-culturing with non-EPS and EPS starter cultures and supplementation with WPC, *Aus. J. Dairy Technol.*, 60, 238–243, 2005.
68. Amatayakul, T., Halmos, A.L., Sherkat, F., and Shah, N.P., Physical characteristics of yoghurts made using exopolysaccharide-producing starter cultures and varying casein to whey protein ratios, *Int. Dairy J.*, 16, 40–51, 2006.
69. Wilcox, C.P. and Swaisgood, H.E., Modification of the rheological properties of whey protein isolate through the use of an immobilized microbial transglutaminase, *J. Agric. Food Chem.*, 50, 5546–5551, 2002.
70. Sodini, I., Lucas, A., Oliviera, M.N., Remeuf, F., and Corrieu, G., Effect of milk base and starter culture on acidification, texture, and probiotic cell counts in fermented milk processing, *J. Dairy Sci.*, 85, 2479–2488, 2002.
71. Greef-Trial, N. and Queguiner, C., French Patent Application, WO/2003/070011, 2003.
72. Antunes, A.E.C., Cazetto, F.L., and Bolini, H.M.A., Viability of probiotic microorganisms during storage, postacidification and sensory analysis of fat-free yogurts with added whey protein concentrate, *Int. J. Dairy Technol.*, 58, 169–173, 2005.
73. Renner, E. and Abd-El Salam, M.H., *Application of Ultrafiltration in the Dairy Industry*, Elsevier Applied Science, London, p. 132, 1991.
74. Brazuelo, A., Suarez, E., Riera, F.A., Alvarez, R., Iglesia, J.R., and Granada, J., Protein enriched yoghurt by ultrafiltration of skim milk, *J. Sci. Food Agric.*, 69, 283–290, 1995.
75. Nakazawa, Y., Furusawa, M., Hohno, H., and Shida, T., Manufacture and proteolytic properties of yoghurt from milk concentrated by ultrafiltration, *Lebensmit. Wiss. Technol.*, 24, 491–494, 1991.
76. Alvarez, F., Arguello, M., Cabero, M., Riera, F.A., Alvarez, R., Iglesias, J.R., and Granada, J., Fermentation of concentrated skim-milk. Effects of different protein/lactose ratios obtained by ultrafiltration-diafiltration, *J. Sci. Food Agric.*, 76, 10–16, 1998.
77. Mistry, V.V., Manufacture and application of high milk protein powder, *Le Lait*, 82, 515–522, 2002.
78. de Castro-Morel, M. and Harper, W.J., Effect of retentate heat treatment and spray dryer inlet temperature on the properties of milk protein concentrates (MPCs), *Milchwissenschaft*, 58, 13–15, 2003.
79. Özer, B.H. and Robinson, R.K., The behaviour of starter cultures in concentrated yoghurt (labneh) produced by different techniques, *Lebensmit. Wiss. Technol.*, 32, 391–395, 1999.
80. Romero, C., Goicoechea, A., and Jiménez Pérez, S., Production of yoghurt from ultrafiltered milk, *Deut. Molk. Ztg*, 109, 1706–1709, 1988.
81. Tamime, A.Y., Davies, G., Chehade, A., and Mahdi, H.A., The production of 'labneh' by ultrafiltration: A new technology, *J. Soc. Dairy Technol.*, 42, 35–39, 1989.
82. El-Samragy, Y.A., El-Sayed, M.M., and Abd-Rabou, N.S., Nutritive value of labneh as affected by processing method, *Egypt. J. Dairy Sci.*, 25, 85–97, 1997.

83. Özer, B.H., Robinson, R.K., Grandison, A.S., and Bell, A.E., Rheological characteristics of labneh (concentrated yoghurt) produced by various concentration techniques, in *Proc. Textural Properties of Fermented Milks and Dairy Desserts*, International Dairy Federation, Brussels, Special Issue 9802, pp. 181–185, 1997.
84. Özer, B.H., Robinson, R.K., Grandison, A.S., and Bell, A.E., Comparison of techniques for measuring the rheological properties of labneh (concentrated yoghurt), *Int. J. Dairy Technol.*, 50, 129–135, 1997.
85. Özer, B.H., Grandison, A.S., Robinson, R.K., and Lewis, M.J., Changes in the physical properties of labneh (concentrated yoghurt) during storage, in *Proc. IFT Annual Meeting*, IFT, Orlando, FL, pp. 117–118, 1997.
86. Özer, B.H., Bell, A.E., Grandison, A.S., and Robinson, R.K., Rheological properties of concentrated yoghurt (labneh), *J. Texture Stud.*, 29, 67–79, 1998.
87. Özer, B.H., Robinson, R.K., Grandison, A.S., and Bell, A.E., Gelation profiles of milks concentrated by different techniques, *Int. Dairy J.*, 8, 793–799, 1998.
88. Özer, B.H., Stenning, R., Grandison, A.S., and Robinson, R.K., Effect of protein concentration and distribution on the rheology of concentrated yoghurt, *Int. J. Dairy Technol.*, 52, 135–138, 1999.
89. Özer, B.H., Stenning, R., Grandison, A.S., and Robinson, R.K., Rheology and microstructure of labneh (concentrated yoghurt), *J. Dairy Sci.*, 82, 682–689, 1999.
90. Özer, B.H., Factors affecting yoghurt gel network. I. Role of thiol-disulphide exchange reactions, *Gida*, 26, 353–358, 2001.
91. Tamime, A.Y., Kalab, M., and Davies, G., Rheology and microstructure of strained yoghurt (labneh) made from cow's milk by three different methods, *Food Microstruct.*, 8, 125–135, 1989.
92. Tamime, A.Y., Kalab, M., and Davies, G., The effect of processing temperatures on the microstructure and firmness of labneh made from cow's milk by the traditional method or by ultrafiltration, *Food Struct.*, 10, 345–352, 1991.
93. Tamime, A.Y., Davies, G., Chehade, A.S., and Mahdi, H.A., The effect of processing temperatures on the quality of labneh made by ultrafiltration, *J. Soc. Dairy Technol.*, 44, 99–103, 1991.
94. Tamime, A.Y., Robinson, R.K., and Latrille, E., Yoghurt and other fermented milks, in *Mechanisation and Automation in Dairy Technology*, A.Y. Tamime and B.A. Law, Eds, Sheffield Academic Press, Sheffield, p. 152, 2001.
95. Özer, B.H., Rheological properties of labneh (concentrated yoghurt), PhD thesis, The University of Reading, Reading, UK, p. 275, 1997.
96. Tamime, A.Y., Kalab, M., Davies, G., and Mahdi, H.A., Microstructure and firmness of labneh (high solids yoghurt) made from cow's, goat's and sheep's milks by a traditional method or by ultrafiltration, *Food Struct.*, 10, 37–44, 1991.
97. Attia, H., Bennasar, M., and de la Fuente, T., Study of the fouling of inorganic membranes by acidified milks using scanning electron microscopy and eletrophoresis, I. Membrane with pore diameter 0.2 μm, *J. Dairy Res.*, 58, 39–50, 1997.
98. Tamime, A.Y., Barclay, M.N.I., Davies, G., and Barrantes, E., Production of low-calorie yogurt using skim milk powder and fat substitute. 1. A review, *Milchwissenschaft*, 49, 85–87, 1994.
99. Barrantes, E., Tamime, A.Y., Davies, G., and Barclay, M.N.I., Production of low calories yogurt using skim milk powder and fat-substitutes. 2. Compositional changes, *Milchwissenschaft*, 49, 135–139, 1994.
100. Barrantes, E., Tamime, A.Y., and Sword, A.M., Production of low calories yogurt using skim milk powder and fat-substitutes. 4. Rheological properties, *Milchwissenschaft*, 49, 263–266, 1994.
101. Lobato-Calleros, C., Torrijos, M.O., Sandoval, C.O., Perez, O.J.P., and Vernon, C.E.J., Flow and creep compliance properties of reduced-fat yoghurts containing protein-based fat replacers, *Int. Dairy J.*, 14, 777–782, 2004.

102. Barrantes, E., Tamime, A.Y., and Sword, A.M., Fat-free yogurt–like or dislike, *Dairy Ind. Int.*, 58, 33–35, 1993.

103. Uysal, H., Kınık, O., Akbulut, N., and Guley, Z., Dusuk kalorili yogurt uretiminde Simplesse®100 kullanimi, *Gida*, 28, 631–635, 2003.

104. Casella, L., Food ingredients Europe, in *Conf. Proc.*, Expoconcult Publishers, Maarsen, The Netherlands, pp. 196–198, 1989.

105. LaBarge, R.G., The search for low calories oil, *Food Technol.*, 42, 84–90, 1988.

106. Murray, P.R., Polydextrose, in *Low Calories Products*, G.G. Birch and M.G. Lindley, Eds, Elsevier Applied Science, London, pp. 83–100, 1988.

107. Barrantes, E., Tamime, A.Y., Sword, A.M., Muir, D.D., and Kaláb, M., The manufacture of set-type natural yoghurt containing different oils–1. Compositional quality, microbiological evaluation and sensory properties, *Int. Dairy J.*, 6, 811–826, 1996.

108. Anonymous, Fat replacers: Food ingredients for healthy eating, http://caloriescontrol.org/fatrepl.html (accessed on 10.08.2008).

109. Iyengar, R. and Gross, A., Fat substitutes, in *Biotechnology and Food Ingredients*, I. Goldberg and R. Williams, Eds, Van Nostrand Reinhold, New York, pp. 287–313, 1991.

110. Yazıcı, F. and Akgun, A., Effect of some protein-based fat replacers on physical, chemical, textural and sensory properties of strained yoghurt, *J. Food Eng.*, 63, 245–254, 2004.

111. Guzel-Seydim, Z., Sarikus, G., and Okur, O.D., Effect of inulin and Dairy-Lo(R) as fat replacers on the quality of set type yogurt, *Milchwissenschaft*, 60, 51–55, 2005.

112. Farooq, K. and Haque, Z.U., Effect of commercial fat replacers on physico-chemical properties of non-fat low calorie set yoghurt, *J. Dairy Sci.*, 78 (Suppl.), 137, 1995.

113. Reineccius, T.A., Reineccius, G.A., and Peppard, T.L., Potential for β-cyclodextrin as partial fat replacer in low-fat foods, *J. Food Sci.*, 69, 334–341, 2004.

114. FAO/WHO, in *Codex Alimentarius Abridged Version*, *Joint FAO/WHO Food Standards Programme-Codex Alimentarus Comission*, B.L. Smith, Ed., FAO, Rome, 1990.

115. Keogh, M.K. and O'Kennedy, B.T., Rheology of stirred yoghurt as affected by added milk fat, protein and hydrocolloids, *J. Food Sci.*, 63, 108–112, 1998.

116. Jung, H.C., Effect of adding various gums on the quality and physico-chemical characteristics of cow's milk yoghurt, *J. Taiwan Livestock Res.*, 35, 351–356, 2002.

117. Guven, M., Stabilizor kullaniminin yogurtlarin bazi kalite kriterleri uzerine etkileri, *Gida*, 23, 133–139, 1998.

118. Atamer, M., Gursel, A., and Yildirim, G., Yogurt yapiminda kullanilan stabilizatorler, in *Proc. III. Milli Sut ve Sut Urunleri Sempozyumu*, M. Demirci, Ed., MPM Yayinlari, Istanbul, pp. 95–110, 1995.

119. Williams, R.P.W., Glakovskaia, O., and Augustin, M.A., Properties of stirred yoghurts with added starch: Effects of alterations in fermentation conditions, *Aus. J. Dairy Technol.*, 58, 228–235, 2003.

120. Anonymous, British Patent Application, GB 1 565006, 1980.

121. Vanderpoorten, R. and Martens, R., Use of starch derivatives in the heat treatment of stirred yoghurt, *Revue de L'Agriculture*, 29, 1509–1523, 1976.

122. Winterton, D. and Meiklejohn, P.G., A modified starch stabiliser for low-cost production of fruit yoghurt, *Aus. J. Dairy Technol.*, 33, 35–36, 1978.

123. Luczynska, A., Bijok, F., Wajnert, T., Kazimerczak, W., Lipinska, W., Kosikowska, M., and Jakubczyk, E., Influence of various stabilizers on the rheological properties of non-heat treated yoghurt, in *Proc. XXth Int. Dairy Congr.*, IE, pp. 836–837, 1978.

124. Pedersen, H.C.A., New pectin type for restoring rheological properties of fruit yogurt, in *Food Ingredients Europe-Conference Proceedings*, Porte de Versailles, 4–6 Octobers, Expoconsult Publishers, Maarsen, pp. 51–54, 1993.

125. Basak, S. and Ramaswamy, H.S., Simultaneous evaluation of shear rate and time dependency of stirred yogurt rheology as influenced by added pectin and strawberry concentrate, *J. Food Eng.*, 21, 385–393, 1994.

126. Gad, A.S., Frank, J.F., Schmidt, K.A., and Abd-El Samh, M.M., Microstructure and some physical properties of yogurt stabilized with pectin, *J. Dairy Sci.*, 78, 127, 1995.
127. Gonc, S., Possibility of using additives to improve characteristics of yogurt, *Ege Univ. Ziraat Fak. Derg.*, 26, 187–194, 1989.
128. Katz, F., Natural and modified starches, in *Biotechnology and Food Ingredients*, I. Goldberg and R. Williams, Eds, Van Nostrand Reinhold, New York, p. 315, 1991.
129. Lo, C.G., Lee, K.D., Richter, R.L., and Dill, C.W., Influence of guar gum on the distribution of some flavor compounds in acidified milk products, *J. Dairy Sci.*, 79, 2081–2090, 1996.
130. Saldamli, I. and Babacan, S., Addition of dietary fiber to yoghurt, in *9th World Congr. of Food Science and Technology*, Budapest, p. 553, 1995.
131. Mehenna, N.M. and Mehenna, A.S., On the use of stabilizer for improving some properties of cow's milk yoghurt, *Egypt. J. Dairy Sci.*, 17, 289–296, 1989.
132. Jogdand, S.B., Lembhe, A.K., Ambadkar, R.K., and Chopade, S.S., Incorporation of additives to improve the quality of dahi, *Ind. J. Dairy Sci.*, 44, 459–460, 1991.
133. Jiang, J.X., Zhu, S.V., Zhu, Y., and Chen, B.Q., Improving the flavour and rheology of biprotein yoghurt, *Dairy Sci. Abstr.*, 57, 345, 1995.
134. Chandan, R.C. and O'Rell, K.R., Principles of yogurt processing, in *Manufacturing Yogurt and Fermented Milks*, R. Chandan, C. White, A. Kilara, and Y.H. Hui, Eds, Blackwell Publishing, Iowa, p. 192, 2006.
135. Chandan, R.C., Dairy: Yogurt, in *Food Processing: Principles and Applications*, J.S. Smith and Y.H. Hui, Eds, Blackwell Publishing, Ames, IA, p. 297, 2004.
136. El-Sayed, E.M., El-Gawad, I.A.A., Murad, H.A., and Salah, S.H., Utilization of laboratory-produced xanthan gum in the manufacture of yogurt and soy yogurt, *Eur. Food Res. Technol.*, 215, 298–304, 2002.
137. Harby, S. and El-Sabie, W., Studies of skim milk yogurt using some stabilizers, in *Proc. 8th Egyptian Conf. for Dairy Science and Technology*, Cairo, Egypt, pp. 537–549, 2001.
138. Schmidt, K.A., Herald, T.J., and Khatib, K.A., Modified wheat starches used as stabilizers in set-style yogurt, *J. Food Qual.*, 24, 421–434, 2001.
139. Fayed, E., Magdoub, M.N., Hammad, A.A., and Meleigi, S.A., Use of microbial gellan gum in some dairy products in *Proc. 8th Egyptian Conf. for Dairy Science and Technology*, Cairo, Egypt, pp. 481–493, 2001.
140. Kebary, K.M.K., Hussein, S.A., and Badawi, R.M., Impact of fortification of cow's milk with a modified starch on yoghurt quality, *Egypt. J. Dairy Sci.*, 32, 111–124, 2004.
141. Huang, C.J., Effect of adding various gums on the quality and physico-chemical characteristics of cow's milk yoghurt, *J. Taiwan Livestock Res.*, 35, 351–356, 2002.
142. Khalafalla, S.M. and Rousdhy, I.M., Effect of stabilizers on rheological and sensory properties of low fat buffalo's yoghurt, *Egypt. J. Food Sci.*, 24, 199–215, 1996.
143. Unal B., Metin, S., and Isikli, N.D., Use of response surface methodology to describe the combined effect of storage time, locust bean gum and dry matter of milk on the physical properties of low-fat set yoghurt, *Int. Dairy J.*, 13, 909–916, 2003.
144. Decourcelle, N., Lubbers, S., Vallet, N., Rondeau, P., and Guichard, E., Effect of thickeners and sweeteners on the release of blended aroma compounds in fat-free stirred yoghurt during shear conditions, *Int. Dairy J.*, 14, 783–789, 2004.
145. Kora, E.P., Souchon, I., Latrille, E., Martin, N., and Marin, M., Composition rather than viscosity modifies the aroma compound retention of flavoured yoghurt, *J. Agric. Food Chem.*, 52, 3048–3056, 2004.
146. McGlinchey, N., The right replacement, *Dairy Ind. Int.*, 60, 29–30, 1995.
147. Everett, D.W. and McLeod, R.E., Interactions of polysaccharide stabilisers with casein aggregates in stirred skim-milk yoghurt, *Int. Dairy J.*, 15, 1175–1183, 2005.

148. Sagdic, O., Simsek, B., Orhan, H., and Dogan, M., Effect of λ-carrageenan on bacteria and some characteristics of yoghurt, *Milchwissenschaft*, 59, 45–49, 2004.
149. Yaygın, H., *Yogurt Teknolojisi*, Akdeniz Universitesi Basimevi, Antalya, p. 331, 1999.
150. Kim, Y.J., Baick, S.C., and Yu, J.H., Effect of oligosaccharides and *Bifidobacterium* growth promoting materials in yogurt base made by *Bifidobacterium infantis* 420, *Korean J. Dairy Sci.*, 17, 167–173, 1995.
151. Fennema, O.R., *Food Chemistry*, Marcel Dekker, New York, p. 991, 1985.
152. Haque, Z.Z. and Aryana, K.J., Effect of sweeteners on the microstructure of yogurt, *Food Sci. Technol. Res.*, 8, 21–23, 2002.
153. Fellows, J.W., Chang, S.W., and Shazer, W.H., Stability of aspartame in fruit preparations used in yogurt, *J. Food Sci.*, 56, 689–695, 1991.
154. Andres, C., Fruit flavoured concentrates provide food flavour systems, *Food Process.*, 48, 24–26, 1987.
155. Robinson, R.K. and Tamime, A., Recent development in yogurt manufacture, in *Modern Dairy Technology*, B.J.F. Hudson, Ed., Elsevier Applied Science, London, pp. 1–34, 1986.
156. Fleet, G.H., Yeasts in dairy products, *J. Appl. Bacteriol.*, 68, 199–211, 1990.
157. Mihyar, G.F. Yamani, M.I., and Al-Sa'ed, A.K., Resistance of yeast flora of labaneh to potassium sorbate and sodium benzoate, *J. Dairy Sci.*, 80, 2304–2309, 1997.
158. Penney, V., Henderson, G., Blum, C., and Gren, J.P., The potential of phytopreservatives and nisin to control microbial spoilage of minimally processed fruit yogurts, *Innov. Foods Sci. Emerg. Technol.*, 5, 369–375, 2004.
159. Song, T.B., Kim, Y.H., Shin, J.H., Lee, Y.K., Cha, K.J., Whang, J.H., and Yu, J.H., Effects of types and sweetness intensity of low calorie sweeteners on growth and lactic acid producing *Lactobacillus bulgaricus* and *Streptococcus thermophilus*, *Dairy Sci. Abstr.*, 58, 243, 1996.
160. Hyvonen, L. and Slotte, M., Alternative sweetening of yogurt, *Int. J. Food Sci. Technol.*, 18, 97–112, 1983.
161. Ohashi, S. and Ochi, T., Flavor enhancing effect of the protein sweetener, thaumatin on fermented milk, *New Food Ind.*, 24, 1, 1982.
162. King, S.C., Lawler, P.J., and Adams, J.K., Effect of aspartame and fat on sweetness perception in yogurt, *J. Food Sci.*, 65, 1056–1059, 2000.
163. Keating, K.R. and White, C.H., Effect of alternative sweeteners in plain and fruit yogurts, *J. Dairy Sci.*, 73, 54–62, 1990.
164. McGregor, J.U. and White, C.H., Effect of sweeteners on major volatile compounds and flavor of yogurt, *J. Dairy Sci.*, 70, 1828–1834, 1987.
165. Monjitano, H. and Borrego, F., Sweet selection, *Dairy Ind. Int.*, 61, 41–43, 1996.
166. Thiriet, B., Actilight, a low calorie sweetener, in *Proc. Food Ingredients Europe*, Expoconsult Publishers, Maarsen, p. 267, 1989.
167. Nelson, A.L., Properties of high intensity sweeteners, in *Sweeteners: Alternative Practical Guide for the Food Industry*, American Association of Cereal Chemists, Eagan Press, Minnesota, pp. 17–30, 2000.
168. Pinheiro, M.V.S., Castro, L.P., Hoffman, F.L., and Penna, A.L.B., Estudo comparativo de edulcorantes em iogurtes probioticos, *Revis. Ins. Laticinos Candido Tostes*, 57, 142–150, 2002.
169. Pinheiro, M.V.S., Oliviera, M.N., Pena, A.L.B., and Tamime, A.Y., The effect of different sweeteners in low-calorie yogurts–A review, *Int. J. Dairy Technol.*, 58, 193–199, 2005.
170. Neves, L., Pampulha, M.E., and Loureiro-Dias, M.C., Resistance of spoilage yeasts to sorbic acid, *Lett. Appl. Microbiol.*, 19, 8–11, 1994.

171. Rajmohan, S. and Prasad, V., Potassium sorbate as an antimycotic agent in enhancing the keeping quality of dahi, *Cheiron*, 23, 26–31, 1994.

172. Benkerroum, N., Oubel, H., and Sandine, W.E., Effect of nisin on yogurt starter, and, on growth and survival of *Listeria monocytogenes* during fermentation and storage of yogurt, *Int. J. Food Saf.*, 1, 1–9, 2008.

173. Kebary, K.M.K. and Kamaly, K.M., Susceptibility of starter and non-starter organisms to nisin in stirred yoghurt during storage, *Egypt. J. Dairy Sci.*, 19, 157–167, 1991.

174. Bossi, M.G., Giraffa, G., Carminati, D., and Neviani, E., Action of nisin on lactic acid bacteria: Conductance measurements, *Dairy Sci. Abstr.*, 51, 135, 1989.

175. Var, I., The effects of natamycin on the shelf-life of yoghurt, *Arch. Lebensmit.*, 55, 7–9, 2004.

176. Sahan, N., Guven, M., and Kacar, A., Farkli asitlikteki yogurtlardan torba yoğurdu uretimi ve natamisinin torba yogurdunun raf omru uzerine etkisi, *Gida*, 29, 9–15, 2004.

177. Baranova, M., Burdova, O., Mal'a, P., and Zezula, I., Variation in titratable acidity of yoghurt culture after addition of $NaNO_3$ and $NaNO_2$, *Dairy Sci. Abstr.*, 59, 58, 1997.

178. Kontova, M. and Prekoppova, J., Influence of lysozyme and KNO_3 on growth of clostridia and lactic acid bacteria in milk, in *Proc. XXIII Int. Dairy Congr.*, Vol. II, p. 352, 1990.

179. Salih, M.A. and Sandine, W.E., Inhibitory effects of Microgard™ on yogurt and cottage cheese spoilage organisms, *J. Dairy Sci.*, 73, 887–893, 1990.

180. Atamer, M., Yildirim, Z., and Sezgin, E., Farkli basinclarda uygulanan homojenizasyon isleminin set yoğurtların bazı nitelikleri üzerine etkisi, *Gida*, 17, 255–258, 1992.

181. Fox, P.F. and McSweeney, P.L.H., *Dairy Chemistry and Biochemistry*, Blackie Academic and Professionals, London, p. 477, 1998.

182. Schkoda, P., Hechler, A., and Hinrichs, J., Influence of the protein content on structural characteristics of stirred fermented milk, *Milchwissenschaft*, 56, 19–22, 2001.

183. Celestino, E., Iyer, M., and Roginski, H., The effects of refrigerated storage of raw milk on the quality of whole milk powder stored for different periods, *Int. Dairy J.*, 7, 119–127, 1997.

184. Driessen, F.M., Modern trends in the manufacture of yogurt, *Fermented Milks*, *IDF Bull.*, 179, 107, 1984.

185. Fox, P.F., *Advanced Dairy Chemistry*, I. *Proteins*, 1st edition, Elsevier Applied Sciences, New York, p. 781, 1992.

186. Hill, A.R., The β-lactoglobulin-κ-casein complex, *Can. Inst. Food Sci. Technol. J.*, 22, 120–123, 1989.

187. Cho, Y., Singh, H., and Lawrence, K.C., Heat-induced interactions of β-lactoglobulin and κ-casein B in a model system, *J. Dairy Res.*, 70, 61–71, 2003.

188. Pearce, R.J., Thermal denaturation of whey proteins, *IDF Bull.*, 238, 17, 1989.

189. Otte, J., Ipsen, R., and Qvist, K.B., Isolation of two tryptic fragments from bovine beta-lactoglobulin and assessment of their thermal gelation ability, *Milchwissenschaft*, 55, 197–200, 2000.

190. Parris, N., Anema, S.G., Singh, H., and Creamer, L.K., Aggregation of whey proteins in heated sweet whey, *J. Agric. Food Chem.*, 41, 460–464, 1993.

191. Mottar, J., Bassier, A., Joniau, M., and Baert, J., Effect of heat-induced association of whey proteins and casein micelles on yoghurt structure, *J. Dairy Sci.*, 72, 2247–2256, 1989.

192. Dannenberg, F. and Kessler, H.G., Effect of denaturation of ß-lactoglobulin on texture properties of set-style non-fat yoghurt. 2. Firmness and flow properties, *Milchwissenschaft*, 43, 700–704, 1988.

193. Labropoulous, A.E., Palmer, J.K., and Lopez, A., Whey protein denaturation of UHT processed milk and its effect on rheology of yoghurt, *J. Texture Stud.*, 12, 365–374, 1981.

194. Labropoulous, A.E., Collins, W.F., and Stone, W.K., Effect of UHT treatment and vat processes on heat-induced rheological properties of yoghurt, *J. Dairy Sci.*, 67, 405–409, 1984.

195. Krasaekoopt, W., Bhandari, B., and Deeth, C.H., Yoghurt from UHT milk: A review, *Aus. J. Dairy Technol.*, 58, 26–29, 2003.

196. Krasaekoopt, W., Bhandari, B., and Deeth, C.H., Comparison of texture of yogurt made from conventionally treated milk and UHT milk fortified with low-heat skim milk powder, *J. Food Sci.*, 69, 276–280, 2004.

197. Parnell-Cluiness, E.M., Kakuda, Y., and Smith, A.K., Microstructure of yoghurt as affected by heat treatment of milk, *Milchwissenschaft*, 42, 413–417, 1987.

198. Anonymous, *Dairy Processing, Handbook*, 2nd revision, Tetra Pak Processing Systems AB, Lund, Sweden, 2003.

199. Robinson, R.K. and Tamime, A.Y., Manufacture of yoghurt and other fermented milks, in *Modern Dairy Technology*, R.K. Robinson, Ed., Elsevier Applied Science, London, p. 1, 1993.

200. Robinson, R.K., Lucey, J.A., and Tamime, A.Y., Manufacture of yoghurt, in *Fermented Milks*, A.Y. Tamime, Ed., Blackwell Publishing, London, pp. 53–75, 2006.

201. Lucey, J.A., Formation and physical properties of milk protein gels, *J. Dairy Sci.*, 85, 281–294, 2002.

202. Lee, W. and Lucey, J.A., Rheological properties, whey separation and microstructure in set-style yoghurt: Effects of heating temperature and gelation temperature, *J. Texture Stud.*, 34, 515–536, 2003.

203. Fira, D., Kojic, M., Banina, A., Spasojevic, I., Strahinic, I., and Topisirovic, L., Characterization of cell envelope-associated proteinases of thermophilic lactobacilli, *J. Appl. Microbiol.*, 90, 123–130, 2001.

204. Abu-Tarboush, H.M., Comparison of associative growth and proteolytic activity of yogurt starters in whole milk from camels and cows, *J. Dairy Sci.*, 79, 366–371, 1996.

205. Roefs, S.P.F.M., Structure of acid casein gels, PhD thesis, Agricultural University, Wagenningen, The Netherlands, 1986.

206. Dickinson, E., Particle gels, *Chem. Ind.*, 19, 595–599, 1990.

207. Rohm, H. and Kovac, A., Effects starter cultures on linear viscoelastic and physical properties of yoghurt gels, *J. Texture Stud.*, 25, 311–329, 1994.

208. Steventon, A.J., Parkinson, J., Fryer, P.J., and Bottomley, R.C., The rheology of yoghurt, in *Rheology of Food, Pharmaceutical and Biological Materials with General Rheology*, R.E. Carter, Ed., Elsevier Applied Science, London, pp. 196–210, 1990.

209. Heertje, I., Visser, J., and Smits, P., Structure formation in acid milk gels, *Food Microstruct.*, 4, 267–277, 1985.

210. Walstra, P. and Jennes, R., *Dairy Chemistry and Physics*, John Wiley and Sons Inc., Canada, p. 467, 1984.

211. Kristo, E., Biliaderis, C.G., and Tzanetakis, N., Modelling of the acidification process and rheological properties of milk fermented with a starter culture using response surface methodology, *Food Chem.*, 83, 437–446, 2003.

212. Hardi, J. and Slacanac, V., Examination of coagulation kinetics and rheological properties of fermented milk products: Influence of starter culture, milk fat and addition of inulin. *Mljekarstvo*, 50, 217–226, 2000.

213. White, C.H., Manufacture of high quality yogurt, *Cult. Dairy Prod. J.*, 30, 18–26, 1995.

214. Guilbert, S. and Gontard, N., Edible and biodegradable food packaging, in *Foods and Packaging Materials-Chemical Interactions*, P. Ackermann, M. Jagerstad, and T. Ohlsson, Eds, The Royal Society of Chemistry, London, pp. 159–168, 1995.

215. Cuq, B., Gontard, N., and Guilbert, S., Edible films and coatings as active layers, in *Active Food Packaging*, M.L. Rooney, Ed., Blackie Academic and Professional, London, pp. 111–142, 1995.

216. Frederiksen, C.S., Haugard, K.V., Poll, L., and Becker, M.E., Light-induced quality changes in plain yoghurt packed in polylactate and polystyrene, *Eur. Food Res. Technol.*, 217, 61–69, 2003.
217. Bastioli, C., Global status of the production of biobased packaging materials. in *Proc. Food Biopack Conf.*, C. Weber, Ed., Copenhagen, Denmark, p. 2, 2000.
218. Ucuncu, M., *Gidalarin Ambalajlanmasi*, Ege Universitesi Basimevi, Izmir, p. 689, 2000.
219. Thomsen, S.B. and Stenaa, D., Migration of monomers and additives from food packaging materials to foods, *Maelkeritidende*, 98, 10–13, 1985.
220. Hinrichs, J. and Fertsch, B., Pretreatments of yogurt with hydrostatic pressure, *Deutsche Milchwirt.*, 50, 875, 2000.
221. Huppertz, T., Fox, P.F., and Kelly, A.L., High pressure treatment of bovine milk: Effects on casein micelles and whey proteins, *Int. Dairy J.*, 71, 97–106, 2004.
222. de Ancos, B., Pilar-Cano, M., and Gomez, R., Characteristics of stirred low-fat yogurt as affected by high pressure, *Int. Dairy J.*, 10, 105–111, 2000.
223. Özer, B.H., Kırmacı, H.A., Öztekin, Ş., Hayaloğlu, A., and Atamer, M., Incorporation of microbial transglutaminase into non-fat yogurt production, *Int. Dairy J.*, 17, 199–207, 2007.

3 Yogurt Microbiology and Biochemistry

G. Candan Gürakan and Neslihan Altay

CONTENTS

3.1   INTRODUCTION

There are many fermented dairy products, including yogurt, kefir, and koumiss, based on lactic acid bacteria (LAB) species and strains. They are developed in regional areas and have various flavors, textures, and fermentation products depending on the fermenting organisms.

It is known that yogurt originated in the Middle East [1,2] may have originated in Turkey [2,3]. It is also a popular product in Europe and America for a long time. *Lactobacillus delbrueckii* ssp. *bulgaricus* (*L. bulgaricus*) and *Streptococcus thermophilus* (*S. thermophilus*) are the most common commercial cultures used in yogurt manufacturing. The microorganisms used in the production of yogurt accomplish briefly two tasks: production of lactic acid and flavor components. Although the consistency, flavor, and aroma may vary from one region to another, the basic ingredients and manufacturing techniques are essentially consistent. Therefore, production of flavor and aroma compounds by different strains of yogurt starter cultures has become a challenging area for many researchers for a long time. Moreover, it is known that the main factor causing differences in the final product is the strain diversity of yogurt cultures. Therefore, various molecular techniques have also been developed as important tools for differentiation of strains of yogurt cultures and probiotic strains. This has been facilitated to recognize and patent strains with important industrial characteristics. Many studies have reported the beneficial effects of yogurt cultures *L. bulgaricus* and *S. thermophilus* on human health. However, the acceptance of yogurt bacteria as probiotics is still under discussion.

3.2 YOGURT PRODUCTION

3.2.1 TRADITIONAL APPROACH

Many fermented foods are still produced either by natural (spontaneous) fermentation or by back-slopping and the active cultures may be poorly defined [4]. Natural fermentation is the process initiated without the use of starter inoculum. Natural fermentation results from competitive activities of contaminating organisms. In small-scale fermentations and in rural (regional) areas in the countries where yogurt is originated, material from a previous successful batch is added to facilitate the initiation of a new process for the production of traditional yogurt called back-slopping. Through this repeated practice of back-slopping [5,6], selection of best-adapted strains can naturally be achieved.

However, spontaneous food fermentations are neither predictable nor controllable, particularly in large-scale production. Therefore, in the industry, commercially produced starter cultures are preferred for standardization and safety reasons during yogurt production.

3.2.2 USE OF STARTER CULTURES

Hassan and Frank [7] described a starter culture as "any active microbial preparation intentionally added during product manufacture to initiate desirable changes."

There are two types of plain yogurt:

- Stirred style yogurt
- Set style yogurt

The milk is usually clarified and separated into cream and skim milk and then *standardized* to achieve the desired fat content before the addition of starter cultures. The various ingredients are then blended together in a mix tank equipped with a powder funnel and an agitation system. Pasteurization using a continuous plate heat exchanger for 30 min at 85°C or for 10 min at 95°C is the next step. A higher temperature than heat treatment of fluid milk pasteurization is used to produce a relatively sterile and conducive environment for the starter culture and to denature and coagulate whey proteins to enhance the viscosity and texture. The mix is then *homogenized* at high pressures of 2000–2500 psi in stirred style yogurt. Besides thoroughly mixing the stabilizers and other ingredients, homogenization also prevents creaming and wheying off during incubation and storage. Stability, consistency, and body are enhanced by homogenization [8]. The yogurt starter culture is added when the homogenized mix has cooled to an optimum growth temperature. Yogurt is usually produced by using a 1:1 mixture [9,10] of *S. thermophilus* and *L. bulgaricus* as the starter culture.

In set style, the yogurt is packaged immediately after inoculation with the starter and is incubated in the packages. Drinking yogurt is stirred yogurt with total solid content not higher than 11% and has undergone further homogenization to reduce the viscosity.

3.3   MICROORGANISMS AS YOGURT STARTER CULTURES

3.3.1   *LACTOBACILLUS DELBRUECKII* SSP. *BULGARICUS*

Genus *Lactobacillus* is characterized as Gram-positive, nonspore forming, rod-shaped, catalase negative, and microaerophilic cells. Their growth is generally enhanced by 5% CO_2. *L. bulgaricus* is one of the three subspecies of *L. delbrueckii* ssp. [11] that belongs to the genus *Lactobacillus*. The other two subspecies are *Lactobacillus delbrueckii* ssp. *lactis* (*L. lactis*) and *Lactobacillus delbrueckii* ssp. *delbrueckii*. *L. bulgaricus* and *L. lactis* are present in milk and milk products. The genus *Lactobacillus* is divided into three groups: obligately homofermentative, facultatively heterofermentative, and obligately heterofermentative. *L. bulgaricus* belongs to the obligately homofermentative group together with *Lactobacillus acidophilus*, *L. lactis*, and *Lactobacillus helveticus* [12]. The optimum temperature of *L. bulgaricus* for growth is 45°C [13].

Recently, genomes of two *L. bulgaricus* strains were completely sequenced, that is, *Lactobacillus bulgaricus* ATCC 11842 and *Lactobacillus bulgaricus* ATCC BAA-365 [14,15].

3.3.2   *STREPTOCOCCUS THERMOPHILUS*

Farrow and Collins [16] proposed to reclassify *S. thermophilus* as a subspecies of *Streptococcus salivarius*, namely *Streptococcus salivarius* subsp. *thermophilus*, and this reclassification was accepted and valid until Schleifer et al. [17] showed that *S. thermophilus* is a distinct species, based on their DNA–DNA hybridization studies under stringent conditions.

S. thermophilus belongs to the viridians streptococci. There are five major groups under viridians streptococci, namely the mutants group, the anginosus group, the sanguinus group, the mitis group, and the salivarius group, which includes *S. thermophilus*, *S. salivarius*, and *Streptococcus vestibularis* [18].

It is a Gram-positive, spherical-shaped bacterium with an optimum growth temperature of 37°C. However, some metabolic activities such as the polysaccharide production or synthesis of acetaldehyde may take place at different temperatures [13]. Its growth ceases at 10°C.

3.3.3   BLEND OF MICROORGANISMS AS STARTER CULTURE
IN YOGURT PRODUCTION

The commercial starter cultures for yogurt production are composed of a symbiotic mixed culture of *S. thermophilus* and *L. bulgaricus*. These starter organisms are ultimately responsible for the formation of typical yogurt flavor and texture. Although they can grow independently, the rate of acid production is much higher when used together than either of the two organisms grown individually. In general, a ratio of 1:1, *S. thermophilus* to *L. bulgaricus*, inoculation is added to the jacketed fermentation tank. A temperature of 42°C is maintained for 4–6 h under the conditions without agitation. This temperature is a compromise between the optimums for the two microorganisms (*S. thermophilus* 37°C; *L. bulgaricus* 45°C) [13]. After the inoculation of milk with starter cultures, *S. thermophilus* grows faster until it accounts for 90% of the total bacterial cells. Over the next 2 h, *S. thermophilus*, by the release of lactic acid, carbon dioxide, and formic acid, synergistically stimulates *L. bulgaricus* to grow faster. The streptococci reduce the initial pH drop of the yogurt mix to approximately 5. Thus, *L. bulgaricus* grows after acidification of the milk, whereas *S. thermophilus* is inhibited as the lactic acid is accumulated. The lactobacilli are responsible for a further decrease to pH 4. On the other hand, the proteolytic activity of *L. bulgaricus* produces stimulatory peptides and amino acids for use by *S. thermophilus*. The yogurt mixture coagulates during fermentation due to the drop in pH. After 4 h, the balance between the populations will be reached. At the end of fermentation, the acidity reaches to 1.2–1.4% lactic acid (pH 4.2–4.3) and the cell count to higher than 2×10^7 cells/mL for each starter organism [13]. Acidity of 1.2–1.4% lactic acid is the preferred level of most consumers. The titratable acidity (TA) is carefully monitored until it is 0.85–0.90%. At this time the jacket is replaced with cool water and agitation begins, both of which stop the fermentation. The fermentation process is usually completed within 3–4 h by both species converting lactose to lactic acid. In fact, the same amount of acidification would take 12–16 h with the same amount of only one single species. When the desired acidity is reached, yogurt is quickly cooled to stop further fermentation and metabolic activity. The coagulated product is cooled to 5–22°C, depending on the product. The product is then cooled and stored at refrigeration temperatures (5°C) to slow down the physical, chemical, and microbiological degradation.

The range of temperature for proper fermentation is quite small, that is, from 42°C to 44°C. In general, as the temperature is raised up to 44°C, the rate of culture metabolism is higher, and the yogurt is sweeter. Faster growth also causes the yogurt to set faster. When the desired acidity is reached, yogurt is quickly cooled to stop further fermentation and metabolic activity. This cooling step is crucial in industrial yogurt production; it must be done quickly to control tightly the acidity of the yogurt, which has a profound effect on the taste.

3.4 FERMENTATION PRODUCTS OF YOGURT BACTERIA

Many volatile organic compounds in yogurt have previously been listed. However, studies have shown that only a few of them with relatively higher concentration have the influence to give the characteristic aroma of yogurt [19].

Both yogurt bacteria have a β-galactosidase system (Ray) [20] so that lactose is hydrolyzed to glucose and galactose. The glucose is metabolized to pyruvate via the Embden–Meyerhoff Pathway (EMP), and then pyruvate is converted to lactic acid by lactate dehydrogenase enzymes. On the other hand, galactose is partly metabolized by *L. delbrueckii* subsp. *bulgaricus* strains, while most strains of *S. thermophilus* do not have the enzymes for metabolizing galactose. Therefore, galactose and lactic acid leave the cell and are accumulated in the yogurt medium.

After the hydrolysis of lactose, the following fermentation products contribute to flavor:

- Lactic acid
- Acetaldehyde
- Acetic acid
- Diacetyl

3.4.1 LACTIC ACID

Lactic acid is the major metabolite that inhibits many other microorganisms present in the same environment due to the decrease in pH level. Acid-forming activity is dependent on the strains in the association [18]. During fermentation of milk to yogurt, lactose is metabolized to 1.2–1.4% lactic acid with a pH of about 4.2–4.3. At this acidity, milk proteins are coagulated to form a firm gel and the overacidification must be avoided by cooling the product.

3.4.2 ACETALDEHYDE

Acetaldehyde at levels of up to $40\,mg\,kg^{-1}$ is the main flavoring component of yogurt [13]. The desirable level is accepted as 25 ppm [20]. Different pathways for acetaldehyde production in LAB are shown in Figure 3.1.

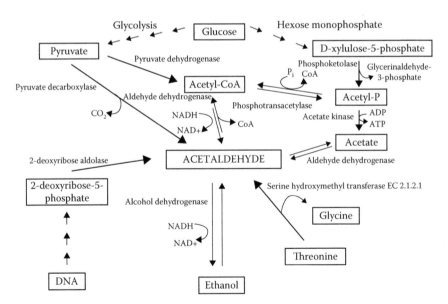

FIGURE 3.1 Overview of the different metabolic pathways in LAB that could lead to acetaldehyde formation. Acetyl-CoA: acetyl coenzyme A. (Reproduced from Chaves, A.C.S.D., et al., *Appl. Environ. Microbiol.*, 68, 5656–5662, 2002. American Society for Microbiology. With permission.)

During yogurt fermentation, acetaldehyde can be produced from

i. Glucose directly via pyruvate
ii. Glucose through the formation of pyruvate and then acetyl coenzyme A
iii. Glucose through the formation of D-xylulose-5-phosphate, then acetyl-P, and then acetate
iv. Degradation of thymidine
v. Threonine

In fact, operation of more than one metabolic pathway is also possible [21]. Threonine is produced through proteolysis in milk. Threonine aldolase catalyzes the reaction of acetaldehyde and glycine production from threonine and this is the direct pathway responsible for acetaldehyde production by LAB. The lower content of acetaldehyde in goat's yogurt compared to cow's yogurt is due to a higher glycine level, which acts as an inhibitor of threonine aldolase [22]. In yogurt, contradictory results were obtained in threonine aldolase activity and the level of acetaldehyde production of *S. thermophilus* and *L. bulgaricus*. Conversion of threonine to acetaldehyde is achieved by production of threonine aldolase as catalyst only in *L. bulgaricus* [23]. Robinson [13] has reported that the activity of this enzyme in *S. thermophilus* is temperature dependent and its activity decreases at temperatures higher than 30°C, whereas the same enzyme in *L. bulgaricus* is not affected by higher temperature of yogurt manufacturing. Thus, *L. bulgaricus* was considered and represented as the major acetaldehyde producer during yogurt manufacturing in many studies. However, lately acetaldehyde production by the activity of this enzyme was found in both yogurt cultures [24]. Furthermore, Chaves et al. [21] indicated that serine hydroxymethyltransferase, which is the enzyme displaying threonine aldolase activity as a secondary activity, constitutes the main pathway for acetaldehyde formation in *S. thermophilus* even at 42°C (Figure 3.1).

3.4.3 ACETIC ACID

Acetic acid is known as a flavor compound produced from pyruvate by *S. thermophilus*. Beshkova et al. [19] detected acetic acid in both *S. thermophilus* and *L. bulgaricus* pure cultures grown in whole cow's milk. Within the free volatile fatty acids examined by Beshkova et al. [19], acetic acid had the highest concentration and the production of acetic acid by *L. bulgaricus* was found to be higher than the amount produced by *S. thermophilus*.

Bifidobacteria, which are heterofermentative, produce acetic acid besides lactic acid and the ratio of lactic acid to acetic acid is 2:3 [7]. Acetic acid causes harshness in the product and also in high levels it gives a "vinegary" taste that decreases the acceptability of the product by consumers [25].

3.4.4 DIACETYL

Diacetyl is considered as the major aroma and flavor component of butter. Citrate is converted to diacetyl via pyruvate metabolism. Diacetyl is also a flavor compound with 0.5 ppm amount in yogurt. Controversial results were also given about the yogurt bacteria producing a major diacetyl in yogurt. *S. thermophilus* was presented as solely responsible for the presence of diacetyl in yogurt in some studies, whereas *L. bulgaricus* was reported as a producer of high amount of diacetyl in other studies [19].

3.4.5 FORMATE

Formate is produced by *S. thermophilus* from pyruvate [20] after lactose utilization. Its production by *S. thermophilus* stimulates the growth of *L. bulgaricus*.

3.5 FAT CONTENT

In addition to fermentation products, the percentage of fat in the final yogurt has a significant effect on yogurt quality. It develops an effect on "mouthfeel." The normal range of fat content is from 0.5% to about 3.5%; however, levels as low as 0% and as high as 10% are found in special products.

3.6 INDUSTRIAL STARTER CULTURE PRODUCTION

Starter cultures are produced in the industrial scale for the manufacture of yogurt. Traditionally, when a suitable starter organism had been found, a large quantity would be grown in a suitable nutrient medium (traditionally milk, but commercial blends of nutrients are also available), and small quantities would be used to inoculate each new batch of yogurt. This technique with a main batch of starter culture is often referred to as using "bulk starter." The use of a bulk starter is becoming increasingly uncommon among commercial producers, mainly because of the risk of "phage" attack on the bulk starter, and the subsequent loss of time while a new batch of starter organisms is prepared. A technique often referred to as direct vat inoculation (DVI) is becoming the industry norm. DVI involves inoculating the yogurt mix directly with a very large number of frozen or freeze-dried starter organisms. Although a slightly longer incubation time is required with the DVI technique, resistance to phage attack will be achieved.

3.6.1 STARTER CULTURE PRODUCERS WORLDWIDE

Major commercial starter culture producers of the dairy industry throughout the world are listed in Table 3.1.

3.6.2 DIFFERENT FORMS OF COMMERCIAL STARTER CULTURES

Storage methods of starter cultures and starter culture production technologies before their inoculation into the milk at dairy plants have been changed during time. Different methods are used for the production of starter cultures. According to these methods, starter cultures can be divided basically into two groups: the cultures that require preliminary preparation steps before inoculation and direct-to-vat or direct-vat-set (DVS) cultures, which are inoculated with the DVI technique. Dairy companies can purchase cultures suitable for bulk starter preparation or DVS cultures (Table 3.2).

TABLE 3.1

Some Commercial Dairy Starter Culture Producers throughout the World

Producer	Country	Website
Christian and Hansen	Denmark	http://www.chr-hansen.com
Danisco	Denmark	http://danisco.com
DSM	The Netherlands	http://www.dsm.com
Alce	Italy	http://www.mofinalce.it
Centro Sperimenti del Latte	Italy	http://www.csl.it
Valio	Finland	http://www.valio.fi
BioSource Flavors, Inc.	United States	http://www.biosourceflavors.com
CSK Food Enrichment	The Netherlands	http://www.cskfood.com
BIOPROX	France	http://www.bioprox.com

3.6.2.1 Bulk Starter Cultures

3.6.2.1.1 Daily Propagated Cultures

In this culture type, the first step is to prepare mother culture having a volume of approximately 100 mL from a stock culture. Then, the amount of culture is increased by sequential inoculations of larger volumes of medium [7]. Finally, bulk starter culture having a volume of 500–1000 L is prepared and is used to inoculate milk. The inoculum ratio of bulk starter culture should be 2–5% of the milk. Liquid or freeze-dried cultures can be used to prepare mother culture in this system [26]. In the case of bulk culture production, the dairy will be responsible for purity and performance. Poor texture, high postacidification, and sourness are some problems that might be encountered after the manufacture of yogurt. However, the main disadvantages of this type of starter cultures are the subsequent loss of time while a new batch of starter organisms is prepared and the high risk of phage contamination.

3.6.2.1.2 Deep-Frozen Cultures

These cultures are inoculated into the bottles of reconstituted skim milk and then frozen by the supplier. Bulk starter is prepared inoculating these cultures in milk

TABLE 3.2

Bulk Cultures and DVS Cultures

Bulk Cultures	DVS Cultures
Daily propagated cultures	Deep-frozen DVS cultures
Deep-frozen cultures	Lyophilized DVS cultures
Deep-frozen concentrated cultures	
Lyophilized concentrated cultures	

into bulk starter medium after thawing and clotting it overnight. Daily propagation by the food manufacturer is eliminated in this culture system.

3.6.2.1.3   Deep-Frozen Concentrated Cultures

Bulk starter is prepared by thawing the contents and using them for inoculation without clotting. These cultures are packed with 70–125 mL content in insulated boxes containing solid CO_2 for maintenance at −70°C. Their shelf life is about 3 months during storage at −50°C [27].

3.6.2.1.4   Lyophilized Concentrated Cultures

Bulk starter is prepared by adding the contents of lyophilized concentrated culture over the surface of the bulk starter medium.

3.6.2.2   DVS Cultures: Deep-Frozen DVS Cultures and Lyophilized DVS Cultures

On the other hand, DVS cultures are defined as the strains mixed to convenient blends for direct inoculation into milk for the fermentation process. They are mostly packed with the weight according to the size of the batch to be fermented. Suppliers sometimes may provide DVS cultures to fulfill the need of the customer [27]. Ratio of blending was defined in order to achieve the desired functionality. DVS cultures are highly concentrated, and culture producers guarantee purity and performance of DVS cultures. Application of DVS cultures reduces the risk of phage infection as the propagation step is eliminated. This resistance to phage attack may also be due to the use of phage-hardened (isolated spontaneous phage-resistant mutants) starter cultures. This allows the use of starter cultures without requiring culture rotation. Therefore, most dairy companies prefer to use commercial starter cultures although preparation of the inoculum at plants is still a valid method for small manufacturers. Therefore, while classifying starter cultures, the first property used is whether the culture is DVS or bulk, the second is if the bulk culture is prepared from a concentrated culture, and the third is the format of the culture (liquid, frozen, or freeze-dried). Since direct-to-vat starter culture usage provides higher flexibility and safety than bulk starter preparation [28], they become the first choice of the big dairy companies even though they have higher prices.

These commercial DVS cultures are supplied in the form of frozen or freeze-dried (lyophilized) for preservation of their activity. Deep-frozen DVS cultures should be stored at −50°C or below, whereas lyophilized DVS cultures have the advantage of easier storage at temperature 4°C.

3.7   STRAIN SELECTION AND/OR TECHNOLOGICAL PROPERTIES OF STRAINS (CULTURE CHARACTERIZATION)

In the yogurt production, one of the most important factors determining the product quality is the type of the starter culture used. That is why the strain selection as yogurt starter culture is crucial. A good strain of starter culture not only affects the flavor and aroma, but it can also speed up the process and thus reduces the effective equipment cost. Therefore, selection of strains to be used as a yogurt starter culture is a very important, but challenging process. While deciding whether a strain is a good candidate to be a yogurt starter culture, some properties of the strain should be examined carefully. Selection of strains can be based on the analysis of phenotypic properties or genetic material [analysis of specific genes, e.g., exopolysaccharide (EPS) genes]. Microarray studies for analysis of gene expression [29] may provide an efficient tool for strain selection. The most important technological properties that are related to yogurt starter cultures may be listed as follows:

Acidification profiles
- Acidification rate
- Postacidification

Flavor
- Proteolytic activity
- Acetaldehyde production

Texture
- EPS production
- Syneresis
- Ropiness
- Gel firmness
- Mouth thickness

Other properties
- Phage resistance
- Rheological properties

3.7.1 ACIDIFICATION RATE

Since acidification leads coagulation of casein and hence formation of the yogurt gel [30], acidification rate is the most important technological property of a yogurt starter culture. Therefore, pH measurement is used to control the process in the industry and is measured discontinuously [31]. A fast acidification is essential for the aroma, texture, and flavor of the product [25]. The characteristic sharp and acidic taste of yogurt was gained by lactic acid [30] produced during the growth of *S. thermophilus* and *L. bulgaricus* in milk. Many researchers used acidification activity as an important tool to be able to select good starter culture candidates for both yogurt production and also other fermented dairy products [32–34]. Ayad et al. [32] classified more than 700 LAB belonging to different genera including *Streptococcus* and *Lactobacillus* based on acidification rate calculated as $\Delta pH = pH_{\text{zero time}} - pH_{\text{at time}}$. In their study, cultures were grouped as fast, medium, or slow acidifying cultures when the incubation time to reach a ΔpH of 0.4 units was 3 h, 3–5 h, and longer than 5 h, respectively, and the fast acidifying cultures were claimed to be good starter culture candidates for dairy fermentations [32]. Although the ranges used in this classification are useful to get preliminary information, particularly about *L. bulgaricus*, *S. thermophilus* as a yogurt culture should be faster than this and might reach a ΔpH of about 0.6 unit after 3 h incubation at 42°C (N. Altay and G.C. Gurakan, unpublished data).

Fast acidification is probably one of the most demanded futures of a yogurt culture. However, further acidification after production of yogurt is known as postacidification and decreases the acceptability of yogurt by consumers. Postacidification leads to the acid and bitter taste. Excessive acidification is mainly due to uncontrollable growth of strains of *L. bulgaricus* at low pH values and refrigerated temperatures [35]. Overacidification could be prevented using cultures with low overacidification behavior [36]. Lactose-negative mutants of *L. bulgaricus* growing with lactose fermenting *S. thermophilus* can be a solution for the postacidification problem [37].

3.7.2   PROTEOLYTIC ACTIVITY

Proteolytic activity in strain selection for yogurt production is not as important as in the strain selection to be used in cheese production, but still has a secondary importance [30]. The difference between the proteolytic activities of *L. bulgaricus* and *S. thermophilus* forms the keystone of the associative growth of these two organisms. Therefore, proteolytic activity may have an important role while combining different strains of *L. bulgaricus* and *S. thermophilus*.

L. bulgaricus has a higher proteolytic activity than *S. thermophilus*, although statistically significant differences were reported between the proteolytic activities of the strains that belong to the same species [38]. Slocum et al. [38] reported that proteolysis was affected by total milk solid percentage, incubated time, and preheating of milk, besides the strains used. In their study, increase at proteolysis was observed by increasing total milk solid to the maximum level (14%); however, further increase in total milk solid caused a decrease in proteolytic activity [38].

Milk proteins, the main nitrogen source for the starter culture, were processed by exocellular proteinases, membrane-bound aminopeptidases and intracellular exopeptidases and proteinases [39].

3.7.3   ACETALDEHYDE PRODUCTION

Yogurt aroma is formed by the combined effects of different compounds. Ott et al. [40] identified 21 volatile compounds having major effects on yogurt aroma out of 91 compounds determined. This outcome also shows the complexity of yogurt aroma. However, acetaldehyde is claimed to be the major aroma compound giving typical yogurt flavor [30]. Therefore, while selecting strains as yogurt culture, acetaldehyde can be accepted as a representative compound of yogurt aroma and can be examined to define the strains capable of improving the characteristic aroma of yogurt.

The acetaldehyde amount produced when *L. bulgaricus* and *S. thermophilus* are inoculated together is much greater than the amount produced by any one of these species alone. It was also reported that the amount of acetaldehyde in yogurt decreases or maintains during storage at 4°C depending on cultures used. Therefore the strains that are capable of producing a high amount of acetaldehyde and utilizing it slowly during storage of the product may be selected to produce desirable yogurt aroma in the end product [41].

3.7.4 EPS Production

EPS produced by LAB during fermentation has a major textural impact on fermented milk products. Yogurts produced using highly EPS-producing cultures exhibit higher viscosity, smooth texture, and creaminess, low syneresis as well as a ropy character. Strains are variable according to the amount of their EPS production. Some strains of *L. bulgaricus* and *S. thermophilus* produce a ropy EPS. This mucoid structure of EPS increases the viscosity of yogurts. The use of EPS-producing cultures rather than additives as fat replacers is suggested to provide a better texture for low-fat yogurts [42].

EPS are the polysaccharides found outside of the cell wall. They are either attached to the cell wall as capsules or secreted into the extracellular environment [43]. Their role has not been well established. EPS do not seem to serve as food sources, since generally slime-forming bacteria cannot catabolize the EPS, which they secrete. However, it was thought that EPS may have several functions such as protecting the bacteria against desicating, phagocytosis, and phage attack, providing higher oxygen tension, participating in metal ions uptake, and functioning as adhesive agents [44].

The functions of EPS are to improve the rheology of a fermented dairy product as natural biothickening agents and to bind water and hence limit syneresis as physical stabilizers. The composition, structure, and interaction of EPS with ions and proteins in milk affect the functionality. Even though EPS have no taste, they contribute to the taste perception by increasing the viscosity of the product and hence increasing the residence time in the mouth and contact time with palate and taste receptors [45].

EPS produced by LAB can be divided mainly into two groups as homopolysaccharides and heteropolysaccharides. Homopolysaccharides are composed of a single type of monosaccharide. On the other hand, heteropolysaccharides consist of multiple types of monosaccharides. Thermophilic LAB strains including *L. bulgaricus* and *S. thermophilus* produce heteropolysaccharides [46].

Cerning et al. [47] showed that ropy strains of *L. bulgaricus* produce water-soluble EPS composed of galactose, glucose, and rhamnose in an approximate molar ratio of 4:1:1. In this study, skim milk was used as a growth medium and growth conditions were selected as close to yogurt manufacture [47]. The molecular weight of EPS produced by *L. bulgaricus* is approximately 5×10^5 [47]. It was also shown [48] that ropy strains of *S. thermophilus* grown on skim milk produce water-soluble EPS composed of glucose, galactose, and *N*-acetyl-D-galactosamine in a ratio of 1:2:1. Cerning et al. [49] determined that EPS produced by *S. thermophilus* contains also small amounts of xylose, arabinose, rhamnose, and mannose. Molecular weight of the heteropolysaccharide produced by *S. thermophilus* was determined as 1×10^6 [48].

3.7.5 Rheological Properties

Yogurt is a thixotropic fluid and slowly develops a three-dimensional network after being manufactured and placed in a container. When shear is applied to these kinds of fluids by, say, mixing with a spoon, the structure is broken down and the material reaches the minimum thickness. Rotational viscometers have been very useful to assess time-dependent fluid behavior like thixotropic fluids [50]. For many years, especially European yogurt manufacturers use starter cultures for improving the textural properties of yogurt since the addition of stabilizers is not allowed. Even in the countries such as United States where using food additives in yogurt manufacturing is not prohibited, these kinds of starter cultures having a positive effect on texture are used to produce more natural and additive-free products [51]. Starter cultures that improve the textural properties of yogurt are EPS-producing cultures (see the EPS section). The chemical structure of the polymer produced by different starters has an effect on the rheological properties of yogurt [52]. A number of other factors have been determined as influencing the rheological properties and so the quality of yogurt. These properties are [53]

- Milk composition (such as dry mater content)
- The amount and properties of the starter culture used
- Incubation temperature
- Storage time

Whey separation is another criterion for rheological properties.

3.7.6 PHAGE RESISTANCE

The search for strains having high acidification rate and flavor with phage resistance is the main goal of starter culture producers and the dairy industry.

3.8 TECHNOLOGICAL PROBLEMS RELATED TO STARTER CULTURE ACTIVITY

3.8.1 CHANGES IN CULTURE ACTIVITY

Routine subculturing may cause changes in culture activity such as rate of acid production and/or level of flavor compounds after certain generations. The reasons for these changes are still not well known. The loss of plasmids encoding these kinds of technological properties such as proteolytic activity, antibiotic resistance, and secretion of glycoproteins for *Lactococcus* spp. is well documented. However, *L. bulgaricus* and *S. thermophilus* strains having plasmids with metabolic significance were not reported yet, while the presence of some cryptic plasmids were shown [13,39]. On the other hand, in the study of Aslim and Beyatli [54], correlation with the resistance to antibiotics in some *S. thermophilus* strains with the occurrence of plasmids was implied.

3.8.2 BACTERIOPHAGE INFECTION OF STARTER CULTURES

Bacteriophages are a group of viruses that attack bacteria. Bacteriophages are normally referred to as "phages." Phages are usually found in the drains and floor gullies of a dairy producing any cultured product. Poor hygiene and a lack of general housekeeping increase the risk. They attack the yogurt starter organisms. They might cause long or never-ending incubations.

In the dairy industry, cheese manufacturing and the subsequent whey handling are prime sources of "phage."

3.8.2.1 Natural Mechanisms of Phage Resistance

Fortunately, there are some starter culture organisms having phage resistance naturally.

Four major groups of natural phage resistance mechanisms are known:

- Inhibition of adsorption (due to a modification or complete absence of phage receptor)
- Prevention of phage DNA injection (injection of DNA into the cell is inhibited)
- Restriction and modification (R/M) systems. (The phage DNA is digested by a specific endonuclease following the entry into the cell, and host DNA is protected by modification by a methylase enzyme)
- Abortive infection (the cell dies without release of phage)

3.8.2.2 Industrial Methods for Inhibition of Phage Infection

An environmental sanitation is the prerequisite for effective control of bacteriophages. Thus, all environmental areas such as floors, ceilings, surfaces, walls doors as well as tank equipments and utensils should be cleaned and sanitized regularly. Air filters should be regularly changed since phages might be airborne. Moreover, culture activity should be monitored and phage activity should be checked.

3.8.2.2.1 Phage Inhibitory Media

These media are formulated to protect starter culture cells from phage attack in the bulk starter culture vessel. All free calcium are chelated by ammonium and sodium phosphates that would prevent phage infection [27].

3.8.2.2.2 Culture Rotation

An effective culture rotation program is another strategy to eliminate the phage problem. Phages are host-specific so that they die out when the culture is changed. Many producers use two different cultures rotating alternating days [27].

3.9 IMPROVEMENT OF THE PROPERTIES IN YOGURT STARTER CULTURES AND GENETICALLY MODIFIED MICROORGANISMS (GMMs)

The microorganism might gain new desirable characteristics or eliminate undesirable properties by insertion or deletion of corresponding genes. Some important genetic changes carried out until now on LAB are shown in Table 3.3.

Among these genetic alterations acquired, phage resistance is particularly important for the prevention of industrial losses during yogurt and/or cheese manufacturing.

TABLE 3.3

Some Important Possible Genetic Alterations in LAB

New Phenotypes	Related Organism	Added Property	Reference
Phage resistance	Lc. lactis	Lethal gene upon infection	Djordjevic [55]
Bacteriophage resistance	Lc. lactis	Antisense mRNA-mediated	Kim [56]
EPS	Lc. lactis	Thickening	Stringele [57]
β-Galactosidase	L. casei	Decrease in lactose content	Pouwels [58]
Bacteriocin	Lc. lactis	Bacteriocin production	Martinez [59]
Proteolytic activity	Lc. lactis	Transfer of peptidase gene	Wegman [60]
Starch degrading ability	Lactobacillus plantarum	Amylase production	Fitzsimons [61]

3.9.1 MECHANISMS FOR PROVIDING PHAGE RESISTANCE TO YOGURT CULTURES

Many naturally occurring strains are lysogenic for bacteriophages. A prophage can enter the lytic cycle spontaneously or it can be induced by some treatments such as UV light or elevated temperature. Phage-insensitive starter cultures, hygienic conditions, or culture rotation systems will also reduce the risk of bacteriophage contamination.

In *Lactococcus* species, phage resistance mechanisms are often located on the plasmid. The plasmids can then be transferred from cell to cell by a mechanism called conjugation. This enables the fast transfer of phage resistance mechanisms within a bacterial population.

Yogurt cultures are also susceptible to phage attack. *S. thermophilus* and *L. bulgaricus* strains during yogurt or cheese manufacturing may be attacked by specific phages [39]. *Lactococcus lactis* (*Lc. lactis*) and *S. thermophilus* are particularly the more sensitive starters causing greatest industrial loss during dairy fermentations due to phage infection [62]. Strain selection for bacteriophage resistance is the method for starter producers. This is achieved by isolation of the phage-resistant mutant of the mother strain as a single colony on an agar plate during the propagation of a phage on this host (phage hardening).

Another strategy for the development of phage-resistant starter bacteria for consumer products is the transfer of natural phage resistance gene-containing plasmid to another strain through a natural mechanism called conjugation [63].

The phage-resistant strains that were developed by phage hardening or conjugation [64] are accepted to be nongenetically modified organisms (GMOs) according to European Union (EU) directives [65] and have been in commercial use for many years [62].

3.9.2 LEGISLATIONS ON GMMS FOR YOGURT CULTURES

The organisms in which genetic material has been altered in a way that does not occur naturally such as by point mutations or deletions are considered to be GMOs [65]. GMOs are defined within the EU legislation according to two Directives: 90/219/EEC on contained use and 2001/18/EC on deliberate release into the environment repealing Council Directive 90/220/EC. Directive 2001/18/EC came into force in

EU member states on October 17, 2002 [66]. A GMM is also considered as GMO and is also subjected to a novel food regulation (258/97/EC) [67]. Labeling requirements of novel foods and genetically modified foods are in place.

World Health Organization (WHO)/Food and Agriculture Organization of the United Nations (FAO) expert consultation has also suggested the use of the concept of substantial equivalence by case-by-case studies [68].

On the other hand, in United States, there are no labeling requirements for products according to GMO status. Products are assessed with respect to their safety in general. The Food and Drug Agency (FDA), United States Department of Agriculture (USDA), and the Environmental Protection Agency (EPA) Toxic Substance Control Act are the main agencies for regulating biotechnology in United States [69,70].

3.9.3 SELF-CLONING

Self-cloning is the reintroduction of DNA from a host that is modified or from a closely related strain of the same species [71]. In this system no heterologous DNA (DNA from other species) is introduced into the strain. This strategy was also defined as "The removal of nucleic acid from a cell or organism, followed by the re-insertion of all or part of that nucleic acid—with or without further enzymatic, chemical or mechanical steps—into the same cell type (or cell-line) or into a phylogenetically closely related species which can naturally exchange genetic material with the donor species. Accordingly, the temporary introduction of plasmids, the deletion of specific DNA sequences, or introduction of DNA from another micro-organism belonging to the same species fall within the definition of self-cloning" by Council Directive 98/81/EC amending 90/219/EC [72]. In case the host is not pathogenic, self-cloning is not considered as GM according to the EU directive on the contained use of GMMs (219/EC) [72]. However, it is not excluded from the EU Directive on the deliberate release of GMMs [73]. Although in many studies [65,74,75] GM-LAB, particularly the ones produced by self-cloning strategies, are recommended for use in foods, in the European Union still no modified LAB have been commercialized yet.

3.10 IDENTIFICATION STRATEGIES FOR YOGURT CULTURES

3.10.1 CONVENTIONAL METHODS

The critical experiments for the identification of yogurt cultures will be listed in this section. Putative *S. thermophilus* and *L. bulgaricus* isolates should be subjected to biochemical identification experiments and the isolates selected according to biochemical tests should be genotypically confirmed. Type strains of *S. thermophilus* and *L. bulgaricus* should be used as positive controls in all experiments performed for identification.

As a first step of identification, the morphologies of all isolates on agar medium and under a microscope should be checked. Since the morphologies on agar vary based on the medium used, the isolate could be compared to the colony morphology of the type strain grown on the same medium. However, the purpose of this test is mainly to get more information about the isolate rather than eliminating the isolate having atypical colony morphology, since difference in colony morphologies can be observed within the same species. Morphology under a microscope will be much more important, since putative *L. bulgaricus* and *S. thermophilus* isolates should appear as long rods and ovoid coccus shaped, respectively.

Since both *S. thermophilus* and *L. bulgaricus* are Gram-positive, catalase–negative, and homofermentative, Gram and catalase reactions and CO_2 production from glucose should be checked and after each of these tests the isolates having different results from those given above must be eliminated.

Checking the growth at 10°C and 45°C is a very simple but powerful way of differentiating yogurt cultures from some species that may share the same environment with yogurt cultures. Both *L. bulgaricus* and *S. thermophilus* do not grow at 10°C, but grow at 45°C (Figure 3.2).

Selective identification can conventionally be achieved using biochemical tests such as API, carbohydrate fermentation tests, electrophoretic mobility and/or genetic tests such as GC% ratio determination and DNA–DNA homology.

It should be noted that the pH of the medium used for isolation of *S. thermophilus* is crucial and should be about 6.8. Generally, M17 medium is used for the growth of *S. thermophilus* and the pH of M17 is slightly changed from manufacturer to manufacturer and even these small changes may affect the growth of this bacterium. If the pH of the medium is different from 6.8, especially greater than this pH, adjusting it to 6.8 may decrease the risk of facing problems in growth.

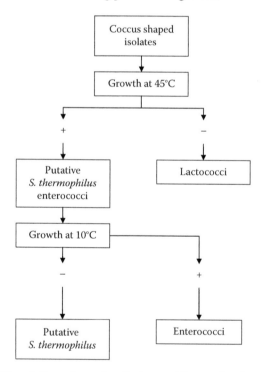

FIGURE 3.2 Differentiation of putative *S. thermophilus* strains from strains of closely related genera. +, growth observed; –, no growth.

3.10.2 MOLECULAR METHODS

Molecular biology techniques have facilitated the identification of yogurt or probiotic bacteria. Sensitivity and speed make molecular methods more efficient compared to conventional methods. Cebeci and Gurakan [76] have recently reported rapid identification of both yogurt cultures, *S. thermophilus* and *L. bulgaricus*, using methionine biosynthesis and 16S ribosomal ribonucleic acid (rRNA) genes.

Denaturing gradient gel electrophoresis (DGGE) was recognized as a useful tool to observe changes in the structure of microbial communities over time and/or following different treatments [77]. This method can have lots of application areas in both starter culture and probiotic culture studies such as confirmation of declared organisms in commercial probiotic products [78] and identification of *Lactobacillus* species of gastrointestinal origin by combining DGGE with species-specific polymerase chain reaction (PCR) primers [79]. A new technique, genome probing microarray, has been developed for quantitative monitoring of community dynamics in LAB at species-specific level during the fermentation process [80]. Both techniques could also be used for the community during yogurt fermentation.

3.10.3 SUBTYPING OF YOGURT CULTURES AND STRAIN DIVERSITY

Molecular fingerprinting methods have also allowed recognizing and tracking individual strains [81]. Strain selection is an important issue for yogurts with better taste, flavor, texture, and long shelf life. Various methods are used for typing strains of a species and indicating genetic diversity among yogurt species. The methods that are widely used to study the strain diversity include ribotyping, amplified fragment length polymorphism (AFLP), amplified restriction digestion of ribosomal DNA analysis (ARDRA), random amplified polymorphic DNA (RAPD), pulsed field gel electrophoresis (PFGE), multiplex PCR and analyzing clustered regularly interspaced short palindromic repeats (CRISPR) [82] loci are also suggested as potentially valuable methods for typing [83]. CRISPR loci are generally characterized by 21–48 bp partially palindromic and highly conserved direct repeats interspaced by usually 20–58 bp sequences [83–85]. It was recently shown that CRISPR provides acquired phage resistance in *S. thermophilus* [86]. CRISPR studies of LAB in the literature are mainly focused on *S. thermophilus*. Therefore, analyzing CRISPR loci may be helpful for having information about typing and phage resistance of especially *S. thermophilus* strains.

3.11 PROBIOTIC PROPERTIES OF YOGURT BACTERIA

Probiotics are usually of human origin, while both *S. thermophilus* and *L. bulgaricus* occur in the dairy environment. Therefore, yogurt bacteria *L. bulgaricus* and *S. thermophilus* are not considered as probiotic organisms as they are not natural inhabitants of the intestine, so they cannot implant themselves in the intestine, and do not survive under acidic conditions and bile concentrations encountered in the gastrointestinal tract [87]. In many studies, better adherence of probiotic lactobacilli such as *L. acidophilus* than *L. bulgaricus* and *S. thermophilus* to human epithelial cells (Coco2 intestinal cells) was reported [88,89]. Additionally, it was suggested that yogurt bacteria are not highly resistant to exposure to gastric acidic conditions [90]. However, with the appearance of recent studies [90] in the literature, the dilemma has become more complicated. Mater et al. [90] and Elli et al. [91] in their study have pointed out that commercial yogurt bacteria *S. thermophilus* and *L. bulgaricus* could survive transit in the gastrointestinal tract. Another analysis reported in a molecular analysis study has supported this result [92]. Microbiota density in groups after consumption of fresh and heat-treated yogurt containing *L. bulgaricus* and *S. thermophilus* was investigated and it was found that LAB was significantly higher in the fresh yogurt group.

3.12   SOME SPECIAL PRODUCTS

3.12.1   Bioyogurt

The application of probiotics to yogurt is commonly referred to as bioyogurt. Yogurt has recently been reformulated to include live strains of *L. acidophilus* and species of *Bifidobacterium* (named as AB cultures) in addition to conventional yogurt bacteria *S. thermophilus* and *L. bulgaricus*. Thus, they contain live probiotic microorganisms to develop health benefits [93]. Regular consumption of 400–500 g/week of AB-yogurt with 10^6 viable cells per mL would be satisfactory to develop a therapeutic minimum of 10^8 live probiotic cells per day [94].

3.12.2   Lactose Reduced Milk

Lactose-intolerant people are unable to digest lactose properly due to the absence of β-D-galactosidase (lactase) in their intestine. Starter cultures used in fermentation and probiotic bacteria produce β-galactosidase. However, for the consumption of milk by lactose-intolerant people, lactose reduced milk has been commercially produced as an alternative to yogurt or probiotic products. β-Galactosidase is added into milk for this product. Purified lactase produced on an industrial scale by the yeast *Kluyveromyces lactis* is widely used for the reduction of lactose in milk [95].

REFERENCES

1. Tamime, A.Y. and Deeth, H.C., Yogurt: Technology and biochemistry, *J. Food. Protect.*, 43, 939–977, 1980.
2. Hayaloglu, A.A., Karabulut, I., Alpaslan, M., and Kelbaliyev, G., Mathematical modelling of drying characteristics of strained yogurt in a convective type tray-dryer, *J. Food Eng.*, 78, 109–117, 2007.
3. Encyclopædia Britannica, 2008, Internet: http://www.britannica.com/EBchecked/topic/653449/yogurt (accessed on October 2008).
4. European Food Safety Authority Scientific Colloquium on Microorganisms in Food and Feed: Qualified Presumption of Safety, 2004, Internet: http://www.isapp.net/docs/heimbachrptEFSAjan05.pdf (accessed on October 2008).
5. Holzapfel, W.H., Appropriate starter culture technologies for small-scale fermentation in developing countries, *Int. J Food Microbiol.*, 75, 197–212, 2002.

6. Giraffa, G., Studying the dynamics of microbial populations during food fermentation, *FEMS Microbiol. Rev.*, 28, 251–260, 2004.
7. Hassan, A.N. and Frank J.F., Starter cultures and their use, in *Applied Dairy Microbiology*, E.H. Marth and J.L.Steele, Eds, Marcel Dekker, New York, pp. 151–206, 2001.
8. Goff, D., *Dairy Science and Technology Education*, University of Guelph, Canada, www.foodsci.uoguelph.ca/dairyedu/home.html (accessed on October 2008).
9. Jay, M.J., *Modern Food Microbiology*, 6th edition, Aspen Publishers, Maryland, 2000.
10. Wouters, J.T.M., Ayad, E.H.E., Hugenholtz, J., and Smith, G., Microbes from raw milk for fermented dairy products, *Int Dairy J.*, 12, 91–109, 2002.
11. Holt, J.G., Krieg, N.R., Sneath, P.H.A., Staley, J.T., and. Williams, S.T., *Bergey's Manual of Determinative Bacteriology*, 9th edition, Williams & Wilkins, Baltimore, 1994.
12. Stiles, M.E. and Holzapfel, W.H., Lactic acid bacteria of foods and their current taxonomy, *Int. J. Food Microbiol.*, 36, 1–29, 1997.
13. Robinson, R.K., Fermented milks, yogurt, in *Encyclopedia of Food Microbiology*, Richard Robinson, Carl Batt, and Pradip D. Patel, Eds, Academic Press, London, 1997.
14. van de Guchte, M., Penaud, S., Grimaldi, C., Barbe, V., Bryson, K., Nicolas, P., Robert, C., et al., The complete genome sequence of *Lactobacillus bulgaricus* reveals extensive and ongoing reductive evolution, *PNAS*, 103 (24), 9274–9279, 2006.
15. Makarova, K., Slesarev, A., Wolf, Y., Sorokin, A., Mirkin, B., Koonin, E., Pavlov, A., et al., Comparative genomics of the lactic acid bacteria, *PNAS*, 103 (42), 15611–15616, 2006.
16. Farrow, J.A.E., Collins, M.D., DNA base composition, DNA–DNA homology and long-chain fatty acid studies on *Streptococcus thermophilus* and *Streptococcus salivarius*, *J. General Microbiol.*, 130, 357–362, 1984.
17. Schleifer, K.H., Ehrmann, M., Krusch, U., Neve, H., Revival of the species *Streptococcus thermophilus* (Ex Orla-Jensen, 1919) *Nom. Rev. Syst. Appl. Microbiol.*, 14, 386–388, 1991.
18. Facklam, R., What happened to the streptococci: Overview of taxonomic and nomenclature changes, *Clin. Microbiol. Rev.*, 15, 613–630, 2002.
19. Beshkova, D., Simova, E., Frengova, G., and Simov, Z., Production of flavour compounds by yogurt starter cultures, *J. Ind. Microbiol. Biot.*, 20, 180–186, 1998.
20. Ray, B., *Fundamental Food Microbiology*, CRC Press, Boca Raton, FL, 1996.
21. Chaves, A.C.S.D., Fernandez, M., Lerayer, A.L.S., Mierau, I., Kleerebezem, M., and Hugenholz, J., Metabolic enginnering of acetaldehyde production by Streptococcus thermophilus, *Appl. Environ. Microbiol.*, 68, 5656–5662, 2002. American Society for Microbiology.
22. Rysstad, G., Knutsen, W., and Abrahamsen, R., Effect of threonine and glycine on acetaldehyde formation in goats' milk yogurt, *J. Dairy Res.*, 57, 401–411, 1990.
23. Raya, R.R., de Nadra, M.C., De Ruiz Halgado, A., and Oliver, G., Acetaldehyde metabolism in lactic acid bacteria, *Milchwissenchaft*, 41, 397–399, 1986.
24. Ott, A., Germond, J.E., and Chaintreau, A., Origin of acetaldehyde during milk fermentation using 13C-labeled precursors, *J. Agric. Food Chem.*, 48, 1512–1517, 2000.
25. De Vuyst, L., Technology aspects related to the application of functional starter cultures, *Food Technol. Biotechnol.*, 38, 2, 105–112, 2000.
26. Mayra-Makinen, A., and Bigret, M., Industrial use and production of lactic acid bacteria, in *Lactic Acid Bacteria Microbiology and Functional Aspects*, S. Salminen, A. von Wright, Eds, Marcel Dekker, New York, pp. 73–102, 1998.
27. Wigley, R.C., Starter cultures/uses in the food industry, in *Encyclopedia of Food Microbiology. Richard Robinson*, Carl Batt, and Pradip D. Patel, Eds, Academic Press, London, 1999.
28. Hansen, E.B., Commercial bacterial starter cultures for fermented foods of the future, *Int. J. Food Microbiol.*,78, 119– 131, 2002.
29. Ahmed, F., Genetically modified probiotics in foods, *Trends Biotechnol.*, 21, 491–497, 2003.

30. Tamime, A.Y. and Robinson, R.K., *Yogurt Science and Technology*, 2nd edition, Woodhead Publishing Limited, England, 2000.
31. De Brabandere, A.G. and De Baerdemaeker J.G., Effects of process conditions on the pH development during yogurt fermentation, *J. Food Eng.*, 41, 221–227, 1999.
32. Ayad, E.H.E., Nashat, S., El-Sadek, N. Metwaly, H., and El-Soda, M., Selection of wild lactic acid bacteria isolated from traditional Egyptian dairy products according to production and technological criteria, *Food Microbiol.*, 21, 715–725, 2004.
33. Ayhan, K., Durulu-Özkaya, F., and Tunail, N., Commercially important characteristics of Turkish origin domestic strains of *Streptococcus thermophilus* and *Lactobacillus delbrueckii* ssp. *Bulgaricus*, *Int. J. Dairy Technol.*, 58 (3), 150–157, 2005.
34. Chammas, G.I., Saliba, R., Corrieu, G., and Beal, C., Characterization of lactic acid bacteria isolated from fermented milk "laBAN", *Int. J. Food Microbiol.*, 110, 52–61, 2006.
35. Lourence-Hattingh, A and Viljoen, B.C., Yogurt as probiotic carrier food, *Int. Dairy J.*, 11, 1–17, 2001.
36. Kneifel, W., Jaros, D., and Erhard, F., Microflora and acidification properties of yogurt and yogurt-related products fermented with commercially available starter cultures, *Int. J. Food Microbiol.*, 18, 179–189, 1993.
37. Mollet, B., New technologies in fermented milk, *Cerevisia*, 21, 63–65, 1996.
38. Slocum, S.A., Jasinski, E. M., and Kilara, A., Processing variables affecting proteolysis in yogurt during incubation, *J. Dairy Sci.*, 71, 596–603, 1988.
39. Zourari, A, Accolas, J.P., and Desmazeaud, M.J., Metabolism and biochemical characteristics of yogurt bacteria. A review, *Lait*, 72, 1–34, 1992.
40. Ott, A., Fay, L.B., and Chaintreau, A., Determination and origin of the aroma impact compounds of yogurt flavor, *J. Agric. Food Chem.*, 45, 850–858, 1997.
41. Hamdan, I.Y., Kunsman, Jr. J.E., and Deane, D.D., Acetaldehyde production by combined yogurt cultures, *J.Dairy Sci.*, 4 (7), 1080–1082, 1971.
42. Guzel-Seydim, Z.B., Sezgin, E., and Seydim, A.C., Influences of exopolysaccharide producing cultures on the quality of plain set type yogurt, *Food Control*, 16, 205–209, 2005.
43. Bubb, W.A., Urashima, T., Fujiwara, R., Shinnai, T., and Ariga, H., Structural characterization of the exocellular polysaccharide produced by *Streptococcus thermophilus* OR 901, *Carbohydr. Res.*, 301, 41–50, 1997.
44. Cerning, J., Exocellular polysaccharides produced by lactic acid bacteria, *FEMS Microbiol. Rev.*, 87, 113–130, 1990.
45. Duboc, P. and Mollet, B., Applications of exopolysaccharides in the dairy industry, *Int. Dairy*, 11, 759–768, 2001.
46. De vuyst, L., and Degeest, B., Heteropolysaccharides from lactic acid bacteria, *FEMS Microbiol. Rev.*, 23, 153–177, 1999.
47. Cerning, J., Bouillanne, C. Desmazeaud, M.J., and Landon, M., Isolation and characterization of exocellular polysaccharide produced by *Lactobacillus bulgaricus*, *Biotechnol. Lett.*, 8, 625–628, 1986.
48. Doco, T., Wieruszeski, J.M., Fournet, B., Carcano, D., Ramos, P., and Loones, A., Structure of an exocellular polysaccharide produced by *Streptococcus thermophilus*, *Carbohydr. Res.*, 198 (2), 313–321, 1990.
49. Cerning, J., Bouillanne, C. Desmazeaud, M.J., and Landon, M., Exocellular polysaccharide production by *Streptococcus thermophilus*, *Biotechnol. Lett.*, 10 (4), 255–260, 1988.
50. Steffe, J.F., *Rhelogical Methods in Food Process Engineering*, 2nd edition, Freeman Press, USA, 1996.
51. Marshall, V.M., Rawson, H.L., Effects of exopolysaccharide-producing strains of thermophilic lactic acid bacteria on the texture of stirred yoghurt, *Int. J. Food Sci. Technol.*, 34, 137–143, 1999.

52. Ruas-Madiedo, Hugenholz, J., and Zoon, P., An overview of the functionality of exopoly-saccharides produced by lactic acid bacteria, *Int. Dairy J.*, 12, 163–171, 2002.
53. Kristo, E., Biliaderis, C.G., and Tzanetakis, N., Modelling of the acidification process and rheological properties of milk fermented with a yogurt starter culture using response surface methodology, *Food Chem.*, 83, 437–446, 2003.
54. Aslim, B. and Beyatli, Y., Antibiotic resistance and plasmid DNA contents of *Streptococcus thermophilus* strains isolated from Turkish yogurts, *Turk. J. Vet. Anim. Sci.*, 28, 257–263, 2004.
55. Djordjevic, G.M., O'sullivan, D.J., Walker, S.A., Conkling, M.A., and Klaenhammer, T.R., A triggered-suicide system designed as a defence against bacteriophages, *J. Bacteriol.*, 179, 6741–6748, 1997.
56. Kim, S.G. and Batt, C.A., Antisense messenger RNA-mediated bacteriophage resistance in *Lactococcus lactis* subsp. *lactis*, *Appl. Environ. Microbiol.*, 57 1109–1113, 1991.
57. Stringele, F., Vincent, S.J., Faber, E.J., Newell, J.W., Kamerling, J.P., and Neeser, J.R., Introduction of the exopolysaccharide gene cluster from *Streptococcus thermophilus* sfi6 into *Lactococcus lactis* MG1363: Production and characterization of an altered polysaccharide, *Mol. Microbiol.*, 32, 1287–1295, 1999.
58. Pouwels, P.H. and Leer, R.J., Genetics of lactobacilli: Plasmid and gene expression, *Antonie van Leeuwenhoek*, 64, 85–107, 1993.
59. Martinez-Cuesta, M.C., Reguena, T., and Pelaez, C., Use of bacteriocin-producing transconjugant as starter in acceleration of cheese ripening, *Int. J. Food Microbiol.*, 70, 79–88, 2001.
60. Wegman, U., Klein J.R., Drumm, I., Kuipers, O.P., and Henrich, B., Introduction of peptidase genes from *Lactobacillus delbrueckii* subsp. *lactis* into *Lactococcus lactis* and controlled expression, *Appl. Environ. Microbiol.*, 65, 4729–4733, 1999.
61. Fitzsimons, A., Hols, P., Jore, J., Leer, R.J., Oconnel, M., and Delcour, J., Development of an amylolytic *Lactobacillus plantarum* silage strain expressing the *Lactobacillus amylovorous* alpha-amylase gene, *Appl. Environ. Microbiol.*, 60, 3529–3535, 1994.
62. Cogan, T.M., Beresford, T.P., Steele, J., Broadbent, J., Shah, N.P. and Ustunol, Z., Advances in starter cultures and cultured foods, *J. Dairy Sci.*, 90, 4005–4021, 2007.
63. Coffey, A., Fitzgerald, G.F., and Ross, R.P. Biotechnology of cheese starter cultures, *The Biochemist*, 19, 20–25, 1997.
64. Beresford, T., What are the bacteriophage and what strategies should be used to avoid phage infection, in *Cheese Problems*, P.L.H. McSweeney, Ed., CRC Press, Boca Raton, FL, 2007.
65. Sybesma, W., Hugenholtz, J., de Vos, W.M., and Smid, E.J., Safe use of genetically modified lactic acid bacteria in food. Bridging the gap between consumers, green groups, and industry, *Electron. J. Biotechnol.*, 9 (4), 424–447, 2006.
66. (http://www.gmfreeireland.org/resources/documents/IRL/EPA/GMOlicensing.php#MainChanges).
67. von Wright, A. and Bruce, A., Genetically modified microorganisms and their potential effects on human health and nutrition, *Trends Food Sci.*, 14, 254–276, 2003.
68. FAO/WHO, Safety assessment of foods derived from genetically modified micro-organisms, Report of a joint FAO/WHO Expert consultation on foods derived from bio-technology, World Health Organization, Geneva, 2001. http://www.who.dk/foodsafety/Publications/mtgrpt http://www.who.int/fsf/Gmfood/index.htm
69. Nap, J.P., Metz, L.J., Escaler, M., and Conner, A.J., The release of genetically modified crops into the environment, *Plant J.*, 33, 1–18, 2003.
70. Davidson, J., Towards safer vectors for the field release of recombinant bacteria, *Environ. Biosaf. Res.*, 1, 9–18, 2002.
71. De Vos, W., Safe and sustainable systems for food-grade fermentations by genetically modified lactic acid bacteria, *Int. Dairy J.*, 9, 3–10, 1999.

72. European Commission (EU) Council Directive 90/219/EC of 23 April 1990 on the contained use of genetically modified micro-organisms.

73. European Commission (EU) Council Directive 2001/18/EC of 12 March 201 on the deliberate release into the environment of genetically modified organisms (repealing Council Directive 90/220/EC).

74. Lindgren, S., Biosafety aspects of genetically modified lactic acid bacteria in EU legislation, *Int. Dairy J.*, 9, 37–41, 1999.

75. Renault, P., Genetically modified lactic acid bacteria: Applications to food or health and risk assessment, *Biochimie*, 84, 1073–1087, 2002.

76. Cebeci, A. and Gürakan, G.C., Molecular methods for identification of *Lactobacillus delbrueckii* subsp. bulgaricus and *Streptococcus thermophilus* using methionine biosynthesis and 16S rRNA genes, *J. Dairy Res.*, 75, 392–398, 2008.

77. Amor, K. B., Vaughan E.E., and de Vos W.M., Advanced molecular tools for the identification of lactic acid bacteria, *J. Nutr.*, 137 (3), 741–747, 2007.

78. Fasoli, S., Marzotto, M., Rizzotti, L., Rossi, F., Dellaglio, F., and Torriani, S., Bacterial composition of commercial probiotic products as evaluated by PCR-DGGE analysis, *Int. J. Food Microbiol.*, 82, 59–70, 2003.

79. Walter, J., Tannock, G.W., Tilsala-Timisjarvi, A., Rodtong, S., Loach, D.M., Munro, K., and Alassatova, T., Detection and identification of gastrointestinal Lactobacillus species by using denaturing gradient gel electrophoresis and species specific primers, *Appl. Environ. Microbiol.*, 66, 297– 303, 2000.

80. Bae, J.W., Rhee, S.K., Park, J.R., Chung, W.H., Nam, Y.D., Lee, I., Kim, H., and Park, Y.H., Development and evaluation of genome-probing microarrays for monitoring lactic acid bacteria, *Appl. Environ. Microbiol.*, 71, 8825–8835, 2005.

81. Ventura, M. and Zink, R., Specific identification and molecular typing of *Lactobacillus* johnsonii by using PCR-based methods and pulse-field gel electrophoresi, *FEMS Microbiol. Lett.*, 219, 141–154, 2002.

82. Jansen, R., van Embden J.D.A., Gaastra, W., and Schouls, L.M., Identification of genes that are associated with DNA repeats in prokaryotes, *Mol. Microbiol.*, 43 (6), 1565–1575, 2002.

83. Horvath, P., Romero, D.A., Coute-Monvoisin, A., Richards, M., Deveau, H., Moineau, S., Boyaval, P., Fremaux, C., and Barrangou, R., Diversity, activity, and evolution of CRISPR loci in Streptococcus thermophilus, *J. Bacteriol.*, 190, 1401–1412, 2008.

84. Mojica, F.J.M., Diez-Villasenor, C., Soria, E., and Juez, G., Biological significance of a family of regularly spaced repeats in the genom of Archaea, Bacteria and mitochondria, *Mol. Microbiol.*, 36, 244–246, 2000.

85. Deveau, H., Barrangou, R., Garneau, J.E., Labonte, J., Fremaux, C., Boyaval, P., Romero, D.A., Horvath, P., and Moineau, S., Phage response to CRISPR-encoded Resistance in *Streptococcus thermophilus*, *J. Bacteriol.*, 190, 1390–1400, 2008.

86. Barrangou, R., Fremaux, C., Deveau, H., Richards, M., Boyaval, P., Moineau, S., Romero, D.A., and Horvath, P., CRISPR provides acquired resistance against viruses in prokaryotes, *Science*, 315, 1709–1712, 2007.

87. Shah, N.P., Functional foods from probiotics and prebiotics, *Food Technol.*, 55 (11), 46–53, 2001.

88. Greene, J.D. and Klaenhammer, T.R., Factors involved in adherence of lactobacilli to human Caco-2 cells, *Appl. Environ. Microbiol.*, 60 (12), 4478–4494, 1994.

89. Conway, P.L., Gorbach, S.L., and Golin, B.R., Survival of lactic acid bacteria in the human stomach and adhesion to intestinal cells, *J. Dairy Sci.*, 70, 1–12, 1987.

90. Mater, D.D., Bretigny, L., Firmesse, O., Flores M.J., Mogenet A., Bresson J.L., and Corthier, G., *Streptococcus thermophilus* and *Lactobacillus delbrueckii* subsp. *bulgaricus* survive gastrointestinal transit of healthy volunteers consuming yogurt, *FEMS Microbiol. Lett.*, 250, 185–187, 2005.

91. Elli, M., Callegari, L.M., Ferrari, S., Bessi, E., Cativelli, D., Soldi, S., Morelli, L., Feuillerat, N.G., and Antoine, J.M., Survival of yogurt bacteria in human gut, *Appl. Environ. Microbiol.*, 72, 7, 5113–5117, 2006.
92. Garcia-Albiach, R., Jose, M., de Flipe, P., Angulo, S., Morosini, M.I, Bravo, D., Baquero, F., and del Campo, R., Molecular analysis of yogurt containing *Lactobacillus delbruckeii* subsp. bulgaricus and *Streptococcus thermophilus* in human intestinal microbiota, *Am. J. Clin. Nutr.*, 87, 91–96, 2008.
93. Lourens-Hattingh, A. and Vilojen, B.C., Yogurt as probiotic carrier food, *Int. Dairy J.*, 11, 1–17, 2001.
94. Tammime, A.Y., Marschall, V.M.E., and Robinson, R.K., Microbiological and technological aspects of milks fermented by bifidobacteria, *J. Dairy Res.*, 62, 151–187, 1995.
95. Hussein, L., El Sayed, S., and Foda, S., Reduction of lactose in milk by purified lactase produced by *Kluyveromyces lactis*, *J Food Protect.*, 52, 30–34, 1989.

4 Ayran: Microbiology and Technology

Celalettin Koçak and Yahya Kemal Avşar

CONTENTS

4.1 INTRODUCTION

Yogurt and yogurt-like fermented dairy products are produced in almost every country in the world. They can be classified by their microflora content as well as their textural properties [1]. By textural classification, drinkable fermented dairy products have an important place and can be classified into three groups as follows [2]:

a. Viscous products
b. Diluted or beverage products
c. Carbonated products

These products can also be further grouped as those consumed fresh or those with a prolonged shelf life. Fermented milk products are very popular in many countries in Asia, in Middle East and Arab countries (with different names such as lassi, doogh, mast, and ayran), and in Scandinavian countries (such as acidophilus milk, viili, täfil, and filmjölk).

In Turkey, ayran is the most popular drinkable fermented product. According to the above given classifications, it can be placed in diluted or beverage products. It is claimed that ayran was discovered by Göktürks while on a war, where yogurt was diluted with water to reduce its sour taste [3]. Then, ayran has made its journey from Central Asia to Anatolia, Balkans, and the Middle East. However, ayran has different properties from those drinking yogurt produced in other countries for its production technique and flavor [4]. Unlike ayran, other products usually contain sugar, fruit syrup, sweeteners, aroma compounds, and colorings to attract consumers [2].

Basically, ayran is known as a fermented dairy product produced by the addition of water to yogurt. By taking its discovery and history into account, this may sound an acceptable definition. However, when ayran production in Turkey is taken into consideration, the above definition appears to be insufficient. According to Turkish Food Codex [5], ayran is defined as "drinkable fermented product prepared by the addition of water to yogurt or by the addition of yogurt culture to standardized milk." The Codex also covers the specifications for ayran's gross and microbiological composition (Table 4.1) [5]. In ayran production, table salt is used as an additive. Upon completion of fermentation, table salt is added to yogurt gel at the level of 0.5–1.0%. The yogurt gel is mixed until a homogeneous and drinkable product is obtained.

Ayran is also obtained as a by-product during traditional production of butter from yogurt. In this case, yogurt is produced, diluted with water, and churned for butter production [6]. After removal of butter, the remaining liquid part is known as *Turkish buttermilk* or *yayık ayranı* (in Turkish) [4,7,8].

To sum up, production of ayran in Turkey can be realized by two ways:

a. Homemade ayran
b. Industrially produced ayran

Homemade ayran is obtained either during the traditional production of butter or prepared by the dilution of yogurt, which is either homemade or purchased from the market. Production of butter from yogurt is a traditional way of Turkish and it is much enjoyed in the rural areas [9].

TABLE 4.1
Production Specifications for Ayran According to Turkish Food Codex

Specifications	Values
Protein (g/100 mL)	Not lower than 2.8
Titratable acidity (g lactic acid/100 mL)	Not lower than 0.6
Fat-free solid matter (g/100 mL)	Not lower than 6
Fat (g/100 mL)	Not lower than 1.8% full fat
	Not lower than 0.8% half fat
	Not higher than 0.15% fat free
Total microbial count (cfu/mL)	$>10^{-7}$
Yeast (cfu/mL)	<100
Mold (cfu/g)	<100
Coliform (cfu/mL)	<100
Escherichia coli (cfu/mL)	0

Source: Modified from Turkish Food Codex, *Communiqué on Fermented Milk*, Communication no. 2001/21, 2001, http://www.kkgm.gov.tr/TFC/2001-21.html (accessed on 8.12.2008).

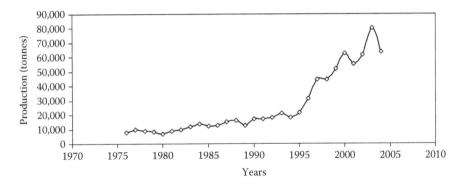

FIGURE 4.1 Consumption of ayran, carbonated beverages with fruit aroma, plain, and cola between 1970 and 2005. (From Avşar, Y.K., *Süt Dünyası, Süt Ürünleri ve Teknolojileri Dergisi*, 9, 28–29, 2007. With permission.)

Turkey produces about 10 millions tons of milk annually. Twenty-three percent of this amount is used for yogurt and ayran production [10]. It is estimated that ayran consumption in Turkey is about 1 million ton annually [11]. As ayran preparation at home is easy, a major part of this amount is estimated to be homemade ayran. Industrially produced ayran is estimated to be 15–20% of total consumption and has been increasing (Figure 4.1) [12].

Since there is no accurate statistic about ayran production and consumption, one has to be cautious with the above given figures. As a matter of fact, it is more likely that ayran production in Turkey is much higher than the given data. Ayran consumption fluctuates throughout a year. In general, its consumption in summer months is higher by 75–80% than that in winter months as it is preferred as a refreshment [10,13,14].

4.2 MICROBIOLOGY

Yogurt bacteria (*Streptococcus thermophilus* and *Lactobacillus delbrueckii* subsp. *bulgaricus*) are used in the fermentation of ayran milk. The flavor formation and textural properties are strongly dependent on the activities of these bacteria. For these reasons, selection of starter bacteria seems to be a crucial step. Some starter culture-producing companies (Christian Hansen, Denmark) have been developing new starter cultures particularly for ayran.

In ayran production, mixed strain yogurt cultures are used widely. Low-viscosity culture strains and slow fermenting starter cultures should be preferred. This can help for the production of a stable product [2]. The pH of ayran at the end of fermentation is important [15–17]. The incubation temperature and starter culture activity should be optimized as they directly affect the final pH. Özer [17] reported that fermentation of stirred-type fermented product should be terminated at pH 4.2–4.4 rather than at pH 4.7–4.8 to obtain an increased viscosity. Similarly, Özdemir and Kilic [15] showed that low pH (4.3) positively contributed to the better textural

TABLE 4.2

Effect of Incubation End pHs on the Serum Separation and Viscosity Values of Ayran Samples ($n = 3$)

	Storage Period					
	Day 1		Day 7		Day 14	
Ayran Samples	Serum Separation (mL)	Viscosity (cP)	Serum Separation (mL)	Viscosity (cP)	Serum Separation (mL)	Viscosity (cP)
G	3.2	71	18.7	69	26.2	65
H	1.8	92	11.9	99	14.8	96
K	0.0	132	1.7	131	2.5	136

Source: Tamuçay-Özünlü, B., Ayran kalitesinde etkili bazı parametreler üzerine araştırmalar, PhD thesis, Ankara University, 2005.

Notes: G: incubation end pH is 4.6, H: incubation end pH is 4.3, and K: incubation end pH is 4.0.

properties of ayran compared to those with high pH (4.6). As shown in Table 4.2, lowering the incubation end pH of the product decreased the serum separation while increasing the viscosity ($P < 0.01$) [16]. However, one should be careful that low pH (4.0) may have a negative effect on the product during storage due to postacidification or excess sourness.

Physiology of yogurt bacteria is the subject of another chapter of this book where detailed information is given (Chapter 3). It should be kept in mind that the microflora of ayran is similar to the microflora of the yogurt from which it is produced. In the case of industrially produced ayran, the composition of ayran microflora is more stable. That is, industrially produced ayran contains only the yogurt bacteria. In the case of homemade ayran, however, the risk of contamination is very high and yeasts, particularly *Kluyveromyces* and *Saccharomyces*, are often present in the final product [17,18]. In addition, the number of yogurt bacteria in ayran produced from milk is higher than that of those produced from yogurt [19].

In yogurt production, starter cultures that are capable of producing exopolysaccharides (EPS) and thus bonding water are also employed [20]. These bacteria are also known as ropy bacteria and are used in the production of drinking yogurt in order to increase the product stability [2], ayran is not an exception. However, it should be noted that not all types of EPS-producing starter cultures increase viscosity or decrease serum separation. The amount, chemical structure, and degree of interaction with milk proteins of EPS play important roles [21]. As shown in Table 4.3, some ropy starter cultures may not improve the textural properties of ayran [22]. Alternatively, EPS-producing bacteria may not give satisfactory results in ayran as they do in other fermented products such as stirred yogurts. This can be explained by the reduction in protein contents and interactions arising from dilutions, mechanical applications (pumping, etc.) after fermentation and salt addition, which reduce protein–water interactions.

TABLE 4.3

Textural Properties of Ayran Produced with Ropy and Nonropy Cultures

Culture	Consistency Coefficient (K) (mPa s^n)	Flow Behavior Index (n)	Apparent Viscosity at 50 s^{-1} (mPa s)	Thixotropy at (Pa s^{-1})	Serum Separation after 10 Days (mL/50 mL)
Nonropy	114.9	0.596	25.3	57.3	16
Ropy	58.6	0.680	18.2	34.4	17

Source: Kılıç, M., Köksoy, A., and Özdemir, Ü., in *Proc. Int. Dairy Symp.*, Z.G. Seydim, F.Y. Ekinci-Kitiş, and A.C. Seydim, Eds, Isparta Suleyman Demirel University, Isparta, pp. 191–194, 2004.

Recently, use of probiotics in ayran production is the subject of some researches [23,24]. Owing to its low pH (<4.5), pathogen bacteria like *Escherichia coli* O157:H7 did not survive in ayran for a long time. Researches showed that the number of *E. coli* O157:H7 inoculated to ayran samples at the level of 7 log cfu/mL decreased to below 1 log cfu/mL ayran within a 2-week storage period under refrigeration conditions [25,26]. Survival of *E. coli* O157:H7 is also dependent on storage temperature. At room temperature, survival of *E. coli* O157:H7 increases compared to those stored at refrigerator conditions [25].

4.3 TECHNOLOGY

As briefly mentioned earlier, ayran is traditionally produced by two methods (Figure 4.2). Homemade ayran is simply prepared by mixing water (*c.* 50%), yogurt (*c.* 50%), and salt (0.5–1.0%) (Figure 4.2a). The mixture is mixed until it has become homogeneous and drinkable. Homemade ayran is produced daily and consumed fresh. Each person prepares it for his/her desire. Ayran is not only consumed as it is, but is also used for preparation of some side dish like "cacik." Cacik is another traditional Turkish side dish prepared with ayran and chopped or grated cucumber.

Ayran is also obtained as a by-product of buttermaking called *yayık ayranı* or "Turkish buttermilk" (Figure 4.2b). Mostly, villagers produce it when they make butter out of yogurt for their home consumption. Before being churned, yogurt is diluted with water by 50% in churns. After churning, butter is removed. The remaining part is called *yayık ayranı*. In general, yogurt for butter production is kept longer than normal for extra acid development. Therefore, *yayık ayranı* has a strong sour taste. In addition, the amount of water for dilution varies, resulting in *yayık ayranı* with different viscosities. Unfortunately, butter production from yogurt in Turkey has been decreasing.

Different materials such as animal skin, wood, earth, and metal are used for traditional churns. For a skin bag churn, a goatskin or a sheepskin is used. A goat or a sheepskin is dried, kept in hot water, and hairs are removed. Following second time drying, fatty tissue is removed. The cleaned and dried skin is kept in boiling water

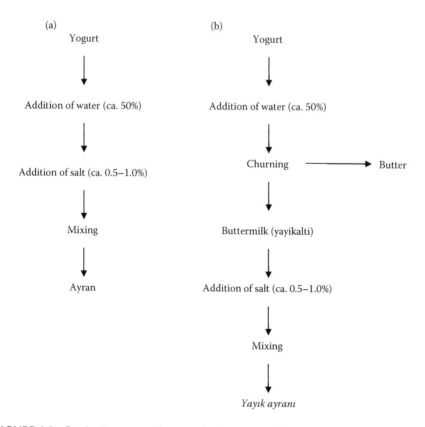

FIGURE 4.2   Production steps of homemade (a) ayran and (b) *yayık ayranı*.

containing pomegranate skins, and dried for the last time. This procedure takes about a week. Finally, the openings of the skin are tied up with threats and hung down vertically from a wooden stand with ropes (Figure 4.3a). Churning is a tedious process as it requires manpower. The skin bag churn is shaken backward and forward by a person until butter is separated from serum. In another form of skin bag, the skin is prepared as a big cloth with a big opening on the top (Figure 4.3b). It is hung vertically. A hand-operated long wooden plunger is used for mechanical agitation. In this case, the plunger is moved up and down until butter is produced.

In some regions, wooden barrel churn is used for butter and *yayık ayranı* production (Figure 4.4). Similar to skin bag ones, two types of wooden barrel churns (horizontal and vertical types) are used. A wooden plunger is used for mechanical agitation in the vertical type, whereas the horizontal type is to be shaken.

Wooden barrel churns are also engraved and painted for decorative look (Figure 4.5).

In some regions, earthenware churns are used (Figure 4.6a). In this case, half-filled churn is rolled on the ground to create a mechanical effect. In some regions, metallic churns are used (Figure 4.6b). Today, electrically driven churns have become popular for traditional butter and *yayık ayranı* production (Figure 4.6c).

(a)   (b)

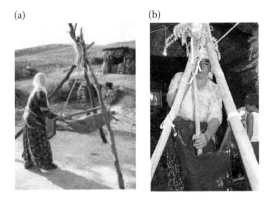

FIGURE 4.3   Skin bag churns: (a) horizontal type and (b) vertical type.

(a)   (b)

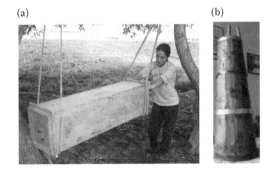

FIGURE 4.4   Wooden barrel churns: (a) horizontal type and (b) vertical type.

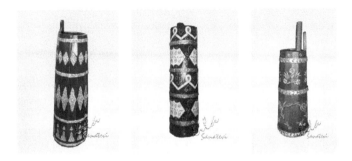

FIGURE 4.5   Painted wooden churns.

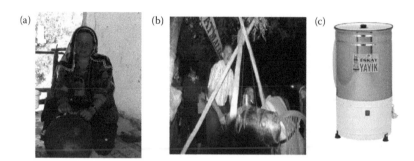

FIGURE 4.6   Different churn types: (a) earthen, (b) metallic, and (c) electrically driven.

Yayık ayran is not available at gross markets as it is not produced at the industrial scale. It is sold at local or open markets. When heated, some acid curd cheeses like Çökelek are obtained from ayran. Ayran is also used for Tarhana, a traditional Turkish dairy product containing dough, tomato paste, some herbs, and spices.

Şenel [27] reported the chemical composition of *yayık ayranı* produced from yogurt with different compositions (Table 4.4). Due to the churning and butter production, the remaining *yayık ayranı* contain a little amount of fat (<0.5% fat). The lower the pH of yogurts used for production, the lower the pH of *yayık ayranı* obtained.

Consumption of traditionally produced ayran is decreasing in contrast to increase in industrially produced ayran [11]. Owing to the changing life style, consumer preference toward fast food preference has been inclining. Not only traditional fast food restaurants that serve doner kebap, meat ball, and so on, most famous fast ones in Turkey that serve burger, pizza, and so on, have already included ayran in their

TABLE 4.4
Some Properties of *yayık ayranı*

Yayık ayranı	Total Solids (g/100 g)	Fat (g/100 g)	pH	Lactic Acid (mg/100 g)
A	5.81	0.37	4.37	0.45
B	6.17	0.30	4.27	0.50
C	6.11	0.25	3.99	0.58
D	5.83	0.33	4.03	0.51

Source: Şenel, E., Bazı üretim parametrelerinin yoğurttan üretilen yayık tereyağının nitelikleri üzerine etkisi, PhD thesis, Ankara Üniversitesi Ziraat Fakültesi Süt Teknolojisi Bölümü, Ankara, 2006.

Notes: A: produced from yogurt with 14% fat and pH 4.6, B: produced from yogurt with 7% fat and pH 4.6, C: produced from yogurt with 14% fat and pH 4.0, and D: produced from yogurt with 7% fat and pH 4.0.

standard menu. For these reasons, improvement of ayran's functional and other properties has been mentioned in the current national development plan of Turkey [28,29].

Like yogurt, ayran can be manufactured from cow's, sheep's, goat's milk, or their mixture. Mostly cow's milk is used. In an attempt to use milk from different goat breeds in ayran production, it was shown that ayran from Turkish Saanen breed had a more goaty flavor than those made from Turkish Hair and Maltese goat breeds [23]. The criteria required for raw material is similar to those for yogurt production as described elsewhere in this book.

Unfortunately, there is no standard ayran production method in Turkey. As raw material and production methods vary, ayran available in the market may be a different one from another [30–36]. Ayran manufacture at the industrial scale is realized by two methods [5]. As shown in Figure 4.7, it is produced either by the addition of water to yogurt or by the addition of starter culture to milk that is previously diluted with water and standardized for total solids and fat content. In both cases, the water to be added should be drinkable and free from contaminants. Preprocessing of raw milk (clarification and deodorization) and main processing steps (standardization for fat and nonfat total solids, homogenization, heat treatment, incubation, etc.) are very similar to those applied in yogurt processing (Figure 4.8).

Both production methods do not yield significant differences in the major composition of the final product (Table 4.5) [37]. However, acetaldehyde content of ayran produced by the dilution of yogurt was found to be lower than that of ayran produced by dilution of milk. Even during storage at 5°C, lactic acid content, pH values, viscosity values, and whey separation of ayran samples produced by two different methods underwent the same changes and no significant differences were observed at the end of the storage. Additionally, the panelists did not notice any sensory differences between ayran samples produced by different methods. One should note that the biggest change during storage was serum separation.

Some defects may occur during storage and deteriorate ayran quality. Serum separation, that is, syneresis, low viscosity, and postacidifications are the most common ones [2,34,36,38–41]. Serum separation spontaneously occurs in acid gels [42]. The reason for this phenomenon is simply the destruction of colloidal stability, which results in protein moving downward as they have a higher density than the serum phase [36,40,43]. This is also known as destruction of product stability.

There are several factors acting on serum separation, for example, total solids, protein, and fat contents, as well as heat treatment, homogenization, and acidity [33,44,45]. These factors also govern the quality of other fermented drinking products [2].

The composition and quality of raw milk have a direct effect on ayran quality. High total solids content, more importantly high protein content, is essential for better product stability in terms of serum separation. Interactions of proteins with water (hydration, adsorption, and solubility), other macromolecules (gelation), or gases (froth forming, air retaining, and whipping) are important for product stability [46]. In addition, the ratio of milk proteins (whey proteins/casein) plays an important role in prevention of serum separation. Therefore, increase in total solids particularly in protein will have a positive effect on ayran stability. For this reason, Turkish

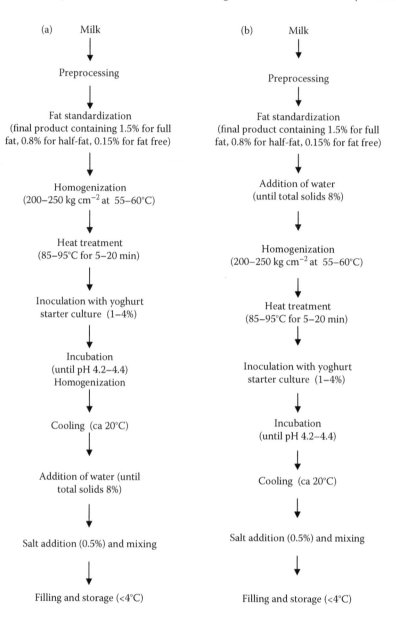

FIGURE 4.7 Industrially ayran production by the addition of water to yogurt (a) or by dilution of milk (b). (From Özer, H.B., *Yoğurt Bilimi ve Teknolojisi*, p. 488, Sidas Medya Ltd, İzmir, 2006. With permission.)

Food Codex [5] particularly emphasis on protein content and set a value that is not lower than 2.8%. As shown in Figure 4.9, increasing the water content of ayran leads to a higher serum separation during storage [34]. This is caused by the increased distance between colloidal proteins and by the decrease in concentration of colloidal particles [17].

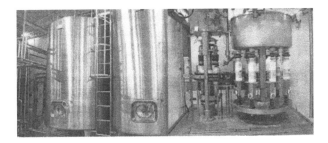

FIGURE 4.8 Industrial ayran production.

Koksoy and Kilic [14] showed that not only increased water content but also increased salt content promotes serum separation due to reduction in the viscosity of ayran (Table 4.6). Ayran has a lower viscosity and a higher acidity than their European counterparts. Therefore, it is prone to textural instability. The main textural defects in ayran are low viscosity and serum separation during separation. Serum separation is a common defect in ayran sold at retail in Turkey (Table 4.7). In addition, due to its low viscosity, ayran has a thin mouthfeel.

TABLE 4.5

Changes in Some Physico-Chemical Properties of Ayran Samples Produced by Two Different Methods During Storage at 5°C for 7 days with Statistical Evaluation ($n = 3$)[a,b]

	Day 1		Day 7	
	Method A[c]	Method B[d]	Method A	Method B
Total solids (g/100 g)	8.3 ± 0.14^A	8.3 ± 0.07^A	—	—
Fat (g/100 g)	1.6 ± 0.03^A	1.6 ± 0.03^A	—	—
Protein (g/100 g)	2.26 ± 0.02^A	2.28 ± 0.03^A	—	—
Salt (g/100 g)	0.65 ± 0.05^A	0.66 ± 0.02^A	—	—
Density (g/mL)	1.0250 ± 0.001^A	1.0255 ± 0.001^A	—	—
Lactic acid (g/100 g)	0.56 ± 0.07^B	0.56 ± 0.05^B	0.61 ± 0.04^A	0.60 ± 0.02^B
pH	4.15 ± 0.02^A	4.17 ± 0.10^A	4.05 ± 0.05^B	4.06 ± 0.02^B
Acetaldehyde (mg/kg)	10.9 ± 0.83^A	7.6 ± 0.22^C	10.8 ± 0.70^A	9.1 ± 0.51^B
Whey separation (mL/100 mL)	3.2 ± 0.63^B	2.9 ± 0.85^B	24.8 ± 3.18^A	22.0 ± 1.74^A
Viscosity (mPa s)	1.7 ± 0.05^A	1.8 ± 0.09^A	1.7 ± 0.07^A	1.9 ± 0.15^A

Source: Koçak, C., Avşar, Y.K., and Tamuçay, B., *Gıda*, 31 (4), 225–231, 2006.

[a] Mean values ± standard deviation.

[b] Means in the same row without a common superscript differ ($P < 0.05$).

[c] Method A: produced by dilution of milk.

[d] Method B: produced by dilution of yogurt.

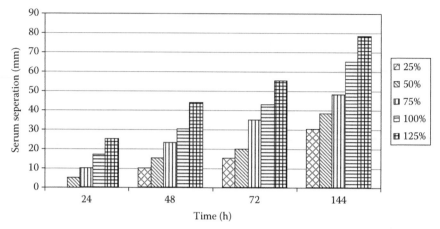

FIGURE 4.9 Serum separation of ayran samples produced from yogurt with different amounts of water addition (25%, 50%, 75%, 100%, and 125%). (From Ergüllü, E. and Demiryol, İ., *Gıda*, 8 (5), 203–208, 1983. With permission.)

To overcome both defects and generate a nice mouthfeel, different applications are employed in ayran production [2,17,36,39,40,41]. Use of different stabilizers is the most common prevention method to prevent serum separation and increase viscosity. Carboxymethyl cellulose (CMC), pectin, gelatin, carragenaan, and locust bean gum (LBG) are commonly used stabilizers. The level of use can vary from 0.3% to 1.0%, depending on stabilizer type [17]. Stabilizers can be used on their own as well as a mixture of two or more stabilizers. For example, positive results on physical stability of ayran have been reported when a mixture of CMC and carragenaan is used [40].

TABLE 4.6

Serum Separation Levels in Ayran Samples Prepared with Different Levels of Added Water and Sodium Chloride during Storage

Ayran Samples		
Added Water (g/100 g)	Added NaCl (g/100 g)	Serum Separation (mL/50 mL)[a]
30	0.0	1
30	0.5	4
30	1.0	5
50	0.0	4
50	0.5	7
50	1.0	13

Source: Koksoy, A. and Kilic, M., *Int. Dairy J.*, 13, 835–839, 2003.

[a] Volume of serum separated from 50 mL of ayran in a graduated cylinder after 15 days of storage, on an average of two replicate trials.

TABLE 4.7
Textural Properties of Ayran Sold at Retail

Sample	Consistency Coefficient (K) (mPa s^n)	Flow Behavior Index (n)	Apparent Viscosity at 55 s^{-1} (mPa s)	Thixotropy at (Pa s^{-1})	Serum Separation after 10 Days (mL/50 mL)
A	889	0.413	84.0	331	10
B	648	0.438	70.4	358	9
C	214	0.725	59.8	654	9
D	188	0.739	64.1	347	12
E	42	0.925	32.4	170	10

Source: Kılıç, M., *Süt Dünyası, Süt ürünleri ve Teknolojisi Dergisi*, 9, 30–32, 2004.

Pectin molecules interact with casein through calcium ions and prevent their aggregation, sedimentation, and hence serum separation by ionic and steric stabilization in acidic milk beverages [47]. Therefore, pectin is used to provide textural stabilization and reduce serum separation in stirred yogurts and drinking yogurts [2,48,49]. Atamer et al. [36] reported that use of pectin at the level of 0.2–0.8% in ayran could be used without causing any off-flavors.

Stabilizers can be used at the optimum level and should be added to the product at the right step. Excess and misuse of stabilizers may mask flavor and cause a sandy structure. For instance, pectin should be added to the fermented product prior to final heat treatment to prevent sedimentation and sandy mouthfeel. Pectin functions best in the pH range 3.7–4.3 [2].

Several attempts have been made to reveal the effect of different stabilizers on ayran stability [36,40,41]. Koksoy and Kilic [41] have compared the separate effects of guar gum, LBG, high-methoxyl pectin (HMP), and gelatin on textural stabilization of ayran (Tables 4.8 and 4.9). As seen from the tables, LBG has yielded the best result concerning textural stabilization and sensory properties. The researchers advised the use of LBG at the level of 0.1%. HMP and gelatin, on the other hand, were unaccepted in the sensory analysis. However, high-ester pectin is in fact one of the stabilizers most commonly used to stabilize acidified milk drink [2]. This controversial result might have arisen from the addition stage of HMP. Unlike its common uses, Koksoy and Kilic [41] added HMP after fermentation of ayran milk.

Homogenization is another important factor affecting ayran stability. It improves the mouthfeel of ayran as it does in yogurt and prevents the formation of cream layer on top of the product. In ayran, homogenization increases the water-holding capacity of milk proteins, and hence it slows down serum separation. Total homogenization of milk is applied in ayran production. The effect of homogenization is best observed when the correct homogenization temperature and pressure is chosen. As seen in Table 4.10, increasing homogenization pressure decreases serum separation while increasing the viscosity [16].

Ayran stability is also affected by the heat treatment of milk. It is well known that heat treatment results in thermal denaturation of whey proteins depending on the

TABLE 4.8

Rheological Properties and Serum Separation of Ayrans Containing Different Types of Stabilizers at Different Levels

Stabilizer (w/w %)	Consistency Coefficient (K) (mPa s[a])	Flow Behavior Index (n)	Apparent Viscosity (mPa s)	Thixotropy[b] (Pa s^{-1})	Serum Separation[c] (mL/50 mL)
No stabilizer	37	0.77	15	50	12
Guar gum					
0.10	94	0.85	48	145	2
0.25	623	0.56	125	271	0
LBG[d]					
0.10	47	0.89	31	59	2
0.25	207	0.75	74	122	0
HMP[e]					
0.25	67	0.78	27	71	6
0.50	153	0.74	50	114	3
Gelatin					
0.25	43	0.78	18	42	9
0.50	148	0.66	37	132	1

Source: Koksoy, A. and Kilic, M., *Food Hydrocoll.*, 18, 593–600, 2004.

[a] Apparent viscosity at shear rate of 55 s^{-1}.

[b] Hysteresis loop area between the upward and downward shear stress/shear rate curves.

[c] Serum separation after 15 days of storage at 4°C.

[d] Locust bean gum.

[e] High-methoxyl pectin.

temperature and time applied. At temperatures above 70°C, denaturation of whey proteins increases with increasing time period. Owing to the denaturation, whey proteins firstly interact with each other and then form a complex with casein micelles. As a result, the water-holding capacity of the proteins increases. Tamuçay-Özünlü [16] reported that heating ayran milk at 95°C for 5 min yielded the lowest serum separation and the highest viscosity values among the other treatments as shown in Table 4.11.

Use of enzymes appears to be an alternative method to improve ayran stability. In these methods, the water-holding capacity of proteins is aimed to be increased by different enzymes. Transglutaminase appears to be a promising enzyme for this purpose [17].

Ayran is a fresh product that has a limited shelf life (10–15 days). According to Turkish Food Codex [5], ayran should contain more than 10^7 cfu of yogurt bacteria per milliliter. Owing to this criterion, it is not possible to further process ayran to prolong its shelf life as any attempt may reduce the bacterial count. When permitted, heat treatments such as pasteurization and ultrahigh temperature processing together with aseptic packaging may be employed for the production of long-life ayran.

TABLE 4.9
Sensory Properties of Ayrans Containing Different Types of Stabilizers[a]

Stabilizer (w/w %)	Odor	Taste	Texture	Consistency	Overall Acceptability
No stabilizer	5.4[A]	5.0[A]	5.0[A]	3.9[A]	4.8[AB]
Guar gum					
0.10	5.1[AB]	4.8[A]	5.0[A]	5.5[B]	4.7[AB]
LBG					
0.10	4.8[AB]	4.6[A]	5.2[A]	5.1[B]	5.0[A]
HMP					
0.25	3.8[C]	3.2[B]	5.2[A]	4.4[A]	3.7[C]
Gelatin					
0.25	4.6[B]	3.8[B]	5.0[A]	4.4[A]	4.1[BC]

Source: Koksoy, A. and Kilic, M., *Food Hydrocoll.*, 18, 593–600, 2004.

[a] Means at the same column with different superscripts are different ($P < 0.05$) by Duncan's multiple comparison test. LBG, locust bean gun; HMP, high-methoxyl pectin. Hedonic scale, like extremely (7), dislike (1).

As stated earlier, plain ayran is produced in Turkey with its characteristic acidic taste unlike its counterparts in Europe and United States where colorings and flavorings are added. However, to increase its competitiveness against carbonated nonalcoholic beverages in the market, carbonated ayran has been designed and produced at the industrial scale recently. In Table 4.12, the results of Avşar et al. [50] on pressurized

TABLE 4.10
Effect of Different Homogenization Pressure on Serum Separation and Viscosity of Ayran Samples Stored at 5°C for 14 days ($n = 3$)

	Storage Period					
	Day 1		Day 7		Day 14	
Ayran Samples[a]	Serum Separation (mL/100 mL)	Viscosity (cP)	Serum Separation (mL/100 mL)	Viscosity (cP)	Serum Separation (mL/100 mL)	Viscosity (cP)
A	3.0	65	13.8	54	18.3	57
B	2.8	123	13.5	149	17.8	138
C	2.5	147	12.5	175	15.8	171

Source: Tamuçay-Özünlü, B., Ayran kalitesinde etkili bazı parametreler üzerine araştırmalar, PhD thesis, Ankara University, 2005.

[a] A, 150 kg/cm²; B, 200 kg/cm²; C, 250 kg/cm².

TABLE 4.11

Effect of Different Heat Treatments of Milk on Serum Separation and Viscosity Values of Ayran Samples ($n = 3$)

	Storage Period					
	Day 1		Day 7		Day 14	
Ayran Samples[a]	Serum Separation (mL/100 mL)	Viscosity (cP)	Serum Separation (mL/100 mL)	Viscosity (cP)	Serum Separation (mL/100 mL)	Viscosity (cP)
A	5.5	66	21.5	58	29.5	65
B	1.9	135	7.6	133	11.8	109
C	0.8	136	5.1	136	8.1	120

Source: Tamuçay-Özünlü, B., Ayran kalitesinde etkili bazı parametreler üzerine araştırmalar, PhD thesis, Ankara University, 2005.

[a] A, 75°C for 5 min; B, 85°C for 5 min; C, 95°C for 5 min.

TABLE 4.12

Effect of Pressurized CO_2 Injection at 0 (control), 0.5 (A5), 1.0 (A10), and 1.5 (A15) MPa for 1 min on the Mean Chemical Properties of Ayran Stored at 5°C for 7 Days ($n = 3$)[a]

	Control		A5		A10		A15	
Composition	Day 1	Day 7	Day 1	Day 7	Day 1	Day 7	Day 1	Day 7
Total solids (g/100 g)	8.3[A]	—	8.2[A]	—	8.3[A]	—	8.2[A]	—
Fat (g/100 g)	1.55[A]	—	1.52[A]	—	1.53[A]	—	1.53[A]	—
Density (g/mL)	1.025[A]	—	1.026[A]	—	1.026[A]	—	1.026[A]	—
Salt (g/100 g)	0.65[A]	—	0.64[A]	—	0.65[A]	—	0.64[A]	—
CO_2 (mg/100 mL)	9.9[D]	11.7[D]	71.5[C]	75.9[C]	136.7[B]	117.9[B]	183.3[A]	199[A]
PH	4.15[C]	4.05[D]	4.28[A]	4.17[C]	4.27[A,B]	4.19[B,C]	4.26[A,B]	4.19[B,C]
SH	31.9[F]	34.9[E]	35.5[E]	37.0[D,E]	39.5[C,D]	40.8[B,C]	43.4[A,B]	45.0[A]
Lactic acid (g/100 g)	0.56[A]	0.61[A]	0.55[A]	0.55[A]	0.55[A]	0.59[A]	0.56[A]	0.57[A]
Acetaldehyde (mg/kg)	10.6[A]	10.8[A]	14.3[A]	14.1[A]	11.7[A]	13.8[A]	13.2[A]	14.2[A]
Serum separation (mL/100 mL)	3.2[C]	24.8[A]	3.1[C]	14.1[B]	4.3[C]	15.2[B]	4.1[C]	27.6[A]

Source: Avşar, Y.K., Koçak, C., and Tamuçay, B., *Gıda*, 33 (1), 3–9, 2008.

[a] Means in the same row without a common superscript differ significantly ($P < 0.05$).

carbonated ayran are presented. CO_2 treatment did not change the gross composition of ayran samples. When whey separation was monitored, however, ayran samples containing *c.* 75.9 mg CO_2/kg (A5) and 117.9 mg CO_2/kg (A10) showed considerably lower whey syneresis at the end of the storage than the control samples and than that containing 199 mg CO_2/kg (A15) ($P < 0.05$). CO_2 bubbles in these samples most likely acted as a physical barrier to a certain extent, thus preventing downward movement of coagulated milk proteins, which would result in phase separation. It could also be possible that denatured milk proteins were adsorbed onto the gas/serum interface, which reduced the amount of dry matter present in the serum phase.

Currently, the reason(s) why a higher CO_2 content in A15 did not improve the serum separation further remains to be explored and accounted for. However, the results clearly indicated that the CO_2 concentration in A5 and A10 reduced whey separation by about 50%.

4.4   FINAL REMARKS

Ayran, as a refreshment, will continue to be popular in Turkey. It is more likely that ayran production at the industrial scale will continue to increase. Therefore, optimization of production parameters, selection of starter cultures, and control of incubation end pHs in order to control the textural stability appear to be crucial in ayran production. High-temperature heat treatment (95°C for 5 min) and high homogenization pressure (250 kg/cm²) are advised to obtain high viscosity and less serum separation. Improvement of hygienic quality and aseptic packaging appear to be two effective means of extending the shelf life of ayran. In addition, a production line, especially designed for the manufacture of ayran with proper and correct equipment, is also crucial for the quality of ayran.

REFERENCES

1. Robinson, R.K. and Tamime, A.Y., Microbiology of fermented milk, in *Dairy Microbiology—The Microbiology of Milk Products*, R.K. Robinson, Ed., Vol 2, 2nd edition, pp. 291–343, Elsevier Applied Science, London, 1990.
2. Nilsson, L.E., Lyck, S., and Tamime, A.Y., Production of drinking products, in *Fermented Milks*, A. Tamime, Ed., Chapter 5, Blackwell Scientific Ltd., Oxford, UK, 2006.
3. Wikipedia, Ayran, http://en.wikipedia.org/wiki/Ayran (retrieved on 8.12.2008).
4. Yaygın, H., *Yoğurt Teknolojisi*, Akdeniz University, Agric. Fac., Publication no. 75, Antalya., p. 331, 1999.
5. Turkish Food Codex, *Communiqué on Fermented Milk*, Communication no. 2001/21, 2001, http://www.kkgm.gov.tr/TFC/2001–21.html (accessed on 8.12.2008).
6. Sagdic, O., Dönmez, M., and Demirci, M., Comparison of characteristics and fatty acid profiles of traditional Turkish yayik butters produced from goats', ewes' or cows' milk, *Food Control*, 15 (6), 485–490, 2004.
7. TSI, *Terms of Milk and Milk Products*, TS 4806, Turkish Standard Institute, Ankara, 1986.
8. Sezgin, E., *Fermente Süt Ürünleri Teknolojisi*, Ankara University, Agri. Fac., Publication no. 1560, Textbook no: 513, pp. 101–136, 2001.
9. Eralp, M., *Tereyağı ve Kaymak Teknolojisi*. Ankara University, Agri. Fac., Publication no. 375, Textbook no. 133, 1969.

10. Özünlü, B., Koçak, C., and Aydemir, S., *Ayran Stabilitesini Etkileyen Faktörler*, Gıda Teknolojisi Derneği Yayın no. 35. Ankara, p. 43, 2007.

11. Anonymous, Ayran pazarı köpürüyor, *Süt Dünyası, Süt Ürünleri ve Teknolojisi Dergisi*, 9, 22, 2007a.

12. Avşar, Y.K., Gazlı Ayran Üretimi, *Süt Dünyası, Süt Ürünleri ve Teknolojileri Dergisi*, 9, 28–29, 2007.

13. Gülmez, M., Güven, A., Sezer, Ç., and Duman, B., Survival of *Escherichia coli* O157:H7, *Listeria monocytogenes* 4b and *Yersinia enterocolitica* O3 in ayran and modified kefir as pre-and postfermentation contaminant, *Vet. Med-Gech.*, 48 (5), 125–132, 2003.

14. Koksoy, A. and Kilic, M., Effects of water and salt level on rheological properties of ayran, a Turkish yoghurt drink, *Int. Dairy J.*, 13, 835–839, 2003.

15. Özdemir, H. and Kilic, M., Influence of fermentation conditions on rheological properties and serum separation of ayran, *J. Texture Stud.*, 35, 415–428, 2004.

16. Tamuçay-Özünlü, B., Ayran kalitesinde etkili bazı parametreler üzerine araştırmalar, PhD thesis, Ankara University, 2005.

17. Özer, H.B., *Yoğurt Bilimi ve Teknolojisi*, p. 488, Sidas Medya Ltd., İzmir, 2006.

18. Topal, Ş., Yoğurdun mikrobiyolojik kontrollerinde karşılaşılan yanılgılar ve sorunlar in *III. Milli Süt ve Süt Ürünleri Sempozyumu(Yoğurt)*, İstanbul, MPM yayınları no. 548, pp. 294–303, 1994.

19. Var, I., Şahan, N., Zorlugenç, B., and Yaşar, K., The effects of using different production methods and commercial cultures on the microbiological properties of ayran, in *Proc. Int. Dairy Symp.*, Z.G. Seydim, F.Y. Ekinci-Kitiş, and A.C. Seydim, Eds, Isparta Suleyman Demirel University, Isparta, p. 369, 2004.

20. De Vuys, L. and Degeest, B., Heteropolysaccharides from lactic acid bacteria, *FEMS Microbiol. Rev.*, 23, 153–177, 1999.

21. Kılıç, M., Ayranın üretim teknolojisi ve yapısal kalitesinin sağlanması. *Süt Dünyası, Süt ürünleri ve Teknolojisi Dergisi*, 9, 30–32, 2004.

22. Kılıç, M., Köksoy, A., and Özdemir, Ü., Factors affecting textural properties of ayran, in *Proc. Int. Dairy Symp.*, Z.G. Seydim, F.Y. Ekinci-Kitiş, and A.C. Seydim, Eds, Isparta Suleyman Demirel University, Isparta, pp. 191–194, 2004.

23. Uysal-Pala, C., Karagul-Yuceer, Y., Pala, A., and Savas, T., Sensory properties of drinkable yoghurt made from milk of different goat breeds, *J. Sens. Stud.*, 21, 520–533, 2006.

24. Tonguç, İ.E., Probiyotik ayran üretimi üzerinde bir araştırma, PhD thesis, Ege University, 2006.

25. Akdemir-Evrendilek, G., Avşar, Y.K., and Karagül-Yüceer, Y., Survival of *Escherichia coli* O157:H7 in different types yoghurt products, in *Proc. Int. Dairy Symp.*, Z.G. Seydim, F.Y. Ekinci-Kitiş, and A.C. Seydim, Eds, Isparta Suleyman Demirel University, Isparta, p. 365, 2004.

26. Simsek, B., Sagdic, O., and Ozcelik, S., Survival of *Escherichia coli* O157:H7 during storage of Ayran produced with different species, *J. Food Eng.*, 78, 676–680, 2007.

27. Şenel, E., Bazı üretim parametrelerinin yoğurttan üretilen yayık tereyağının nitelikleri üzerine etkisi, PhD thesis, Ankara University, Ankara, 2006.

28. Anonymous, *Sekizinci Beş Yıllık Kalkınma Planı Özel İhtisas Komisyonu Raporu, Süt ve Süt Ürünleri Sanayii Alt Komisyonu Rapor*, Devlet Planlama Teşkilatı, Ankara, p.75, 2001.

29. Anonymous, *Dokuzuncu Kalkınma Planı, Gıda Sanayi Özel İhtisas Komisyonu Raporu*, Devlet Planlama Teşkilatı, Ankara, p. 94s, 2007b.

30. Uraz, D. and Aksoy, E., *Ayran*, Çayır Mer'a ve Zootekni Araştırma Enstitüsü, Yayın no. 52, Ankara, 1975.

31. Yaygın, H., Ayranın özellikleri üzerine bir araştırma, *Ege Üni. Zir. Fak. Der. Rauf Cemil Adam Özel sayısı*, 27–32, 1979.

32. Duru, S. and Özgüneş, H., Ankara piyasasında satılan ayran ve yoğurt örneklerinin hijyenik kaliteleri üzerinde araştırmalar, *Gıda*, 6 (4) 19–23, 1982.
33. Yaygın, H. and Gahun, Y., Değişik kaynaklı yoğurtlardan yapılan ayranların bazı özellikleri üzerinde bir araştırma. *Ege Uni. Zir. Fak. Der.*, 20 (3), 83–90, 1983.
34. Ergüllü, E. and Demiryol, İ., Yoğurda değişik oranlarda su katılarak yapılan ayranların bazı özellikleri üzerine araştırma, *Gıda*, 8 (5) 203–208, 1983.
35. Akın, N. and Rice, P., Main yoghurt and related products in Turkey, *Cult. Dairy Prod. J.*, 29 (3), 23–29, 1994.
36. Atamer, M., Gürsel, A., Tamuçay, B., Gençer, N., Yıldırım, G., Odabaşı, S., Karademir, E., Şenel, E., and Kırdar, S., Dayanıklı ayran üretiminde pektin kullanım olanakları üzerine bir araştırma, *Gıda*, 24 (2) 119–126, 1999.
37. Koçak, C., Avşar, Y.K., and Tamuçay, B., A comparative study on the production methods of ayran, *Gıda*, 31 (4), 225–231, 2006.
38. Demir, S., Ankara piyasasındaki ayranların genel nitelikleri üzerine araştırma, Bitirme ödevi, Ankara Üniversity, Agricul. Fac., Dept. Dairy Technol., 1983.
39. Gülümser, N., Karboksimetilselüloz ile ayranın dayanıklı hale getirilmesi üzerine araştırmalar, MSc thesis, Ege University, İzmir, 1986.
40. Şimşek, O., Ayran yapımında farklı stabilizatör kullanımı ve etkileri, Trakya Üniversity, Tekirdağ Ziraat Fak. Yayın no. 229, Tekirdağ, 1995.
41. Koksoy, A. and Kilic, M., Use of hydrocolloids in textural stabilization of a yogurt drink, ayran, *Food Hydrocoll.*, 18, 593–600, 2004.
42. Lucey, A.J., The relationship between rheological parameters and whey separation in milk gels, *Food Hydrocoll.*, 15, 603–608, 2001.
43. Bodyfelt, F.W., Tobias, J., and Trout, G.M., *The Sensory Evaluation of Dairy Products*, Van Nostrand Reinhold, New York, p. 598, 1988.
44. Rasic, J.L.J. and Kurmann, J.A., *Yoghurt*, Vol. I. Technical Dairy Publishing House, Copenhagen, Denmark, p. 427, 1978.
45. Gönç, S., Akbulut, N., Kınık, Ö., and Kılıç, S., Bazı kimyasal koruyucu katkı maddelerinin ayranın dayanıklılığına etkisi üzerine bir araştırma, *Ege Üni. Ziraat Fak. Der.*, 26 (2) 195–206, 1989.
46. Koçak, C. and Aydemir, S., *Süt Proteinlerinin Fonksiyonel Özellikleri*, Gıda Tek. Derneği, Yayın no. 20, Ankara, 1994, 465.
47. Lucey, A.J., Tamehana, M., Singh, H., and Munro, P.A., Stability of model acid milk beverage: effect of pectin concentration, storage temperature and milk heat treatment, *J. Texture Stud.*, 30 (3), 305–318, 1999.
48. Foley, J. and Mulcahy, A.J., Hydrocolloid stabilization and heat treatment for prolonging shelf life of drinking yoghurt and cultured buttermilk. *Irish J. Food Sci. Technol.*, 13 (1), 43–50, 1989.
49. Başak, S. and Ramaswamy, H.S., Simultaneous evaluation of shear rate and time dependency of stirred yoghurt rheology as influenced by added pectin and strawberry concentrate, *J. Food Eng.*, 21 (3), 385–393, 1994.
50. Avşar, Y.K., Koçak, C., and Tamuçay, B., Effect of pressurized carbon dioxide on the quality criteria of ayran, *Gıda*, 33 (1), 3–9, 2008.

5 Kefir and Koumiss: Microbiology and Technology

*Zeynep Guzel-Seydim, Tuğba Kök-Taş,
and Annel K. Greene*

CONTENTS

5.1 KEFIR

5.1.1 HISTORY AND DESCRIPTION OF KEFIR AND KEFIR GRAINS

Kefir is a traditional fermented dairy product originating from the tribes of the Northern Caucasus mountain region in Russia, located between the Black Sea and the Caspian Sea. For many decades, the longevity of the Caucasian people has been attributed to the high consumption of fermented dairy products, especially kefir.

There is no known record concerning the time of origin of the first kefir grains or first kefir product. Historically, kefir was made in sheep skin bags by continuous fermentation under uncontrolled conditions. Fresh milk was added as fermented milk was removed [1,2]. Kefir can be produced from cow's milk, sheep's milk, or goat's milk and also there are studies on kefir made from soymilk.

Kefir contains a diverse range of inherent microorganisms. Kefir is a self-carbonated refreshing fermented milk drink that has a unique flavor due to a mixture of lactic acid, acetaldehyde, acetoin, slight alcohol, and other fermented flavor products. It is produced by fermentative activity of "kefir grains" added to milk. Kefir grains are small, cauliflower-shaped, semihard granules that contain a specific balance of bacterial and yeast microorganisms existing in a complex symbiotic relationship (Figure 5.1). When kefir grains are added to milk, microorganisms are shed from the grains. These organisms continue to proliferate with the production of the acid and other flavor compounds causing physicochemical changes. New kefir grains grow from preexisting grains during the process of kefir fermentation [3,4].

More than two decades ago, Kemp [5] described kefir as the "champagne" of cultured dairy products, and suggested that kefir might be an alternative drink to soft drinks. However, unlike yogurt, kefir consumption has been slow to spread through Europe and the rest of the world. In the past decade, the number of published research studies on kefir has increased along with a slow increase in industrial kefir production. Flavored and unflavored kefir products are on the shelves in the markets in Europe and United States [6].

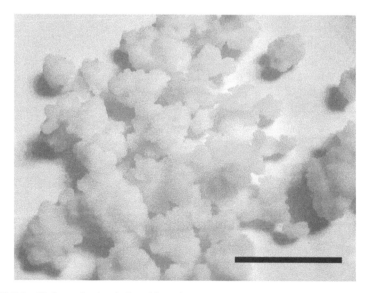

FIGURE 5.1   Kefir grains (scale bar: 15 mm).

5.1.2 PRODUCTION

Fermented dairy products have been classified into three groups based on the metabolites produced [7]:

1. Lactic fermentation
2. Yeast-lactic fermentation
3. Mold-lactic fermentation

Yogurt and buttermilk are grouped in the first category as solely lactic acid fermentations, whereas kefir and koumiss are listed in the second category as a combination of eukaryotic and prokaryotic fermentations [7].

To make authentic kefir, kefir grains are added to previously pasteurized and cooled milk and incubated with stirring for approximately 24 h at 25°C. Upon completion of fermentation, agitation of the kefir curd will cause the kefir grains to float due to the effect of carbon dioxide. A unique feature of authentic kefir that differs from other fermented milk products is that kefir grains are recovered after fermentation for future use in subsequent kefir fermentations [3]. Some authors have claimed that it is necessary to use kefir grains in order to manufacture authentic kefir [8,9]. However, industrial production of kefir using kefir grains is difficult due to postfermentation separation requirements. As a result, much of the kefir produced in industrial practice is not considered authentic kefir because it is not incubated with the grains. These same researchers indicate that the kefir generated by incubation of milk with kefir grains cannot be used as the starter culture for a subsequent batch of kefir [8,9]. However, unpublished results obtained in our laboratory indicate that upon removal of the grains, the resultant kefir can be used as kefir starter culture for the production of kefir [10]. Using this method, the microbial population, especially the number of yeast cells, is slightly decreased but the product manufactured from this technique is acceptable. An advantage of this method is that reduced yeast populations may limit the amount of swelling in the final packages.

Much of the commercial production of kefir involves use of lyophilized starter cultures containing lactic acid bacteria (LAB) and yeast. Using this method, activated starter culture is added to homogenized and pasteurized milk containing 2–5% milk fat (Figure 5.2). After fermentation at 25°C for 20–24 h, the product is stored at refrigeration temperatures. The pH gradually drops to 4.6 and fermentation is completed in approximately 20–24 h, which gives sufficient time for the formation of taste and aroma substances when an inoculation rate of 2–5% kefir culture is used [8,10].

Due to the different production techniques utilized, resultant kefir products are varied. To our knowledge no universal standards for the product exist. In order to guarantee a consistent and authentic product, it is important to define standards for the microbially complex kefir product.

5.1.3 KEFIR CHEMISTRY

The typical final kefir product has lactic acid, ethanol, carbon dioxide, and other flavor products such as acetaldehyde, diacetyl, and acetoin [11]. In the scientific

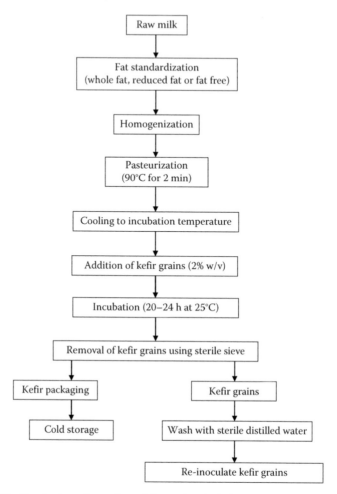

FIGURE 5.2 Production scheme for making authentic kefir.

literature, reports of ethanol content of kefir vary widely: 0.12–0.18% [12], 0.17% [13], 0.035–2% [14–16], and 0.17–0.25% [8,17].

The refreshing taste of traditional kefir has been attributed to the combined yeast and lactic acid fermentation. However, due to the production of carbon dioxide by the yeast, package swelling can occur. To avoid this problem, some companies use starter cultures that lack the yeast flora. However, the flavor of kefir is altered from that of authentic kefir due to lack of alcohol fermentation and little to no production of carbon dioxide. Fontán et al. [18] determined the microbiological and biochemical parameters that occur during fermentation of kefir over a long incubation period (168 h) using a commercial kefir starter culture. The researchers noted that during the first 24 h of incubation, *Lactococcus* spp. were the most abundant strain, but thereafter, *Lactobacillus* spp. predominated. No *Leuconostoc* strains were detected throughout the fermentation period and although yeast counts increased after 48 h of incubation, mean yeast populations were lower than reported by other studies [18].

The microbial quality of kefir grains, the grain to milk ratio, incubation time and temperature, sanitation during handling of kefir grains, and cold storage drastically affect the product quality. All these factors also influence the subsequent microflora of the kefir grains. In the scientific literature, a wide range of grain to milk ratios has been reported: 1 g/L [19], 20–50 g/L [13,20–22], and 50–100 g/L [23,24]. Garrote et al. [25] investigated the effects of different kefir grain to milk ratios on the quality characteristics of the final product. Using kefir grains obtained from private households in Argentina, milk was fermented with different amounts of kefir grains at 20°C for 48 h. The kefir grain to milk ratios used in this study were as follows: 1, 10, 20, 50, and 100 g/L. Results indicated that pH, viscosity, microflora, and carbon dioxide content of the final fermented milk were affected by the different ratios of grains to milk. When the highest ratio was used (100 g/L), a rapid rate of acidification and a large decline in lactococci content were reported.

Irigoyen et al. [26] investigated the importance of inoculation rate of kefir grain. In this study, 1% and 5% ratios (w/w) were used and fermentation proceeded at 25°C for 24 h. Interestingly, pH values and microbial content of kefir samples did not change significantly between the two inoculation ratios. The *Lactobacilli* to *Lactococci* to yeast to acetic acid bacteria ratio was $10^8 : 10^8 : 10^5 : 10^6$ cfu/mL, respectively. During storage there was no significant difference in microbial composition with the exception of the lactic acid bacterial count, which was reduced by almost 2 log. Viscosity values of kefir gradually decreased from 425 to 188 mPa for samples made with 1% kefir grain and from 501 to 357 mPa for samples made with 5% kefir grain.

Kuo and Lin [17] investigated the effect of incubation temperature and the amount of kefir grain addition on weight gain of Taiwanese kefir grains. It was noted that the rate of kefir grain weight increase was reduced when the inoculation amount was greater. The highest rate of kefir grain weight gain occurred with the lowest inoculation rate (1%), and conversely, the lowest weight gain rate occurred with the maximum inoculation rate (10%).

Guzel-Seydim et al. [15,16] determined the content of organic acids and flavor substances of kefir during fermentation and over 21 days of cold storage. The concentration of lactic acid slowly increased during the first 10 h of fermentation, and then rapidly increased from 590 to 3700 μg/g between 10 and 15 h of fermentation. Results indicated that kefir had lower lactic acid content than yogurt, which typically has 8760 μg/g lactic acid [27] and 14,550 μg/g lactic acid [28]. Guzel-Seydim [15,16] noted that acetaldehyde was first detected for 10 h and increased significantly until after 15 h of fermentation. The average final concentration of acetaldehyde was 5 μg/g, whereas plain yogurt was reported to have acetaldehyde content ranging from 23 to 41 μg/g [29]. This may be due to the preferential use of a heterofermentative pathway with a resultant production of carbon dioxide. Studies in other laboratories on yogurt revealed that acetaldehyde can be converted to ethanol by alcohol dehydrogenase [30]. This activity may explain the lower amount of acetaldehyde observed in kefir samples versus yogurt samples. Guzel-Seydim et al. [15,16] noted that acetaldehyde content increased throughout the storage process and kefir samples contained an average of 11 µg/g acetaldehyde at day 21. However, acetoin content decreased from 25 µg/g at day 1 to 16 µg/g at day 21. Rea et al. [19] detected lactate, ethanol, acetate, and acetoin as major metabolites in kefir from Irish grains. Kefir made directly from kefir grains and kefir made from a mother culture generated from culture of kefir grains, both had approximately the same amount (8.2 g/L) of lactic acid [8].

Abraham and Antoni [31] investigated the growth of Argentinean kefir grains in soymilk. Kefir grains were collected from four different households in Argentina. Grains were inoculated at a rate of 1% in soymilk and incubated at 20°C for 48 h. This incubation time was longer than that commonly reported in the literature for kefir grains in cow's milk. The researchers analyzed the microbial composition of soy cultured grains and compared the results with kefir grains grown in cow's milk. The concentration of viable bacteria and yeast in kefir grains, grain composition (water, sugar, and protein content), and protein pattern of kefir grains were determined. Their results indicated that kefir grains were able to ferment soymilk. After 48 h of incubation, pH values of 5.3, 4.9, 4.7, and 4.2 were achieved for the four different kefir grain sources. Chemical and microbiological compositions of kefir grains were different after 20 subcultures in cow's milk versus soymilk. Water and protein concentrations were higher in soymilk, whereas the polysaccharide content of grains was higher after growth in cow's milk. While there was no significant difference between amounts of *Lactobacilli* and *Lactococci* in kefir grains, kefir grains grown in soymilk had higher yeast content. The overall protein profiles of kefir grains had very slight differences. Researchers concluded that soymilk could be used for fermentation of kefir grains instead of cow's milk. Soymilk does not contain cholesterol, has low saturated fatty acid content, and contains important phenolic substances such as genistein, which have been proved to be anticarcinogenic. Therefore soymilk has significant potential as an alternative starting product in the production of a kefir-like product. Since both ethanol and lactic acid content were lower in soymilk-derived kefir, glucose (1%) was added to soymilk. The glucose positively affected LAB and yeast growth and consequently increased the concentration of lactic acid and ethanol to levels similar to cow's milk kefir control samples [32]. Kefir made from soymilk had a lower viscosity than control kefir, and kefir grains grown in soymilk were smaller than bovine milk cultured kefir grains.

Kefir grains were used to experimentally manufacture whey-based fermented beverages [33,34]. Paraskevopoulou et al. [35] successfully used kefir grains to produce single cell protein through aerobic culture of whey. The resultant single cell protein had properties similar to soyflour. Tratnik et al. [34] prepared kefir using goat's milk and cow's milk supplemented with 2% inulin, skimmed milk powder, and whey protein concentrate. They reported that kefir supplemented with whey protein powder had increased viscosity due to interaction of hydrophilic groups of proteins and water. Kefir made from goat's milk had significantly lower viscosities and lower sensory scores regardless of the supplementation [34].

In a study by Assadi [36], different ratios of previously identified LAB (*Lactobacillus kefir*, *Lactobacillus brevis*, *Lactobacillus casei*, *Lactobacillus plantarum*, *Streptococcus lactis*, and *Leuconostoc mesenteroides*), acetic acid bacteria (*Acetobacter aceti*), and yeast (*Candida kefir* and *Saccharomyces lactis*) were used to ferment whey to produce a fermented whey beverage. The resultant fermented whey beverage made with 2.5% (v/v) LAB, 0.5% (v/v) acetic acid bacteria, and 2% (v/v) yeast had a pleasant refreshing taste.

It was determined that an exopolysaccharide produced by a strain of *Lactobacillus kefiranofaciens* had a better emulsifying capability than xanthan gum, guar gum, and locust gum [37].

Yuksekdag et al. [38,39] identified 11 strains of *Lactococcus cremoris*, 4 strains of *Lactococcus lactis*, 3 strains of *Streptococcus thermophilus*, and 3 strains of *Streptococcus durans* from Turkish kefir grains. These strains produced lactic acid and acetaldehyde levels of 2.3–9.9 mg/mL and 0.18–3.96 µg/mL, respectively. The isolated strains did not produce diacetyl.

Kuo and Lin [17] compared the chemical and microbial composition of Taiwanese kefir versus raw milk. No difference in the ash and crude protein content was noted in kefir versus raw milk. However, the amount of lactose in kefir samples was 20–30% lower than in the raw milk since, in kefir, the lactose was converted to lactic acid. A reduction in the kefir pH was observed. Ethanol production in Taiwanese kefir samples varied from 0.01% to 0.25%. *Lactobacilli* and *Streptococci* populations were more prevalent than the yeast in Taiwanese kefir grains.

Guzel-Seydim et al. [40] determined the fatty acid profiles of milk, yogurt, and kefir. A two-step methylation method followed by gas chromatography was used to identify conjugated linoleic acids (CLAs). Fermentation slightly affected fatty acid composition.

5.1.4 Kefir Microbiology

The metabolic activity of a variety of LAB and yeast imparts a unique flavor to kefir. The most frequently reported bacterial genera in kefir grains are homofermentative and heterofermentative *Lactobacillus*, *Lactococcus*, *Leuconostoc*, and acetic acid bacteria [8,19,38,39,41–46]. Species that have been identified include *Lactobacillus brevis* [23,45], *Lactobacillus viridescens*, *Lactobacillus gasseri*, *Lactobacillus fermentum*, *Lactobacillus casei* [45], *Lactobacillus kefir* [23,45,47], *Lactobacillus acidophilus* [45,48], *Leuconostoc* [49], *Lactobacillus kefiranofaciens* [42,50,51], *Lactobacillus kefirgranum*, and *Lactobacillus parakefir* [52]. Garrote et al. [53] identified *Lactobacillus plantarum*, *Lactobacillus lactis* subsp. *lactis*, *Leuconostoc mesenteroides*, *Saccharomyces*, *Acetobacter*, *Lactobacillus parakefir*, *Kluyveromyces marxianus*, and *Lactobacillus lactis* subsp. *lactis* biovar. *diacetylactis* in Argentinean kefir grains.

Four strains of *Lactobacillus kefiranofaciens* were isolated and identified in kefir grains by Fujisawa et al. [54]. *Lactobacillus kefiranofaciens* is a homofermentative, rod-shaped, and slime-forming lactic acid bacterium that is different from other homofermentative species of the genus *Lactobacillus* in pattern of carbohydrate fermentation. Vancanneyt et al. [55] reported that *Lactobacillus kefirgranum* should be reclassified as *Lactobacillus kefiranofaciens* subsp. *kefirgranum* subsp. nov., because the organisms had the same 16S rDNA sequence. Santos et al. [46] identified 19 strains of *Lactobacillus kefir*, 11 strains of *Lactobacillus brevis*, 8 strains of *Lactobacillus paracasei*, 5 strains of *Lactobacillus plantarum*, 6 strains of *Lactobacillus acidophilus*, and 4 strains of *Lactobacillus kefiranofaciens*.

Several researchers have used polymerase chain reaction denaturing gradient gel electrophoresis (PCR-DGGE)-based applications including fingerprinting to determine microbial flora in kefir grains [56–58].

Lin et al. [59] identified and characterized LAB and yeasts isolated from Taiwanese kefir grains. They isolated *Lactobacillus helveticus* and *Leuconostoc mesenteroides*, and yeasts identified as *Kluyveromyces marxianus* and *Pichia fermentans*. They then inoculated those bacteria and yeast individually into skim milk and incubated at 30°C. *Lactobacillus helveticus* had the fastest growth rate with a generation time of 94 min, followed by 210 min for *Kluyveromyces marxianus*, 241 min for *Leuconostoc mesenteroides*, and 300 min for *Pichia fermentans*. *Kluyveromyces marxianus* produced more L-lactic acid than the other species. The D-form of lactic acid was produced by leuconostocs. Both isomers of lactic acid were produced by *Lactobacillus helveticus*. *Kluyveromyces marxianus* produced the highest ethanol production at the end of the incubation.

The yeasts isolated from kefir include *Saccharomyces cerevisiae* [45,60], *Candida kefir*, the imperfect form of *Kluyveromyces lactis* [45,48,61], *Saccharomyces delbruecki* [49,61], *Torulopsis holmii* [62], *Candida holmii* and *Saccharomyces unisporus* [45,61], *Kluyveromyces marxianus* [60], *Torulospora delbrueckii*, *Candida friedricchi* [45], and *Pichia fermentans* [60]. Latorre-Garcia et al. [57] isolated yeast colonies from 10 different homemade and commercial kefir samples. Using DNA purification, PCR amplification, and sequence analysis, it was revealed that the most prevalent yeast species were *Kluyveromyces lactis*, *Issatchenkia orientalis*, *Saccharomyces unisporus*, *Saccharomyces exiguus*, and *Saccharomyces humaticus*. Wang et al. [58] reported that *Kluyveromyces marxianus*, *Saccharomyces turicensis*, and *Pichia fermentans* were isolated and identified using a combination of classic microbiological and PCR methods in Taiwanese kefir grains.

Vedamuthu [63] reported that a symbiotic relationship between LAB and yeast existed in the kefir grains. Koroleva [64] stated that "yeast exert a favorable effect on the activity of the LAB providing them with growth stimulants as well as by metabolizing some of the lactic acid."

Kroger [22] reported that European kefir contained 3×10^5 yeast cfu/mL, 10^8–10^{10} cfu/mL streptococci, 10^5 cfu/mL thermophilic lactobacilli, and 10^2–10^3 cfu/mL mesophilic lactobacilli. In a study by Rea et al. [19], the microbial composition of Irish kefir grains was reported to consist of lactococci (10^9/mL), leuconostocs (10^8/mL), lactobacilli (10^6/mL), acetic acid bacteria (10^5/mL), and yeasts (10^6/mL); in this study, the reported concentration of lactobacilli was lower than reports in the literature for other kefir grains. The numbers of LAB and yeast in South African kefir grains were 10^4–10^8 and 10^5–10^8 g/cfu, respectively [65], and lactobacilli were reported as the most prevalent bacteria in the kefir grain microbial population [66]. Guzel-Seydim et al. [67] reported that the lactococci population in the final product reached 8.64 log cfu/mL by the end of the fermentation. Kefir yeast populations increased significantly throughout the fermentation period from 4.21 log cfu/mL in first 5 h of fermentation to 6.16 log cfu/mL at the end of the fermentation. After 1 day cold storage, LAB and yeast contents were measured as 9.19 and 6.55 log cfu/mL, respectively.

In a number of studies, the microbial composition of various kefir grains was investigated using scanning electron microscopy (SEM). Studies indicated that the interior versus exterior portions of the kefir grain are not uniform in ratios of lactobacilli to yeast, and lactococci have not been generally observed [19,67–69]. Bottazzi and Bianchi [20] used SEM to observe the microorganisms of kefir grains and noted a "spongy fibrillar structure with a reticular lamellar matrix and a fiber mass which, especially in the center of the grain, shows branching and interconnections with long cordons." Marshall et al. [23] also observed "sheet like structures and scroll like forms" in the composition of kefir grains using transmission electron microscopy (TEM) and SEM. Toba et al. [69] used SEM to observe propagable and nonpropagable kefir grains (Chr. Hansen's). The distribution of microorganisms and especially encapsulated bacteria was analyzed in kefir grains. According to their results, long and short lactobacilli and yeast formed separate colonies on the surface of grains. Lactobacilli and yeast colonized separately in a spongy matrix on the inside part of propagable grains, and in this part, lactobacilli had filamentous appendages that implied that encapsulated bacteria were located in the center of the grains. Rea et al. [19] noted that long, short, and curved lactobacilli and yeast were present in all samples. Curved rods were found only in the interior section, whereas lactococci were observed on the surface. Lactococci occurred in pairs and chains only on the surface of one sample. Rea et al. [19] concluded that lactococci were very lightly bound to the kefir grain during growth, and were washed off the grains during sample preparation. Other researchers did not report lactococci present in observations of kefir grains. Lin et al. [59] also used SEM and determined that the outer surface of kefir grains was almost entirely covered with long, rod-shaped bacteria. Yeast colonization was mainly observed on the surface area in close relation to the LAB. Arihara et al. [70] studied the distribution of *Lactobacillus kefiranofaciens* and *Lactobacillus kefir* by applying immunofluorescent staining. Results revealed that *Lactobacillus kefiranofaciens* was dispersed throughout the grain, but *Lactobacillus kefir* was located only in the surface layers. In a study by Guzel-Seydim et al. [67], lactobacilli were observed embedded throughout Turkish kefir grains. The microflora of kefir grains were in a matrix of a fibrillar material (Figures 5.3 through 5.6). The amount of yeast increased toward the center of the grains.

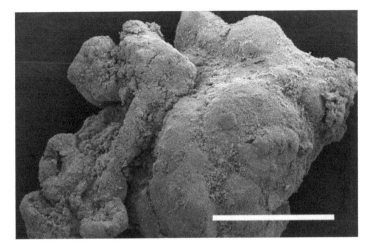

FIGURE 5.3 Scanning electron micrograph of Turkish kefir grain (45 × magnification; scale bar: 1 mm).

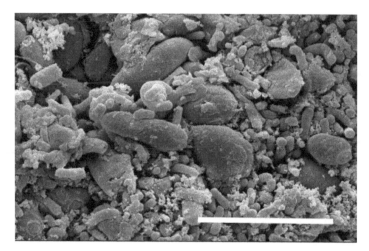

FIGURE 5.4   Scanning electron micrograph of Turkish kefir grain (5000 × magnification; scale bar: 10 μm).

Kefir cultures have been used experimentally as starter cultures for cheese manufacture. Katechaki et al. [71] used freeze-dried kefir culture and freeze-dried kefir immobilized on casein in the manufacture of hard-type cheese. Use of the kefir culture resulted in open cheese texture due to carbon dioxide generation. Sensory results indicated that use of 1 g/L freeze-dried kefir culture had better texture, color, and flavor than the control [71]. Cheese made with kefir culture had higher populations of total aerobic bacteria, yeast, lactococci, and lactobacilli than control cheese. Forty-seven flavor substances were identified. Kefir culture cheese had higher levels of flavor compounds and free fatty acids, benzaldehyde and butanal were significantly

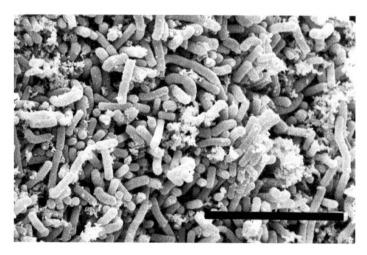

FIGURE 5.5   Scanning electron micrograph of Turkish kefir grain (5000 × magnification; scale bar: 10 μm).

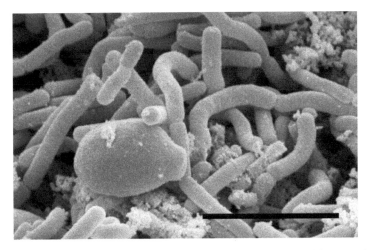

FIGURE 5.6   Scanning electron micrograph of Turkish kefir grain (10,000 × magnification; scale bar: 5 μm).

higher in kefir cheeses. Kourkoutas et al. [72] determined that kefir coculture suppressed spoilage and pathogenic bacteria during ripening of white soft cheese as well as provided good flavor due to increased amounts of esters, free fatty acids, alcohols, and carbonyl compounds.

5.1.5   KEFIRAN

In the kefir grain, LAB, yeast, and sometimes acetic acid bacteria are trapped in a complex matrix. This matrix comprises a polysaccharide known as kefiran, bound water, denatured proteins and a small amount of fat.

The exopolysaccharide in kefir was first named "kefiran" by La Riviere et al. [73]. It is a heteropolysaccharide, composed of equal amounts of glucose and galactose [74]. Early kefir investigators suggested that kefiran was produced by *Lactobacillus kefir* [47], *Streptococcus mutans* [75], *Leuconostoc mesenteroides*, and/or *Streptococcus cremoris* [76–78] since all are capable of producing extracellular polysaccharides. More recent investigations suggest that *Lactobacillus kefiranofaciens* is the major producer of the exopolysaccharide matrix of the kefir grain [46,54].

Food textural properties are very important due to the effect on consumer acceptation. Exopolysaccharides produced by food-grade LAB are of interest to food processors for use as thickening agents in dairy products. Kefiran can be used as a food-grade functional additive for fermented dairy products since it enhances rheological properties [79]. Piermaria et al. [80] obtained high-purity, 107 Da molecular weight kefiran consisting of glucose and galactose. The intrinsic viscosity of kefiran was lower than locust bean gum and guar gum but was higher than the intrinsic viscosity of some dextrans [80]. It was also reported that Newtonian behavior was observed at concentrations below 1 g/L, while a pseudoplastic or shear thinning flow was noted at higher concentrations.

Since kefiran has commercial potential, Maeda et al. [81] investigated the use of a new rice hydrolysate medium to cultivate *Lactobacillus kefiranofaciens* for the production of exopolysaccharide on the industrial scale. The medium used contained rice starch hydrolysate as a carbon source and rice protein hydrolysate as a nitrogen source. The project was successful in generating kefiran using this medium. The resultant kefiran was reported to be identical to kefiran produced by microbial growth on PYG10 medium.

Rimada and Abraham [79] reported that concentrations of exopolysaccharides released into milk or whey were 218 and 247 mg/L, respectively. Kefiran improved the rheological properties of gels made from skim milk directly acidified with glucono-δ-lactone (GDL). The apparent viscosity, elastic modulus, and viscous modulus of milk gels in which kefiran extracts were used were higher than those of gels without kefiran addition [79].

In a study by Piermaria et al. [80], kefiran isolated and purified from kefir grains was successfully used in the production of transparent edible film along with application of glycerol.

5.1.6   KEFIR GRAIN GENERATION

The microorganisms in kefir grains are reactivated by successive incubations in pasteurized or reconstituted milk. During fermentation, the soft kefir grains grow slowly from preexisting kefir grains and new biomass is added slowly. After fermentation in milk, kefir grains are recovered from milk for subsequent inoculation into additional milk.

An important limitation in industrial kefir production is the slow kefir grain growth. Schoevers and Britz [82] conducted a study on the factors that affect kefir grain proliferation. Parameters such as incubation temperature (18, 22, 25, and 30°C), culture medium enrichment with tryptose (20 g/L), and/or yeast extract (20 g/L), as well as cultivation with or without agitation were studied. The largest biomass increase (582%) occurred when grains were cultured in low-fat milk with tryptose enrichment, 130 rpm agitation, and 25°C incubation temperature. However, it was reported that when low-fat or full-fat milk were used without enrichment, kefir grain biomass increased by only 331% and 304%, respectively.

Gorsek and Tramsek [4] used Taguchi experimental design to determine the effect of process parameters on kefir grain mass increase. The researchers determined that the rotational frequency of the stirrer had the greatest relative influence on kefir grain growth, whereas glucose concentration and culture temperature had less effect. Kuo and Lin [17] determined that incubation temperature also affected weight gain of kefir grains and the length of time required to make kefir. When a low incubation temperature (15°C) was used, the time to reach pH 4.7 was 31–35 h, and the total weight increase of kefir grains was 12–16%. When a higher incubation temperature (30°C) was used, the incubation was completed in 14–15 h but the total weight increase was approximately 8–11%.

Guzel-Seydim et al. [83] reported that as low as 2% addition of the commercial fat replacement product Dairy Lo® to reconstituted nonfat milk caused significant rapid increases in kefir grain mass. Dairy Lo is a whey-based product produced by Carbery, Inc. (Cork, Ireland).

5.1.7   ANTIMICROBIAL EFFECT OF KEFIR

Kefir has been reported to have antimicrobial effects against other organisms due to competition for nutrients from kefir microorganisms as well as due to metabolites such as polysaccharides, peptides, bacteriocins, organic acids, and free fatty acids that are produced during fermentation.

Cevikbas et al. [84] determined the antibacterial effects of kefir and kefir grains using the agar diffusion method against *Staphylococcus aureus, Staphylococcus epidermidis, Pseudomonas aeruginosa, Proteus vulgaris, Klebsiella pneumoniae,* and *Bacillus subtilis.* In this study, the greatest antimicrobial activity of kefir was exhibited against Gram-positive microbes. This research team further reported that kefir exhibited inhibitory activity against strains of *Candida, Torulopsis glabrata, Microsporum nanum, Trichopyton mentagrophytes,* and *Trichopyton rubrum.* However, no antifungal effect was observed against *Cryptococcus neoformans* and *Candida parapsilosis.*

Garrote et al. [85] studied the inhibitory power of kefir against Gram-negative microorganisms isolated from human fecal species (*Escherichia coli, Salmonella, Shigella flexneri,* and *Shigella sonnei*), and Gram-positive bacteria isolated from food samples (*Bacillus subtilis* and *Staphylococcus aureus*). To be able to further elucidate the mechanisms of the inhibitory power of kefir, the role of organic acids (lactic acid and acetic acid) was investigated. Kefir grains were inoculated into either sterile skim milk or MRS (*Lactobacillus* agar according to De Man, Rogosa, and Sharpe) broth and incubated at 20°C for 48 h. Following incubation, cultures were centrifuged and the supernatant fractions were collected. Inhibitory activity was determined by either the agar spot test or the agar well diffusion assay. Diameters of the zones of inhibition varied between a maximum of 20.50 mm to a minimum of 11 mm against Gram-positive and Gram-negative microorganisms, respectively. Zones were larger against Gram-positive than Gram-negative species. Authors concluded that the inhibitory effect was due to the undissociated forms of lactic and acetic acids that were produced during fermentation.

In identifying strains from Turkish kefir grains, Yuksekdag et al. [38] noted antimicrobial activity against *Staphylococcus aureus,* as well as *E. coli* and *Pseudomonas aeruginosa.* Powell et al. [86] reported that *Lactobacillus plantarum* ST8KF, isolated from kefir, produced a 35-kDa bacteriocin with a narrow spectrum of activity.

5.1.8   PRESERVATION OF KEFIR GRAINS

To maintain culture stocks, it is necessary to have effective methods of preserving kefir grains. Brialy et al. [87] studied methods for preserving kefir grains by lyophilization followed by submersion in sodium glutamate, ribitol, or glycerol. Kefir grains possess an intrinsic inhibitory activity ("inhibitory power"), which is measured against five microorganisms: *Staphylococcus aureus, Klebsiella pneumoniae, Escherichia coli, Candida albicans,* and *Saccharomyces cerevisiae.* Brialy et al. [87] determined that fresh kefir grains had inhibitory power against the three bacteria but not against the yeast. However, lyophilization of kefir grains without addition of cryoprotective substances caused total loss of inhibitory power. After lyophilization, upon regenerating kefir grains either in milk or in water, Brialy et al. [87]

observed that use of water instead of milk caused total loss of inhibitory power. The use of protective agents produced different results. Sodium glutamate was determined to be inadequate for the cryoprotection of the grains, whereas ribitol and glycerol were recommended as cryoprotective substances for kefir grains to preserve the intrinsic inhibitory power.

Garrote et al. [88] also evaluated different methods for the preservation of kefir grains. Grains were stored at 4°C, −20°C, and −80°C and monitored for metabolic activity. Grains stored at both −20°C and −80°C maintained viable microflora and slightly increased in weight after subsequent culture. Grains stored at 4°C did not increase in weight upon subsequent culture. Kefir made from grains stored at −20°C and −80°C had the same microflora, rheological behavior, acidity, and carbon dioxide content as kefir made from nonstored grains. The kefir product made from grains stored at 4°C did not have the same quality for acidity and viscosity of the standard product. Therefore, it was concluded that storage of kefir grains at −20°C is sufficient to preserve kefir grains.

Papapostolou et al. [89] used conventional, vacuum, and convective drying methods for preserving kefir grains. Cell viability and subsequent fermentation rate were determined. SEM was used to observe dried kefir cells. Results indicated that a conventional drying method at 33°C had promising results. LAB viability was high and subsequent fermentation rates were acceptable for grains stored up to 4 months.

5.2 KOUMISS

5.2.1 HISTORY AND DESCRIPTION OF KOUMISS

Koumiss is a traditional, fermented milk drink originating from the nomadic tribes of Central Asia and Russia and known to be especially popular in Kazakhstan and Krgyzstan [90]. Although a product with a long history, research on koumiss has been limited. The product is unique among dairy foods in that it is made using mare's milk. Starter cultures used include a variety of LAB and yeasts. Similar to kefir, both lactic acid and alcohol fermentations occur in koumiss. However, unlike kefir, there is no grain structure of the koumiss starter. Traditionally, the natural starter culture is the previously fermented koumiss [91]. Danova et al. [92] described three types of koumiss as strong (pH 3.3–3.6), moderate (pH 3.9–4.5), and light (pH 4.5–5) based on the lactic acid content. Different acid content was attributed to different LAB cultures used in the production of koumiss. Koumiss consumption is limited to a specific geographic area and has not been globally commercialized [93]. In areas where it is widely consumed, koumiss has been traditionally considered a health-promoting product that improves metabolism and protects the nervous system and kidneys [90]. Di Cagno et al. [94] cited a reference suggesting use of mare's milk for allergic children. However, supportive scientific data regarding the health-promoting attributes of koumiss are limited. Sun et al. [95] isolated 21 strains of *Lactobacillus* from koumiss and reported that 16 strains produced ACE (angiotension I-converting enzyme) inhibitory activity and 2 strains produced γ-aminobutyric acid (GABA). ACE activity plays an important role in the regulation of blood pressure. ACE inhibitors and GABA have antihypertensive effect.

5.2.2 COMPARATIVE MILK COMPOSITION

Mare's milk is chemically different from cow's milk by having higher lactose and lower fat and protein content [96]. Mare's milk pH is approximately 7. The proteins of mare's milk were purified and it was determined that the β- and α-caseins in mare's milk were more acidic than those in cow's milk [97]. Mare's milk contains less casein but a higher content of immunoglobulins than cow's milk [93]. Higher levels of polyunsaturated fatty acids and phospholipids were measured in mare's milk than cow's milk [93,98]. Mare's milk is translucent, is less white, and, because of a higher lactose content, is sweeter than either cow's milk or goat's milk (Table 5.1).

5.2.3 PRODUCTION

Koumiss is traditionally produced using mare's milk (Figure 5.7). However, several attempts have been made to produce koumiss using cow's milk that has been modified to make it chemically similar to mare's milk. Cow's milk protein content must be decreased and lactose content increased to simulate mare's milk. Kucukcetin et al. [100] used membrane technologies such as ultrafiltration, nanofiltration, and microfiltration to modify the milk composition. In their study, a starter culture consisting of *Kluyveromyces lactis* (ATCC 56498), *Lactobacillus delbrueckii* subsp. *bulgaricus*, and *Lactobacillus acidophilus* was used to manufacture koumiss from modified cow's milk and mare's milk. Chemical and sensory results revealed that modified cow's milk could be used for koumiss production.

In the production of koumiss, pasteurized mare's milk or modified cow's milk is cooled to 25°C (Figure 5.7). Natural starter culture or a starter culture comprising defined, isolated microorganisms from koumiss is added. During fermentation the product is frequently agitated. When koumiss pH reaches 4.6, the fermentation ends. After packaging, koumiss is stored at 4°C [91]. The composition of koumiss is presented in Table 5.2.

TABLE 5.1
Average Composition of Milk of Different Species

Species	Fat %	Protein %	Lactose %	Ash %	Water %
Cow	3.9	3.3	4.7	0.7	87.4
Goat	4.5	3.3	4.6	0.6	87.0
Mare	1.9	2.6	6.2	0.5	88.8
Sheep	7.5	5.6	4.4	0.9	81.6
Zebu	4.8	3.3	4.7	0.7	86.5

Source: Tamime, A.Y. and Robinson, R.K., *Yoghurt: Science and Technology*, 3rd edition, Woodhead Publishing Limited and CRC Press, LLC, Boca Raton, FL, 2007.

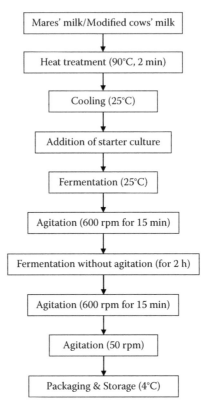

FIGURE 5.7   Production scheme for making koumiss. (Yaygın, H., *Kımız ve özellikleri, Yeni Matbaa*, Antalya, Turkey, 69pp., 1992.)

TABLE 5.2
Composition of Koumiss

Component	Content (g/kg)
Protein	21
Lactose	55
Fat	12
Lactic acid	7–18
Ethanol	6–25
Carbon dioxide	5–9

Source: Litopolou-Tzanetaki, E. and Tzanetakis, N., in *Encyclopaedia of Food Microbiology*, R. Robinson, C. Batt, and P. Patel, Eds, Vol. 2, p. 223, Academic Press, London.

5.2.4 MICROBIOLOGY OF KOUMISS

Danova et al. [92] isolated and characterized homofermentative strains of *Lactobacillus salivarius*, *Lactobacillus buchneri*, and *Lactobacillus plantarum*. Wang et al. [90] identified 12 strains of *Lactobacillus* from homemade koumiss samples. According to physiological, biochemical, and 16S RNA sequence analyses, *Lactobacillus helveticus*, *Lactobacillus fermentum*, *Lactobacillus casei*, and *Lactobacillus plantarum* were identified.

ACKNOWLEDGMENTS

The authors wish to thank Dr. Atif Can Seydim and Ms Rayleen A. Hendrix for their kind assistance.

REFERENCES

1. http://www.liberte.qc.ca/en/page.ch2?uid=Kefir22.
2. http://coproweb.free.fr/kefiranglais.htm.
3. Seydim, Z.B., Studies on fermentation, microbial and biochemical properties of kefir and kefir grains, PhD dissertation, Clemson University, Clemson, 2001.
4. Gorsek, A. and Tramsek, M., Quantitative examination of process parameters during kefir grain biomass production, *Int. J. Chem. React. Eng.*, 5, 1, 2007.
5. Kemp, N., Kefir, the champagne of cultured dairy products, *Cultur. Dairy J.*, XX, 29, 1984.
6. http://wewantorganicfood.com/2008/03/06/kefir-history-information-and-a-kefir-recipe.
7. Robinson, R.K. and Tamime, A.Y., Dairy microbiology, in *The Microbiology of Milk Products*, R.K. Robinson, Ed., Vol.2, p. 291, Elsevier, London, 1990.
8. Simova, E., et al., Lactic acid bacteria and yeasts in kefir grains and kefir made from them, *J. Ind. Microbiol. Biot.*, 28, 1, 2002.
9. Farnworth, E.R. and Mainville, I., Kefir: A fermented milk product, in *Handbook of Fermented Functional Foods*, E.R. Farnworth, Ed., p. 77, CRC, Boca Raton, FL, 2003.
10. Ertekin, B., Effect of using fat replacers on quality criteria of kefir, Master thesis, Suleyman Demirel University, 89 p., 2008.
11. Wood, B.J.B. and Hodge, M.M., Yeast-lactic acid bacteria interactions and their contribution to fermented foodstuffs, in *Microbiology of Fermented Foods*, B.J.B. Wood, Ed., Elsevier, London, Chapter 7, 1985.
12. Duitschaever, C.L., Kemp, N., and Emmons, D., Pure culture formulation and procedure for the production of kefir, *Milchwissenchaft*, 42, 80, 1987.
13. Marshall, V.M. and Cole, W.M., Methods for making kefir and fermented milks based on kefir, *J. Dairy Res.*, 52, 451, 1985.
14. Libudzisz, Z. and Piatkiewicz, A., Kefir production in Poland, *Dairy Ind. Int.*, 55, 31, 1990.
15. Guzel-Seydim, Z.B., et al., Determination of organic acids and volatile flavor substances in kefir during fermentation, *J. Food Comp. Anal.*, 13, 35, 2000.
16. Guzel-Seydim, Z.B., Seydim, A.C., and Greene, A.K., Organic acids and volatile flavor components evolved during refrigerated storage of kefir, *J. Dairy Sci.*, 83, 275, 2000.
17. Kuo, C.Y. and Lin, C.W., Taiwanese kefir grains: Their growth, microbial and chemical composition of fermented milk, *Aus. J. Dairy Technol.*, 54, 19, 1999.

18. Fontán, M.C.G., et al., Microbiological and chemical changes during the manufacture of kefir made from cows' milk, using a commercial starter culture, *Int. Dairy J.*, 16, 762, 2005.
19. Rea, M.C., et al., Irish kefir-like grains: Their structure, microbial composition and fermentation kinetics, *J. Appl. Bacteriol.*, 81, 83, 1996.
20. Bottazzi, V. and Bianchi, F., A note on scanning electron microscopy of micro-organisms associated with the kefir granule, *J. Appl. Bacteriol.*, 48, 265, 1980.
21. Hosono, A., Tanabe, T., and Otani, H., Binding properties of lactic acid bacteria isolated from kefir milk with mutagenic amino acid pyrolyzates, *Milchwissenchaft*, 45, 647, 1990.
22. Kroger, M., Kefir, *Cultured Dairy J.*, 28, 26, 1993.
23. Marshall, V., Cole, W.M., and Brooker, B.E., Observations on the structure of kefir grains and the distribution of the microflora, *J. Appl. Bacteriol.*, 57, 491, 1984.
24. Neve, H., Analysis of kefir grain starter cultures by scanning electron microscopy, *Milchwissenchaft*, 47, 275, 1992.
25. Garrote, G.L., Abraham, A.G., and De Antoni, G.L., Characteristics of kefir prepared with different grain: Milk ratios, *J. Dairy Res.*, 65, 149, 1998.
26. Irigoyen, A., et al., Microbiological, physicochemical and sensory characteristics of kefir during storage, *Food Chem.*, 90, 613, 2005.
27. Fernandez-Garcia, E. and McGregor, J.U., Determination of organic acids during the fermentation and cold storage of yogurt, *J. Dairy Sci.*, 77, 2934, 1994.
28. Marsili, R.T., et al., High performance liquid chromatographic determination of organic acids in dairy products, *J. Food Sci.*, 46, 52, 1981.
29. Gorner F., Palo V., and Seginnova M., Aroma compounds in cultured milks, *Dairy Sci. Abstr.*, 35, 317, 1973.
30. Tamime, A.Y. and Robinson, R.K., *Yogurt Science and Technology*, Pergamon Press, Oxford, 1983.
31. Abraham, A.G. and De Antoni, G.L., Characterization of kefir grains grown in cows' milk and in soya milk, *J. Dairy Res.*, 66, 327, 1999.
32. Liu, J.R. and Lin, C.W., Production of kefir from soymilk with or without added glucose, lactose or sucrose, *J. Food Sci.*, 65, 716, 2000.
33. Athanasiadis, I., et al., Development of a novel beverage by fermentation with kefir granules: Effect of various treatments, *Biotechnol. Progr.*, 20, 1091, 2004.
34. Tratnik, L., et al., The quality of plain and supplemented kefir from goat's and cow's milk, *Int. J. Dairy Technol.*, 59, 40, 2006.
35. Paraskevopoulou, A., et al., Functional properties of single cell protein produced by kefir microflora, *Food Res. Int.*, 36, 431, 2003.
36. Assadi, M.M., Abdolmaleki, F., and Mokarrame, R.R., Application of whey in fermented beverage production using kefir starter culture, *Nutr. Food Sci.*, 38, 121, 2008.
37. Wang, Y., et al., Physicochemical properties of exopolysaccharide produced by *Lactobacillus kefiranofaciens* ZW3 isolated from Tibet kefir, *Int. J. Biol. Macromol.*, 43, 283, 2008.
38. Yuksekdag, Z.N., Beyatlı, Y., and Aslim, B., Metabolic activities of *Lactobacillus* spp. strains isolated from kefir, *Nahrung Food*, 48, 218, 2004.
39. Yuksekdag, Z.N., Beyatli, Y., and Aslim, B., Determination of some characteristic coccoid forms of lactic acid bacteria isolated from Turkish kefirs with natural probiotic, *Lebens. Wiss. Technol.*, 37, 663, 2004.
40. Guzel-Seydim, Z.B., et al., Determination of antimutagenic properties of some fermented milks including changes in the total fatty acid profiles including CLA, *Int. J. Dairy Technol.*, 59, 209, 2006.
41. Ergüllü, E. and Üçüncü, M., Kefir microflorasi uzerinde arastirma, *Gida*, 8, 3, 1983.
42. Toba, T., Abe, S., and Adachi, S., Modification of KPL medium for polysaccharide production by *Lactobacillus* spp. isolated from kefir grain, *Jpn. J. Zootechnol. Sci.*, 58, 987, 1987.

43. Duitschaever, C.L., Kemp, N., and Emmons, D., Comparative evaluation of five procedures for making kefir, *Milchwissenchaft*, 43, 343, 1988.

44. Koroleva, N.S., Technology of kefir and kumys, *Bull. IDF*, 227, 96, 1988.

45. Angulo, L., Lopez, E., and Lema, C., Microflora present in kefir grains of the Galician region (North-West of Spain), *J. Dairy Res.*, 60, 263, 1993.

46. Santos, A., et al., The antimicrobial properties of different strains of *Lactobacillus* spp. isolated from kefir, *Syst. Appl. Microbiol.*, 26, 434, 2003.

47. Kandler, O. and Kunath, P., *Lactobacillus kefir* sp. nov., a component of the microflora of kefir, *Syst. Appl. Micro.*, 4, 286, 1983.

48. Marshall, V.M., Starter cultures for milk fermentation and their characteristics, *Int. J. Dairy Technol.*, 46, 49, 1993.

49. Rosi, J. and Rossi, J., I Microrganismi del kefir: I fermenti lattice, *Scieza e Tecnica Lattiero-Casearia*, 29, 291, 1978.

50. Fujisawa, T., et al., Taxonomic study of the *Lactobacillus gallinarum* sp. nov. and *Lactobacillus johnsonii* sp. nov. and synonymy of *Lactobacillus acidophilus* group A3 with the type strain of *Lactobacillus amylovorus*, *Int. J. Syst. Bacteriol.*, 42, 565, 1992.

51. Mukai, T., et al., Presence of glycerol techoic acid the cell wall of *Lactobacillus kefiranofaciens*, *Lett. Appl. Microbiol.*, 15, 29, 1992.

52. Takizawa, S., et al., *Lactobacillus kefirgranum* sp. nov. and *Lactobacillus parakefir* sp. nov., two new species from kefir grains, *Int. J. Syst. Bacteriol.*, 44, 435, 1994.

53. Garrote, G.L., Abraham, A.G., and De Antoni, G.L., Chemical and microbiological characterization of kefir grains, *J. Dairy Res.*, 68, 639, 2001.

54. Fujisawa, T., et al., *Lactobacillus kefiranofaciens* sp. nov. isolated from kefir grains, *Int. J. Syst. Bacteriol.*, 38, 12, 1988.

55. Vancanneyt, M., et al., Reclassification of *Lactobacillus kefirgranum*, Takizawa et al., 1994 as *Lactobacillus kefiranofaciens* subsp. *kefirgranum* subsp. nov. and amended description of *L. kefiranofaciens*, Fujisawa et al., 1988, *Int. J. Syst. Evol. Microbiol.*, 54, 551, 2004.

56. Garbers, I.M., Britz, T.J., and Witthuhn, R.C., PCR-based denaturing gradient gel electrophoretic typification and identification of the microbial consortium present in kefir grains, *World J. Microbiol. Biotechnol.*, 20, 687, 2004.

57. Latorre-Garcia, L., del Castillo-Agudo, L., and Polaina, J., Taxonomical classification of yeasts isolated from kefir based on the sequence of their ribosomal RNA genes, *World J. Microbiol. Biotechnol.*, 23, 785, 2007.

58. Wang, S.Y., et al., Identification of yeasts and evaluation of their distribution in Taiwanese kefir and Viili starters, *J. Dairy Sci.*, 91, 3798, 2008.

59. Lin, C.W., Chen, H.L., and Liu, J.R., Identification and characterization of lactic acid bacteria and yeasts isolated from kefir grains in Taiwan, *Aus. J. Dairy Technol.*, 54, 14, 1999.

60. Rohm, H., Eliskases-Lechner, F., and Braver, M., Diversity of yeasts in selected dairy products, *J. Appl. Bacteriol.*, 72, 370, 1992.

61. Engel, V.G., Krusch, U., and Teuber, M. Mikrobiologische zusammensetzung von kefir, *Milchwissenchaft*, 41, 418, 1986.

62. Iwasawa, S., et al., Identification and fermentation character of kefir yeast, *Agric. Biol. Chem.*, 46, 263, 1982.

63. Vedamuthu, E.R., Exotic fermented foods, *J. Food Protect.*, 40, 801, 1977.

64. Koroleva, N.S., Starters for fermented milks: Kefir and kumys starter, *Bull. IDF*, 227, 35, 1988.

65. Witthuhn, R.C., Schoeman, T., and Britz, T.J., Isolation and characterization of the microbial population of different South African kefir grains, *Int. J. Dairy Technol.*, 57, 33, 2004.

66. Witthuhn, R.C., Schoeman, T., and Britz, T.J., Characterization of the microbial population at different stages of kefir production and kefir grain mass cultivation, *Int. Dairy J.*, 15, 383, 2005.

67. Guzel-Seydim Z.B., et al., Turkish kefir and kefir grains: Microbial enumeration and electron microscopic observation, *Int. J. Dairy Technol.*, 58, 25, 2005.
68. Duitschaever, C.L., Kemp, N., and Smith, A.K., Microscopic studies of the microflora of kefir grains and of kefir made by different methods, *Milchwissenchaft*, 43, 479, 1988.
69. Toba, T., Arihara, K., and Adachi, S., Distribution of microorganisms with particular reference to encapsulated bacteria in kefir grains, *Int. J. Food Microbiol.*, 10, 219, 1990.
70. Arihara, K., Toba, T., and Adachi, S., Immunofluorescence microscopic studies on distribution of *Lactobacillus kefiranofaciens* and *Lactobacillus kefir* in kefir grains, *Int. J. Food Microbiol.*, 11, 127, 1990.
71. Katechaki E., et al., Production of hard-type cheese using free or immobilized freeze-dried kefir cells as a starter culture, *J. Agric. Food Chem.*, 56, 5316, 2008.
72. Kourkoutas, P.Y., et al., Evaluation of freeze-dried kefir co-culture as starter in Greek Feta-type cheese production, *Appl. Environ. Microbiol.*, 72, 6124, 2006.
73. La Riviére, J.W.M., et al., Kefiran, a novel polysaccharide produced in the kefir grain by *Lactobacillus brevis*, *Arch. Mikrobiol.*, 59, 269, 1967.
74. Yokoi, H., et al., Isolation and characterization of polysaccharide-producing bacteria from kefir grains, *J. Dairy Sci.*, 73, 1684, 1990.
75. Baird, J.K., et al., Water insoluble and soluble glucans produced by extracellular glycosyltransferases from *S. mutans*, *Microbios.*, 8, 143, 1973.
76. Brooker, B.E., Surface coat transformation and capsule formation by *L. mesenteroides* NCDO 523 in the presence of sucrose, *Arch. Microbiol.*, 111, 99, 1976.
77. Brooker, B.E., Cytochemical observations on the extracellular carbohydrate produced by *S. cremoris*, *J. Dairy Res.*, 43, 283, 1976.
78. Brooker, B.E., Ultrastructural surface changes associated with dextran synthesis by *L. mesenteroides*, *J. Bacteriol.*, 131, 288, 1977.
79. Rimada, P.S. and Abraham, A.G., Kefiran improves rheological properties of glucono-delta-lactone induced skim milk gels, *Int. Dairy J.*, 16, 33, 2006.
80. Piermaria, J.A., et al., Gelling properties of kefiran, a food-grade polysaccharide obtained from kefir grain, *Food Hydrocoll.*, 22, 1520, 2008.
81. Maeda, H., et al., Structural characterization and biological activities of an exopolysaccharide kefiran produced by *Lactobacillus kefiranofaciens* WT-2B(T), *J. Agric. Food Chem.*, 52, 5533, 2004.
82. Schoevers, A. and Britz, T.J., Influence of different culturing conditions on kefir grain increase, *Int. J. Dairy Technol.*, 56, 183, 2003.
83. Guzel-Seydim, Z.B., et al., Use of Dairy Lo® significantly increases kefir grain biomass, 2009 (to be submitted).
84. Cevikbas, A., et al., Antitumoural antibacterial and antifungal activities of kefir and kefir grain, *Phytother. Res.*, 8, 78, 1994.
85. Garrote, G.L., Abraham, A.G., and De Antoni, G.L., Inhibitory power of kefir: The role of organic acids, *J. Food Protect.*, 63, 364, 2000.
86. Powell, J.E., et al., Characterization of bacteriocin ST8KF produced by a kefir isolate *Lactobacillus plantarum* ST8KF, *Int. Dairy J.*, 17, 190, 2007.
87. Brially, C., et al., Microbiological study of lyophilized dairy kefir, *Folia Microbiol.*, 40, 198, 1995.
88. Garrote, G.L., Abraham, A.G., and De Antoni, G.L., Preservation of kefir grains, a comparative study, *Lebens. Wiss. Technol.*, 30, 77, 1997.
89. Papapostolou, H., et al., Fermentation efficiency of thermally dried kefir, *Bioresource Technol.*, 99, 6949, 2008.
90. Wang, J., et al., Identification of *Lactobacillus* from koumiss by conventional and molecular methods, *Eur. Food Res. Technol.*, 227, 1555, 2008.
91. Yaygın, H., *Kımız ve özellikleri, Yeni Matbaa*, Antalya, Turkey, 69p., 1992.

92. Danova, S., et al., Isolation and characterization of *Lactobacillus* strains involved in koumiss fermentation, *Int. J. Dairy Technol.*, 58, 100, 2005.
93. Malacarne, M., et al., Protein and fat composition of mare's milk: Some nutritional remarks with reference to human and cow's milk, *Int. Dairy J.*, 12, 869, 2002.
94. Di Cagno, R., et al., Uses of mares' milk in manufacture of fermented milks, *Int. Dairy J.*, 767, 2004.
95. Sun, T., et al., ACE-inhibitory activity and gamma-aminobutyric acid content of fermented skim milks by *Lactobacillus helveticus* isolated from Xinjiang koumiss in China. *Eur. Food Res. Technol.*, 228, 607, 2009.
96. Solaroli, G., Pagliarini, E., and Peri, C., Chemical and physical characteristics of mare's milk, *Ital. J. Food Sci.*, 4, 323, 1993.
97. Egito, A.S., et al., Separation and characterization of mares' milk α_{s1}-, β-, κ-caseins, γ-casein-like, and protease peptone component 5-like peptides, *J. Dairy Sci.*, 85, 697, 2002.
98. Iametti, S., Primary structure of kappa-casein isolated from mares' milk, *J. Dairy Res.*, 68, 53, 2001.
99. Tamime, A.Y. and Robinson, R.K., *Yoghurt: Science and Technology*, 3rd edition, Woodhead Publishing Limited and CRC Press, LLC, Boca Raton, FL, 2007.
100. Kucukcetin, A., et al., Adaptation of bovine milk towards mares' milk composition by means of membrane technology for koumiss manufacture, *Int. Dairy J.*, 13, 945, 2003.
101. Litopolou-Tzanetaki, E. and Tzanetakis, N., Fermented milks, in *Encyclopaedia of Food Microbiology*, R. Robinson, C. Batt, and P. Patel, Eds, Vol. 2, p. 223, Academic Press, London, 2000.

6 Probiotic Dairy Beverages: Microbiology and Technology

*G. Candan Gürakan, Aysun Cebeci,
and Barbaros Özer*

CONTENTS

6.1 INTRODUCTION

Traditionally, lactic acid bacteria (LAB) were used to preserve foods, but in the last decades their use shifted to the field of probiotic products, in order to bring distinct health benefits. As a result of this new direction, product development required the development of special starter cultures delivering specific flavor or health compounds in a selected product [1].

Within LAB, a large strain-to-strain diversity exists with respect to flavor formation and nutraceutical production. With their unique fermentation abilities, LAB strains can be found in diverse environments, and these can provide an important reservoir for industrial strains. These industrial strains were selected according to their probiotic properties such as adhesion to intestinal wall and acid and bile tolerance.

6.2 PROBIOTICS

Probiotics were defined as "live microorganisms which when administered in adequate amounts confer a health benefit on the host" by FAO (Food and Agriculture Organisation of the United Nations) in 2002 [2]. More or less similar definitions are also available [3–5]; however, the above definition points to the most important properties of a probiotic product. The first property is that a probiotic product should contain live microorganisms, and second, the live microorganisms should be provided in a proper amount to exert their health benefits.

The word *probiotic* comes from Greek "pro" and "bios," meaning "for life," and is contrary to the word "antibiotics," meaning "against life." Although the term was used in the mid-1950s, the pioneer of the concept was brought into our lives by Nobel Laureate Elie Metchnikoff at the Institute of Pasteur. Metchnikoff correlated the long lives of Bulgarian peasants with their high consumption of fermented dairy products. His major focus was on LAB, which comprise many of the probiotic bacteria. At the same time, Henry Tissier observed that children with diarrhea had a low number of cells of bifidobacteria in their stools, while healthy children have a high number of cells of these bacteria. Tissier suggested the use of bifidobacteria to restore the healthy gut microflora in children having diarrhea.

Probiotic preparations generally contain LAB (e.g., lactobacilli, enterobacteria, and bifidobacteria), which are normal constituents of the human gastrointestinal microflora. However, use of other microorganisms is also possible, as in the case of

Saccharomyces boulardii, which are not normal inhabitants of the gastrointestinal tract (GIT) [6]. The use of non-GIT origin probiotics suggests that the definition of probiotics could be less strict.

In the dairy industry, probiotic products can be prepared in the form of "shots," called "probiotic shot" (yogurt drink) in a little bottle or in the form of dairy products such as yogurt [7], buttermilk [8], cheese [9], and ice cream [10] into which beneficial probiotic bacteria are added or they can be prepared in the form of capsules or in sachets, and so on.

6.3 CRITERIA FOR SELECTION OF PROBIOTICS/STRAIN SELECTION

Probiotic bacteria must simultaneously survive in the food in high numbers, withstand gastric pH and survive intestinal bile acids, adhere to or interact with the intestinal surface, colonize the intestinal environment, displace pathogenic bacterial competitors, and prevent immune sensitization by the host (Table 6.1) [11].

The criteria to be accomplished by a microorganism to be selected as probiotics are changing. In the last decade, these criteria were well defined [12,13] and included the following.

6.3.1 ORIGIN OF STRAINS

One of the criteria proposed for probiotics included was that probiotic strains for humans should be of human origin. This resulted from the assumption that some health-promoting effects may be species-specific, and human origin strains would already be adapted to the digestive system. However, FAO/WHO [2] suggested reconsidering the human origin as a compulsory property for probiotic bacteria. LAB exist in diverse environments, due to their unique fermentation abilities. In the Expert Consultation report of WHO/FAO [2], it was specified that the resulting action should

TABLE 6.1
General Properties of Probiotic Bacteria as Selection Criteria

Properties	Related to
Origin (of human origin preferred)	Strain property
Well characterized	Strain property
Strain and genus safety	Safety
Able to be active and able to survive in products	Stability
Low pH resistance	Stability
Stomach acid resistant	Stability
Bile resistant	Stability
Able to adhere to the human intestinal surface	Stability
Able to colonize and grow in the human gastrointestinal system (*in vivo*)	Stability
Able to inhibit the growth of pathogenic bacteria	Antagonism

be taken into consideration, not the origin of the species. It was also indicated that the analytical tools cannot discriminate the origin of a species after its primary isolation.

6.3.2 BIOSAFETY

It is known that the pathogenic potential of lactobacilli and bifidobacteria is very low, while some members of the *Enterococcus* genus contain opportunistic pathogens. The use of intestinal isolates of LAB as probiotics has raised the concern of biosafety. The criteria for approval of these organisms are basically based on self-regulation of the manufacturer with the GRAS (generally recognized as safe) status in United States [3] and Novel Foods Regulations (258/97/EC) in some specific cases in Europe [14]. Members of the *Lactococcus* and *Lactobacillus* are the most common organisms in GRAS status. In the European Union, probiotics as food are not governed under specific EU regulatory frameworks [15]. The Novel Foods Regulation is, in fact, for the introduction of the newly discovered strains or genetically modified LAB [14]. However, the European parliament and the Council recently adopted a new regulation on nutrition and health claims of foods, (EC) No. 1924/2006, in December 2006, to harmonize legislation between EU Member States [16]. Under Article 13 of the regulation, Member States were responsible for providing the European Community (EC) with national lists of claims (accompanied by the conditions applying to them and relevant scientific justification) by January 31, 2008. Each claim will be assessed by European Food Safety Authority (EFSA) for inclusion of an approved list of health claims for the EC. From January 2010 onward, the claims on the final EU approved list will be the only health claims permitted on food products on the basis of national lists provided from the Member States [17].

6.3.3 TOLERANCE TO ACID AND BILE SALTS

Probiotic strains were required to be acid and bile tolerant, in order to reach the GIT, which is the main target area of most probiotic strains. In the stomach, where probiotic organisms should survive, the pH can reach as low as 1.5. If the probiotic organisms can survive the harsh acidic conditions of the stomach, resist to digestive enzymes and peristalsis of the stomach, and tolerate bile salts, then they are more likely to reach the colon, where they will present their beneficial action to the host. The probiotic cultures on the market are able to tolerate acid and bile, which enable them to implant in the intestinal tract [18,19]. An exception to this situation is the *Escherichia coli* strain Nissle. This strain is not resistant to acid and bile salts, and can still reach the colon, since they are administered in enteric-coated capsules [4].

An important point is that there exist considerable difference *in vivo* and *in vitro* assays, and a low level of *in vitro* tolerance seems to be enough for *in vivo* resistance. In addition, tolerance to bile salts shows differences in resistance to the bile salts used (from bovine or porcine) [18]. It must also be noted that through the GIT passage, yogurt and milk appear to provide protection to probiotic microorganisms [12].

6.3.4 ADHESION TO INTESTINAL CELLS

Strains should successfully adhere and colonize—at least temporarily—to the intestinal cells. By this way, they can generate their suggested health benefits. *In vitro* adhesion studies generally use Caco-2 cell lines, and the use of colonic or intestinal biopsy samples and mucus glycoproteins has also been studied [20,21]. Nevertheless, the adhesion studies are variable, and even stated as incomplete by some researchers [22]. As a consequence, it was stated that the *in vitro* analyses could only be used as preliminary analysis, that is, in order to differentiate adhesive ones from nonadhesives; however, *in vitro* adhesion constants did not correlate with *in vivo* assays [21].

6.3.5 PRODUCTION OF ANTIMICROBIAL SUBSTANCES

Production of antimicrobial substances may result in inactivation of pathogens in the intestine and normalization of the gut microflora. The antimicrobial substances include lactic acid, hydrogen peroxide, and bacteriocins. Lactic acid and other organic acids produced by lactobacilli contribute to human health by lowering the pH of the medium. Low pH adversely affects pathogenic bacteria present in the colon and in the vagina. Hydrogen peroxide production is particularly desirable for probiotic use in urogenital infections. Production of bacteriocins such as nisin, plantaricin, and so on is another important property.

6.3.6 UTILIZATION OF PREBIOTICS AND FRUCTO-OLIGOSACCHARIDES

Recently, the symbiotic relation of prebiotics and probiotics has become important. Thus, prebiotics such as fructo-oligosaccharides (FOS) utilization by probiotics has been an important criterion during strain selection [23].

Taken as a whole, there is disagreement on the definition of probiotics, and the required criteria for a probiotic strain are changing. Examples of *Saccharomyces boulardii* and *Escherichia coli* Nissle strains do not fulfill the above-mentioned criteria, yet they are considered as probiotic strains. The current concept of probiotics—as in the probiotic definition suggested by WHO/FAO—focuses on two important properties: the microorganisms should be alive at their target site, and they should benefit the health of the consumer. This broadened definition produces the necessary baseline for probiotics.

6.4 SHOULD YOGURT BACTERIA BE CONSIDERED AS PROBIOTICS? SHOULD PLAIN (CLASSICAL) YOGURT BE CONSIDERED AS A PROBIOTIC PRODUCT?

Yogurt contains two starter bacteria *Lactobacillus delbrueckii* subsp. *bulgaricus* and *Streptococcus thermophilus*. These yogurt starter bacteria are not usually considered as probiotics, since they were reported not to proliferate in the intestines [2,24]. They are called "transient," which means that they do not live and colonize in the gastrointestinal system. Although they may have some beneficial activities in the

GIT, it is considered that they do not remain there for a sufficient time to indicate probiotic activities.

On the contrary, in considering yogurt as a probiotic product or not, two main points in the disagreement are raised by some researchers. In the first case, yogurt starter bacteria (all *Streptococcus thermophilus* and most *Lactobacillus delbrueckii* subsp. *bulgaricus*) strains have a high β-galactosidase activity [3]. Studies showed that yogurt consumption improves lactose digestion and eliminates symptoms of lactose intolerance [4]. In addition to their health benefits, yogurt is known to contain high numbers of live starters; hence another property of probiotics has also been accomplished. As a result, in some studies, yogurt was described as a probiotic [4,25]. In the second case, it is accepted worldwide that the properties of probiotics are strain-specific, and yogurt was always considered as if it had been produced with the same starter strains, while certainly this is not the case. Yogurt should not be considered by itself as a product, but its starter strains should be carefully tested by *in vitro* and *in vivo* assays, in order to reach a conclusion. *In vitro* assays to study the probiotic properties of starter and probiotic bacteria show that yogurt starter bacteria contribute to the benefits of probiotic products. Moreover, Elli et al. [26] described yogurt as a probiotic product [26] since the yogurt bacteria they studied survived in the GIT *in vivo* clinical assays. Additionally, the National Yogurt Association (NYA) has published a position statement for probiotics in September 2006 that "live and active yogurt that contains *Lactobacillus delbrueckii* subsp. *bulgaricus* and *Streptococcus thermophilus* is probiotic food as it provides a beneficial effect related to lactose digestion" [27]. Hence their contributions should be evaluated together with probiotic bacteria [28].

6.5   MICROORGANISMS AND THE GUT

Bacteria are normal inhabitants of humans and the overall balance of bacteria can profoundly influence gut ecology and health, since the GIT harbors more than 400 microorganism species, whose numbers are 10-fold the number of tissue cells forming the human body [29]. In healthy individuals, bacteria and human live in symbiosis, from which both the host and the bacteria benefit. Bacterial colonization in humans can be explained in four phases. In the uterine, fetus is in a germ-free environment. Phase 1 includes the delivery, where newborn initially encounters maternal vaginal and colonic microflora. Phase 2 starts with the introduction of oral feeding. The third phase is the weaning period, and the last phase is the acquisition of the complete adult microflora, which is around age 2 [30]. The composition of the intestinal flora is fairly constant within an individual in spite of considerable intraindividual variation in the composition of the diet. Unless disturbed by chronic diseases [colon cancer and inflammatory bowel disease (IBD)] or antibiotic administration, the composition remains constant.

The mechanisms by which bacteria provide advantages to their hosts could be explained as follows [31]:

1. Colonization resistance and production of antimicrobials. Normal flora can protect against the unwanted establishment of pathogenic populations. This

occurs as a result of decrease in nutrient and space. By competing for the available nutrient substrate, beneficial bacteria can inhibit the growth of other, less favorable flora. Competition for bacterial adhesion sites is also a strategic activity. For instance, *Lactobacillus acidophilus* inhibits the adhesion of several enteric pathogens to human intestinal cells. A related activity is enzymatically modifying a toxin receptor. Studies using *Saccharomyces boulardii*, a probiotic yeast, indicate that its interactions with host cell receptors may be important in reducing the pathological effects of infections [32]. Probiotics may also produce various antimicrobial substances. These include production of lactic acid, bacteriocins, and hydrogen peroxide. Lactic acid and acetic acid account for more than 90% of the acids produced. Other acids include citric, hippuric, orotic, and uric acid. By producing these acids, probiotic bacteria lower the pH of the gut, which itself is a way of controlling the growth of unwanted bacteria, especially Gram-positive ones. If organic acids are produced together with hydrogen peroxide, the inhibitory effect is augmented.

2. Second, by providing energy (through fermentation of carbohydrates to organic acids) and vitamins (e.g., vitamin K) [33].

3. The third activity involves a systemic effect. The intestine is the body's largest immune organ (Figure 6.1) and acts as a primary defense against microbial pathogens that have entered our bodies. The effects of probiotics are caused by evoking nonspecific immune response. Probiotic cultures produce γ-interferon by T-cells and stimulate cytokines as represented by TNF-α (tumor necrosis factor) and IL-6 and IL-10 (interleukins 6 or 10) [34].

Probiotics are usually the members of *Lactobacillus* and *Bifidobacterium* (Table 6.2) [35]. However, nonpathogenic *Enterococcus*, yeast [36], and *Bacillus* members are also used as probiotics (Table 6.3).

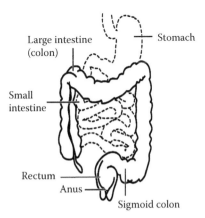

FIGURE 6.1 Front of abdomen, showing the large intestine, with the stomach and small intestine in dashed outline.

TABLE 6.2

Strains of Lactobacilli and Bifidobacteria Used as Probiotic Cultures

Species	Strains
Lactobacillus acidophilus	LA-1/LA-5[a] (Chr. Hansen)
Lactobacillus acidophilus	NCFM[a] (Rhodia)
Lactobacillus acidophilus (Johnsonii)	La1[a] (Nestle)
Lactobacillus acidophilus	DDS-1 (Nebraska Cultures)
Lactobacillus acidophilus	SBT-2062 (Snow Brand Milk Products)
Lactobacillus bulgaricus	Lb12
Lactobacillus lactis	L1A (Essum AB)
Lactobacillus rhamnosus	GG[a] (Valio)
Lactobacillus rhamnosus	GR-1 (Urex Biotech)
Lactobacillus rhamnosus	LB21 (Essum AB)
Lactobacillus rhamnosus	271 (Probi AB)
Lactobacillus plantarum	299v[a], Lp01 (Probi)
Lactobacillus reuteri	SD2112/MM2[a] (Biogaia)
Lactobacillus reuteri	SD2112 (also known as MM2)
Lactobacillus casei	Immunitas (Danone)
Lactobacillus casei	Shirota[a] (Yakult)
Lactobacillus paracasei	CRL 431 (Chr. Hansen)
Lactobacillus fermentum	RC-14 (Urex Biotech)
Lactobacillus helveticus	B02
Bifidobacterium adolescentis	ATCC 15703, 94-BIM
Bifidobacterium longum	BB536[a] (Morinaga Milk Industry)
Bifidobacterium longum	SBT-2928[a] (Snow Brand Milk Products)
Bifidobacterium breve	Yakult
Bifidobacterium bifidus	Bb-11
Bifidobacterium lactis (reclassified as *Bifidobacterium animalis*)	Bb-12[a] (Chr. Hansen)
Bifidobacterium essensis	Danone (Bioactivia)
Bifidobacterium lactis	Bb-02
Bifidobacterium infantis	Shirota
Bifidobacterium infantis	Immunitass
Bifidobacterium infantis	744
Bifidobacterium infantis	01
Bifidobacterium laterosporus	CRL 431
Bifidobacterium lactis	Lafti™[a], B94[a] (DSM)
Bifidobacterium longum	UCC 35624 (UCCork)
Bifidobacterium lactis	DR10/HOWARU[a] (Danisco)

Source: Adapted from Shah, N., *Int. Dairy J.*, 17, 1262–1277, 2007. With permission.

[a] Most common commercial strains.

TABLE 6.3

Probiotic Microorganisms Belonging to Genera Other than Lactobacilli and Bifidobacteria

Species	Strains
Saccharomyces cerevisiae boulardii	Biocodex
Enterococcus faecium (*Gaio*)	PR88
Enterococcus faecium	M-74
Enterococcus faecalis	
Propionibacterium freudenreichii ssp. *shermanii*	JS
Bacillus subtilis	
Bacillus clausii	
Lactobacillus. gasseri	OLL2716(LG21)
Streptococcus thermophilus	TMC 1543
Streptococcus thermophilus	CCRC 14085

Source: Adapted from Shah, N., *Int. Dairy J.*, 17, 1262–1277, 2007. With permission.

6.6   PROBIOTICS AND THEIR HEALTH BENEFITS

Probiotic bacteria can promote health by several activities by several mechanisms. In the 1990s, the suggested health effects of probiotics were quite diverse as listed below [36,37]:

1. Increased nutritional value (better digestibility, increased absorption of minerals, and vitamins)
2. Promotion of intestinal lactose digestion
3. Positive influence on intestinal flora (antibiotics or radiation-induced colitis)
4. Prevention of intestinal tract infections (antagonism against food-borne pathogens)
5. Control of rotavirus and *Clostridium difficile*-induced colitis
6. Prevention of ulcers related to *Helicobacter pylori*
7. Regulation of gut motility (constipation and irritable bowel syndrome)
8. Improvement of the immune system
9. Prevention of colon cancer
10. Reduction of catabolic products eliminated by kidney and liver
11. Prevention of atherosclerosis (reduction of serum cholesterol)
12. Prevention of osteoporosis
13. Better development (growth)
14. Improved well-being
15. Prevention of allergy
16. Prevention and treatment of urogenital tract infections
17. Antihypertensive effect

In contrary to the previous decade, current health benefits of probiotics mainly focus on the following areas; inflammatory diseases [IBD and irritable bowel syndrome (IBS)], diarrhea, and allergy. The following displays brief information about these and some other health benefits of probiotic cultures.

6.6.1 LACTOSE INTOLERANCE

The inability of adults to digest lactose, or milk sugar, is prevalent worldwide. People of northern European descent are unique in retaining the ability to produce the lactose-digesting enzyme, lactase, into adulthood. However, 70–100% of the rest of the adults worldwide are lactose malabsorbers [38]. Consumption of lactose by those lacking adequate levels of lactase can result in symptoms of diarrhea, bloating, abdominal pain, and flatulence. These symptoms are due to the undigested lactose reaching the large intestine and being fermented by the colonic microbes. These microbes can produce gases and products that lead to watery stool.

Dairy product consumption, which is so important for supplying bioavailability and preventing osteoporosis, can be facilitated by managing the symptoms of lactose intolerance. The approach to coping with lactose digestion problems can be multifaceted, including restricting intake of dairy products, ingesting lactase prior to eating dairy products, and consumption of products containing predigested lactose. It has been documented scientifically that many susceptible individuals are better able to consume fermented dairy products, such as yogurt, with fewer symptoms than the same amount of unfermented milk, even though yogurt contains about the same amount of lactose as milk. The traditional cultures used in making yogurt (i.e., *Lactobacillus delbrueckii* subsp. *bulgaricus* and *Streptococcus thermophilus*) contain substantial quantities of β-D-galactosidase [18].

6.6.2 ALLERGY

In a double-blind, randomized, placebo-controlled trial, *Lactobacillus rhamnosus* GG was given to pregnant women for four weeks prior to delivery, then to newborns at high risk of allergy for six months with the result that there was a significant reduction in early atopic disease [39].

6.6.3 PREVENTION OF DIARRHEA CAUSED BY CERTAIN PATHOGENIC BACTERIA AND VIRUSES

Infectious diarrhea is a major world health problem, especially in developing countries responsible for several million deaths each year. While the majority of deaths occur among children in developing countries, it is estimated that up to 30% of the population even in developed countries are affected by food-borne diarrhea each year. Probiotics can potentially provide an important means to reduce these problems.

The strongest evidence of a beneficial effect of defined strains of probiotics has been established using *Lactobacillus rhamnosus* GG and *Bacillus lactis* BB-12 for prevention [40,41] and treatment [42–44] of acute diarrhea mainly caused by rotaviruses in children. Some of these probiotics were administered as a nonfood form.

6.6.4 INFLAMMATORY DISEASES (IBS AND IBD)

The intestinal microflora is likely to play a critical role in inflammatory conditions in the gut, and probiotics could potentially modify such conditions by changing the microflora. The intestines of people with IBD have low numbers of *Lactobacillus* and *Bifidobacterium* and high numbers of coccoids and anaerobes [18]. Other studies support the potential role of probiotics in therapy and prophylaxis [45,46].

6.6.5 CANCER

There is some preliminary evidence that probiotic microorganisms can prevent or delay the onset of certain cancers. *In vitro* studies with *Lactobacillus rhamnosus* GG and bifidobacteria and an *in vivo* study using *Lactobacillus rhamnosus* strains GG and LC-705 as well as *Propionibacterium* spp. showed a decrease in availability of carcinogenic aflatoxin in the lumen [47,48]. Guerin-Danan et al. [49] reported a decrease in bacterial activity of β-glucorinidase and β-glucosidase enzymes, which is implicated in the enterohepatic circulation of toxic and carcinogenic substances, in healthy infants receiving milk fermented with yogurt cultures and *Lactobacillus casei*. Thus, they are considered that they metabolize and detoxify potentially harmful carcinogens. However, in order to make definitive clinical conclusions regarding the efficacy of probiotics in cancer prevention, extensive studies are required.

6.6.6 *H. PYLORI* INFECTION AND COMPLICATIONS

A new development for probiotic applications is activity against *H. pylori*, an opportunistic pathogen responsible for type B gastritis, peptic ulcers, and gastric cancer [18,50]. Detailed studies are needed to discover the effectiveness of probiotic strains against *H. pylori* infections.

6.6.7 DOSAGE

In order to exert their proposed health effects, probiotic bacteria should be consumed at a certain level. The proposed levels differ between 10^8 and 10^{11} day^{-1} [3,18]. Sanders and Huis In't Veld [36] suggested that at least 10^8–10^9 probiotic bacteria as daily intake should reach the small intestine in order to have their beneficial activities. They also stated that it is possible when the total daily dose is about 10^9–10^{10} live probiotic bacteria [36]. Some other authors suggested the level of $>10^7$ and 10^8 cfu mL^{-1} per day as the minimum to achieve such a therapeutic effect [51]. Indeed, the NYA of the United States has developed a criterion that 10^8 cfu g^{-1} of LAB are a prerequisite at the time of manufacture to have the logo of "NYA Live and Active Culture" on the containers of the product [51]. Minimum live bacteria concentrations for the strains declared on the label are also discussed by the Codex Alimentarius Commission. At least 10^7 cfu g^{-1} of the concentration of specific microorganisms (sum of the microorganisms constituting the starter culture in the final product) is suggested by the final codex standard 243-2003 for fermented milks, while the concentration of at least 10^6 cfu g^{-1} should be the labeled microorganisms [52].

Minimum criteria to use the term "probiotic" on the label of a product are described in the FAO guidelines [2]. The efforts to establish standards for probiotic bacteria in commercial products by various organizations such as the FAO/WHO, European Food and Feed Culture Association, International Dairy Federation, Codex Alimentarius, and NYA are summarized in the ISAPP (International Scientific Association for Probiotics and Prebiotics) report published in June 2005 [53].

6.7   SAFETY EVALUATION OF PROBIOTICS

LAB have a long history associated with foods. Members of the genera *Lactobacillus* and *Lactococcus* have been given GRAS status, whereas *Streptococcus* and *Enterococcus* genera include pathogenic species. The intrinsic capacity of *Enterococcus* species for survival and the pathogenicity of some species, coupled with their tendency to transfer genetic material, make their use as probiotics questionable [54]. In the literature, there exist also some reports displaying the disadvantages of probiotics, particularly endocarditis [55].

LAB are intrinsically resistant to many antibiotics [23]. In most cases the resistance is not transferable and the species are also sensitive to antibiotics in clinical use. However, the plasmid associated with antibiotic resistance can be transferred to other species and genera, in particular to enterococci [55].

In order to avoid such undesired effects, each probiotic strain should be assessed for its safety, and special emphasis should be placed on strains from genera that are known to harbor pathogenic species. Prior to the incorporation of novel strains into products, their efficacy and safety should be carefully assessed to evaluate whether they reach the safety status of traditional food-grade organisms. Table 6.4 describes the required safety assessments necessary for probiotic cultures.

TABLE 6.4
Safety Factors to be Assessed for Probiotic Cultures

Property	Safety Factors
Intrinsic properties of LAB	Adhesion factors, antibiotic resistance, plasmid transfer, and enzyme profile
Metabolic products	Concentrations, safety, and other effects
Toxicity	Acute and subacute effects of ingestion of large amounts of culture
Infective properties	*In vitro* with cell lines; *in vivo* with animal models
Dose–response effects	Oral administration in volunteers
Clinical assessment	Potential for side effects and disease-specific effects; careful evaluation in healthy volunteers
Epidemiological studies	Surveillance of large populations following introduction of new strains and products

Source: Reproduced from Gardiner, G.E. et al., *Dairy Microbiology Handbook: The Technology of Milk and Milk Products*, R.K. Robinson, Ed., John Wiley & Sons, Inc., New York, pp. 431–478, 2002. With permission.

Fecal microflora of human, consuming a probiotic product containing *Lactobacillus rhamnosus* DR 20 (daily dose of 1.6×10^9 lactobacilli), was analyzed by Tannock et al. [57]. In their study, they concluded that the *Lactobacillus* and enterococcal contents of the feces of the majority of consumers have been transiently altered by consumption of this milk product.

Additionally, each new strain should be correctly identified in order to assign the correct genera and species name. Identification of LAB can be successfully performed using PCR-based methods, sequencing of the 16S ribosomal DNA gene, and pulsed field gel electrophoresis (PFGE).

6.8 GENETICALLY MODIFIED PROBIOTICS IN FOODS AND LEGISLATIONS

The success of probiotics on health encouraged genetic engineers to develop GM probiotics to improve their characteristics. Through genetic modification or improvement of LAB, it was possible to increase proteolytic activity [58], to develop phage resistance mechanisms [59], to control utilization of lactose [60], to produce bacteriocins [61], and so on. In fact, conjugation is a natural way of transfer that is not considered as genetic modification. Thus, genetically improved LAB by this method bypass most of the sociopolitical and regulatory issues associated with ribosomal DNA (rDNA) technology [62]. However, genetically modified probiotics using other techniques are not introduced into the market due to lack of consumer's acceptance, particularly in Europe [63]. Therefore, they could not enter the food chain. Foods derived from genetically modified microorganisms (GMMs) are not authorized according to the present directive 2001/18/EC on the deliberate release into the environment and Novel Food Regulation of 258/97 EU [64].

6.9 FUNCTIONAL FOODS, PREBIOTICS, PROBIOTICS, AND SYNBIOTICS

Functional foods are the foods that have demonstrated physiological benefits and/or reduce the risk of chronic disease beyond basic nutritional functions and are consumed as a part of the normal diet [7].

Some approaches to produce functional foods are listed below:

1. Use of prebiotics
2. Use of probiotics
3. Mixture of probiotics and prebiotics, called synbiotics
4. Addition of very specific ingredients such as conjugated linoleic acid (CLA)

Prebiotics are nondigestible food ingredients that improve the host health by selectively stimulating the growth of certain beneficial microorganisms in the GIT.

The products that contain both prebiotics and probiotics are referred to as synbiotics [18]. The most thoroughly studied prebiotics are dietary fibers, nondigestible ingredients, in foods such as (i) oligosaccharides including FOS and galacto-oligosaccharides (GOS) and (ii) various polysaccharides including inulin and starch-based materials.

These substances are found in various plants. These carbohydrates as prebiotics are only digestible by some probiotics so that they provide a selective environment for them. Thus, the ability of probiotic bacteria to ferment oligosaccharides has become a crucial property for selection of probiotic strains [65]. The most widely used desirable probiotic bacteria metabolizing prebiotic oligosaccharides are strains of *Lactobacillus* and *Bifidobacterium* spp.

6.10 TECHNOLOGY OF FUNCTIONAL DAIRY BEVERAGES

6.10.1 PROBIOTIC DAIRY BEVERAGES

Functional foods are those foods or food components that are scientifically recognized as having physiological benefits beyond those of basic nutrition. Functional foods are also called nutraceuticals and can include foods that are genetically modified. Dairy products such as yogurt and cheese-containing probiotics and milk-containing Omega-3, phytosterols, isoflavins, CLA, minerals, and vitamins have a prominent position in the development of functional foods. Fermented beverages constitute an important part of human diet because fermentation is an inexpensive technology, which preserves the food, improves its nutritional value, and enhances its sensory properties [66]. Dairy beverages (both fermented and nonfermented) have long been considered as important vehicles for the uptake of probiotics. Intensive efforts have been made to commercialize dairy beverages containing probiotic bacteria. Today, there are numerous commercial dairy-based beverages in which various strains of probiotic bacteria are incorporated that are available for human consumption (Table 6.5).

6.10.1.1 Acidophilus Milk

Lactobacillus acidophilus is an acid-loving bacterium and as a result of its fastidious nature, these bacteria do not rapidly grow in milk [67]. Therefore, in the production of acidophilus milk, it is essential to maintain the inoculum active by daily transfers of mother culture. During fermentation, the pH of the milk often goes beyond the narrow range of optimal pH of *Lactobacillus acidophilus* (pH 5.5–6.0). This eventually leads to decline in the counts of these bacteria. In the traditional acidophilus milk production, the milk (wholly or partly skimmed) is heat-treated at 95°C for 1 h or at 125°C for 15 min (Figure 6.2) [68]. Such a high heat treatment stimulates the growth of *Lactobacillus acidophilus* as these bacteria possess fairly low proteolytic activity and high heat treatment provides *Lactobacillus acidophilus* with nutrients (e.g., denatured proteins and released peptides) essential for its growth. It is a common practice that high-heat-treated milk is cooled to 37°C and kept at this temperature for a period of 3–4 h to allow any spores present to germinate [67]. Then, milk is resterilized to eradicate almost all vegetative cells. Unless skim milk is used, the heat-treated milk is homogenized and cooled down to inoculation temperature (37°C). Since the end product is in liquid form, the possible adverse effects of high heat treatment to textural properties of the product are negligible. Inoculation is achieved by adding active bulk culture of *Lactobacillus acidophilus*. The level of inoculation is usually 2–5% and the inoculated milk is left to ferment until pH 5.5–6.0 or ~1.0% lactic acid is obtained,

TABLE 6.5
Some Commercial Biofermented Dairy Beverages Available in the Market

Product	Starter Organisms
Acidophilus milk	*Lactobacillus acidophilus*
Sweet acidophilus milk	*Lactobacillus acidophilus*
Acidophilin	*Lactobacillus acidophilus, Lactococcus lactis* subsp. *lactis*, kefir yeasts
Nu-Trish A/B	*Lactobacillus acidophilus, Bifidobacterium* spp.
Diphilus milk	*Lactobacillus acidophilus, Bifidobacterium bifidum*
Biomild	*Lactobacillus acidophilus, Bifidobacterium bifidum*
Cultura® or A/B milk	*Lactobacillus acidophilus, Bifidobacterium bifidum*
Bifighurt®	*Bifidobacterium longum* (CKL 1969) or *Bifidobacterium longum* (DSM 2054)
Acidophilus buttermilk	*Lactobacillus acidophilus, Lactococcus lactis* subsp. *lactis*, subsp. *cremoris*, subsp. *lactis* biovar. *diacetylactis*
Acidophilus-yeast milk	*Lactobacillus acidophilus, Saccharomyces lactis*
Bifidus milk	*Bifidobacterium bifidum* or *Bifidobacterium longum*
Yakult	*Lactobacillus paracasei* subsp. *paracasei* Shirota
Yakult Miru-Miru	*Lactobacillus paracasei* subsp. *paracasei, Bifidobacterium bifidum* or *Bifidobacterium bereve, Lactobacillus acidophilus*
A-38 fermented milk	*Lactobacillus acidophilus*, mesophilic lactic cultures
Onaka He GG, Gefilus (Valio Ltd)	*Streptococcus thermophilus, Lactobacillus delbrueckii* subsp. *bulgaricus, Lactobacillus* GG
CHAMYTO	*Lactobacillus johnsonii, Lactobacillus helveticus*
Vitagen	*Lactobacillus acidophilus*
Procult drink	*Bifidobacterium longum* BB536, *Streptococcus thermophilus, Lactobacillus delbrueckii* subsp. *bulgaricus*

Source: After Refs. [69–74].

with no alcohol [70]. The fermentation takes about 18–24 h under quiescent conditions. After the fermentation, the number of viable *Lactobacillus acidophilus* colonies is about $2–3 \times 10^9$ cfu mL^{-1}, but a decline in number up to consumption time is observed. The extended incubation period causes some technical difficulties, that is, reduction in counts of *Lactobacillus acidophilus*. To overcome this handicap, Nahaisi and Robinson [75] proposed the replacement of 25% of *Lactobacillus acidophilus* culture by a mixture of *Streptococcus thermophilus* and *Lactobacillus delbrueckii* subsp. *bulgaricus*. If this is the case, the suppressive effect of hydrogen peroxide produced by *Lactobacillus delbrueckii* subsp. *bulgaricus* on *Lactobacillus acidophilus* should be kept in mind. Following fermentation, the warm product is rapidly cooled to <7°C before agitation and pumped to a filler where it is filled into bottles or cartons [68,76]. Before packaging, stabilizers may be added to reduce the risk of separation in carton and improve the mouth-feel of the product [77].

Basically, there is not much difference between the nutritional values of acidophilus milk and nonfermented milk. Although protein quality and total amino acid content

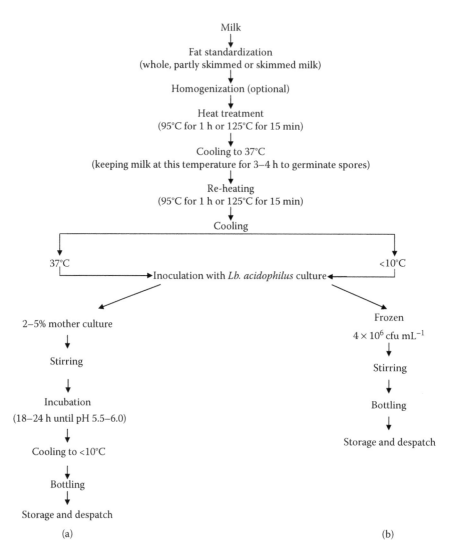

FIGURE 6.2   Flow chart of acidophilus milk (a) and sweet acidophilus milk (b) production.

are similar in both products, acidophilus milk has higher free amino acids than milk. As the milk lactose is hydrolyzed by β-galactosidase of *Lactobacillus acidophilus*, acidophilus milk is more suitable for individuals suffering from lactose intolerance. The uptake of minor milk compounds is enhanced in acidophilus milk. It is also possible to enrich acidophilus milk with minerals (i.e., calcium and iron) and vitamins.

6.10.1.2   Sweet Acidophilus Milk

Despite the well-established therapeutic background of acidophilus milk, this fermented milk product has gained limited popularity in Western society due to its undesirable sour milk flavor. Therefore, attempts have been made to convert acidophilus milk into a product that is more palatable and appealing to consumers [67]. As a result of these attempts, sweet acidophilus milk has been developed and introduced into Western markets. It is a well-known fact that *Lactobacillus acidophilus* does not grow at low temperatures (i.e., <10°C). When *Lactobacillus acidophilus* is incorporated into pasteurized milk at about 5°C and bottled aseptically, these bacteria are able to keep their viability up to 14 days without reducing the pH of milk. It is recommended that the initial load of *Lactobacillus acidophilus* in sweet acidophilus milk should be 4×10^6 cfu mL^{-1} to keep the number of these bacteria above the level of the therapeutic minimum at the end of the "best before date." In case freeze-dried concentrated cultures are used, the bacteria may keep their viability up to 58% after 23 days at 4°C in sweet acidophilus milk [78]. Brashears and Gilliland [79] reported that two or three strains of *Lactobacillus acidophilus* remained viable in sweet acidophilus milk over 28 days at 7°C. According to Vedamuthu [68], addition of 170–200 g of frozen culture concentrate to 2000 L of pasteurized milk is satisfactory to reach the target level of *Lactobacillus acidophilus* in the end product. The nutritional properties of sweet acidophilus milk are fairly similar to milk. As with acidophilus milk, fat standardization and homogenization are optional in sweet acidophilus milk production. In the enumeration of *Lactobacillus acidophilus* in sweet acidophilus milk, de Mann Rogosa Sharpe (MRS) agar or Ragosa agar are widely used. In order to improve the selectivity of the agar media, the addition of 0.15% bile salts is recommended [68]. The petri plates are incubated anaerobically at 35–37°C for 72 h.

6.10.1.3   Bifidus Milk and Acidophilus–Bifidus Milk (A/B Milk)

Methods of manufacture of bifidus milk and A/B milk show similarities to acidophilus milk. In both products, the milk is standardized to desired protein and fat levels. Then, for the manufacture of bifidus milk, the milk is heat-treated at 80–120°C for 5–30 min and rapidly cooled to 37°C. The heat-treated milk is inoculated with frozen culture of *Bifidobacterium bifidum* and *Bifidobacterium longum* at a level of 10% and left to ferment until pH 4.5 is obtained. When the fermentation is stopped, the product is cooled to <10°C and packaged. The final product has a slightly acidic flavor and the ratio of lactic acid to acetic acid is 2:3. The viable bifidobacteria count is about 10^8–10^9 cfu mL^{-1} after 2 weeks of storage.

The milk used for the production of A/B milk is usually enriched with protein prior to fat standardization and homogenization. The standardized milk is heat-treated at 75°C for 15 s (with a plate heat exchanger) or 85°C for 30 min (with the vat system). After cooling the milk to 37°C, frozen cultures of *Lactobacillus acidophilus* and *Bifidobacterium bifidum* are inoculated and fermentation is allowed until pH 4.5–4.6 is reached (~16 h). Following fermentation, the fermented milk is cooled to <10°C. The final product contains both probiotic bacteria at levels of 10^8–10^9 cfu mL^{-1} and the shelf life of the product is about 20 days. A/B milk has a characteristic aroma and slightly acidic flavor. The viscosity of the product is high and in some countries this product is produced in set form. In Denmark, this product is marketed under the name of Cultura AB.

It is also possible to produce probiotic milks by simply adding mix culture of *Lactobacillus acidophilus* and *Bifidobacterium bifidum* to cold pasteurized milk. The flow chart of this type of probiotic product is similar to sweet acidophilus milk production. Bifighurt, another probiotic milk drink, is produced by fermenting milk using *Bifidobacterium bifidum* or *Bifidobacterium longum* CKL 1969 (DSM 2054, a slime-forming variant) and *Streptococcus thermophilus* at 42°C (for human strains, incubation temperature is set at 37°C). The usual inoculation rate of mix culture is 6% and the pH of the final product is 4.7. Bioghurt has a mild acidic flavor and contains L(+) lactic acid at a level of 95%. The number of *Bifidobacterium bifidum* is usually higher than 10^7 cfu mL^{-1} in the fresh product and declines *c.* 2 log during refrigerated storage for 1–2 weeks. Diphilus milk is made from cow's milk and has a specific taste and aroma. This fermented milk drink is widely used in the therapy of intestinal disorders.

6.10.1.4 Mil-Mil

This product is quite similar to A/B milk and is very popular in Japan. In the production of Mil-Mil, pasteurized milk is inoculated with a mix culture of *Lactobacillus acidophilus*, *Bifidobacterium bifidum*, and *Bifidobacterium breve*. In most cases, glucose or fructose is added to balance the taste of the product and carrot juice is added as a colorant [80].

6.10.1.5 Yakult

Yakult is a sweetened and therapeutic milk beverage that is widely popular in Japan and has been known since 1935. It is made from skim milk or skim milk powder, sugar, dextrose, and water. The manufacturing steps of Yakult are outlined in Figure 6.3. Raw ingredients are mixed with filtered sterilized water in a mixing tank to obtain a sweet milky solution. The milk solids and sugar levels of the mixture are 3.7% and 14%, respectively [81]. The solution is sterilized at high temperature for a short time (UHT), destroying any bacteria that may be present. After the mixture is cooled to 37°C, it is pumped into a fermentation tank. Live *Lactobacillus paracasei* subsp. *paracasei* Shirota, which is resistant to gastric juice and bile, is added to the fermentation tank and the solution is allowed to ferment until the number of *Lactobacillus paracasei* subsp. *paracasei* Shirota reaches an ideal concentration. The fermentation takes 16–18 h. The final product contains 10^8 cfu mL^{-1} of *Lactobacillus paracasei* subsp.

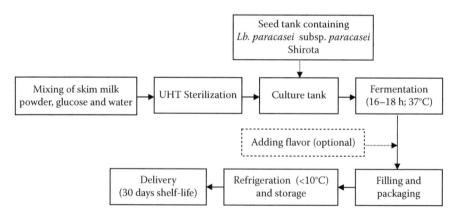

FIGURE 6.3 Flow chart of Yakult production.

paracasei Shirota [70]. High heat treatment of skim milk triggers the Maillard reaction between glucose added to skim milk and milk proteins, resulting in characteristic light coffee color of Yakult [82]. The yield of Yakult is close to 99%, with no by-products. The product is also flavored with nature-identical flavors (e.g., tomato, celery, carrot, cabbage, parsley, and a number of other vegetable juices). Yakult can be added to cereals, smoothies, milkshakes, cheesecakes, and any other cold foods. The shelf life of Yakult is about 30 days under refrigerated conditions.

Yakult Miru-Miru, a Yakult-related product, is a milk-base functional dairy beverage and has a broadly similar composition to cow's milk, that is, 3.1% fat, 3.1% protein, and 4.5% lactose. It also contains other saccharides. Yakult Miru-Miru is manufactured by incorporation of *Bifidobacterium bifidum*, *Bifidobacterium breve*, and *Lactobacillus acidophilus* [81]. The product is marketed in Japan under the names of Miru-Miru, Miru-Miru E, and Bifiru.

6.10.1.6 Miscellaneous Dairy-Based Probiotic Beverages

Acidophilus-yeast milk is very common in the former Republic of Soviet Union. Whole or skimmed milk is heat-treated at 90–95°C for 10–15 min, and cooled down to 35°C. Inoculation is achieved with mix culture of *Lactobacillus acidophilus* and *Saccharomyces lactis* until 0.8% lactic acid and 0.5% ethanol is produced. The product is described as viscous, slightly acidic, and yeasty taste [70]. Acidophilin, a sweetened milk beverage, is another fermented dairy drink that is similar to acidophilus-yeast milk. Acidophilin is made from whole or skimmed milk inoculated with *Lactobacillus acidophilus*, *Lactococcus lactis* subsp. *lactis*, and kefir yeasts or kefir starter [83]. Fortification of the milk with skim milk powder, sucrose, and/or cream provided improved sensory properties of this product. Acidophilin has been used to treat colitis, enterocolitis, dysenteria, and other intestinal diseases [84]. Macedo et al. [85] described a dairy-based probiotic beverage fermented by a mix culture of *Lactobacillus casei* Shirota and *Bifidobacterium adolescentis*. The product contains 35% buffalo cheese whey, 30% soy milk, and 35% cow's milk. Gefilus® developed by Valio Ltd (Finland) contain a large amount of *Lactobacillus* GG. This product range includes yogurt, milk, buttermilk, and drinks.

6.10.2 Nondairy Probiotic Beverages

Most of the probiotic research to date has focused on dairy-based products. Currently, fresh milk, fermented milk, and yogurt seem to be the most common vehicles for the uptake of probiotics. In recent years, since the vegetarianism has become a common trend throughout the developed countries, the popularity of probiotic nondairy foods has tremendously increased. Vegetarian probiotic foods, by definition, must be free from all animal-derived ingredients. It has been suggested that fruit/vegetable juices and cereal-based foods/beverages containing microorganisms can also serve as probiotics [86–88]. Fruits and vegetables are recognized as healthy foods, because they are rich in antioxidants, vitamins, dietary fibers, and minerals [89]. Furthermore, fruits and vegetables do not contain any dairy allergens that might prevent usage by certain segments of the population [89,90]. Some commercial and/or traditional nondairy probiotic beverages are listed in Table 6.6.

TABLE 6.6
Some Examples of Nondairy Fermented Probiotic Beverages

Product	Organisms Isolated or Used as Starter	Remarks
Boza	*Lactobacillus plantarum*, *Lactobacillus acidophilus*, *Lactobacillus fermentum*, *Lactobacillus caprophilus*, *Leuconostoc raffinolactis*, *Leuconostoc mesenteroides*, *Lactobacillus brevis*, *Saccharomyces. cerevisiae*, *Candida tropicalis*, *Candida glabrata*, *Geotrichum penicillatum*, and *Geotrichum candidum*	Traditional fermented product native to Turkey, Romania, Albania, and Bulgaria. Ratio of LAB to yeast is 2.4. Made from maize, wheat, rye, millet, and other cereals. The product has a light to dark beige color and slightly sharp to slightly sour/sweet taste
Fermented cassava flour	*Lactobacillus plantarum* A6	The product contains cassava flour at a level of 20%. Inoculum rate of probiotic bacteria is 8%. Incubation is carried out at 35°C for 16 h. The level of probiotic bacteria is 2.3×10^9 cfu mL^{-1}. Storage period of the product is 28–30 days
Probiotic oats drink	*Lactobacillus plantarum* B28	Fermentation period is about 8 h. The number of probiotic bacteria is 7×10^{10} cfu mL^{-1} and additives (aspartame, cyclamate, and saccharine) has no adverse effect on probiotic strain used. Shelf life of the product is 21 days at 4°C
Fermented soybean drinks	*Bifidobacterium* spp.	For a better growth of probiotic bacteria, the raw material is recommended to be heat-treated at 65°C for 10 min or over 100°C. At 85°C for 5–30 min is unsuitable for the growth of *Bifidobacterium* spp. Higher protein level in soybean increases the buffering capacity and growth of probiotic strains
Fruit juice-based probiotic drinks	*Bifidobacterium* spp., *Lactobacillus acidophilus*	A wide range of fruit juices are added to milk. Sensory properties of the product are pleasing to all the age groups

continued

TABLE 6.6   (continued)

Product	Organisms Isolated or Used as Starter	Remarks
Probiotic fermented beet juice	*Lactobacillus acidophilus* LA39, *Lactobacillus plantarum* C3, *Lactobacillus casei* A4, *Lactobacillus delbrueckii* D7	Fermentation continued until pH 4.5 was reached (about 48 h). *Lactobacillus acidophilus* remained active up to 4 weeks at 4°C
Probiotic tomato juice	*Lactobacillus acidophilus* LA39, *Lactobacillus plantarum* C3, *Lactobacillus casei* A4, *Lactobacillus delbrueckii* D7	Fermentation was carried out at 30°C for 72 h. Total viable probiotic count was $1–9 \times 10^9$ cfu mL^{-1} after 72 h fermentation and $10^6–10^8$ cfu mL^{-1} after 4 weeks of storage at 4°C
Probiotic cabbage juice	*Lactobacillus plantarum* C3, *Lactobacillus casei* A4, *Lactobacillus delbrueckii* D7	Fermentation was achieved with 24-h-old culture at 30°C. After 48 h fermentation, the counts of *Lactobacillus plantarum* C3, *Lactobacillus casei* A4, and *Lactobacillus delbrueckii* D7 reached 10^9 cfu mL^{-1}
Probiotic fermented carrot and beetroot juice	*Lactobacillus acidophilus*, yeast autolysate	Yeast autolysate stimulated the growth of *Lactobacillus acidophilus*. Amino acids, vitamins, minerals, and antioxidants reduced the fermentation time
Probiotic blackcurrent juice	Probiotic cultures	The product received high sensory scores from the panelists. The product was regarded as "healthy"
Probiotic orange juice	Probiotic cultures	The product was described as possessing perceptible "dairy," "medicinal," and "dirty" flavors, distinguishing them from the conventional orange juice
Commercial products		
Grainfields Whole Grain Probiotic Liquid®	*Lactobacillus acidophilus*, *Lactobacillus delbrueckii*, *Saccharomyces boulardii*, *Saccharomyces cerevisiae*	The product is made from organic ingredients including the grains, beans, and seeds such as pearl barley, linseed, maize, rice, alfalfa seed, mung beans, rye grains, wheat, and millet. It is a dairy-free effervescent product with no added sugar

continued

TABLE 6.6   (continued)

Product	Organisms Isolated or Used as Starter	Remarks
Vita Biosa® by Live Superfoods (USA)	Probiotic cultures	Vita Biosa is made by fermenting aromatic herbs and other plants byLAB. The product contains no sugar and can produce CO_2. The pH of the product can drop to 3.5 after fermentation and contains high amount of antioxidants
Proviva® by Skane Dairy (Sweden)	*Lactobacillus plantarum* 299v	This is the first probiotic food that does not contain milk or milk constituents. The active component of the product is fermented oatmeal gruel. Malted barley is added to enhance the liquefaction. The final product contains *Lactobacillus plantarum* at a level of *ca.* 10^{10} cfu mL^{-1}
Bioprofit® by Valio Ltd (Finland)	*Lactobacillus rhamnosus* GG, *P. freudenreichii* subsp. *shermanii* JS	It is a fruit juice-based product
Biola® by Tine BA (Norway) under the license from Valio Ltd	*Lactobacillus rhamnosus* GG	It is a probiotic fruit juice containing 95% fruit juice, with no added sugar. Orange–mango and apple–pear flavors are available
Rela® by Biogaia (Sweden)	*Lactobacillus reuteri* MM53	

Source: After Refs. [88–112].

6.10.3   FUNCTIONAL NONPROBIOTIC DAIRY BEVERAGES WITH ADDED BIOACTIVE COMPONENTS

Consumer interest in the relationship between diet and health has increased the demand for information about functional foods. Rapid advances in science and technology, increasing healthcare costs, changes in food law affecting label and product claims, an aging population, and rising interest in attaining wellness through diet are among the factors fuelling overall interest in functional foods [113]. Credible scientific research indicates that there are many clinically demonstrated and potential health benefits from food components. A large body of credible scientific research has confirmed the positive effects of nutraceuticals (i.e., Omega-3 fatty acids), isoflavones, and phytosterols on human health. Among the nutraceuticals, the importance of Omega-3 fatty acids has been widely investigated. Omega-3 is considered as an essential nutrient since it is the precursor of eicosapentaenoic acid (EPA) and docosahexanoic acid (DHA), which cannot be synthesized in the human body [114]. The latter fatty acids are essential for development of brain, concentration, and learning ability of children as well as promoting heart health in the general population [115]. The major sources of Omega-3 fatty acids are fatty fishes, flaxseed oils, and other vegetable oils including canola and corn oils. Omega-3 consumption has been rising since 2004 as dairy manufacturers launched Omega-3 mix, ice creams, cheeses, and yogurts. The potential handicaps of incorporation of Omega-3 into functional dairy beverages are that this fatty acid is sensitive to heat, light, and air, and may cause undesirable flavor in the end product [116].

Isoflavones are secondary vegetable substances that can act as estrogens in the body and have protective functions. Isoflavones can be found in many foods but the best known source is the soybean [117]. Red clover is another source of isoflavones. Since red clover is not suitable for direct consumption, the isoflavones extracted from red clover are used as supplement in food industry. Isoflavones have potent antioxidant properties, comparable to that of the well-known antioxidant vitamin E. The antioxidant powers of isoflavones can reduce the long-term risk of cancer by preventing free radical damage to DNA. Genistein is the most potent antioxidant among the soy isoflavones, followed by daidzein. In nature, isoflavones usually occur as glycosides and, once deconjugated by the intestinal microflora, the isoflavone can be adsorbed into the blood [114]. The potential health benefits of the isoflavones are as follows:

i. Ease menopause symptoms
ii. Reduce heart disease risk
iii. Protect against prostate problems
iv. Improve bone health
v. Reduce cancer risk

It should be borne in mind that most of the isoflavones show poor solubility in water and lead to flavor defects such as bitterness and beany taste.

Phytosterols (or plant sterols) are a group of steroid alcohols, photochemicals naturally occurring in plants. Phytosterols have many applications as food additives and, as a food ingredient or additive, phytosterols have cholesterol-lowering properties (reducing cholesterol absorption in intestines) [118]. Jones et al. [119] demonstrated that inclusion of 1.7 g day^{-1} of phytosterols into the diet of hypercholesterolemic men had the effect of lowering blood cholesterol. As consumer awareness has increased, the number of products containing plant sterols or plant stanols and their esters has increased. In this respect, milk-based beverages containing phytosterols have gained a distinct place among the functional foods. Phytosterols dissolve in water rather poorly and may cause technological problems in low- or no-fat dairy beverages [116].

CLA is found almost exclusively in animal products. Dairy products high in CLA such as milk allow consumers to obtain the therapeutic health benefits of CLA by consuming a natural food product. Since dairy products high in CLA have tremendous potential within the emerging nutraceutical and functional food markets, there is growing interest in CLA-related research work across the world. As a result of these efforts, some dairy-based products containing CLA have been introduced into the market. Yogurt is the major functional dairy product containing added CLA. The functional dairy beverages containing CLA, phytosterols, or Omega-3 fatty acids are also gaining popularity and, today, a number of milk-based functional beverages (fermented or non-fermented) are marketed under the commercial brands (Table 6.7).

TABLE 6.7

Some Commercial Functional Dairy Beverages with Added Bioactive Components

Functional Dairy Beverage	Brand	Manufacturer	Source of Bioactive	Comments
		Nonfermented Products		
Low-fat milk	Lactantia nature addition	Lactantia Parmalat Canada	Omega-3 (flaxseed oil)	300 mg 250 mL^{-1} serve, mainly Alanine (ALA)
Low-fat milk	Heart Plus	PB Food Australia	Omega-3 (fish oil)	200 mg 250 mL^{-1} serve, mostly DHA and EPA
Low-fat milk	Natrel Omega-3	Natrel Canada	Omega-3 (organic flaxseed oil)	300 mg 250 mL^{-1} serve
Low-fat milk (fresh)	Dawn Omega Milk	Dawn Dairy Ireland	Omega-3 (fish oil)	150 mg 250 mL^{-1} serving. Europe's first, fresh pasteurized Omega-3 milk. DSM supplied Omega-3 is added at final stage of production using Tetra Pak-developed dosing system
Low-fat milk	Farmers Best	Dairy Farmers Australia	Omega-3 (vegetable oils)	33 mg 250 mL^{-1} serve. First product to be made from fresh milk where almost all saturated fat has been replaced with the healthier monounsaturated and Omega-3 fats
Low-fat milk	Flora Pro-Activ	Unilever, UK	Phytosterol	Carries the health claim "helps to reduce cholesterol"
Low-fat milk	Night-Time Milk	Cricketer Farm, UK	Melatonin	Promoted as a natural solution for good night sleep
Low-fat milk (UHT)	Omega Plus	Nestle Malaysia and Singapore	Omega-3 (vegetable oil-canola and corn oil)	UHT and powdered milk

continued

TABLE 6.7 (continued)

Functional Dairy Beverage	Brand	Manufacturer	Source of Bioactive	Comments
Milk	Meiji Love	Meiji Milk-Japan	Calcium and iron	350 mg calcium and 3 mg iron per 200 mL serve
Fresh milk	St. Ivel Advance	Dairy Crest UK	Omega-3	
Premium milk	Neilson Dairy Oh!	Neilson Dairy Ltd Canada	DHA, Omega-3	
Premium milk	Dairyland Milk-2-Go	Saputo Canada	Calcium, Omega-3, vitamins	
Chocolate milk	Beatrice	Parmalat Canada	Omega-3	
Milk–fruit juice drink	Natural Linea	Corporacion Alimentaria Penanata S.A. Spain	CLA (Tonalin brand from Cognis)	Carries the health claim "helps to reduce body fat"
Fermented Products				
Yogurt drink	Flora Pro-Activ	Unilever, UK	Phytosterol	Claims "clinically proven to reduce cholesterol"
Yogurt drink	Benecol	Mc Neil Nutritionals, UK	Phytosterol	Licensed technology from Raiso, Finland. Contains 3% phytosterol esters
Low-fat dairy drink	Danacol	Danone	Phytosterol	1.6 g phytosterols 100 mL^{-1} bottle. Claims that "consuming 1.6 g of plant sterols per day, as part of a healthy diet, is proven to reduce cholesterol"
Fermented milk drink	Zen	Danone Belgium	Mg	
Fermented dairy fruit beverage	Evolus	Valio Finland	Bioactive peptides obtained by milk fermentation	Evolus claims to be the first European functional food to help in lowering blood pressure
Probiotic fermented milk	*Lactobacillus casei* + lactoferrin	Kyodo Milk Japan	*Lactobacillus casei*, lactoferrin	Promoted as antibacterial and preventing infections

Source: After Sharma, R., *Aus. J. Dairy Technol.*, 60, 196–199, 2005.

Apart from the nutraceuticals mentioned earlier, vitamins and minerals are also added into fermented and nonfermented dairy beverages and the market share of these products is rapidly increasing. In recent years, scientific studies on the incorporation of bioactive peptides, protein hydolysate, and prebiotics (or dietary fibers) into functional dairy beverages have been intensified and a few commercial products have been introduced into the market.

REFERENCES

1. Hansen, E.B., Commercial bacterial starter cultures for fermented foods of the future, *Int. J. Food Microbiol.*, 78, 119–131, 2002.
2. FAO, *Food and Nutrition Paper, Probiotics in food, Health and Nutritional Properties of Probiotics and Guidelines for Evaluation*, World Health Organization, Food and Agriculture Organization of the United Nations, Rome, 2006, ftp://ftp.fao.org/es/esn/food/wgreport2.pdf.
3. Sanders, M.E., Probiotics, *Food Technol.*, 53, 67–75, 1999.
4. Guarner, F., Perdigo, G., Corthier, G., Salminen, S., Koletzko, B., and Morelli, L., Should yoghurt cultures be considered probiotic? *Br. J. Nutr.*, 93, 783–786, 2005.
5. Huis int' Veld, J.H.J., Havenaar, R., and Marteau, P., Establishing a scientific basis for probiotic R&D, *Tibtech*, 12, 6–8, 1994.
6. Penner, R., Fedorak, R.N., and Madsen, K.L., Probiotics and nutraceuticals: Non-medicinal treatments of gastrointestinal diseases, *Curr. Opin. Pharmacol.*, 5, 596–603, 2005.
7. Katan, M.B., The probiotic yogurt activia: Accelerated intestinal transit has been established, but not stimulation of bowel movements, *Netherlans Tijdschrift voor Geneskunde*, 152, 846–847, 2008.
8. Antunes, A.E.C., Marasca, E.T.G., Moreno, I., Dourado, F.M., Rodrigues, L.G., and Lerayer, A.L.S., Development of probiotic buttermilk, *Ciencia e Tehnologia de Alimentos*, 27, 83–90, 2007.
9. Ong, L. and Shah, N.P., Influence of probiotic *Lactobacillus acidophilus* and *L. helveticus* on proteolysis, organic acid profiles, and ACE-inhibitory activity of cheddar cheeses ripened at 4, 8, and 12C, *J. Food Sci.*, 73, M111–M120, 2008.
10. Hagen, M. and Narvhus, J.A., Production of ice cream containing probiotic bacteria, *Milchwissenchaft*, 54, 265–268, 1999.
11. German, B., Schiffrin, E.J., Reniero, R., Mollet, B., Pfeifer, A., and Neeser, J.R., The development of functional foods: Lessons from the gut, *Trend Biotechnol.*, 17, 492–499, 1999.
12. Salminen, S., Isolauri, E., and Salminen, E., Clinical uses of probiotics for stabilizing the gut mucosal barrier: Successful strains and future challenges, *Anton. van Leeuw.*, 70, 347–358, 1996.
13. Vaughan, E.E. and Mollet, B., Probiotics in the new millennium, *Nahrung*, 43, 148–153, 1999.
14. Wright, A.V., Regulating the safety of probiotics—The European Approach. *Curr. Pharmaceut. Des.*, 11, 17–23, 2005.
15. Feord, J., Lactic acid bacteria in a changing legislative environment, *Anton. van Leeuw.*, 82, 353–360, 2002.
16. *Official J. Eur. Union* L 404 of 30 December 2006, Internet: http://eurlex.europa.eu/LexUriServ/site/en/oj/2007/l_012/l_01220070118en00030018.pdf
17. Newsletter of SYNDIFRAIS science committee, 2007, Internet: http://www.isapp.net/docs/Probiotics_Reference_syndifrais.pdf (accessed on September 2008).

18. Shah, N., Functional cultures and health benefits, *Int. Dairy J.*, 17, 1262–1277, 2007.
19. Lankaputhra, W.E.V. and Shah, N.P., Survival of *Lactobacillus acidophilus* and *Bifidobacterium* spp. in the presence of acid and bile salts, *Cult. Dairy Prod. J.*, 30, 2–7, 1995.
20. Tuomola, E., Crittenden, R., Playne, M., Isolauri, E., and Salminen, S., Quality assurance criteria for probiotic bacteria, *Am. J. Clin. Nutr.*, 73, 393S–398S, 2001.
21. Morelli, L., *In vitro* assessment of probiotic bacteria: From survival to functionality, *Int. Dairy J.*, 17, 1278–1283, 2007.
22. Blum, S., Reniero, R., Schiffrin, E.J, Crittenden, R., Mattila-Sandholm, T., Ouwehand, A.C, Salminen, S., and Morelli, L., Adhesion studies for probiotics: Need for validation and refinement, *Trend Food Sci. Technol.*, 10, 405–410, 1999.
23. Cebeci, A. and Gurakan, C., Properties of potential probiotic *Lactobacillus plantarum* strains, *Food Microbiol.*, 20, 511–518, 2003.
24. Klein, G., Pack, A., Bonnaperte, C., and Reuter, G., Taxonomy and physiology of lactic acid bacteria. *Int. J. Food Microbiol.*, 41, 103–125, 1998.
25. Guglielmotti, D., Marcó, M.B., Vinderola, C., de los Reyes Gavilán, C., Reinheimer, J., and Quiberoni, A., Spontaneous *Lactobacillus delbrueckii* phage-resistant mutants with acquired bile tolerance, *Int. J. Food Microbiol.*, 119, 236–242, 2007.
26. Elli M., Callegari M.L., and Ferrari, S., Survival of yogurt bacteria in human gut, *Appl. Environ. Microbiol.*, 72, 5113–5117, 2006.
27. National Yogurt Association, Position statement for probiotics, September 2006, http://www.aboutyogurt.com/lacYogurt/Probiotics.pdf (accessed on August 2008).
28. Vinderola, C.G. and Reinheimer, J.A., Lactic acid starter and probiotic bacteria: A comparative "*in vitro*" study of probiotic characteristics and biological barrier resistance, *Food Res. Int.*, 36, 895–904, 2003.
29. Tannock, G.W., Probiotic properties of lactic acid bacteria: Plenty of scope for fundamental R&D, *Tibtech*, 15, 270–274, 1997.
30. Bousvaros, A., Probiotics: Overview and Rationale: Use in Inflammatory Bowel Disease, The Health Impact of Active Cultures: Probiotics, Harvard Medical School Division of Nutrition, 2005, Internet: http://www.presentme.com/harvard/oct2005.htm (accessed on May 2008).
31. Tuohy, K.M., Probert, H.M., Smejkal, C.W., and Gibson, G.R., Using probiotics and prebiotics to improve gut health, *Drug Discov. Today*, 8, 692–701, 2003.
32. Lukaczer, D., Schiltz, B., and Liska, D.J., A pilot trial evaluating the effect of an inflammatory-modulating medical food in patients with fibromyalgia, *Clin. Pract. Alternative Med.*, 1, 148–156, 2000.
33. Hugenholtz, J., The lactic acid bacterium as a cell factory for food ingredient production, *Int. Dairy J.*, 18, 466–475, 2008.
34. Wikipedia, Internet: http://en.wikipedia.org/wiki/Image:Intestine.png (accessed on July/August 2008).
35. Shah, N.P., Ali, J.F., and Ravula, R.R., Populations of *L. acidophilus, Bifidobacterium* spp., and *L. casei* in commercial fermented milk products, *Biosci. Microflora*, 19, 35–39, 2000.
36. Sanders, M.E. and Huis In't Veld, J., Bringing a probiotic-containing functional food to the market: Microbiological, product, regulatory and labeling issues, *Anton. van Leeuw., Int. J. Gen. Mol. Microbiol.*, 76, 293–315, 1999.
37. Dugas, B., Mercenier, A., Lenoir-Wijnkoop, I., Arnaud, C., Dugas, N., and Postaire, E., Immunity and probiotics, *Trend Immunol. Today*, 20, 387–390, 1999.
38. de Vrese, M., Stagelmann, A., Richter, B., Fenselau, S., Laue, C., and Schrezenmeir, J., Probiotics-compensation for lactase insufficiency, *Am. J. Clin. Nutr.*, 73, 421S–429S, 2001.

39. Kalliomaki, M., Salminen, S., Arvilommi, H., Kero, P., Koskinen, P., and Isolauri, E., Probiotics in primary prevention of atopic disease: A randomised placebo-controlled trial, *Lancet*, 357, 1076–1079, 2001.

40. Saavedra, J.M., Bauman, N.A., Oung, I., Perman, J.A., and Yolken, R.H., Feeding of *Bifidobacterium bifidum* and *Streptococcus thermophilus* to infants in hospital for prevention of diarrhea and shedding of rotavirus, *Lancet*, 344, 1046–1049, 1994.

41. Szajewska, H., Kotowska, M., Mrukowicz, J.Z., Armanska, M., and Mikolajczyk, W., Efficacy of *Lactobacillus* GG in prevention of nosocomial diarrhea in infants, *J. Pediatr.*, 138, 361–365, 1999.

42. Majamaa, H. and Isolauri, E., Probiotics: A novel approach in the management of food allergy, *J. Allergy Clin. Immunol.*, 99, 179–85, 1997.

43. Shornikova, A.V., Isolauri, E., Burkanova, L., Lukovnikova, S., and Vesikari, T., A trial in the Korelian Republic of oral rehydration and *Lactobacillus* GG for treatment of acute diarrhea, *Acta Paediatr.*, 86, 460–465, 1997.

44. Guandalini, S., Pensabene, L., Zikri, M.A., Dias, J.A., Casali, L.G., Hoekstra, H., Kolacek, S., Massar, K., Micetic-Turk, D., Papadopoulou, A., de Sousa, J. S., Sandhu, B., Szajewska, H., and Weizman, Z., *Lactobacillus* GG administered in oral rehydration solution to children with acute diarrhea: A multicenter European trial, *J. Pediatr. Gastroenterol. Nutr.*, 30, 54–60, 2000.

45. McFarland, L.V., Meta-analysis of probiotics for the prevention of antibiotic associated diarrhea and the treatment of *Clostridium difficile* disease, *Am. J. Gastroenterol.*, 101, 812–822, 2006.

46. Nobaek, S., Johansson, M.L., and Molin, G., Alteration of intestinal microflora is associated with reduction in abdominal bloating and pain in patients with irritable bowel syndrome. *Am. J. Gastroenterol.*, 95, 1231–1238, 2000.

47. El-Nezami, H., Mykkanen, H., Kankaanpaa, P., Salminen, S., and Ahokas, J., Ability of *Lactobacillus* and *Propionibacterium* strains to remove aflatoxin B1 from chicken duodenum, *J. Food Protect.*, 63, 549–552, 2000.

48. Oatley, J.T., Rarick, M.D., Ji, G.E., and Linz, J.E., Binding of aflatoxin B1 to bifidobacteria in vitro, *J. Food Protect.*, 63, 1133–1136, 2000.

49. Guerin-Danan, C., Chabanet, C., Pedone, C. Popot, F., Vaissade, P., Bouley, C., Szylit, O., and Andrieux, C. 1998. Milk fermented with yogurt cultures and *Lactobacillus casei* compared with yogurt and gelled milk: Influence on intestinal microflora in healthy infants, *Am J. Clin. Nutr.*, 67, 111–117, 1998.

50. Cats, A., Kulpers, E.J., Bosschaert, M.A., Pot, R.G., Vandenbroucke-Gauls, C.M., and Kusters, J.G., Effect of frequent consumption of *Lactobacillus casei*-containing milk drink in *Helicobacter pylori* colonized subjects, *Pharmacol. Therap.*, 17, 429–435, 2003.

51. Rybka, S. and Kailasapathy, K., *Lb. acidophilus* and *Bifidobacterium* spp.—their therapeutic potential and survival in yogurt, *Aus. J. Dairy Technol.*, 52, 28–35, 1997.

52. Codex Alimentarius, http://www.codexalimentarius.net/download/standards/400/CXS_243e.pdf (accessed on June 2008).

53. ISAPP, International Scientific Association for Probiotics and Prebiotics: Report, June 2005, Internet: http://www.isapp.net/activities.asp#2006, http://www.isapp.net/docs/probiotic%20standards%20justification.pdf (accessed on August 2008).

54. Donohue, D.C., Safety of novel probiotic bacteria, in *Lactic Acid Bacteria—Microbiology and Functional Aspects*, 3rd edition, S. Salminen, A. von Wright, and A. Ouwehand, Eds, Marcel Dekker Inc., New York, pp. 531–546, 2004.

55. Adams, M.R., Safety of industrial lactic acid bacteria, *J. Biotechnol.*, 68, 171–178, 1999.

56. Gardiner, G.E., Ross, R.P., Kelly, P.M., Stanton, C., Collins, J.K., and Fitzgerald, G., Microbiology of therapeutic milks, in *Dairy Microbiology Handbook: The Technology of Milk and Milk Products,* 3rd edition, R.K. Robinson, Ed., John Wiley & Sons Inc., New York, pp. 431–478, 2002.

57. Tannock G.W., Munro, K., Harmsen, H.J.M., Welling, G.W., Smart, J., and Gopal, P.K., Analysis of the fecal microflora of human subjects consuming a probiotic product containing *Lactobacillus rhamnosus* DR 20, *Appl. Environ. Microbiol.*, 66, 2578–2588, 2000.
58. Kok, J. and de Vos W.M., The proteolytic system of lactic acid bacteria, in *Genetics and Biotechnology of Lactic Acid Bacteria*. M.J. Gasson, and W.M. De Vos, Eds, Blackie Academic and Professional, London, UK, pp. 169–210, 1994.
59. Klaenhammer, T.R. and Fitzgerald, G.F. Bacterophages and bacteriophage resistance, in *Genetics and Biotechnology of Lactic Acid Bacteria*, M.J. Gasson, and W.M. De Vos, Eds, Blackie Academic and Professional, London, UK, pp. 106–168, 1994.
60. de Vos, W.M. and Simons, G.F.M., Gene cloning and expression systems in lactococci, in *Genetics and Biotechnology of Lactic Acid Bacteria*, M.J. Gasson, and W.M. de Vos, Eds, Blackie Academic and Professional, London, UK, pp. 52–97, 1994.
61. Dodd, H.M. and Gasson, M.J. Bacteriocins of lactic acid bacteria, in *Genetics and Biotechnology of Lactic Acid Bacteria*, M.J. Gasson, and W.M. de Vos, Eds, Blackie Academic and Professional, London, UK, pp. 211–251, 1994.
62. Cogan, T.M., Beresford, T.P., Steele, J., Broadbent, J., Shah, N.P., and Ustunol, Z., Invited review: Advances in starter cultures and cultured foods, *J. Dairy Sci.*, 90, 4005–4021, 2007.
63. Ahmed, F.E., Genetically modified probiotics in foods, *Trend Biotechnol.*, 21, 491–497, 2003.
64. von Wright, A. and Bruce, A., Genetically modified microorganisms and their potential effects on human health and nutrition, *Trend Food Sci. Technol.*, 24, 264–276, 2003.
65. Kaplan, H. and Hutkins, R.W., Metabolism of fructooligosaccharides by *Lactobacillus paracasei* 1195, *Appl. Environ. Microbiol.*, 2217–2222, 2003.
66. Gagada, T.H., Mutukumira, A.N., Narvhus, J.A., and Feresu, S.B., A review of traditional fermented foods and beverages of Zimbabwe, *Int. J. Food Microbiol.*, 53, 1–11, 1999.
67. Salji, J., Acidophilus milk products: Food with a third dimension, in *Encyclopaedia of Food Science, Food Technology and Nutrition*, R. Macrae, R.K. Robinson, and M.J. Sadler, Eds, Academic Press, London, pp. 3–7, 1993.
68. Vedamuthu, E.R., Other fermented and culture-containing milks, in *Manufacturing Yogurt and Fermented Milks*, R. Chandan, C.H. White, A. Kilara, and Y.H. Hui, Eds, Blackwell Publishing, pp. 295–308, 2006.
69. Lee, Y.K., Nomoto, K., Salminen, S., and Gorbach, S.L., *Handbook of Probiotics*, Wiley, New York, pp. 13–17, 1999.
70. Surono, I.S. and Hosono, A., Fermented milks: Types and standards of identity, in *Encyclopedia of Dairy Microbiology*, H. Roginski, J. Fuquay, and P.F. Fox, Eds, pp. 1018–1023, 2002.
71. Sellars, R.L., Acidophilus products, in *Therapeutic Properties of Fermented Milks*, R.K. Robinson, Ed., Elsevier Applied Science, London, pp. 81–116, 1991.
72. Kurmann, J.A. and Rasic, J.L., Technology of fermented special foods, in *Fermented Milks: Science and Technology*, International Dairy Federation Bulletin, no. 227, IDF, Brussels, pp. 101–109, 1988.
73. Lee, Y.K. and Wong, S.F., Stability of lactic acid bacteria in fermented milk, in *Lactic Acid Bacteria*, S. Salminen and von A. Wright, Eds, Marcel Dekker, New York, pp. 103–114, 1993.
74. Temmerman, R., Pot, B., Huys, G., and Swings, J., Identification and antibiotic susceptibility of bacterial isolates from probiotic products, *Int. J. Food Microbiol.*, 81, 1–10, 2002.
75. Nahaisi, M.H. and Robinson, R.K., Acidophilus drinks: The potential for developing countries, *Dairy Ind. Int.*, 50, 16–17, 1985.
76. Kosikowski, F.V. and Mistry, V.V., Cheese and fermented milk foods, in *Origin and Principles: Fermented Milks*, F.V. Kosikowski, Ed., LLC, Westport, pp. 57–74, 1997.

77. Tamime, A.Y. and Robinson, R.K., Fermented milks and their future trends, Part 2: Technological aspects, *J. Dairy Sci.*, 55, 281–307, 1988.

78. Mitchell, S.L. and Gilliland, S.E., Pepsinized sweet whey medium for growing *Lactobacillus acidophilus* for frozen concentrated cultures, *J. Dairy Sci.*, 66, 4712–4718, 1983.

79. Brashears, M.M. and Gilliland, S.E., Survival during frozen and subsequent refrigerated storage of *Lactobacillus acidophilus* cells as influenced by the growth phase, *J. Dairy Sci.*, 78, 2326–2335, 1995.

80. Kurman, J.A., Rasic, J.L., and Kroger, M., *Encyclopedia of Fermented Fresh Milk Products*, AVI Publishing, New York, p. 203, 1992.

81. Tamime, A.Y. and Robinson, R.K., Technology of manufacture of thermophilic milks, International Dairy Federation, Bulletin No. 227, IDF, Brussels, pp. 82–96, 1988.

82. Akuzawa, R. and Surono, I.S., Fermented milks: Asia, in *Encyclopedia of Dairy Microbiology*, H. Roginski, J. Fuquay, and P.F. Fox, Eds, pp. 1045–1049, 2002.

83. Tamime, A.Y. and Marshall, V.E., Microbiology and technology of fermented milks, in *Microbiology and Biochemistry of Cheese and Fermented Milk*, B.A. Law, Ed., Blackie Academic and Professional Publication, London, pp. 57–154, 1997.

84. Koroleva, N.S., Products prepared with lactic acid bacteria, in *Fermented Milks-Science and Technology*, International Dairy Federation Bulletin, No. 227, IDF, Brussels, pp. 159–179, 1991.

85. Macedo, R.F., Soccol, C.R., and Freitas, R.J.S., Production of low cost beverage with soya milk, buffalo cheese whey and cow milk fermented by *Lactobacillus casei* Shirota and *Bifidobacterium adolescentis*, *J. Sci. Ind. Res.*, 57, 679–685, 1998.

86. Brown, A., Shovic, A., Salam, I., Holck, P., and Huang, A., Non-dairy probiotic's (poi) influence on changing the gastrointestinal tract's microflora environment, *Altern. Ther. Health Med.*, 11, 58–64, 2005.

87. Mattila-Sandholm, T., Myllarinen, P., Crittenden, R., Mogensen, G., Fonden, R., and Saarela, M., Technological challanges of future probiotic foods, *Int. Dairy J.*, 12, 173–182, 2002.

88. Prado, F., Parada, J.L., Pandey, A., and Soccol, C.R., Trends in non-dairy probiotic beverages, *Food Res. Int.*, 41, 111–123, 2008.

89. Yoon, Y.K., Woodams, E.E., and Hang, Y.D., Probiotication of tomato juice by lactic acid bacteria, *J. Microbiol.*, 42, 315–318, 2004.

90. Luckow, T. and Delahunty, C., Which juice is healthier? A consumer study of probiotic non-dairy juice drink, *Food Qual. Pref.*, 15, 751–759, 2004.

91. Blandino, A., Al-Aseeri, M.E., Pandiella, S.S., Cantero, D., and Webb, C., Cereal based fermented foods and beverages, *Food Res. Int.*, 36, 527–543, 2003.

92. Gotcheva, V., Pandiella, S.S., Angelov, A., Roshkova, Z.G., and Webb, C., Microflora identification of the Bulgarian cereal-based fermented beverage boza, *Process Biochem.*, 36, 127–130, 2000.

93. Santos, M.C.R., Desenvoltimento de bebida e farinha lactea fermentada de acão probiotica a base de soro de leite e farinha de mandioca por cultura mista de *Lactobacillus plantarum* A6, *Lactobacillus casei* Shirota e *Lactobacillus acidophilus*, M.Sc. thesis, UFPR, pp. 106, 2001.

94. Stark, A. and Madar, Z., Dietary fibre, in *Functional Foods: Designer Foods, Pharmafoods, Nutraceuticals*, I. Goldberg, Ed., Chapman & Hall, New York, pp. 183–201, 1994.

95. Wrick, K.L., Potential role of functional foods in medicine and public health, in *Functional Foods: Designer Foods, Pharmafoods, Nutraceuticals*, I. Goldberg, Ed., Chapman & Hall, New York, pp. 480–494, 1994.

96. Fuchs, R.H., Borsato, D., Bona, E,. and Hauly, M.C.O., "Iogurte" de soja suplementado com oligofrutose e inulina, *Ciencia e Technologia de Alimentos*, 25, 175–181, 2005.

97. Shimakawa, Y., Matsubara, S., Yuki, N., Ikeda, M., and Ishikawa, F., Evaluation of *Bifidobacterium breve* strain Yakult-fermented soy milk as a probiotic food, *Int. J. Food Microbiol.*, 81, 131–136, 2003.

98. Wang, Y.C., Yu, R.C., and Chou, C.C., Growth and survival of bifidobacteria and lactic acid bacteria during the fermentation and storage of cultured soymilk drinks, *Food Microbiol.*, 19, 501–508, 2002.

99. Chou, C.C. and Hou, J.W., Growth of bifidobacteria in soy milk and survival in the fermented soy milk drink during storage, *Int. J. Food Microbiol.*, 56, 113–121, 2000.

100. Matsuyama, J., Hirata, H., Yamagisi, T., Hayashi, K., Hirano, Y., Kuwata, K., Kiyasawa, I., and Nagasawa, T., Fermenttaion profiles and utilization of sugars of bifidobacteria soy milk, *Nippon Shokuhin Kogyo Gakkaishi*, 39, 887–893, 1992.

101. Chang, C.Y. and Stone, M.B., Effect of total soymilk solids on acid production by selected lactobacilli, *J. Food Sci.*, 55, 1643–1646, 1990.

102. Mital, B.K. and Steinkraus, K.H., Fermentation of soy milk by lactic acid bacteria: A review, *J. Food Protect.*, 42, 895–899, 1979.

103. Young Tae, K. and Mi Hwa, O., Freeze-drying of fermented milk prepared from milk and fruit juices, *Korean J. Food Sci. Technol.*, 30, 1448–1455, 1999.

104. Tourilla, H. and Cardello, A.V., Consumer responses to an off-flavour in juice in the presence of specific health claims, *Food Qual. Pref.*, 13, 561–569, 2002.

105. Rakin, M., Vukasinovic, M., Siler-Marinkovic, S., and Maksimovic, M., Contribution of lactic acid fermentation to improved nutritive quality vegetable juices enriched with brewer's yeast autolysate, *Food Chem.*, 100, 599–602, 2007.

106. Chae, H.J., Joo, H., and In, M.J., Utilization of brewer's yeast cells for the production of food grade yeast extract: Part I: Effects of different enzymatic treatments on solid and protein recovery and flavor characteristics, *Biosource Technol.*, 76, 253–258, 2001.

107. Luckow, T. and Delahunty, C., Consumer acceptance of orange juice containing functional ingredients, *Food Res. Int.*, 37, 805–814, 2004.

108. Superfoods, 2006, www.livesuperfoods.com, (accessed on November 1, 2008).

109. Molin, G., Probiotics in foods not containing milk or milk constituents, with special reference to *Lactobacillus plantarum* 299v, *Am. J. Clin. Nutr.*, 73 (Suppl.), 380S–385S, 2001.

110. Leporanta, K., Probiotics for juice-based products. Case Valio Gefilus®, International sales, www.valio.fi (accessed on November 1, 2008).

111. Leporanta, K., Tine is using LGG under licence from Valio Ltd., Valio Today's-News, www.valio.fi (accessed on November 1, 2008).

112. Daniells, S., Valio continues research into probiotic fruit juices. Nutraingradients, available at www.nutraingredients.com (accessed on November 1, 2008).

113. IFIC, Functional foods, International Food Information Council Foundation, available at http://ific.org (accessed on November 1, 2008).

114. Awaisheh, S.S., Haddadin, M.S.Y., and Robinson, R.K., Incorporation of selected nutraceuticals and probiotic bacteria into a fermented milk, *Int. Dairy J.*, 15, 1184–1190, 2004.

115. Milner, J.A. and Alison, R.G., The role of dietary fat in child nutrition and development, *J. Nutr.*, 129, 2094–2105, 1999.

116. Sharma, R., Market trends and opportunities for functional dairy beverages, *Aus. J. Dairy Technol.*, 60, 196–199, 2005.

117. Messina, M.J., Legumes and soybeans: Overview of their nutritional profiles and health effects, *Am. J. Clin. Nutr.*, 70, 439S–450S, 1999.

118. Ostlund, R.E., Racette, S.B., and Stenson, W.F. Inhibition of cholesterol absorption by phytosterol-replete wheat germ compared with phytosterol-depleted wheat germ, *Am. J. Clin. Nutr.*, 77, 1385–1589, 2003.

119. Jones, P.J., Ntanios, F.Y., Raeini-Sarjaz, M., and Vanstone, C.A., Cholesterol-lowering efficiacy of a sitostanol-containing phytosterol mixture with a prodent diet in hyperlipidemic men, *Am. J. Clin. Nutr.*, 69, 1144–1150, 1999.

7 Functional Bioactive Dairy Ingredients

Theodoras H. Varzakas and
Ioannas S. Arvanitoyannis

CONTENTS

7.1 INTRODUCTION

Functional foods stand for a new category of remarkably promising foods bearing properties (i.e., low cholesterol, antioxidant, antiaging, anticancer, etc.), which have already rendered them quite appealing. There are many classes of functional foods (pro- and prebiotics, dietary fiber, low fat, etc.) and their definition is occasionally confused with that of nutraceuticals and novel foods. Functional dairy ingredients include dairy propionibacteria as probiotics and synbiotics: a combination of the effect of probiotics and prebiotics, plant sterols and stanols, hypoallergenic (HA) hydrolysates for prevention and treatment of cow's milk allergy (CMA), oligosaccharides, caseinophosphopeptides (CPPs), and conjugated linoleic acid (CLA).

Consumers' main skepticism vis-à-vis functional foods resides in the veracity of health claims and in the low and often inadequate control of their claimed properties. Legislation concerning this matter is progressing at an extremely low pace and currently only Japan, the United Kingdom, the United States, and Scandinavian countries have managed to make notable progress. Moreover, labeling of functional foods is far from informative, providing scanty information about nutritional value, storage, and cooking recipe. It is anticipated that technological advances in the food industry in conjunction with extensive clinical trials and thorough governmental control will eventually guarantee the credibility of health claims and ensure consumers' confidence in functional foods. The realization that attention to diet, as part of a healthy lifestyle, can reduce considerably disease risk and promote health has created a lucrative market for a whole range of new products called "functional foods" or functional dairy ingredients.

The main factors that led to the endorsement of the "functional food" concept are increasing life expectancy in the developed countries (often entailing longer hospital care); high health care costs; advances in food and ingredients technology; the need for publicly funded research institutions to publicize their findings; and the greater media coverage given to these findings and to health issues.

The food industry is expecting that consumers, after years of being bombarded with negative health messages to reduce the intake of fat, cholesterol, and sodium, are ready to welcome foods that emphasize the positive benefits of newly added dairy ingredients, even if the scientific community has not yet clearly concluded their real benefits. Despite the continuously growing popularity of functional foods and more specifically dairy ingredients, scientists have identified a few specific substances, or combinations of substances, that proved to reduce the risk of disease. Moreover, the category of functional foods comprises nutraceuticals, designer foods, pharmafoods, and dairy ingredients.

Therefore, it is doubtful whether the consumer will actually manage to benefit from this trend. Some products might lead to significant public health advances and it makes sense to foster their development, marketing, and consumption. However, on the other hand, the absence of convincing scientific research and inadequate regulatory controls may create a situation in which the marketplace is flooded with products of exaggerated claims. In brief, if governments do not require functional ingredients to be proven effective (and safe) before they become part of the food supply; if functional ingredients are simply added to foods high in fat, cholesterol, sodium, or sugar, then dubious functional foods may be just added to the plethora of foods already manufactured.

This chapter aims at examining current trends in the regulation of functional foods in the United States and the European Union, the largest markets for such products, and pointing out the possible pros and cons for the consumer. Moreover, the different functional dairy ingredients are examined as well as the effect of their action.

7.2   DAIRY PROPIONIBACTERIA AS PROBIOTICS

At the end of the 19th century, propionibacteria were described as microorganisms involved in the fermentation of lactate into acetate and propionate with the simultaneous production of carbon dioxide during the ripening of Emmental cheese.

Propionibacteria are pleomorphic rods, 0.5–0.8 µm in diameter and 1–5 µm in length, often club-shaped or coccoid, bifid, or even branched. They are nonmotile, nonsporing bacteria, anaerobic to aerotolerant, and generally catalase positive, growing in the temperature range 15–40°C, in the pH range 5.1–8.5, with an optimum at 30°C and neutral pH. They are heterofermentative and metabolize different carbohydrates, various alcohols, and organic acids to a mixture of propionate, acetate, succinate, and carbon dioxide. Propionic fermentation involves the Wood–Werkman cycle [1] and requires the enzyme methylmalonyl-CoA carboxyl transferase that catalyzes the reversible transfer of a carboxyl group from methylmalonyl-CoA to pyruvate to form propionyl-CoA and oxaloacetate [2].

7.2.1   PRODUCTION OF ANTIMICROBIAL COMPOUNDS

Propionic acid and its salts are used as antifungal agents in the food industry. Propionate produced during food fermentation by dairy propionibacteria shows inhibitory actions toward undesirable microorganisms. Propionibacteria cultures are also considered biopreservatives. Microgard commercial product is a pasteurized skimmed milk product fermented by *Propionibacterium freudenreichii* subsp. *shermanii* showing inhibitory activity toward several Gram-negative bacteria and fungi but not Gram-positive bacteria [3]. Cocultures of lactic acid bacteria and propionibacteria were found to be more effective in avoiding food spoilage yeasts as described by Schwenninger and Meile [4].

7.2.2   PRODUCTION OF VITAMINS

Dairy propionibacteria have been used in the industrial production of vitamin B_{12} by fermentation [5]. Propionibacteria allow the production of food-grade vitamin, either during fermentation or as a food additive. B_9 is naturally present in milk but its concentration can be enhanced in fermented milks. The yogurt starter *Streptococcus thermophilus* produced B_9, which is consumed by lactobacilli [6].

7.2.3   USE IN FERMENTED FOOD PRODUCTS

Propionibacteria participate not only in ripening but also in microbiological safety (increase shelf life) and nutritional cheese quality. The main fermented food product containing propionibacteria is a Swiss-type cheese.

Babuchowski et al. [7] reported the use of dairy propionibacteria in fermented vegetables such as sauerkraut, red beet juice, and vegetable salads. This resulted in increase of propionic and acetic acids and B_9 and B_{12} contents and increase in the shelf life of the products.

Propionibacterium freudenreichii NIZO B2336, producing large amounts of riboflavin, was incorporated into joghurts and ingested by rats that were fed with a riboflavin-deficient diet as shown by LeBlanc et al. [8]. The resulting fermented milk had an enhanced concentration of riboflavin suppressing the symptoms of ariboflavinosis in rats, whereas the conventional joghurt without propionibacteria did not show such a health effect. Moreover, *Propionibacterium freudenreichii* converts free linoleic acid, added to skimmed milk by incorporation of hydrolyzed soil oil, during fermented milk production and storage [9]. Rumenic acid is the main isomer produced with anticarcinogenic effects.

7.3   SYNBIOTICS: COMBINATION OF THE EFFECTS OF PROBIOTICS AND PREBIOTICS

Probiotics and prebiotics are the main products that influence the composition and activity of the intestinal microbiota.

Probiotics according to FAO/WHO [10] are defined as live microorganisms that, when administered in adequate amounts, confer a health benefit on the host.

Prebiotics are defined as nondigestible food ingredients that, when consumed in sufficient amounts, selectively stimulate the growth and activity of one or a limited number of microbes in the colon, resulting in documented health benefits [11].

The two can be mixed and may reinforce each other's effect creating a symbiotic: a mixture of probiotics and prebiotics that beneficially affects the host by improving the survival and implantation of live microbial dietary supplements in the gastrointestinal tract, by selectively stimulating the growth and/or activating the metabolism of one or a limited number of health-promoting bacteria and thus improving host welfare [12,13].

7.3.1   SAFETY OF SYNBIOTICS: FUNCTIONAL BENEFITS

Prebiotics have been part of the human diet for a long time. Fructosyl-type ingredients are natural components of edible plants [14].

Polydextrose is another novel prebiotic used as a food ingredient for years.

The prebiotic part of a symbiotic combination tries to improve the transient colonization of the probiotic part.

Concern is raised about prebiotics regarding their tolerability, which varies between different prebiotic compounds. Moreover, sensitivity to side effects varies. Excessive consumption of prebiotics can lead to gastrointestinal symptoms such as bloating and laxation. Osmotic diarrhea is caused by a high luminal concentration of low-molecular-weight compounds such as polyols [13]. Highly fermentable prebiotics may lead to the production of gases that cause abdominal distension and produce flatus. The excessive fermentation in the proximal colon may also decrease the available carbohydrates for microbes in the distal colon with the possibility of protein fermentation by microbes and the production of harmful metabolites such as indoles and phenols.

Most members of the genera *Lactobacillus* and *Bifidobacterium* are used as probiotics and are recognized as safe. They are used safely especially in fermented dairy products and are rarely associated with disease. The frequency of bacteraemia caused by these organisms is very low.

Anderson et al. [15] did not observe any translocation by the probiotics fed in elective surgical patients showing that the prebiotic inulin did not cause any translocation of the strains.

Synbiotics can improve gastrointestinal health reducing susceptibility to infections. Consistent with the reports on anti-inflammatory effects of bifidobacteria in *in vitro* studies, bifidobacteria reduce the expression of selected inflammatory markers also *in vivo* [16]. Liu et al. [17] showed that synbiotics or fermentable fiber can be used as an alternative treatment to lactulose in minimal hepatic encephalopathy patients with cirrhosis. Treatment with a combination of prebiotics such as β-glucan, inulin, pectin, and resistant starch, and nonurease-producing probiotics such as *Pediococcus pentosus*, *Leuconostoc mesenteroides*, *Lactobacillus paracasei*, and *Lactobacillus plantarum* modified the fecal microbiota composition.

Prebiotics not only play a protective role within a symbiotic but also provide a source of fermentable energy to the probiotic component of the symbiotic. Adding prebiotics to probiotic yogurts has been observed to improve the storage stability of the probiotic [18].

The protection of a probiotic by a prebiotic could be used in encapsulation techniques. Many probiotic encapsulation techniques rely on the use of carbohydrates as either carrier (e.g., resistant starch) and/or coating materials. Certain strains of bifidobacteria have been observed to have an affinity for resistant starch [19].

Prebiotics have also been shown to protect a probiotic such as *Lactobacillus rhamnosus* GG during spray-drying. However, Capela et al. [18] observed reduced survival of probiotics during freeze-drying of synbiotic yogurt.

7.4 PLANT STEROLS AND STANOLS AS FUNCTIONAL DAIRY INGREDIENTS

The Scientific Committee on Food (SCF) in its opinion "General view on the long-term effects of the intake of elevated levels of phytosterols from multiple dietary sources, with particular attention to the effects on β-carotene" of September 26, 2002, indicated that there was no evidence of additional benefits at intakes higher than 3 g/day and that high intakes may induce undesirable effects and that it was therefore prudent to avoid plant sterol intakes exceeding 3 g/day. Furthermore, the European Food Safety Authority's (EFSA) Panel on Dietetic Products, Nutrition, and Allergies in its opinion "on a request from the Commission related to a Novel Food application from Forbes Medi-Tech for approval of plant sterol-containing milk-based beverages" of November 25, 2003, agreed with the conclusions of the SCF, in its opinion on applications for approval of a variety of plant sterol-enriched foods of March 5, 2003, came to the conclusion that the addition of phytosterols is safe, provided that the daily consumption does not exceed 3 g.

Commission Regulation (EC) No. 608/2004 [20] concerning the labeling of foods and food ingredients with added phytostanol esters ensures that consumers receive the information necessary in order to avoid excessive intake of added phytosterols/phytostanols.

Phytosterols and phytostanols are sterols and stanols that are extracted from plants and may be presented as free sterols and stanols or esterified with food-grade fatty acids. Phytosterols and phytostanols extracted from sources other than vegetable oil suitable for food have to be free from contaminants, best ensured by a purity of more than 99% of the phytosterol/phytostanol ingredient.

Phytosterols or plant sterols are lipophilic naturally occurring compounds that are structurally related to cholesterol, but they differ in their side chain substitutions at the C-24 position. Over 40 plant sterols have been identified so far in nature. The major phytosterols are β-sitosterol, campesterol, stigmasterol, and avenasterol. Rapeseed oil contains a small amount of brassicasterol. Other phytosterols are the so-called stanols (plant stanols or phytostanols), which are saturated phytosterols that are less abundant in nature but can be produced by 5-α hydrogenation of the corresponding phytosterols (e.g., sitostanol and campestanol) [21].

Sterols in plants are found in the free form or esterified to fatty acids or as steryl glycosides. Plant sterols are present in Western diets in amounts similar to those of dietary cholesterol (150–400 mg/day), with vegetarian diets containing about 50% higher amounts. The main dietary source of plant sterols is vegetable oils such as corn, sunflower, soybean, and rapeseed oils [22]. Phytosterols are not endogenously synthesized in humans and are derived solely from the diet. There is no known role for phytosterols in human nutrition.

It has been recently reported that phytosterols that are naturally present in commercial corn oil significantly reduce cholesterol absorption in humans [23] and there is some evidence that naturally occurring plant sterols might reduce blood cholesterol to a small degree [21].

Margarines and butter appear as ideal vehicles for plant sterols because of their strong lipophilic nature. Actually, the first food fortified with phytosterols was a margarine, Benecol, already in 1995; stanols were added because the evidence available suggested that they had a greater blood cholesterol-lowering potential than sterols and because the amount of stanols absorbed from the gut was very low [24]. However, cream cheese, mayonnaises, salad dressings, yogurts, and other foods are also intended as phytosterol-enriched foods.

Esterification of phytosterols with long-chain fatty acids increases their lipid solubility and facilitates their incorporation into these foods [25].

7.4.1   EFFICACY OF PLANT STANOL ESTERS VERSUS PLANT STEROL ESTERS: DAIRY PRODUCTS FORTIFIED WITH STEROLS AND STANOLS

First studies indicated that sitostanol was more effective than sitosterol in displacing cholesterol from micelles *in vivo* [26] and in reducing blood total cholesterol (Tc) and low-density lipoprotein cholesterol (LDLc) levels [27]. This has also been observed more recently [28].

Weststrate and Meijer [29] included normolipidemic subjects in their study following their habitual diet except that their habitual spreads were replaced by test margarine-containing plant stanols (Benecol), soybean oil distillate sterols (Henkel Corporation, LaGrange, GA, USA), rice bran sterols (Tsuno, Wakayama, Japan), or sheanut sterols (Loders Croklaan, Wormerveer, the Netherlands). It was shown that unhydrogenated soy sterols were as effective as a stanol ester margarine in lowering blood cholesterol concentrations.

Trautwein et al. [30] reported that 4,4'-dimethylsterol esters (of both sterols and stanols) caused a weaker cholesterol-lowering effect compared with the 4-desmethylsterols.

However, plant sterols and stanols interfere with the absorption of carotenoids as deduced from the reduction of carotenoid blood levels. Other fat-soluble vitamins, such as vitamin E and tocopherols, may also be affected, although to a lesser extent than β-carotene. This problem, the observed effects and the likely mechanisms implicated, has to be considered for an appropriate assessment of the risks associated with consumption of phytosterol-enriched products, particularly in a long-term perspective. The decreases in blood carotenoids appear to plateau when doses of sterols or stanols reached 2.2 g/day and amounted to a reduction of 33% after 1-year consumption of an enriched margarine providing 3 g/day [25].

The Committee has very recently expressed an opinion on three other applications for products based on phytosterols and phytosterol esters [31]. These included submissions by "Oy Karl Fazer AB" (plant sterol-enriched bakery products, grain-based snack products, and gum arabicum pills), "Pouttu Ltd" (meat products that are plant sterol-enriched frankfurters, sausages and cold cuts), and "Teriaka Ltd" (plant sterol-enriched fat ingredient Diminicol planned to be added to yogurts, fresh cheese, margarine, and fruit–milk drinks).

The early recommendation of the Committee for the phytosterol profile of phytosterol esters of fatty acids was updated and extended to unesterified phytosterols/phytostanols resulting in the following phytosterol/phytostanol profile acceptable in general [31]: up to 80% β-sitosterol, 15% β-sitostanol, 40% campesterol, 5% campestanol, 30% stigmasterol, 3% brassicasterol, and 3% other phytosterols.

Plant sterols of vegetable oil origin are derived from deodorized distillate from one or more of the following vegetable sources: soybean, corn, canola, sunflower seed, cottonseed, and peanut.

The esterification is made through *trans*-esterification with food-grade fatty acid esters and free sterols. Food-grade oil is methylated with methanol using sodium methylate as a catalyst. The resulting methyl ester is used to *trans*-esterify free sterols under mild vacuum and 100°C.

The application describes (as an example) the manufacturing process of bakery products, snacks, yogurt, ketchup, and dressing [32]. During the manufacture of the final product, sterols will not be exposed to especially high temperatures, high air pressure, or vigorous stirring. It can be stated that phytosterols are relatively stable compounds due to their chemical structure. The applicant presents examples of the effect of the production method on the concentration and the stability of phytosterols in final products. In bakery products, baking in the oven has not been proved to have any marked effects on the concentration or the composition of phytosterols when the sterol concentration is at the desired level of 1–5%. However, enrichment at higher concentrations (10–15%) is technologically problematic and results in significant losses during the process. No changes in the concentration of sterols were detected in toasted rye bread or wheat rolls, either when flour was kept in a cold store or when bread was kept in a freezer over a 2–3-month period.

Plant sterol-enriched food (Benecol margarine, containing esterified stanols) was first retailed in 1995 in Finland. Later on, other Benecol products (fresh cheese, snack bars, salad dressing, and yogurt) were launched on the market in Finland, Benelux, the United Kingdom, Ireland, Sweden, Denmark, and the United States. The recommended intake is based on 2 g/day of plant stanols. Yearly about 200,000 Finns eat Benecol products every day. By the year 2001, more than 12.5 million Benecol product packages with either Benecol margarine or fresh cheese have been sold in Finland [25].

Raisio introduced stanol-containing spreads into Finland in 1995. Raisio of Finland produces esterified stanol derived from soy and tall oil sterols and this has been added into milk, butter milk, yogurt, drinking yogurt, single shot drink, and cheese spread by various dairy companies. These products are sold under the Benecol brand with distribution of at least one of these products in 16 countries. Benecol is marketed in the United States and the European Union excluding the Scandinavian countries by McNeil.

Unilever produces a semiskimmed milk drink containing plant sterols derived from soy and other vegetable oils as well as yogurt and a mini drink as Flora Pro. Activ brands and Lipton Take control.

Suppliers of vegetable oil sterol esters include Cargill (Corowise), Cognis (Vegapure), and Archer Daniels Midland (Cardioaid). MultiBene produces free and esterified sterols for a wide variety of dairy (e.g., Yoplait yogurt sold by Glanbia) and nondairy products including ketchup and spicy sauces. Other dairy products include a low-fat cheese containing Corowise phytosterol esters. Danone sells sterol containing yogurt under the Danacol brand. Triple Crown AB sells free sterols from vegetable oils and tall oil [33].

Teriaka from Finland sells sterols in a special formulation of free sterols or stanols partly dissolved in fat and in semicrystalline form and is approved in Europe, the United States, and Mexico. Adumin is a small Israeli company marketing encapsulated free sterols in cooking oil.

The Canadian company Forbes Meditech produces pine-derived free sterols and stanols (tall oil) under Reducol brand sold by many dairy companies such as Fayrefield Foods sold by Tesco in the United Kingdom and Pirkka brand sold by Kesko in Finland.

The largest supplier of tall oil in the United States is Arboris LLC, followed by Cargill that supplies wood-derived sterols. However, particular attention has to be paid on the identity of genetically modified (GM) soy. Prime Pharma derives its tall oil sterols from Derives Resiniques et Terpeniques (DRT), the largest European supplier of tall oil.

7.4.2 PLANT STEROLS AND STANOLS IN CHOLESTEROL REDUCTION

Plant sterols and stanols lower LDL cholesterol by 5–10% in dairy products and spreads. Volpe et al. [34] showed the effect of low-fat yogurt containing 1 g/day of soybean-derived sterols in 30 men and women with elevated LDL cholesterol. LDL cholesterol was lowered by 6.2% after 4 weeks compared with placebo. Eleven of the volunteers continued for another month on 2 g/day of sterols and achieved a lowering of LDL by 15.6%, although there was no comparison with placebo.

Clifton et al. [35] studied 58 people who ate 1.6 g/day of esterified sterols in either milk, yogurt, bread, or breakfast cereals for 3 weeks each. Serum total and LDL cholesterol levels were significantly lowered by consumption of phytosterol-enriched foods: milk (8.7% and 15.9%) and yogurt (5.6% and 8.6%). Serum LDL cholesterol levels fell significantly by 6.5% with bread and 5.4% with cereal.

Mensink et al. [36] added a 1 g/day of esterified plant stanols in a low-fat yogurt in 60 subjects in a 4-week placebo-controlled randomized study. LDL cholesterol fell by 13.7% compared with placebo. β-Carotene/LDL cholesterol ratio fell by 14.4%, whereas the total tocopherol/LDL cholesterol level increased.

Korpela et al. [37] added nonesterified sterols (2 g/day) in low-fat yogurt, low-fat hard cheeses, and low-fat fresh soft cheeses and lowered the LDL cholesterol by 9.8% compared with sterol-free products.

Doornbos et al. [38] studied 185 people and showed that LDL cholesterol was lowered by 9.4% when a single shot yogurt drink containing 2 g plant sterols was taken with a meal compared with 5.1–6.9% when taken without a meal. Varying the fat content of the drink from 2.2% to 3.3% had no effect.

Noakes et al. [39] fed 40 subjects either a sterol-enriched yogurt (1.7 g/day) or a stanol-enriched yogurt (1.8 g/day) or a placebo yogurt and showed a 5–6% lowering of LDL cholesterol after 3 weeks.

Jauhiainen et al. [40] conducted a randomized double-blind parallel group in 67 mildly hypercholesterolemic volunteers. The subjects in the stanol group consumed a hard cheese enriched with 2 g of plant sterols per day for 5 weeks. The LDL/cholesterol ratio decreased by 10.3% in the stanol group compared with the control group that did not consume any plant stanols. There were no significant changes in HDL, triglycerides, or apolipoprotein B concentrations between the two groups. The lack of change in the latter shows that LDL particles have become smaller and contain less cholesterol but are not reduced in number.

7.5 HA HYDROLYSATES FOR PREVENTION AND TREATMENT OF CMA

HA protein hydrolysates are used as functional ingredients in infant formulas and are of high nutritional and therapeutic value.

HA cow's milk-based formulas are administered during the first 6 months of life in infants at risk that are partially breastfed or not breast-fed at all [41].

They are added to prevent CMA, mainly an IgE-mediated hypersensitivity reaction. They are classified as extensively hydrolyzed formulas (eHF) and partially hydrolyzed formulas (pHF) based on the degree of proteolysis [42].

Depending on primary or secondary prevention of CMA, the HA formulas used are different. When infants are already sensitized to cow's milk proteins (CMPs), low amounts of cow's milk may trigger an allergic reaction and only eHF or amino acids formulas should be used for infants with established CMA, whereas pHF should be used for primary prevention of CMA in nonsensitized at-risk infants [43]. pHF may be of benefit in long-term protection against CMA. Such formulas are sufficiently reduced in allergenicity [44].

These protein hydrolysates should be rich in low-molecular-weight peptides, especially di- and tripeptides, with the least possible quantity of free amino acids. Quality control of these products includes degree of hydrolysis (percentage of peptide bonds released by enzymatic hydrolysis), *in vitro* characterization of peptide size, and determination of allergenicity. The safety and efficacy of these formulas can only be determined by clinical trials using appropriate standards. The presence of reactive epitopes in the hydrolysates, very important for the suitability of these HA products, is determined by *in vitro* immunochemical assays such as enzyme-linked immunosorbent assay (ELISA), radioallergosorbent (RAST) and enzyme allergosorbent (EAST) tests, and Western blotting techniques.

Enzymatic proteolysis and heat treatment are normally used to reduce the content of β-lactoglobulin and other intact proteins and therefore reduce the antigenicity of milk proteins in the production of pHP or eHF from cow's milk. These techniques are also used to prepare HA formulas based on protein hydrolysates from other sources [45].

Ultrafiltration is used as a posthydrolysis process to remove residual high-molecular-weight peptides and proteins and the enzymes used in the digestion. The residual antigenicity of infant formulas will depend on the hydrolysis grade obtained, the enzyme specificity, and the filtration technique used. However, residual allergenicity has been reported in several commercial preparations [46], which could be due to inaccessibility of some epitopes to proteases even in the denatured protein.

Most recently there has been great interest in the development of new HA hydrolysates with limited hydrolysis using high-pressure and microwave irradiation techniques. Excess hydrolysis might cause low palatability, off flavor, bitterness, and loss of nutritional value.

7.6   OLIGOSACCHARIDES

According to IUB-IUPAC terminology [47], oligosaccharides have been defined as carbohydrates with a degree of polymerization up to 10. Oligosaccharides have also been defined as ranging from a degree of polymerization of 2 up to 20 and more [48].

Free oligosaccharides are natural constituents of all placental mammals' milk and can be found in bacteria, fungi, and plants [49]. They are derived from hydrolysis of dietary polymers during digestion. They can be extracted from natural sources and can be synthesized from monomers and/or small oligosaccharides, or derived from hydrolysis of natural polymers.

Nondigestible oligosaccharides such as fructo-oligosaccharides, lactulose, and *trans*-galacto-oliogosaccharides are effective prebiotics since they confer the degree of selective fermentation required. Other prebiotics are xylo-oligosaccharides, soybean oligosaccharides, and isomalto-oligosaccharides. Lactulose, the lactose derivative, is a very well-known laxative also displaying prebiotic behavior in the colon at sublaxative doses.

Human milk contains considerable amounts of oligosaccharides showing that they play an important role during postnatal period. Human milk oligosaccharides contribute to the establishment of specific intestinal flora dominated by bifidobacteria, the postnatal stimulation of the immune system, the defense activity of human milk against viral and bacterial infections, and the enhancement of the bioavailability of minerals.

Human milk contains 0.7–1.2 g oligosaccharides/L, making the oligosaccharide fraction the major component of human milk [48]. The monomers of human milk oligosaccharides are D-glucose, D-galactose, *N*-acetylglucosamine, L-fucose, and sialic acid (*N*-acetyl neuraminic acid). All core molecules carry lactose at their reducing end with few exceptions. The activity of several fucosyltransferases and sialyltransferases results in an attachment at a different position in the core molecule in different linkages [49]. Fucosylated oligosaccharides, representing the majority of oligosaccharides in human milk, could not be detected in cow's milk, goat's milk, or sheep's milk. On the other hand, 3′- and 6′-galactosyl-lactose and 3′- and 6′-sialyl-lactose could be detected in both animal milks and human milk [50].

Moreover, oligosaccharides of more simple structures than human milk oligosaccharides have been used as components in several dietary products to mimic the beneficial effect of human milk oligosaccharides [51].

The most important prebiotic oligosaccharides, larger than disaccharides, of nonmilk origin, which show significant bifidogenic effect in human feces, are galacto-oligosaccharides prepared using the enzymatic synthesis of lactose; fructo-oligosaccharides/inulin extracted from natural sources are prepared using the enzymatic hydrolysis of natural polymers and the enzymatic synthesis of sucrose. Palatinose/isomaltulose are also prepared by the enzymatic synthesis of sucrose. Soybean oligosaccharide is extracted from natural sources, lactosucrose is prepared using the enzymatic synthesis of lactose, and xylo-oligosaccharides are prepared by the enzymatic hydrolysis of corncob xylan.

Polysaccharide hydrolysis used to manufacture fructo- and xylo-oligosaccharides as prebiotics gives a higher degree of control over the molecular weight distribution of the products influencing the rheological properties and leading to persistent selective fermentation toward distal regions of the colon. Endoglucanases in enzyme membrane reactors can be used in the controlled hydrolysis of polysaccharides. Controlling factors such as residence time and the ratio of enzyme to substrate, dextran was converted into different oligodextran preparations with average molecular weight varying from trisaccharide up to 12,000 Da. These are proved to be very effective in gut model systems with selective fermentation extending through to the third vessel (mimicking the distal colon) [52]. This approach has been extended to the system of bacterial extracellular polysaccharides (EPS). Suitable enzymes for the degradation of these polysaccharides can be isolated from bacteriophages. Phage enzymes in conjunction with other glycosidases to remodel the resultant oligosaccharides could generate a huge diversity of oligosaccharide structures.

The most extensive studies exist for fructans, which are linear or branched fructose polymers and are either β2-1-linked inulins or β2-6-linked levans. Inulin-type fructans can be easily extracted from plant sources such as asparagus, garlic, leek, onion, artichoke, and chicory roots and thus have been widely used as a functional ingredient in dietary products.

Galacto-oligosaccharides are synthesized from lactose via enzymatic *trans*-galactosylation using β-galactosidases of bacterial origin (*Bacillus circulans*) [53].

Oligosaccharides are involved in many functional effects related to the gastrointestinal tract and the systemic processes. According to Loo et al. [54], oligosaccharides affect intestinal flora and bowel habit. They also reported that they might affect mineral absorption and lipid metabolism and the end products of bacterial metabolism might play a role in colon cancer prevention.

The prebiotic concept is based on the fact that these dietary ingredients are nondigestible, reach the colon, and can be utilized by health-promoting bacteria such as bifidobacteria and lactobacilli. The human intestine lacks enzymes able to hydrolyze β-glycosidic linkages with the exception of lactose.

Several nonmilk oligosaccharides such as galacto-oligosaccharides and fructans stimulate bifidobacteria and lactobacilli, as shown by clinical trials in human infants and adults. A mixture of galacto-oligosaccharides and fructans is very effective in the stimulation of bifidobacteriae and changes the stool characteristics to become closer to those found in breastfed infants [55,56]. Hence, these show that they can partially mimic the effects of human milk oligosaccharides.

Finally, according to Lidestri et al. [57], an infant formula supplemented with a mixture of galacto-oligosaccharides (90%) and inulin (10%) resulted in higher renal excretion of calcium compared to that found in infants fed with a nonsupplemented formula indicating calcium absorption.

Prebiotics added to the diet are characterized by techniques such as DNA probing and molecular fingerprinting including fluorescent *in situ* hybridization (FISH), restriction fragment length polymorphism (RFLP), ribosomal DNA sequencing, ribotyping, and direct amplification.

Second-generation prebiotics have started to appear. These include higher molecular weight oligomers with targeted activities in the distal colon where colonic disorder usually takes place [58]. There are several ways in which they reach the distal colon. It is assumed that the longer the oligosaccharide, the slower the fermentation and the further the prebiotic effect will penetrate through the colon. Long-chain inulin, for example, may exert a prebiotic effect in more distal colonic regions than the lower molecular weight fructo-oligosaccharide, which may be more quickly fermented in the saccharolytic proximal bowel. This approach has led to industrial forms of inulin/FOS mixtures with controlled chain length distributions (Synergie II by Oraft, Belgium). Moreover, plant-derived inulin is intrinsically limited in its degree polymerization (DP), microbial fructans such as levan (a polysaccharide with molecular weight measured in millions) might be a better starting point for oligosaccharide generation. This polysaccharide will be probably more persistent through the distal colon since it will take longer to be digested in the colon.

Moreover, modification of a proportion of the residues in an inulin or isomalto-oligosaccharide chain might lead to partial resistance to enzymic attack. Modification might also bring changes in physicochemical properties such as a fatty mouthfeel from starch acylation.

The most prevalent cancer in humans is colon cancer. Prebiotics may protect against the development of colon cancer through the production of protective metabolites such as butyrate, a common fermentation end product stimulating apoptosis in colonic cancer cell lines, produced in the gut by clostridia and eubacteria [59].

Another mechanism by which prebiotics may protect against the development of colon cancer is subversion of colonic metabolism away from protein and lipid metabolism. Prebiotics might induce a shift in bacterial metabolism in the colon toward more benign end products, for example, shift the metabolism of clostridia and bacteroides away from proteolysis to saccharolysis.

One of the most strong health benefits proposed for prebiotics is the barrier function against invasion of gastrointestinal pathogens. There are many ways by which lactobacilli and bifidobacteria can inhibit pathogens. Fermentation of carbohydrates results in the production of short-chain fatty acids (SCFAs) [60]. These reduce luminal pH in the colon to levels below those at which pathogens such as *Escherichia coli* can effectively multiply. Moreover, bifidobacteria and lactobacilli can inhibit pathogens by producing antimicrobial agents active against salmonellae, campylobacters, and *E. coli*.

Glycobiology is developing antiadhesive prebiotics incorporating receptor sites for common gut pathogens. Many intestinal pathogens utilize monosaccharides or short oligosaccharide sequences as receptors, and knowledge of these receptor sites has relevance for biologically enhanced prebiotics. The colonization process includes binding of pathogens to these receptors as a first step. These agents are multivalent derivatives of the sugars and act as blocking factors removing the adherent pathogen [61]. These molecules should have enough antiadhesive activity to inhibit the binding of low levels of pathogens. Such multifunctional prebiotics thought of as decoy oligosaccharides should increase host resistance to infection.

7.7   CPPs AS FUNCTIONAL INGREDIENTS

CPPs are casein-derived peptides that have phosphorous bound via monoester linkages to seryl residues [62].

CPPs have the ability to bind to a range of macroelements such as calcium, magnesium, and iron and trace elements such as zinc, barium, chromium, nickel, cobalt, and selenium. Moreover, the enhanced dietary bioavailability of calcium from milk and dairy products may be attributed to the presence of CPPs. This is due to the fact that *in vitro* CPPs possess the ability to bind and solubilize calcium at high pH, corresponding to the alkaline conditions occurring in the small intestine where maximal massive vitamin D-independent calcium absorption takes place. Many companies market CPP-containing/enriched milk protein hydrolysate products.

CPPs are produced by enzymatic digestion of whole casein or fractions enriched in specific individual caseins. Hydrolysis is carried out at neutral to alkaline pH (7.0–8.0). CPPs present in the resulting clarified hydrolysate supernatants can be aggregated on inclusion of a range of mineral salts around neutral pH with calcium used as the major aggregating agent. The aggregated CPPs can be precipitated with hydrophilic solvents such as ethanol, methanol, propanol, butanol, and acetone and have been collected by centrifugation. Ultrafiltration through defined molecular mass cut-off membranes has been used at pilot scale to separate aggregated CPPs from nonphosphorylated peptides [63]. Alternatively, CPPs have been isolated/enriched from calcium/ethanol-precipitated aggregates using many ion-exchange techniques. Fractions containing isolated/enriched CPPs are then subjected to spray-drying or freeze-drying.

CPPs bind and solubilize minerals such as calcium. The highly anionic phosphorylated regions in CPPs are responsible for mineral binding. However, the amino acid sequence around this anionic hydrophilic domain also seems to play a significant role in mineral binding [64].

The calcium-binding properties of CPPs have been studied using calcium selective electrodes, microultrafiltration methods in combination with atomic absorption, competitive assays with Chelex resin, and capillary zone electrophoresis.

CPPs show protective effects in cancer development. The most probable target site for the cytomodulatory action seems to be the gastrointestinal tract. The antipro-liferative effect of milk-protein-derived peptides as well as other minor milk compo-nents in colon cancer cell lines suggests that they could have a role in the prevention of colon cancer by blocking hyperproliferation of the epithelium and by promoting apoptosis [65].

Cytochemical experiments carried out on CPP preparations using a variety of human cell culture model systems did not show a cytotoxic response of CPPs toward human cells, provided that the orally ingested doses correspond to reasonable con-centrations for use in functional foods.

It should also be noted that the allergenic potential of CPPs, following their con-sumption by the human population that shows allergenic reactions to caseins, should be considered in the use of CPPs as functional food ingredients/neutraceuticals. More specifically, IgE displays a higher binding affinity for phosphorylated caseins than the corresponding dephosphorylated derivatives.

Potential applications of CPPs include prevention of osteoporosis, recalcification of bones after fracture, hypertension, prevention of dental caries, Mg deficiency in pregnancy and old age, anemia, oligoelement supplementation, and humanization of bovine milk by increasing phosphorus levels [66].

7.8 CLA AS A FUNCTIONAL DAIRY INGREDIENT

CLA is usually found in dairy products and meat from ruminants. Pariza and Hargraves [67] found a fraction isolated from grilled minced beef that contained isomers of octadecadienoic acid having two conjugated double bonds and could inhibit carcinogenesis.

Out of many positional and geometrical isomers of CLA, the 9 *cis*, 11 *trans*-octadecadienoic acid (or 9c,11t-18:2) predominates in food products.

Milk and dairy products (butter, cheese, and yogurt) seem to contain the highest amounts of CLA [68]. For dairy products, CLA contents up to 30.0 mg/g fat were reported [69].

Plant oils or margarine contain only small amounts of CLA. CLAs are formed as a result of industrial processing—oil refining processes (mainly deodorization) and catalytic process of hydrogenation to produce margarine. Otherwise they appear in oils due to high-temperature treatments.

The naturally occurring CLA in milk is formed using two different pathways. In the first pathway, the bioconversion of polyunsaturated fatty acids (PUFA) takes place in the rumen. The ingested dietary unsaturated fatty acids, for example, lino-leic acid, are metabolized by enzymes of different bacteria present in the rumen [70]. Various *trans* fatty acids appear in this biohydrogenation pathway as intermediates. 9c,11t-18:2 is formed during this bacterial transformation. Kepler and Tove [71] iso-lated a linoleate isomerase from the rumen bacterium *Butyrivibrio fibrisolvens*, responsible for the isomerization of linoleic acid into 9c,11t-18:2 in a first step. Then the double bond in position $\Delta 9$ is hydrogenated to form vaccenic acid. The last step includes hydrogenation of vaccenic acid into stearic acid. The intermediates (9c,11t-18:2 and vaccenic acid) accumulate and are absorbed into the intestine.

Vaccenic acid also leads to the formation of 9c,11t-18:2. Moreover, following Δ9 desaturation in adipose tissue and in the mammary gland of the lactating cow, 9c,11t-18:2 is produced. The endogenous synthesis in the mammary gland is very important as ~60% of CLA in milk fat is formed via this pathway in the lactating cow. Regarding the second most important CLA isomer in milk fat, the 7t, 9c-18:2, it is only formed via the Δ9 desaturation pathway of 9t-18:1 [72].

Various factors influence the CLA content in milk such as the food of the ruminant, the season (decreased CLA content during winter, with the lowest level in March and increased level in the summer, positively correlated to the grazing period), the animal breeding type, the number of lactation times, and the current lactation state [73]. The lactation stage can affect CLA content in milk since body fat stores of the cow are mobilized at the beginning of lactation. Pasture in spring time contains higher amounts of PUFAs, which caused a higher bacterial biohydrogenation in the rumen [74].

Commercial production of CLAs is carried out by alkali isomerization of linoleic acid-producing complex CLA mixtures containing two predominant isomers.

Dehydration of hydroxyl fatty acids has been used to prepare conjugated fatty acids. For example, dehydration of ricinoleic acid, an expensive starting material, can prepare 9c,11t-18:2.

Zinc in aqueous n-propanol is very selective in the reduction of the acetylenic bond to the z-olefinic bond to prepare 9c,11t-18:2.

Pure CLA isomers can also be produced by total stereoselective multiple step synthesis in small quantities; the isomeric purity can be higher than 98%. Stereoselective synthesis guarantees the exact chemical structure of the final molecule and limits the formation of by-products due to several purification procedures carried out during the synthesis. These syntheses could allow the preparation of labeled molecules of CLA with deuterium, C^{13}, or C^{14}.

Functional benefits of CLA include high anticarcinogenic effects, decreased LDL cholesterol in rabbits, decrease in atherosclerotic lesions, protection against immune-induced cachexia (growth suppression or weight loss), and questionable antidiabetic effects. Human long-term experiments need to be carried out. The only experiments carried out today in humans have investigated the influence on body composition with controversial results.

More experiments using isolated isomers to evaluate the effects of each CLA isomer are required. Finally, toxicological risks need to be evaluated since little data on the safety aspects of CLAs are available.

Finally, CLAs, due to the conjugated double bond system, are seen as more sensitive to oxidation, or isomerization during heat treatment than linoleic acid. It has been demonstrated that food processing methods such as frying, baking, boiling, or microwaving did not affect or change CLA content in grilled hamburger beef patties [75]. Only intensive heating for 15 min, using temperatures higher than 200°C, could lead to isomerization of CLA in milk [76].

The influence of storage on the CLA content was also tested in butter, yogurt, and sour cream with no modification of CLA content detected [77]. However, the use of different fermentation cultures, processing temperatures, or ripening periods could affect the CLA level in the final food product.

7.9   LEGISLATION RELATED TO FOODSTUFFS INTENDED FOR SPECIFIC NUTRITIONAL USES IN THE EUROPEAN UNION

According to the Directive 89/398/EEC (entry into force 16/5/1990), foodstuffs for particular nutritional uses are foodstuffs that, owing to their special composition or manufacturing process, should be clearly distinguishable from foodstuffs for normal consumption. A particular nutritional use must fulfill the particular nutritional requirements (i) of certain categories of persons whose digestive processes or metabolism are disturbed, (ii) of certain categories of persons who are in a special physiological condition, and (iii) of infants or young children in good health. Such specific Directives may cover in particular essential requirements as to the nature or the composition of the products, provisions regarding the quality of raw materials, hygiene requirements, permitted changes, a list of additives, provisions regarding labeling, presentation, and advertising, sampling procedures, and methods of analysis for checking compliance with the requirements. To permit efficient official monitoring of those foodstuffs, the following specific provisions shall apply: (i) when a product is placed on the market for the first time, the manufacturer or the importer shall notify the competent authority of the Member State where the product is being marketed by forwarding it a model of a label used for the product; (ii) in the case where the same product is subsequently placed on the market in another Member State, the manufacturer or the importer shall provide the competent authority with the same information together with a notification of the recipient of the first notification; (iii) where necessary, the competent authority shall be empowered to require the manufacturer or the importer to produce the scientific work and the data establishing the product's compliance with the Directive; (iv) Member States shall communicate to the Commission the identity of the competent authorities and any other useful information on them; and (v) 4 years after notification of this Directive, the Commission shall send the Council a report.

The Directive 91/321/EEC (entry into force 30/5/1991) laid down compositional and labeling requirements for infant formulas and follow-on formulas intended for use by infants in good health in the Community. It also provides for Member States to give effect to the principles and aims of the International Code of Marketing of Breast-Milk Substitutes dealing with marketing, information, and responsibilities of health authorities. The essential composition of infant formulas when reconstituted as instructed by the manufacturer comprises (1) energy (minimum: 250 kJ, maximum: 315 kJ), (2) proteins: (a) formulas manufactured from unmodified CMPs (minimum: 0.56 g/100 kJ, maximum: 0.7 g/100 kJ), (b) formulas manufactured from modified CMPs (minimum: 0.45 g/100 kJ, maximum: 0.7 g/100 kJ), (c) formulas manufactured from soya protein isolates, alone or in a mixture with CMPs (minimum: 0.56 g/100 kJ, maximum: 0.7 g/100 kJ), (d) in all cases, the addition of amino acids is permitted solely for the purpose of improving the nutritional value of the proteins, and only in the proportions necessary for that purpose. (3) Lipids (minimum: 0.8 g/100 kJ, maximum: 1.5 g/100 kJ). The use of the following substances is prohibited: (a) sesame seed oil, cotton seed oil, fats containing more than 8% *trans* isomers of fatty acids; (b) lauric acid; (c) myristic acid; and (d) linoleic acid. (4) Carbohydrates (minimum: 1.7 g/100 kJ, maximum: 3.4 g/100 kJ). Only the following carbohydrates may be

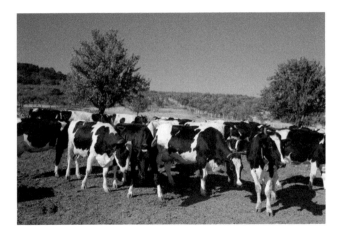

FIGURE 1.1 Holstein cows before milking.

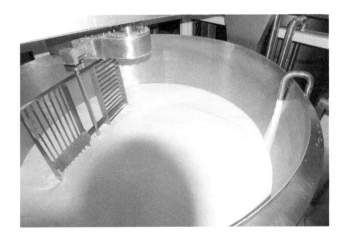

FIGURE 1.2 Yogurt culture addition in a tank.

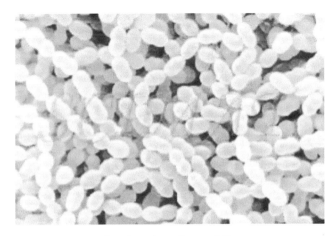

FIGURE 1.3 *Streptococcus salivarius* subsp. *thermophilus.*

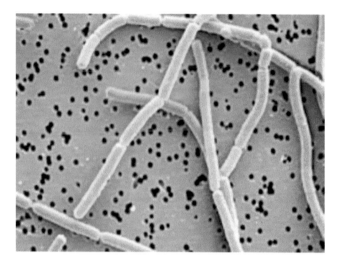

FIGURE 1.4 *Lactobacillus delbrueckii* subsp. *bulgaricus.*

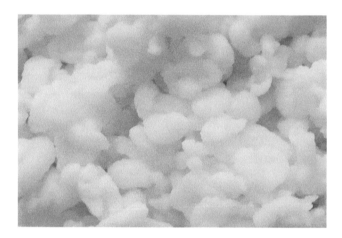

FIGURE 1.5 *Lactobacillus delbrueckii* subsp. *bulgaricus* in coagulated milk.

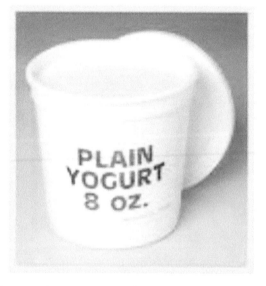

FIGURE 1.6 Plain yogurt in consumer container.

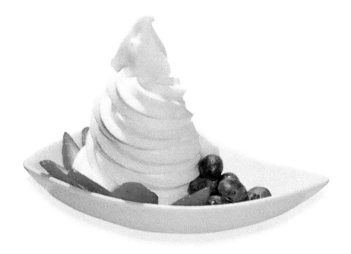

FIGURE 1.7 Low fat frozen yogurt with fruits.

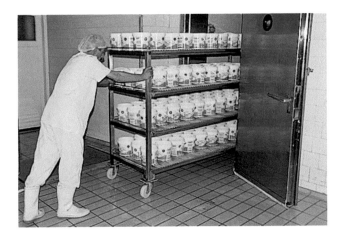

FIGURE 1.8 Yogurt containers on the shelves of an incubation room at 42–43°C.

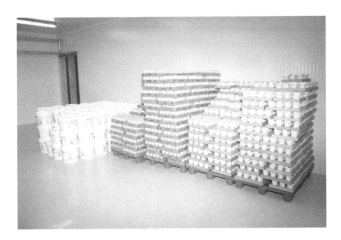

FIGURE 1.9 Yogurt in cold storage room after incubation at 5–22°C.

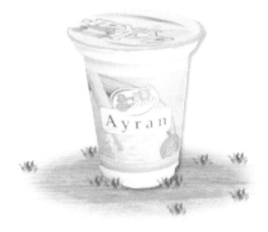

FIGURE 1.10   Single serve ayran package.

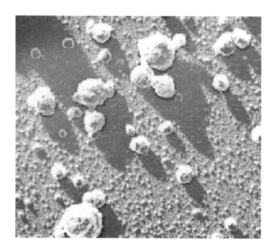

FIGURE 1.11   Casein micelles in milk.

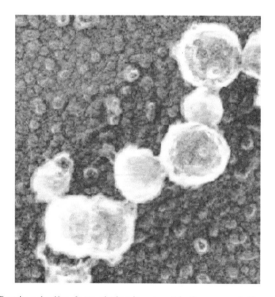

FIGURE 1.12   Casein micelles form chains in yogurt before coagulation.

used: lactose, maltose, sucrose, malto-dextrins, glucose syrup or dried glucose syrup, precooked starch, and gelatinized starch naturally free of gluten. (5) Mineral substances: formulas manufactured from CMPs per 100 kJ sodium, potassium, chloride, calcium, phosphorus, magnesium, iron, zinc, copper, and iodine.

Directive 96/5/EC (entry into force 8/3/1996) covers foodstuffs for particular nutritional use fulfilling the particular requirements of infants and young children in good health in the Community and are intended for use by infants while they are being weaned, and by young children as a supplement to their diet and/or for their progressive adaptation to ordinary food. They comprise (a) "processed cereal-based foods" that are divided into the following four categories: simple cereals that are or have to be reconstituted with milk or other appropriate nutritious liquids, cereals with an added high-protein food that are or have to be reconstituted with water or other protein-free liquid, pastas that are to be used after cooking in boiling water or other appropriate liquids, rusks, and biscuits that are to be used either directly or, after pulverization, with the addition of water, milk, or other suitable liquids, and (b) "baby foods" other than processed cereal-based foods. There should be an arrangement of the quantities of cereal content, protein, carbohydrates, lipids, minerals, and vitamins.

In Directive 96/8/EC (entry into force 17/3/1997), foods for use in energy-restricted diets for weight reduction are specially formulated foods that, when used as instructed by the manufacturer, replace the whole or part of the total daily diet. They are divided into two categories: (a) products presented as a replacement for the whole of the daily diet and (b) products presented as a replacement for one or more meals of the daily diet. The labeling of the products concerned shall bear the following mandatory particulars: (a) the available energy value expressed in kilojoule and kilocalorie, and the content of proteins, carbohydrates, and fat, expressed in numerical form, per specified quantity of the product ready for use as proposed for consumption; (b) the average quantity of each mineral and each vitamin, expressed in numerical form, per specified quantity of the product ready for use as proposed for consumption; (c) instructions for appropriate preparation, when necessary, and a statement as to the importance of following those instructions; (d) if a product, when used as instructed by the manufacturer, provides a daily intake of polyols in excess of 20 g/day, there shall be a statement to the effect that the food may have a laxative effect; (e) a statement on the importance of maintaining an adequate daily fluid intake; and (f) for products for diets: a statement that the product provides adequate amounts of all essential nutrients for the day and a statement that the product should not be used for more than 3 weeks without medical advice shall be included. There should be an arrangement of the quantities of: energy, protein, fat, dietary fiber, vitamins, and minerals.

Directive 1999/21/EC (entry into force 27/4/1999) applies to "dietary foods for special medical purposes," which are a category of foods for particular nutritional uses specially processed or formulated and intended for the dietary management of patients and to be used under medical supervision. They are intended for the exclusive or the partial feeding of patients with a limited impaired or disturbed capacity to take, digest, absorb, metabolize or excrete ordinary foodstuffs or certain nutrients contained therein or metabolites, or with other medically determined nutrient requirements, whose dietary management cannot be achieved only by notification of the normal diet, by other foods for particular nutritional uses, or by a combination of the two. Those foods are classified into the following three categories: (a) nutritionally complete foods with a standard nutrient formulation, which, used in accordance with the manufacturer's instructions, may constitute the sole source of nourishment for the persons for whom they are intended; (b) nutritionally complete foods with a nutrient-adapted formulation specific for a disease, disorder, or medical condition, which, used in accordance with the manufacturer's instructions, may constitute the sole source of nourishment for the persons for whom they are intended; and (c) nutritional incomplete foods with a standard formulation or a nutrient-adapted formulation specific for a disease, disorder, or medical condition, which are not suitable to be used as the sole source of nourishment. The labeling shall bear the following mandatory particulars: (a) the name under which these products are sold as "foods for special medical purposes"; (b) the available energy value and the content of protein, carbohydrate, and fat; (c) the average quantity of each mineral and vitamin; (d) the content of components of protein, carbohydrate, and fat, and of other nutrients and their components; (e) information on the osmolality or osmolarity of the product where appropriate; and (f) information on the origin and nature of the protein and/or protein hydrolysates contained in the product. The labelling shall in addition bear the following particulars, preceded by the words "important notice" or their equivalent: (a) a statement that the product must be used under medical supervision, (b) a statement whether the product is suitable for use as the sole source of nourishment, (c) a statement that the product is intended for a specific age group, (d) where appropriate, a statement that the product poses a health hazard when consumed by persons who do not have the diseases, disorders, or medical conditions for which the product is intended.

Following Directive 2002/46/EC (entry into force 12/7/2002), "food supplements" are foodstuffs, the purpose of which is to supplement the normal diet and which are concentrated sources of nutrients or other substances with a nutritional or physiological effect, alone or in combination, marketed in dose form, namely forms such as capsules, pastilles, tablets, pills, and other similar forms, sachets of powder, ampoules of liquids, drop dispensing bottles, and other similar forms of liquids and powders designed to be taken in measured small unit quantities. Maximum amounts of vitamins and minerals present in food supplements per daily portion of consumption as recommended by the manufacturer shall be set, taking the following into account: (a) upper safe levels of vitamins and minerals established by scientific risk assessment based on generally accepted scientific data, taking into account, as appropriate, the varying degrees of sensitivity of different consumer groups and (b) intake of vitamins and minerals from other dietary sources. Substances that can be used in the manufacture of food supplements are vitamins, minerals, vitamin substances, and mineral substances. The labeling shall bear the following particulars: (a) the names of the categories of nutrients or substances that characterize the product or an indication of the nature of those nutrients or substances, (b) the portion of the product recommended for daily consumption, (c) a warning not to exceed the stated recommended daily dose, (d) a statement to the effect that food supplements should not be used as a substitute for a varied diet, (e) a statement to the effect that the products should be stored out of the reach of young children.

The titles, main points, and comments of the Directives for foodstuffs intended for specific nutritional uses are summarized in Table 7.1.

TABLE 7.1
Directives (Main Points and Comments) Focused on Foodstuffs Intended for Specific Nutritional Uses

Directive—Title	Main Points	Comments
Directive 89/398/EEC (entry into force 16/5/1990) Approximation of the laws of the Member States related to foodstuffs intended for particular nutritional uses	• Concerns the particular nutritional requirements of certain categories of persons • The use of the adjectives "dietetic" or "dietary" is prohibited in the labeling, presentation, and advertising of foodstuffs for normal consumption • Disposal on the retail market in prepackaged form	• Directive 77/94/EEC is repealed by this one amendments • Directives 96/84/EC (entry into force 11/3/1997) and 1999/41/EC (entry into force 8/7/2000) amend this one
Directive 91/321/EEC (entry into force 30/5/1991) Infant formulas and follow-on formulas	• Rules for the marketing of infant formulas and follow-on formulas intended for use by infants in good health in the Community and also provides for Member States to give effect to the principles and aims of the International Code of Marketing of Breast-Milk Substitutes • Stipulation of authorized food ingredients, compositional criteria, substances that may be used in the manufacture of the formulas concerned, sales names, compulsory label information, etc. • Advertising is restricted to publications specializing in baby care and scientific publications	• Directives 96/4/EC (rules for labeling infant formulas and follow-on formulas) 1999/50/EC (reduction of the maximum level of pesticide residues in infant formulas and follow-on formulas to 0.01 mg/kg) (entry into force 22/6/1999), and 2003/14/EC (strengthening of the protection of infants by introducing stronger detective controls for a small number of particularly dangerous pesticides or metabolites of pesticides amend this Directive)
Directive 96/5/EC (entry into force 8/3/1996) Processed cereal-based foods and baby foods for infants and young children	• Applicable for foodstuffs for particular nutritional use that fulfill the particular requirements of infants and young children in good health • Not applicable to milks intended for young children • Processed cereal-based foods and baby foods shall be manufactured from ingredients whose suitability for particular nutritional use by infants and	• Directives 98/36/EC (entry into force 22/6/1998) and 1999/39/EC (entry into force 28/5/1999) amend this one

continued

TABLE 7.1   (continued)

Directive—Title	Main Points	Comments
	young children has been established by generally accepted scientific data • Specific labeling	
Directive 96/8/EC (entry into force 17/3/1997) On foods intended for use in energy-restricted diets for weight reduction	• Foods for use in energy-restricted diets for weight reduction are specially formulated foods that, when used as instructed by the manufacturer, replace the whole or part of the total daily diet • Specific labeling, advertising, and presentation	
Directive 1999/21/EC (entry into force 27/4/1999)	• The formulation of dietary foods for special medical purposes shall be based on sound medical and nutritional principles	
Dietary foodstuffs for special medical purposes	• Specification of the name under which these foodstuffs are sold in the 11 official languages of the European Union • Specific labeling and official monitoring	
Directive 2002/46/EC (entry into force 12/7/2002) Approximation of the laws of the Member States relating to food supplements	• Applicable to concentrated sources of nutrients marketed in dose form in order to supplement nutrient intake in a normal diet • Not applicable to medicinal products • Food supplements may only contain specific vitamins and mineral salts • Specific labeling and monitoring system	

7.9.1   REGULATORY PERSPECTIVE IN THE UNITED STATES

Since functional foods do not possess a legal definition, there are no straightforward regulations (Tables 7.2 and 7.3) apart from some published in the European Union. As a result, it is rather ambiguous whether a new product should be labeled as food, supplement, or drug. Functional foods exist at the interface between foods and drugs. There is no provision in the existing food regulations for foods intended to be consumed to prevent disease. As the current situation stands, dietary supplements will

TABLE 7.2
Applicable Legislation, Regulations, and Guidelines
(www.scisoc.org/aacc/funcfood)

Jurisdiction	1. Legislation	2. Regulations	3. Guidelines
EU	Adopted Legislation agreed at EU level may not be implemented within Member States (countries), published in "L" series of EU Official Journal. Proposal for a directive on claims has been under review for several years but appears stalled	Regulation exists (optional implementation by Member States) in the form of directives	n.a.
U.S.	Nutrition Labeling and Education Act (NLEA) Separate law exists for dietary supplements— Dietary Supplement Health Education Act	Seven-page NLEA Act accessible through the Internet Some allowable label claims under DSHEA remain to be defined	Three publications exist, in addition to the Federal Register. Further advice is available from the Food and Drug Administration (FDA) Office of Food Labeling and the Office of Special Nutritionals
Japan	Sale of FOSHU ("functional foods") is governed by the Nutrition Improvement Act, which also regulates the conduct of a National Nutrition Survey, established a Nutrition Consultation Office and appointment/ certification of Nutrition Instructors. Act provides for approval and labeling of special nutritive foods, enriched foods, and foods for special dietary uses	FOSHU (foods for specified health use) exists under regulatory umbrella of "Special Nutritive Foods," enabling manufacturers to establish basis for functional (health benefit) claims	Japan Health Food and Nutrition Food Association is authorized by Japan's Ministry of Health and Welfare to provide guidance to the food industry in assembling data for formal submission for licensing of new FOSHU to the Ministry of Health and Welfare (MHW)
Canada	Primary statute is Food and Drugs Act and Regulations, defining "food" and "drug," prohibitions governing sale of foods	Extensive regulations to the Food and Drugs Act can be amended without reference to Parliament as necessary to prevent deception or to injury to the health of the	Guide for food manufacturers and advertisers, guidelines for nutritional labeling, guidelines for safety assessment of novel foods and others.

continued

TABLE 7.2   (continued)

Jurisdiction	1. Legislation	2. Regulations	3. Guidelines
		consumer. However, matters pertaining to health promotion and disease prevention are considered to be beyond the reach of the F&D Act, originally passed for, among other things, food safety and food integrity	Requirements also exist for premarket review of food additives, infant formulas, and irradiated foods

be marketed under the Dietary Supplement Health and Education Act and foods will be marketed under the Nutrition Labeling and Education Act [78].

The concept of "substantial equivalence" was developed as a practical approach for evaluating the safety of foods that contained or were produced from genetically modified organisms. This approach is focused on whether the novel food is substantially equivalent or sufficiently similar to its traditional counterpart. This concept was not intended to be applied to other types of novel foods but appears to be increasingly used by various regulatory agencies. The idea is to focus on the differences between a novel food and a traditional food; the safety assessment can zero in on the differences and thereby minimize the expense and time required for the assessment. An International Life Sciences Institute-Europe Technical Committee established three different classes of equivalence and set up guidelines for safety assessments of novel foods (http://www.fda.gov/cdrh/ode/guidance/1131.html):

- Class I: foods or food ingredients substantially equivalent to a traditional reference food/ingredient
- Class II: foods sufficiently similar to a traditional reference food
- Class III: foods neither substantially equivalent nor sufficiently similar to a traditional reference food or ingredient

In order to establish the appropriate equivalency class, extensive background information about the food is required, which ranges from the raw material source and its origins to methods of production and expected use of the novel food. Class I foods would not be subjected to safety assessment, Class II foods would be but the testing should focus on the differences between it and the respective traditional food or ingredient, and Class III foods would be subjected to rigorous safety assessment on a case-by-case basis. Provided the food or ingredient passes the rigorous safety considerations, any health claim should be subjected to scientific evaluation as well. However, this is quite a lengthy process requiring several years for its completion.

TABLE 7.3
Compliance, Enforcement, and Penalties (www.scisoc.org/aacc/funcfood)

Jurisdiction	1. Jurisprudence	2. Level of Enforcement	3. Penalties
EU	A body of jurisprudence in many areas is evolving as a result of decisions made by the European Court of Justice	Adopted legislation is in the form of Commission or Council directives or regulations, which have been agreed upon at the Community level and published in the "L" series of the Official Journal. Such legislation may or may not be implemented in all of the 15 Member States. Challenges respecting implementation are ultimately resolved by the European Court of Justice	
U.S.	Pertinent court rulings and discussions of constitutional issues concerning the NLEA are contained in a number of Federal Register regulations	High level of voluntary compliance. Enforcement measures are not clearly declared by FDA, which relies primarily upon field inspections and consumer/industry complaints to identify noncompliant products	Imprisonment and fines
Japan	n.a.	Industry self-regulation as government has delegated the determination of standards, licensing of certain products, and review of labeling, nutritional, and health claims to industry bodies	n.a.
Canada	Limited. Most prosecutions have involved the alleged adulteration of food products with prohibited substances and the manufacture of foods under unsanitary conditions.	Encouragement of voluntary compliance with regulation and guidelines. Compliance is monitored by periodic field inspection and related product analysis.	Liability on summary conviction or on conviction upon indictment, for fines and/or imprisonment

continued

TABLE 7.3   (continued)

Jurisdiction	1. Jurisprudence	2. Level of Enforcement	3. Penalties
	Compositional and identity standards for food products in the Food and Drug Regulations have been enforceable only when the standardized product crosses an interprovincial or international border	Enforcement is normally achieved through "voluntary" measures encouraged by federal authorities. Enforcement can be achieved through product recalls and seizures and, in rare cases, prosecution under the Food and Drugs Act	

7.9.2 RECOMMENDATIONS

Requirements for the type of scientific evidence that must be submitted to obtain a functional food label should be upgraded. While double-blinded clinical trials are not necessarily required in all cases, rigorous scientific testing should be one of the main elements of approval. An approval should be granted only in cases where there is significant agreement within the scientific community regarding the benefit of a specific ingredient. Directives or regulations should ensure that health claims may only be permitted for foods that can reasonably be expected to make a significant overall contribution to a healthy diet, and claims should be based on sound scientific evidence. It is highly advisable to adopt a diet rich in healthy conventional foods, especially fruits, vegetables, and fish. In many cases, there may be no need for consumers to purchase functional foods with added ingredients. Sound nutrition based on conventional dietary changes should serve as the foundation to reduce the incidence of chronic disease.

If the term "functional food" is to have any real meaning to consumers, then product labels should clearly disclose the amount of the functional ingredient and the extent to which the product supplies the amount of the functional ingredient required to provide a health benefit. Labels should also clearly describe the population for whom the product is intended for (e.g., elderly and diabetics); the length of time within which the product must be used; the minimum and maximum amounts to be consumed on a daily basis; whether particular cooking methods (e.g., microwave and boiling) enhance or destroy the potency of the product; whether the product should be consumed in conjunction with another product for best performance; and whether certain other products should be avoided while the functional food is consumed. The consumer should also be informed of any side effects and provided with guidance as to warning signs that use of the product should be discontinued and that an expert should be consulted [78].

The task of raising awareness and educating consumers is vitally important if functional foods are to fulfill their potential [79], but the question of who provides that education needs to be carefully addressed. For many people, the media, especially television, are a major source of information about health and functional foods. The other important source is the product label itself. Health professionals are less important sources of information for most people, but the credibility of that information is high. In contrast, most consumers do not believe marketing claims from food companies and many people doubt that scientists themselves understand what good nutrition really is. Since government credibility in relation to food issues tends to remain low, scientists are advised to communicate much more effectively (and without the use of jargon) with the general public. They should explain to consumers that understanding the effects of foods on health is an evolving knowledge and they should make efforts, wherever possible, to be more quantitative in their messages about the beneficial effects of foods (e.g., how much is beneficial and how much is likely to be harmful) [80].

The marketing of such products would increase the legitimacy of functional foods and help fuel a demand for such products. Thus, both the consumer and the food industry are anticipated to benefit from such reforms. Experience—in the United Kingdom and the United States—has proved that it would be advantageous to establish requirements for premarket approval of claims. Prohibition of therapeutic claims for foods and marketing of unlicensed medicines are inadequate to deal with the new generation of foods that blur the distinction between food and medicine. Under a premarket approval approach, no health claim could be made unless the government determined, based on a review of the totality of the reliable scientific evidence, that there is, at least, significant scientific convergence by experts in the field that the claim is really valid [78].

7.9.3 FUTURE OF FUNCTIONAL FOODS

Children stand for a rich market despite the increase in childhood obesity incidents. Although no single functional food can erase the effects of a poor diet, foods with genuine health benefits could make life a little easier for the many people struggling to eat well consume the appropriate food at the appropriate dosage. Functional foods deliver the positive message of "eating well," rather than the old messages of "reduce" and "avoid." Another aspect of flavoring fortified and functional foods is that consumers sometimes expect them to have a certain level of off-taste or they may not feel they are "getting the real thing."

Customized functional foods are the term with the greatest long-term potential [81]. The most typical target groups are infants and menopausal and perimenopausal women. Products enriched with calcium, iron, and phytoestrogens have flooded the market and are preferred to medication. It is expected that a wider range of female preventive products will emerge after the approval of the FDA to pursue heart and cancer prevention claims. Another strategy is targeting toward preventing/treating a specific condition or providing products to individual population segments that have specific deficiencies or needs for specific nutrients.

The pharmacy–food store interface is gradually emerging and more shoppers feel comfortable asking nutrition advice from pharmacists some of whom have been specially trained on such issues. Major companies have been aggressively supporting the "Whole Health Initiatives for Retail Pharmacists Program" on continuing-education programs, which include nutrition and disease management components for more than a decade [82]. Thus, the lines between food store and pharmacy are likely to disappear, thereby leading to marriage of food and pharmaceutical industries.

Genomics is another key factor that might lead to truly individualized nutrition. The future grocery stores will have a mini clinic with the ability to perform a quick blood test and provide a genome printout that includes the person's top disease risks and a recommended shopping list [83].

The worldwide opportunity for future growth and development of novel functional foods is overwhelming. Advances in medical research, in conjunction with continuous new food technology developments, are anticipated to provide many more opportunities for manufacturers to produce cutting-edge functional foods.

7.10 CONCLUSIONS

It has been substantiated that functional foods containing physiologically active components, either from plant or animal sources, may have a beneficial effect on health and longevity. However, functional foods are not a universal panacea for poor health habits. The perception of "deficient" versus "adequate" diets is gradually moving toward the concept of "optimal" nutrition. The evolving concept of functional foods is closely linked to that of optimal nutrition. Functional foods must be safe and claimed benefits must be real and their taste and convenience must not be compromised or they will not sell. The merit of such products can be appreciated only by educated consumers who must also be able to afford them. The regulations governing the scientific evidence required to support claims must protect the consumer while not obstructing innovation. It will be difficult to achieve a regulatory formula that pleases everyone, but the consumer's rights must have a priority over any other involved issue. Provided that these hurdles are eventually overcome, potential markets for functional foods are bound to become a success. Innovation in science results in more and more products with proven efficacy, helping improving and maintaining the health and vitality of the greater part of the world's population, not just the affluent few in developed countries. However, it is clear that a great deal of further research is required, including development of valid disease biomarkers and clinical trials, before most of these numerous benefits are properly measured and substantiated.

REFERENCES

1. Wood, H.G., Metabolic cycles in the fermentation of propionic acid bacteria, in *Current Topics in Cellular Regulation*, R.W. Eastbrook and P. Srera, Eds, pp. 255–287, Academic Press, New York, 1981.
2. Deborde, C., *Propionibacterium* spp., in *Encyclopedia of Dairy Sciences*, H. Roginski, J.W. Fuquay, and P.F. Fox, Eds, pp. 2330–2339, Academic Press, Elsevier Science, Kent, UK, 2002.
3. Al-Zoreky, N., Ayres, J.W., and Sandrine, W.E., Antimicrobial activity of microgard™ against food spoilage and pathogenic microorganisms, *J. Dairy Sci.*, 74, 758–763, 1991.
4. Schwenninger, S.M. and Meile, L., A mixed culture of *Propionibacterium jensenii* and *Lactobacillus paracasei* subsp. *paracasei* inhibits food spoilage yeasts, *System. Appl. Microbiol.*, 27, 229–237, 2004.

5. Jan, G., Lan, A., and Leverrier, P., Dairy propionibacteria as probiotics, in Functional Dairy Products, M. Saarela, Ed., Vol. 2, pp. 165–194, Woodhead Publishing Ltd., Cambridge, UK and CRC Press, Boca Raton, 2007.
6. Crittenden, R.G., Martinez, N.R., and Playne, M.J., Synthesis and utilization of folate by joghurt starter cultures and probiotic bacteria, Int. J. Food Microbiol., 80, 217–222, 2003.
7. Babuchowski, A., Laniewska-Moroz, L., and Warminska-Radyko, I., Propionibacteria in fermented vegetables, Lait, 79, 113–124, 1999.
8. LeBlanc, J.G., Rutten, G., Bruinenberg, P., Sesma, F., De Giori, G.S., and Smid, E.J., A novel dairy product fermented with Propionibacterium freudenreichii improves the riboflavin status of deficient rats, Nutrition, 22, 645–651, 2006.
9. Xu, S., Boylston, T.D., and Glatz, B.A., Conjugated linoleic acid content and organoleptic attributes of fermented milk products produced with probiotic bacteria, J. Agric. Food Chem., 53, 9064–9072, 2005.
10. FAO/WHO, Guidelines for the evaluation of probiotics in food, pp. 1–11, 2002, http://www.who.int/foodsafety/publications/fs_management/probiotics2/en/ (accessed on 10/10/2008).
11. Ouwehand, A.C., Makelainen, H., Tiihonen, K., and Rautonen, N., Digestive health, in Sweeteners and Sugar Alternatives in Food Technology, 1st edition, Blackwell Publishing Ltd., India, 2006.
12. Gibson, G.R. and Roberfroid, M.B., Dietary modulation of the human colonic microbiota: Introducing the concept of prebiotics, J. Nutr., 125, 1401–1412, 1995.
13. Ouwehand, A.C., Tiihonen, K., Makivuokko, H., and Rautonen, N., Synbiotics: Combining the benefits of pre- and probiotics, in Functional Dairy Products, M. Saarela, Ed., Vol. 2, pp. 195–213, Woodhead Publishing Ltd., Cambridge, UK and CRC Press, Boca Raton, 2007.
14. Van Loo, J., Coussement, P., De Leenheer, L., Hoebregs, H., and Smits, G., On the presence of inulin and oligofructose as natural ingredients in the western diet, Crit. Rev. Food Sci. Nutr., 35, 525–552, 1995.
15. Anderson, A.D.G., McNaught, C.E., Jain, P.K., and MacFie, J., Randomised clinical trial of symbiotic therapy in elective surgical patients, Gut, 53, 241–245, 2004.
16. Furrie, E., MacFarlane, S., Kennedy, A., Cummings, J.H., Walsh, S.V., O'Neill, D.A., and Macfarlane, G.T., Synbiotic therapy (Bifidobacterium longum/Synergy 1) initiates resolution of inflammation in patients with active ulcerative colitis: A randomized controlled pilot trial, Gut, 54 (2), 242–249, 2005.
17. Liu, Q., Duan, Z.P., Ha, D.K., Bengmark, S., Kurtovic, J., and Rioordan, S.M., Synbiotic modulation of gut flora: Effect on minimal hepatic encephalopathy in patients with cirrhosis, Hepatology, 39 (5), 1441–1449, 2005.
18. Capela, P., Hay, T.K.C., and Shah, N.P., Effect of cryoprotectants, prebiotics and microencapsulation on survival of probiotic organisms in yoghurt and freeze-dried yoghurt, Food Res. Int., 39, 203–211, 2006.
19. Crittenden, R.G., Morris, L.F., Harvey, M.L., Tran, L.T., Mitchell, H.L., and Playne, M.J., Selection of a Bifidobacterium strain to complement resistant starch in a symbiotic joghurt, J. Appl. Microbiol., 90, 268–278, 2001.
20. European Commission Regulation (EC) No. 608/2004OJ L 97, 1.4., p. 44, 2004.
21. Gurr, M., Plant sterols in the diet, Lipid Technol., 8, 114–117, 1996.
22. Ling, W.H. and Jones, P.J., Dietary phytosterols: A review of metabolism, benefits and side effects, Life Sci., 57, 195–206, 1995.
23. Ostlund, R.E., Jr., Racette, S.B., Okeke, A., and Stenson, W.F., Phytosterols that are naturally present in commercial corn oil significantly reduce cholesterol absorption in humans, Am. J. Clin. Nutr., 75, 1000–1004, 2002a.
24. Law, M., Plant sterol and stanol margarines and health, BMJ, 320, 861–864, 2000.

25. Scientific Committee on Food, SCF/CS/NF/DOS/20 ADD 1 Final October 3, 2000, General view of the Scientific Committee on Food on the long-term effects of the intake of elevated levels of phytosterols from multiple dietary sources, with particular attention to the effects on β-carotene (expressed on September 26, 2002).

26. Ikeda, I, Tanabe, Y., and Sugano, M., Effects of sitosterol and sitostanol on micellar solubility of cholesterol, *J. Nutr. Sci. Vitaminol.*, (Tokyo), 35, 361–369, 1989.

27. Heinemann, T, Leiss, O., and von Bergmann, K., Effect of low-dose sitostanol on serum cholesterol in patients with hypercholesterolemia, *Atherosclerosis*, 61, 219–223, 1986.

28. Jones, P.J., Raeini-Sarjaz, M., Ntanios, F.Y., Vanstone, C.A., Feng, J.Y., and Parsons, W.E., Modulation of plasma lipid levels and cholesterol kinetics by phytosterol versus phytostanol esters, *J. Lipid Res.*, 41, 697–705, 2000.

29. Weststrate, J.A. and Meijer, G.W., Plant sterol-enriched margarines and reduction of plasma total- and LDL-cholesterol concentrations in normocholesterolaemic and mildly hypercholesterolaemic subjects, *Eur. J. Clin. Nutr.*, 52, 334–343, 1998.

30. Trautwein, E.A., Schulz, C., Rieckhoff, D., Kunath-Rau, A., Erbersdobler, H.F., de Groot, W.A., and Meijer, G.W., Effect of esterified 4-desmethylsterols and -stanols or 4,4′-dimethylsterols on cholesterol and bile acid metabolism in hamsters. *Br. J. Nutr.*, 87, 227–237, 2002.

31. SCF (Scientific Committee on Food), *Opinion on Applications for Approval of a Variety of Plant Sterol-enriched Foods*. Opinion adopted by the Scientific Committee on Food on March 5, 2003, available online at: 2003, http://europa.eu.int/comm/food/fs/sc/scf/out174_en.pdf. (accessed on 10/11/2008).

32. Dossier from MB MultiBene Health Oy Ltd., Finland, 2001. www.multibene.com

33. Clifton, P., Plant sterols and stanols as functional ingredients in dairy products, in *Functional Dairy Products*, M. Saarela, Ed., Vol. 2, pp. 165–194, Woodhead Publishing Ltd., Cambridge, UK and CRC Press, Boca Raton, 2007.

34. Volpe, R., Niittynen, L., Korpela, R., Sirtori, C., Bucci, A., Fraone, N., and Pazzucconi, F., Effects of yoghurt enriched with plant sterols on serum lipids in patients with moderate hypercholesterolaemia, *Br. J. Nutr.*, 86 (2), 233–239, 2001.

35. Clifton, P.M., Noakes, M., Sullivan, D., Erichsen, N., Ross, D., Annison, G., Fassoulakis, A., Cehun, M., and Nestel, P., Cholesterol lowering effects of plant sterol esters differ in milk, yoghurt, bread and cereal, *Eur. J. Clin. Nutr.*, 58 (3), 503–509, 2004.

36. Mensink, R.P., Ebbing, S., Lindhout, M., Plat, J., and van Heugten, M.M., Effects of plant stanol esters supplied in low-fat yoghurt on serum lipids and lipoproteins, non-cholesterol esters and fat soluble antioxidant concentrations, *Atherosclerosis*, 160 (1), 205–213, 2002.

37. Korpela, R., Tuomilehto, J., Hogstrom, P., Seppo, L., Piironen, V., Salo-Vaananen, P., Toivo, J., Lamberg-Allardt, C., Karkkainen, M., Outila, T., Sundvall, J., Vilkkila, S., and Tikkanen, M.J., Safety aspects and cholesterol-lowering efficacy of low fat dairy products containing plant sterols, *Eur. J. Clin. Nutr.*, 60 (5), 633–642, 2006.

38. Doornbos, A.M., Meynen, E.M., Duchateau, G.S., van der Knaap, H.C., and Trautwein, E.A., Intake occasion affects the serum cholesterol lowering of a plant sterol-enriched single-dose yoghurt drink in mildly hypercholesterolaemic subjects, *Eur. J. Clin. Nutr.*, 60 (3), 325–333, 2006.

39. Noakes, M., Clifton, P.M., Doornbos, A.M., and Trautwein, E.A., Plant sterol ester-enriched milk and yoghurt effectively reduce serum cholesterol in modestly hypercholesterolemic subjects, *Eur. J. Nutr.*, 44 (4), 214–222, 2005.

40. Jauhiainen, T., Salo, P., Niittynen, L., Poussa, T., and Korpela, R., Effects of low-fat hard cheese enriched with plant stanol esters on serum lipids and apolipoprotein B in mildly hypercholesterolaemic subjects, *Eur. J. Clin. Nutr.*, 60 (11), 1253–1257, 2006.

41. Penas, E. and Gomez, R., In *Functional Dairy Products*, M. Saarela, Ed., Vol. 2, pp. 214–254, Woodhead Publishing Ltd., Cambridge, UK and CRC Press, Boca Raton, 2007.

42. Businco, L., Dreeborg, S., Einarsson, R., Giampetro, P.G., Host, A., Keller, K.M., Strobel, S., and Wahn, U., Hydrolysed cow's milk formulae. Allergenicity and use for treatment and prevention, *Pediatr. Allergy Immunol.*, 4, 101–111, 1993.
43. Host, A., Kiletzko, B., Dreborg, S., Muraro, A., Wahn, U., Aggett, P., Bresson, J.L., Hernell, O., Lafeber, H., Michaelsen, K.F., Micheli, J.L., Rigo, J., Weaver, L., Heymans, H., Strobel, S., and Vandenplas, Y., Dietary products used in infants for treatment and prevention of food allergy. Joint statement of the *European society for Paediatric Allergology and Clinical Immunology (ESPACI)*, Committee on Hypoallergenic formulas and the European Society Gastroenterology, Hepatology and Nutrition (ESPGHAN). Committee on Nutrition, 1999.
44. Clemente, A., Enzymatic protein hydrolysates in human nutrition, *Trend Food Sci. Technol.*, 11, 254–262, 2000.
45. Wahn, U., 1995. Role of hydrolysates in prophylactic and therapeutic diets for food allergy, in *Intestinal Immunology and Food Allergy*, de Wech Al and H.A. Sampson, Eds, Vol. 34, pp. 289–295, Nestel Nutrition Workshop Series, New York, Nestec Ltd., Raven Press, Vevey, 2002.
46. Calvo, M.M. and Gomez, R., Peptidic profile, molecular mass distribution and immunological properties of commercial hypoallergenic infant formulas, *Milchwissenshaft*, 57 (4), 187–190, 2002.
47. IUB-IUPAC Joint Commission on Biochemical Nomenclature (JCBN), Abbreviated terminology of oligosaccharide chains. Recommendations, *J. Biol. Chem.*, 257, 334, 1980.
48. Kunz, C., Rudloff, S., Baier, W., Klein, N., and Strobel, S., Oligosaccharides in human milk: structural, functional and metabolic aspects, *Ann. Rev. Nutr.*, 20, 699–722. 2000.
49. Boehm, G. and Stahl, B., Oligosaccharides. in *Functional Dairy Products*, T. Mattila-Sandholm, and M. Saarela, Eds, pp. 203–243, Woodhead Publishing Ltd., Cambridge, UK and CRC Press, Boca Raton, 2003.
50. Finke, B., Isolierung and charakterisierung von oligosacchariden aus humanen und tierischen Milchen, PhD thesis, University of Giessen, Shaker Verlag Aachen, Germany, 2000.
51. Gibson, G.R., Dietary modulation of the human gut microflora using the prebiotics oligofructose and inulin, *J. Nutr.*, 129, 1438S-1441S, 1999.
52. Olano-Martin, E., Mountzouris, K.C., Gibson, G.R., and Rastall, R.A., *In vitro* fermentability of dextran, oligodextran, and maltodextrin by human gut bacteria, *Br. J. Nutr.*, 83, 247–255, 2000.
53. Tanaka, R. and Matsumoto, K., Recent progress on prebiotics in Japan, including galactooligosaccharides, *Bull IDF*, 336, 21–27, 1998.
54. Loo, J.V., Cummings, J., Delzenne, N., Englyst, H., Frank, A., Hopkins, M., Kok, N., MacFarlane, G., Newton, D., Quingley, M., Roberfroid, M., Vliet, T., and Heuvel, E., Functional food properties of non-digestible oligosaccharides: A consensus report from the ENDO project (DGXII AIRII-CT94–1095), *Br. J. Nutr.*, 81, 121–132, 1999.
55. Moro, G., Minoli, I., Mosca, M., Fanaro, S., Jelinek, J., Stahl, B., and Boehm, G., Dosage-related bifidogenic effects of galacto- and fructooligosaccharides in formula-fed term infants, *J. Pediatr. Gastroenterol. Nutr.*, 34, 291–295, 2002.
56. Boehm, D., Lidestri, M., Casetta, P., Jelinek, J., Negretti, F., Stahl, B., and Marini, A., Supplementation of a bovine milk formula with an oligosaccharide mixture increases counts of faecal bifidobacteria in preterm infants, *Arch. Dis. Child*, 86, F0–F4, 2002.
57. Lidestri, M., Agosti, M., Marini, A., and Boehm, G., Oligosaccharides might stimulate calcium absorption in formula-fed preterm infants, *Acta Paediatr.*, 92 (s441), 91–92, 2003.
58. Rastall, R.A. and Gibson, G.R., Prebiotic oligosaccharides: Evaluation of biological activities and potential future developments, in *Probiotics and Prebiotics: Where Are We Going?* Chap. 5, G.W. Tannock, Ed., pp. 107–148, Caister Academic Press, Wymondham, UK, 2002.

59. Cummings, J.H. and Macfarlane, G.T., The control and consequences of bacterial fermentation in the human colon, *J. Appl. Bacteriol.*, 70, 443–459, 1991.

60. Gibson, G.R. and Roberfroid, M.B., Dietary modulation of the human colonic microflora: Introducing the concept of prebiotics, *J. Nutr.*, 125, 1401–1412, 1995.

61. Jayaraman, N., Nepogodiev, S.A., and Stoddart, J.F., Synthetic carbohydrate-containing dendimers, *Chem. Eur. J.*, 3, 1193–1199, 1997.

62. Fitzgerald, R.J. and Meisel, H., Caseinophosphopeptides (CPPs) as functional ingredients, in *Functional Dairy Products*, T. Mattila-Sandholm and M. Saarela, Eds, Chapter 8, pp. 187–202, Woodhead Publishing Ltd., Cambridge, UK and CRC Press, Boca Raton, 2003.

63. Brule, G., Roger, L., Fauquant, J., and Piot, M., Nutrient composition containing non-phosphorylated peptides from casein-based material, US Patent no. 5, 334, 408. 1994.

64. McDonagh, D. and Fitzgerald, R.J., Production of caseinophosphopeptides (CPPs) from sodium caseinate using a range of commercial proteases, *Int. Dairy J.*, 8, 39–45, 1998.

65. Meisel, H., Gunther, S., Martin, D., and Schlimme, E., Apoptosis induced my modified ribonucleosides in human cell culture systems, *FEBS Lett.*, 433, 265–268. 1998.

66. Fitzgerald, R.J., Potential uses of caseinophosphopeptides, *Int. Dairy J.*, 8, 451–457, 1998.

67. Pariza, M.W. and Hargraves, W.A., A beef-derived mutagenesis modulator inhibits initiation of mouse epidermal tumours by 7,12-dimethylbenz(a)anthracene, *Carcinogenesis*, 6, 591–593, 1985.

68. Gnadig, S., Xue, Y., Berdeaux, O., Chardigny, J.M., and Sebedio, J.-L., Conjugated linoleic acid (CLA) as a functional ingredient, in *Functional Dairy Products*, T. Mattila-Sandholm, and M. Saarela, Eds, Chapter 11, pp. 263–298, Woodhead Publishing Ltd., Cambridge, UK and CRC Press, Boca Raton, 2003.

69. O'shea, M., Lawless, F., Stanton, C., and Devery, R., Conjugated linoleic acid in bovine milk fat: A food-based approach to cancer chemoprevention, *Trend Food Sci. Technol.*, 9, 192–196, 1998.

70. Harfoot, C.G. and Hazelwood, G.P., Lipid metabolism in the rumen, in *The Rumen Microbial Ecosystem*, P. Hobson, Ed., London, Elsevier Science Publishers, pp. 285–322, 1998.

71. Kepler, C.R. and Tove, S.B., Biohydrogenation of unsaturated fatty acids, *J. Biol. Chem.*, 242, 5686–5692, 1967.

72. Corl, B., Baumgard, L., Griinari, J., Delmonte, P., Morehouse, K., Yurawecz, M., and Bauman, D., *trans-7, cis9CLA* is endogenously synthesized by D-9 desaturation in lactating dairy cows, AOCS Annual Meeting, Montreal, 2002.

73. Sebedio, J.L., Gnadig, S., and Chardigny, J.M., Recent advances in conjugated linoleic acid, *Curr. Opin. Clin. Nutr. Metab. Care*, 2, 499–506, 1999.

74. Jahreis, G., Ftitsche, J., and Steinhart, H., Conjugated linoleic acid in milk fat-high variation depnding on production system, *Nutr. Res.*, 17, 1479–1484, 1997.

75. Shantha, N.C., Crum, A.D., and Decker, E.A, Evaluation of conjugated linoleic acid concentrations in cooked beef, *J. Agric. Food Chem.*, 42, 1757–1760, 1994.

76. Precht, D., Molkentin, J., and Vahlendick, M., Influence of the heating temperature on the fat composition of milk fat with the emphasis on *cis/trans*-isomerization, *Nahrung Food*, 43, 25–33, 1999.

77. Shantha, N.C., Ram, L.N., O'Leary, J., Hicks, C.L., and Decker, E.A., Conjugated linoleic acid concentrations in dairy products as affected by processing and storage, *J. Food Res.*, 60, 695–720, 1995.

78. Arvanitoyannis, I.S. and Van Houwelingen-Koukaliaroglou, M., Functional foods: A survey of health claims, pros and cons and current legislation, *Crit. Rev. Food Sci. Nutr.*, 445 (5), 385–404, 2005.

79. Leatherhead Functional foods and the consumer Survey, Leatherhead Food Res. Assn. Leatherhead, Surrey, UK.mhilliam@ifra.co.uk, 1999.

80. McNutt, K.W., Consumers' views on functional foods, in *Functional Foods; Designer Foods, Pharmafoods, Nutraceuticals*, I. Goldberg, Ed., pp. 523–534, Chapman & Hall, London, 1994.
81. Sloan A.E., Fortification frenzy: The new wellness mindset, *Food Technol.*, 54 (2), 20, 2000.
82. White, R., Bringing supermarket pharmacies into the whole health loop., *Supermarket Bus.*, 54 (10), 50–51, 1999.
83. Van der Meer, I.M., Bovy A.G., and Bosch, D., Plant-based raw material: Improved food quality for better nutrition via plant genomics, *Curr. Opin. Biotechnol.*, 12, 488–492, 2001.

REFERENCES ON LEGISLATION

Directive 89/398/EEC (http://europa.eu.int/smartapi/cgi/sga_doc?smartapi!celexplus!prod!DocNumber&lg=en&type_doc=Directive&an_doc=1989&nu_doc=398).
Directive 91/321/EEC (http://europa.eu.int/smartapi/cgi/sga_doc?smartapi!celexplus!prod!DocNumber&lg=en&type_doc=Directive&an_doc=1991&nu_doc=321).
Directive 96/5/EC (http://europa.eu.int/smartapi/cgi/sga_doc?smartapi!celexplus!prod!DocNumber&lg=en&type_doc=Directive&an_doc=1996&nu_doc=5).
Directive 96/8/EC (http://europa.eu.int/smartapi/cgi/sga_doc?smartapi!celexplus!prod!DocNumber&lg=en&type_doc=Directive&an_doc=1996&nu_doc=8).
Directive 1999/21/EC (http://europa.eu.int/smartapi/cgi/sga_doc?smartapi!celexplus!prod!DocNumber&lg=en&type_doc=Directive&an_doc=1999&nu_doc=21).
Directive 2002/46/EC (http://europa.eu.int/smartapi/cgi/sga_doc?smartapi!celexplus!prod!DocNumber&lg=en&type_doc=Directive&an_doc=2002&nu_doc=46).

E-REFERENCES

http://www.fda.gov/cdrh/ode/guidance/1131.html.
www.scisoc.org/aacc/funcfood (accessed on 10/11/2008).

8 Quality Attributes of Yogurt and Functional Dairy Products

Barbaros Özer and Hüseyin Avni Kırmacı

CONTENTS

8.1 INTRODUCTION

The increasing awareness and demand of consumers for safe and high-quality food have led many dairy companies to undertake a comprehensive evaluation and reorganization of their food control systems in order to improve efficiency, rationalization of human resources, and to harmonize approaches. This evaluation in food control systems has resulted in the necessity to shift from the traditional approach that relied heavily on end product sampling and inspection and to move toward the implementation of a preventive safety and quality approach, based on risk analysis and on the principles of the hazard analysis critical control point (HACCP) system [1]. The HACCP technique for the identification, evaluation, and control of food safety hazards was developed in the mid-1960s and publicly presented in the early 1970s. Since then it has been progressively adopted by the food industry and enforced by regulators [2]. Owing to its nature, fermented milks are regarded as perishable products. Therefore, implementation of the HACCP system is of critical importance in ensuring a high-quality and safe end-product. HACCP has seven principles [3]:

1. Hazard analysis
2. Identify critical control points (CCPs)
3. Establish critical limits
4. Monitor the CCPs
5. Establish corrective actions
6. Record keeping
7. Verification

For a safe production of fermented milks, hazards that may present risk for the consumers must be carefully analyzed and effective measures must be taken to eliminate these sources of risks completely or to reduce the total assessed risk of that hazard to an acceptable level. For the efficiency of the HACCP system, some prerequisites must be met. These prerequisites have been indicated in European Council Directive 92/46/EEC [4]. According to the directive, the possible microbial contamination sources in dairy plants are as follows:

i. External (raw material and additives, water, packaging, and small insects)
ii. Internal (wet flour, equipment, construction, and vehicles)
iii. Air
iv. Staff

For the success of the HACCP program, all these points must be controlled strictly [5]. There are three potential hazard sources of a fermented milk processing plant: (i) microbial, (ii) chemical, and (iii) physical hazards. Microbiological sources of hazard can be divided into three subgroups: severe, medium-severe with high risk of epidemics, and medium-severe with limited risk of epidemics (Table 8.1).

TABLE 8.1

Microorganisms Carrying Potential Risk for the Consumer's Health in the Production of Fermented Milks

Severe	Severe with High Risk of Epidemics	Severe with Limited Risk of Epidemics
Brucella spp.	*Salmonella* spp.	*Bacillus cereus*
Clostridium botulinum	Enterotoxigenic *E. coli*	*Campylobacter jejuni*
Listeria monocytogenes	*E. coli* O157:H7	*Clostridium perfringens*
Salmonella typhi	*Shigella* spp.	*Staphylococcus aureus*
Salmonella paratyphi	Viruses	*Aeromonas* spp.
Salmonella dublin	*Cryptosporidium* spp.	*Yersinia enterocolitica*
Shigella dysanteria		Parasites
Hepatitis A and B		

Potential sources of physical contamination in fermented milks manufacturing are metal and/or glass pieces, insects, wooden pieces, human sources physical materials, plastics, and other physical materials that make consumption of fermented milks unsafe.

Natural toxics, metal ions, veterinary drug residues, residual detergents, pesticides, and some food additives are among the possible chemical contamination sources in production of fermented milks. Particularly, mycotoxins can cause acute or chronic mycotoxicosis. The most common acute mycotoxins are ochratoxin, trichotecene, zearalenone, and aflatoxin.

Copper, cadmium, and mercury are the metal ions that are most likely found in traditional yogurts. β-Lactam, sulfonamides, and tetracyclines are the most common drug residues in yogurt and other fermented milks [6].

In order to prevent the contamination of the above-mentioned potential hazards, the HACCP system must be operated efficiently. It is of crucial importance to create a quality team before starting the build-up of a quality control system. Analyzing the CCPs and establishing the verification parameters for control points (CPs) are the most critical steps of an HACCP program (Table 8.2).

Another factor affecting the success of an HACCP program is the establishment of the critical limits for potential hazards. There are decision trees available to help identify a CCP. Figures 8.1 and 8.2 illustrate decision trees for raw milk and yogurt processing line. Depending on the production model, CCPs show differences. For example, in the continuous yogurt production, the fermentation step is not considered as a CCP; however, in the discontinuous yogurt production this processing step is a critical point (Figure 8.3). Similarly, if raw milk contains antibiotic residues, raw milk should be evaluated as a CCP as this carries a risk for the people who suffer from allergy against antibiotics. The HACCP program is not only applied during the processing of foods, but the production sites can also be subjected to the HACCP program. In most cases, processing lines and production sites are evaluated together in the HACCP system. Bacterial load of the surfaces contacting with foods is considered as a criterion for the efficiency of the HACCP program in processing areas (Table 8.3).

In recent years, with the increasing in-site cleaning programs (C.I.P. or C.O.P.), in some countries, the critical limit for total bacteria has been reduced to <200 cfu 100 cm^{-2}.

8.2 CONTROL OF CHEMICAL COMPOSITION

The majority of regulations covering yogurt (and bioyogurt) include a section on chemical composition, where a minimum percentage of milk solids nonfat (SNF) and/or fat is stipulated [8]. These standards are essential both in terms of consumer expectations and in terms of nutritional quality. In the USA and the EU, the SNF and fat contents of yogurt-type fermented milks range between 8.2–8.65% and 2.25–5.0%, respectively. In the Netherlands, the SNF content of yogurt varies in a wider range (8.2–12.6%).

For the determination of totals solids, the modified standard gravimetric method is widely employed. In this method, the products with an acidity of 2% lactic acid

TABLE 8.2
Determination of Hazard Analysis and CCP in Fermented Milk Production

Processing Steps	Hazards	Preventive Measurement	Critical Limit	Monitoring/ Frequency	Recording	Staff-in-Charge	Evaluation	Verification
Milk reception	Microbiological	Temperature, Total mesophilic bacteria count	≤7°C, <100,000 cfu mL^{-1}	Every day, Each milk tanker	Quality control office records	Staff in-charge of milk reception	Reject milk if not complaint to microbiological limits	Calibration of thermometer and test kits
	Residual drugs	β-Lactam	Negative	Each milk tanker	Quality control office records	Staff in-charge on milk reception	Reject	Calibration of test kits
	Foreign material	In-line filter, Inspect tanker before off-loading	No damaged gaskets	Each milk tanker	Quality control office records	Staff in-charge on milk reception	Filtering or clarifying milk	Daily tanker inspection
Raw milk and cream storage	Microbiological	Temperature, Time	≤7°C, ≤72 h	Four times a day	Quality control office records	Quality control engineer	Pre-evaluation and decision	Calibration of thermometer
Heat treatment	Microbiological	Temperature, Time	≥72°C/15 s (plate heat exchanger), ≥85°C/20 min (VAT heating)	After each heat treatment	Processing office records	Staff in-charge of processing	Reheating	Calibration of thermometer and timer; Testing pasteurization efficiency

Fermentation	Microbiological	pH and fermentation period	pH ≤ 4.6 ≥3.5–5 h ≤	During each production	Processing office records	Staff in-charge of processing	Reject or accept after microbiological evaluations	Calibration of pH-meter and thermometer
Fruits/ sweeteners addition	Microbiological	Yeasts/molds counts; Coliform counts; Fruit storage temperature	Yeasts ≤ 10 g^{-1}; Molds ≤ 10 g^{-1}; Negative; $\leq 7^\circ$C	During each production	Processing office records	Staff in-charge of processing	Reject or accept after microbiological evaluations	Calibration of microbiological test methods; Calibration of thermometer
Packaging	Physical	Presence of physical objects	Negative	After each production	Quality control office records	Staff in-charge of processing	Reject if positive	Visual inspection; Infrared inspector (if available)
Storage	Microbiological	Yeasts/molds counts; Coliform counts; Storage temperature	Yeasts ≤ 10 g^{-1}; Molds ≤ 10 g^{-1}; Negative; $\leq 7^\circ$C	After each production	Processing office records	Staff in-charge of processing	Reject or accept after microbiological evaluations	Calibration of microbiological test methods; Calibration of thermometer

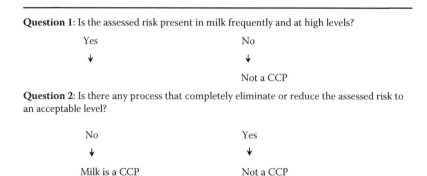

FIGURE 8.1   Decision tree for raw milk used for yogurt production.

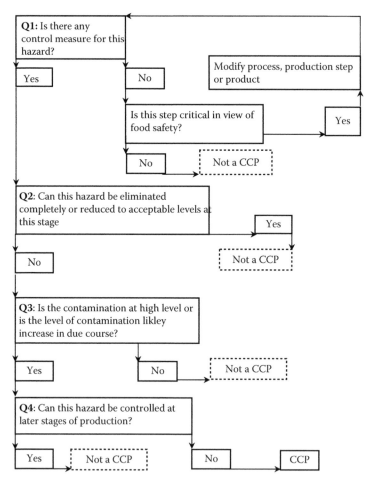

FIGURE 8.2   Decision tree for yogurt production. (Based on Karaali, A., *Gida Isletmelerinde HACCP Uygulamalari ve Denetimi*, p. 196, Saglik Bakanligi Temel Saglik Hizmetleri Genel Mudurlugu Yayinlari, Ankara, 2003.)

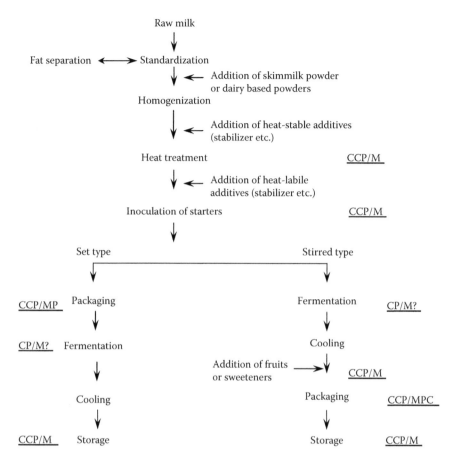

FIGURE 8.3 CCPs and CPs in set- and stirred-type yogurt productions. M: microbial hazards, P: physical hazards, C: chemical hazards. ?: CCP only for discontinued yogurt production. (Based on Varnam, A.H. and Sutherland, J.P., *Milk and Milk Products. Technology, Chemistry and Microbiology*, p. 451, Chapman & Hall, London, 1994.)

TABLE 8.3

Evaluation of Microbiological Quality of Milk Processing Plants According to the Load of Bacteria on the Surfaces Contacting with Milk

Total Mesophilic Bacteria	Total Coliform Bacteria	Evaluation
500 cfu/100 cm^2	<10/100 cm^2	Satisfactory
500–2500 cfu/100 cm^2	10–100/100 cm^2	Doubtful
>2500 cfu/100 cm^2	>100/100 cm^2	Insufficient

Source: Adapted from Harringan, W.F. and McCance, M.E., *Laboratory Methods in Food and Dairy Microbiology*, p. 452, Academic Press, London, 1993.

should be neutralized before drying with 0.1 N strontium hydroxide, and a factor of 0.0048 g mL^{-1} of alkali deducted from the dry weight of the sample [11]. The micro-wave oven drying of yogurt samples has proved to be unsatisfactory [12]. For a desired textural and organoleptic quality set yogurt, the total solids content should be about 15.0–16.0% [6]. Yogurt and yogurt-type fermented products fall into four groups on the basis of fat content: (i) very low fat, (ii) low fat, (iii) regular fat, and (iv) full fat (including strained yogurt and luxury yogurt). Milk fat is one of the major milk components affecting the consumer's palate and attempts have been made to compensate for the sensory quality loss in very low-fat and low-fat yogurts and other fermented milk products. In this respect, protein and starch-based fat substitutes have been developed [13,14]. Nevertheless, the success of fat substitutes in providing luxury mouthfeel yogurt that is quite unique for milk fat is still debatable [15,16]. Determination of milk fat is not only important to meet legal requirements, but also the milk fat has a major impact on the mouthfeel of yogurt [17]. Overall, 1% milk fat is regarded as the minimum to produce the desired response from the consumer [17]. In most cases, the fat content of fermented products is adjusted to produce "light" or "low-fat" yogurt. In this case, the milk fat content should be declared in a manner acceptable in the country of sale to the final consumer, either as (i) a percentage of mass or volume, or (ii) in grams per serving as qualified in the label, provided that the number of servings is stated [18]. Fat determination can be achieved by employ-ing either volumetric methods (e.g., the Babcock or Gerber methods) or gravimetric methods (e.g., the Röse Gottlieb method). The gravimetric methods tend to be regarded as more accurate, but the volumetric methods are less time consuming and require rather less-skilled personnel. For rapid determination of fat, an infrared detection system using a homogenized sample of yogurt (~50 g) is more suitable, if the number of samples being analyzed is high [19]. Before measuring milk fat using the infrared detection method, the yogurt samples should be neutralized with 0.5 M sodium hydroxide and, for fruit yogurts, measurements should be carried out prior to fruit addition [8].

The acidity is one of the most important quality parameters for yogurt with regard to palatability, consumer acceptance, and shelf life of the product. Development of lactic acid under controlled conditions during fermentation is essential for the for-mation of yogurt gel network. On the contrary, development of acidity after the fer-mentation is not desired since it leads to wheying off, textural defects, and excess sourness, which masks the perception of aroma compounds by the consumers. Therefore, it is desirable that the control of the acidity should be accurate and effec-tive, and the consumers are assured of a product of predictable quality. In the retail product, a minimum of 0.7% lactic acid has been suggested by the International Dairy Federation (IDF) [20]. Codex Alimentarius suggests a minimum of 0.6% lac-tic acid for yogurt, alternate culture yogurt, kefir, and acidophilus milk, >0.7% for kumys, and >0.3% for other fermented milks (Table 8.4) [18]. The titration acidity is measured by various techniques in various countries. The most common method is based on the titration of a mixture of 10 g of the product and 10 mL of distilled water with 0.1 N NaOH in the presence of phenolphthalein (1 mL) as indicator. The titration is ended when the color of the mixture turns to pinkish, and the results are expressed

TABLE 8.4
Chemical Composition of Fermented Milk Products

	Fermented Milk	Yogurt, Alternate Yogurt, and Acidophilus Milk	Kefir	Koumiss
Milk protein[a] (% m/m)	2.7 min	2.7 min	2.7 min	
Milk fat (% m/m)	less than 10	less than 15	less than 10	less than 10
Titratable acidity, expressed as % lactic acid (% m/m)	0.3 min	0.6 min	0.6 min	0.7 min
Ethanol (% vol./w)				0.5 min
Sum of microorganisms constituting the starter culture (cfu/g)	10^7 min	10^7 min	10^7 min	10^7 min
Labeled microorganisms (cfu/g)	10^6 min	10^6 min	ND	ND
Yeasts (cfu/g)	ND	ND	10^4 min	10^4 min

Source: Adapted from Anonymous, *Codex Standards for Fermented Milks*, Codex Stan 243, 2003.
[a] Protein content is calculated by multiplying the total Kjeldahl nitrogen determined by 6.38.

as °SH (Soxhelet Henkel) or % lactic acid. In some countries, alternative titration methods including Thorner (°T) or Dornic (°D) are used. The concentrations of the results of these methods are converted to % lactic acid as follows:

$$1 \text{ SH} = 0.0225\% \text{ lactic acid} = 2.5°\text{T} = 2.25°\text{D}.$$

The pH value of yogurt or fermented milks represents the true (present) acidity. It is widely recognized that with a highly buffered system like yogurt, the relationship between titratable acidity and pH is by no means straightforward [11]. On the other hand, the monitoring of pH during the manufacture of yogurt and other fermented milks is a routine practice. Therefore, the effectiveness of pH measurement should be monitored regularly by other means.

Determination of other milk compounds (i.e., protein, lactose, and ash) in view of routine quality control is not a common practice. However, determination of the level of protein will help the manufacturers to closely control the effectiveness of their total solids fortification methods. Although yogurt and yogurt-type fermented milk products are usually not considered as vitamin sources, these products have detectable quantities of riboflavin, thiamine, folic acid, panthotenic acid, and vitamin A [21]. Except for the fortified yogurts, the vitamin contents of fermented milks are not monitored routinely [22].

8.3 PHYSICAL ASSESSMENT OF YOGURT AND FERMENTED MILKS

Understanding the physical properties of yogurt and other fermented milks is important in the following steps during manufacturing: (i) quality control of ingredients and finished products; (ii) design and evaluation of processing equipment, unit operations, and process parameters; (iii) adjustment of time × temperature × flow rate selection of fluid dairy products; and (iv) characterization and development of dairy products for consumer acceptability, and elucidation of the structure and relationship among structure and textural properties [23,24]. The yogurt gel is a heat-induced acid casein gel, and consists of a permanent network composed mainly of noncovalent protein bonds (e.g., hydrophobic and electrostatic bindings) as well as covalent thiol–disulfide bonds [25–27]. There are many factors that affect the physical properties of yogurt, such as the type and number of the protein interactions, the size and shape of the protein network, and the distribution of whey proteins and caseins over the gel network. All these factors are affected by the technical applications, such as heat treatment, incubation temperature and pH, type of starter culture, methods of manufacture, and the type of milk [28].

Conventional techniques, such as the Plummet device, the Posthumus funnel, the falling ball, the Namatre vibrator, and the Rheomat, have been almost universally accepted for the measurement of the physical properties of set or stirred yogurts, and rotational viscometers, such as the Haake and the Brookfield, have become widely used as well [29]. For set products, different types of penetrometers/consistometers, such as the curd tension-meter, Instron testing machine, Stevens Texture Analyzer, and the SUR penetrometer PNR, have been widely used to assess the firmness of the body/gel. Measurement of gel firmness in yogurt is achieved by means of constant speed penetration on universal testing machines or similar instruments, using cylindrical plungers and crosshead speed values ranging between 10 and 100 mm min^{-1} at <10°C. The force-response is monitored as a function of penetration depth [30]. The plunger size and the penetration depth affect the force-response.

Gel firmness can be measured either at a predefined period of time or at a predefined depth [31]. A large variety of probes, penetration rates, penetration depths, and temperatures are used. Consequently, it is hardly possible to compare the results between laboratories.

From the rheological point of view, the stirred yogurt can be classified as a non-Newtonian fluid that shows a yield stress, and exhibits shear-thinning and time-dependent properties. Viscosity of the stirred yogurt is usually determined by means of rotational geometry. In single-spindle instruments, which have been frequently used for this purpose, only the rotating part is geometrically defined. In this case, for the non-Newtonian fluids, it is not possible to convert the measured torque into viscosity units [32]. Similar to the destructive gel firmness techniques, the single-point viscosity measurements can be achieved either at a predefined period of time or at a predefined shear rate [33].

Yogurt is a typical example of a weak viscoelastic gel [34]. In a viscoelastic gel, the physical parameters can only be determined by measuring its viscous and elastic moduli [35–37]. Dynamic rheological measurements of yogurt and other gel-based fermented milk products are of interest as they are directly related to its viscous and solids properties, which can be measured in such experiments. Yogurt has a highly complex rheology, and it is not possible to obtain a complete understanding using traditional viscometers and/or consistometers of the type commonly used in quality assurance in the yogurt industry. The main drawbacks of the conventional methods are as follows: (i) they effectively measure the remnants of the gel after disruption, (ii) give a single-point measurement (fixed rate, strain, or both), which do not reflect the actual physical properties of yogurt, and (iii) it is impossible to calculate the exact shear rate/strain [38].

A dynamic study involves subjecting the material to an oscillating strain/stress and measuring the resulting stress/strain (Figure 8.4). From the dynamic rheological testing, two shear moduli can be defined: the storage and the loss moduli, which represent the elastic and viscous contributions of the material, respectively [39–41]. Viscoelastic material under dynamic testing shows a linear viscoelastic region in which both shear moduli of the gel are independent of strain or stress. The linear viscoelastic region ends at some applied strain where the material begins to break down and the elastic modulus decreases with increasing shear. To avoid the use of complex nonlinear theories, gel characterization is usually made in the linear viscoelastic region for the analysis of the results, which are greatly facilitated if the viscoelastic behavior is linear [28,34,36]. Generally, mechanical spectra obtained within the linear viscoelastic region, that is, a strain lower than ~1–3%, reveal a response typical of biopolymer gels, with the storage (elastic) modulus, G', exceeding the loss (viscous) modulus, G'', by a factor of about 5–7 [30]. Qualitatively, the mechanical spectra of the stirred yogurt resemble those of set yogurt, with the moduli being 8–10 times lower. The rheological properties of an acid casein gel-like yogurt are closely related to the casein concentration, enthalphic/entrophic nature of the gel, and the extent of repulsion/attraction forces between casein particles and gelation mechanism [42]. In addition, the size and distribution of macromolecules

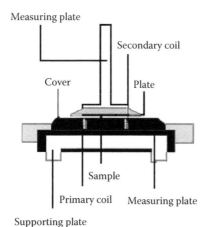

FIGURE 8.4   Working principle of a dynamic oscillatory rheometer.

(e.g., caseins) and the number of protein contact points also influence the rheology of a gel. In general, the rheological properties of a viscoelastic gel are determined by measuring the resistance of permanent protein bonds against the force applied. Additionally, nonpermanent and weak protein bonds also play a role in determining the rheological properties of a weak viscoelastic gel [43]. In other words, the balance between the strong and permanent protein bonds, and the weak and nonpermanent bonds, determines the rheological characteristics of an acid casein gel. Viscoelastic gels are metastable and have a rather low minimum Helmholtz energy level, defined as the minimum energy level required to keep a gel in its metastable position and characterized by the following equation:

$$dA = dU - T\,dS,$$

where A is the Helmholtz energy, U is the integral energy, S is the entrophy, and T is the temperature.

Generally, acid casein gels are not able to regain their original structure after being destroyed.

With deformation, the internal energy (U) of the system increases, but the decrease in entrophy is limited. This eventually leads to an increase in the Helmholtz energy level and to a permanent loss of structural unity [44]. This point is schematized in Figure 8.5. In conclusion, rheological measurements are only reliable if gel properties do not alter, at least within the period of observation; to keep the structural integrity of a test material, the selected parameters must be so small that the material is not destroyed. In order to obtain data that mirror the actual rheological characteristics of the gel in question, the selection of rheological methods is of primary importance. In this respect, the recent developments in dynamic rheological testings have

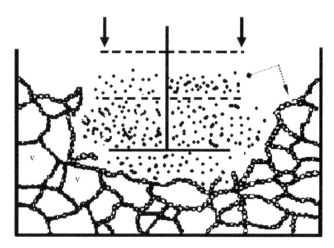

FIGURE 8.5   Schematic illustration of destructive effect of empirical viscosimeters on a weak viscoelastic gel. (Adapted from Özer, B.H., *Turkish J. Agric, Forestry*, 28, 19–23, 2004.)

enabled more precise and objective evaluation and characterization of the physical properties of weak viscoelastic materials such as yogurt [45].

Syneresis is another rheological quality parameter and is considered to be a defect in yogurt-type acid casein gels. Susceptibility of yogurt-type gels to syneresis depends on several factors, particularly on the preheat treatment of milk, the total solids content, and the acidity [46–48]. In general, too slow or too fast acidity development during fermentation stimulates whey separation in yogurt. Mechanical disturbance of the product, especially before it has fully set, readily causes whey separation. Too severe shearing during pumping the stirred yogurt from cooling tanks to the packaging unit also leads to whey separation in the final product. There are several ways of measuring the level of whey separated in yogurt-type gels. In the most common method, a certain amount of yogurt (i.e., 25 g) is filtered through a filter paper at <7°C for 2 h and the amount of whey collected in a cylinder is measured at 5 min intervals. Harwalkar and Kalab [49] proposed an alternative method that is based on centrifugation of yogurt and measuring the whey separated after centrifugation. In this method, the yogurt samples are made in 15 mL calibrated tubes and are centrifuged at 6°C for 10 min at centrifugal forces ranging from 30 to 2000 g. The volume of the whey separated is plotted against the centrifugal force applied. g-force values of inflection points obtained on S-shaped curves are used as arbitrary measures of the susceptibility to syneresis.

8.4   MICROBIOLOGICAL QUALITY CONTROL

Microbiological quality control of fermented milk products is of primary importance in ensuring food safety as well as conforming to the existing standards and/or regulations in the country of sale. For this purpose, monitoring the numbers of specific microorganisms (starter cultures and/or adjuncts), and indicator and pathogenic microorganisms in the product, is a routine practice. Additionally, determination of the level of microbial metabolites in the fermented milks is a common microbial quality control tool.

As stated in Table 8.4, according to Codex Alimentarius Standard for Fermented Milks [18], the number of specific microorganisms (starter culture) in yogurt, alternate yogurt, kefir, and koumiss should be >10^7 cfu g^{-1}, at the time of consumption. As the numbers of starter microorganisms likely decrease during the cold storage as a result of the development of acidity, one should bear in mind that the initial inoculation level of fermented milk should be high enough to meet the target level in the end product. Too high counts of specific microorganisms in fermented milk may lead to development of atypical aroma/flavor in the final product. Especially, *Lactobacillus delbrueckii* subsp. *bulgaricus* grows rapidly in yogurt during storage at high temperatures, leading to development of overacidification in yogurt. Overall, it is ideal that the starter microflora should be abundant and viable in the retail product at the end of "best before" date [8]. A number of specific growth media are available in counting specific microorganisms in fermented milks. Some of these media allow differentiation of more than one group of bacteria in one petri plate. Tables 8.5 through 8.7 summarize the growth media commonly used in counting starter bacteria used in yogurt and bioyogurt.

TABLE 8.5

Growth Media Used in Counting *Lactobacillus delbrueckii* subsp. *bulgaricus* and *Streptococcus thermophilus* on the Same Plate

Medium	Separating Agent	*Lactobacillus delbrueckii* subsp. *bulgaricus*	*Streptococcus thermophilus*	Incubation Conditions	Reference
Elliker's agar	—	Growth	Growth	Anaerobic, 37°C/48 h	[65]
LAB agar	Double pour plate method	Rough, irregular colonies	Small, round, or lenticular colonies	Anaerobic, 42°C/48 h	[66]
Hansen's yogurt agar	Sugar	Colonies (2–10 mm in diameter)	Colonies (1–3 mm in diameter)	Anaerobic, 37°C/48 h	[67]
Lee's agar	Sugar + BCP[a]	Large white colonies	Small yellow colonies	Anaerobic, 37°C/ 48 h	[68]
M17 agar	β-Glycerophosphate	No growth	Growth	Aerobic, 37°C/48 h	[69]
L-S agar	TTC[b]	Irregular, red colonies with opaque zone	Circular red colonies with clear zone	Aerobic, 42°C/48 h	[70]
TPPY-eriochrome agar	Erichrome Black T	Irregular, transparent colonies	Opaque white-red colonies with a dark center	Anaerobic, 42°C/48 h	[71]
Modified lactic agar	TTC[b]	Large white colonies	Small red colonies	Anaerobic, 37°C/48 h	[72]
Acidified MRS agar	Acetic acid (pH 5.4)	Growth	No growth	Anaerobic, 37°C/72 h	[69]
TPY-HGME agar	Eriglaucine + HGME	Large dark blue colonies	Small light blue colonies	Anaerobic, 37°C/72 h	[73]
YGLP-YLA agar	Skimmed milk	Large white colonies	Small bright white colonies	Anaerobic, 37°C/48 h	[74]
RCPB agar	Prussian blue	Small white-blue colonies with wide blue zones	Large white-blue colonies with small blue zones	Anaerobic, 37°C/48 h	[75]

TPY-HGME: trypticase phytone yeast-hydrophobic grid membrane filter.

[a] Bromocresol red.

[b] Trizolium tetra chloride.

Owing to its acidic nature, fermented milks limit the growth of pathogenic microorganisms. Especially, some pathogens including *Listeria monocytogenes*, *Salmonella* spp., coliforms, and *Staphylococcus aureus* are rarely present in yogurt and other fermented milks [50]. These pathogens are rapidly inhibited within 24 h after

TABLE 8.6
Growth Medium Used in Counting *Lactobacillus acidophilus* and *Bifidobacterium* spp. in Yogurt and Fermented Milk Products

Growth Medium	Separating Agent	*Lactobacillus acidophilus*	*Bifidobacterium bifidum*	*Bifidobacterium infantis*	*Bifidobacterium breve*	*Bifidobacterium longum*	Incubation Conditions
MRS-LP agar	Lithium propionate	−	+	+	+	+	Anaerobic, 37°C/48–72 h
MRS-salicin agar	Salicin 0.5%	+	−	−	−	−	Anaerobic, 37°C/48 h
MRS-NNLP agar[a]	NNLP or NNLP + 0.05% cystein-HCl	−	+	+	+	+	Anaerobic, 37°C/48–72 h
LC agar	Lithium chloride 0.1% Sodium phosphate 0.3%	−	−	−	−	+	Anaerobic, 40°C/72 h
MRS-C agar	Lithium chloride 0.2% Sodium propionate 0.3%	−	−	−	+	+	Anaerobic, 37°C/48 h
Acidified MRS agar	pH 5.6 (M HCl)	+	−	−	−	−	Aerobic, 37°C/48 h
MRS-bile agar	—	+	−	−	−	−	Aerobic, 37°C/72 h
CAB agar[b]	0.05% Cystein 0.2% Lithium chloride 0.3% Sodium propionate	−	+	+	+	+	Anaerobic, 37°C/48 h

continued

TABLE 8.6 (continued)

Growth Medium	Separating Agent	Lactobacillus acidophilus	Bifidobacterium bifidum	Bifidobacterium infantis	Bifidobacterium breve	Bifidobacterium longum	Incubation Conditions
CAB-NNLP agar	5% NNLP	–	+	–	–	–	Anaerobic, 37°C/48 h
mMRS agar[c]	0.5% Lactose 0.05% Cystein-HCl	–	+	–	–	–	Anaerobic, 37°C/48 h
Beerens' agar		–	+	+	+	+	Anaerobic, 37°C/96 h
TPY-NNLP agar		–	–	–	–	+	Anaerobic, 37°C/48 h
RCM agar[d]	0.03% Aniline blue, 2 ppm dicloxacillin	–	+	+	+	+	Anaerobic, 37°C/72 h
BLA-NNLP[e]		–	+	–	–	–	Anaerobic, 37°C/72 h
Rogosa agar	Xglu[f]	–	+	–	–	–	Anaerobic, 37°C/72 h

Sources: Adapted from [76–87].

[a] NNLP: neomycine sulfate (100 mg l^{-1}), nalidixic acid (50 mg l^{-1}), paramycin sulfate (200 mg l^{-1}), lithium chloride (3000 mg l^{-1}).

[b] CAB: California Agar Base.

[c] Modified agar: 0.05% ((κ-casein + β-glycerophosphate + α-lactalbumin) + 0.5% yeast extract) or (0.5% yeast extract + 0.1% β-glycerophosphate).

[d] RCM: reinforced clostridial agar.

[e] BLA: blood liver agar.

[f] Xglu: 5-bromo-4-chloro-3-indolyl-β-D-gluco-pyranosidase.

TABLE 8.7
Growth Medium Used in Counting Yogurt Starter Bacteria and Probiotic Bacteria on the Same Petri Plate

Bacteria	mMRS Agar[a]	RCPB Agar[b]	RCPB Agar, pH 5	mLA[c]	TPPY Agar[d]	M 17 Agar
Lactobacillus acidophilus	Creamy colonies (2–2.5 mm in diameter)	No growth	No growth	Red colonies (1 mm in diameter)	No growth	No growth
Lactobacillus delbrueckii subsp. *bulgaricus*	No growth	Colonies with white-blue center and wide blue zone (1 mm in diameter)	Colonies with white center and blue zone (1 mm in diameter)	White colonies (2 mm in diameter)	Smooth and irregular transparent colonies (2 mm in diameter)	No growth
Bifidobacterium spp.	Cream colonies (1 mm in diameter)	Shiny white colonies (2 mm in diameter)	Shiny white colonies (2 mm in diameter)	Red colonies (1 mm in diameter)	Oval gray colonies (1 mm in diameter)	No growth
Streptococcus thermophilus	No growth	Colonies with blue center and blue zone (2 mm in diameter)	No growth	Red colonies (1 mm in diameter)	Opaque colonies with circular and dark center (2 mm in diameter)	Creamy colonies (1.5 mm in diameter)

Source: Adapted from Rybka, S. and Kailasapthy, K., *Int. Dairy J.*, 6, 839–850, 1996.

[a] mMRS: Modified MRS agar.
[b] RCPB: reinforced clostridial Prussian blue agar.
[c] mLA: modified lactic agar.
[d] TPPY: tryptose proteose peptone yeast extract agar.

the manufacture [17]. The level of survivability of the pathogenic organisms in fermented milk depends on the severity of contamination and the pH of the product [51,52]. Mild yogurts with pH values of >4.5 can allow the survival of salmonellae for up to 10 days [53]. Yogurt starter bacteria can prevent the growth of *Staphylococcus aureus* to some extent; the enterotoxin A synthesized by this organism can remain in yogurt throughout storage [54,55]. Similarly, yogurt starter bacteria show a strong antagonistic effect against *Listeria monocytogenes*; however, some strains of this organism are able to develop an acid adaptation and remain in yogurt during storage period [56,57]. Depending on the level of contamination, *Yersinia enterocolitica* is partly or completely inhibited in yogurt and other fermented milk products [58–60]. *Campylobacter jejuni* and *Salmonella* spp. (except *Salmonella infantis*) rarely remain viable in fermented milk products [61].

The presence of coliforms indicates the poor sanitary conditions during production of fermented milk products. In general, coliforms cannot stand high acidity and, therefore, are rarely present in fermented milk products with low pH values. However, Massa et al. [62] reported that *Escherichia coli* can survive in yogurt with pH values higher than 4.5 for up to 7 days. Additionally, coliform group microorganisms usually do not show resistance against the antibiotics produced by the yogurt starter bacteria. On the contrary, postfermentation contamination of verotoxigenic *Escherichia coli* O157:H7 carries a high risk for consumers' health [63]. Although *E. coli* O157:H7 is negatively affected by high acidity, it can survive in yogurt during cold storage [62]. Monitoring the viablity of pathogenic microorganisms in yogurt and fermented milk products is not a routine practice. However, in order to test the efficiency of the preventive measures against pathogenic contamination, it is recommended to monitor the viability of coliforms and *E. coli* in yogurt routinely [64]. Acid and gas production from lactose are the essential indicators of presence of coliform microorganisms. In the counting the number of coliform group bacteria, the violet red bile agar (VRBA), lauryl sulfate tryptose broth (LSTB), brilliant green lactose bile broth (BGLB), and MacConkey's broth are widely employed. On VRBA, the lactose-positive (lac$^+$) purple colonies with a diameter of <0.5–2.0 mm are recognized as coliform bacteria. In case the same colonies generate fluorescent light under a UV lamb at 360 nm wavelength, they are considered as *E. coli* [89]. For the rapid identification of coliform bacteria and *E. coli*, the modified LSTB agar added with 4-methyl-umbelliferyl *p*-D-glucuronide (MUG), culture media containing chromogene (*E. coli*/coliform medium, tryptone bile *X*-glucronide medium) and Petrifilm™ are used [90–92].

Despite the low risk of pathogenic microorganisms in yogurt and fermented milk products, the yeasts and molds present cause serious problems in fruit yogurts and fruit bioyogurts in terms of product quality and food safety [93]. In normal practice, the number of yeasts should not exceed the level of <1 g^{-1} of the product [94]. At low storage temperatures, the shelf life of fruit yogurt can be extended up to 30 days. In contrast, at higher temperatures, the growth of yeasts is stimulated, leading to the gas production and aroma/flavor defects in the end product [95]. If the number of yeasts exceeds the level of 10^5–10^6 g^{-1}, these defects are clearly evident [96]. Especially, galactose-positive (gal$^+$) yeasts can cause blowing in the fruit yogurt packages [97].

The most commonly isolated yeasts from fruit yogurt are *Kluyveromyces* spp. and *Saccharomyces* spp. (particularly, *Kluyveromyces marxianus* var. *marxianus* and *Saccharomyces cerevisiae*) [97,98]. In addition, *Saccharomyces exiguous*, *Rhodotorula glutinis*, *Yarrowia lipolytica*, and *Debaryomyces hansenii* likely cause quality problems in fruit yogurts stored at relatively high temperatures (e.g., 15–20°C) [99]. The major sources of yeasts in fruit yogurt are the fruit and additives that are added into the product after heat treatment [96]. Additionally, the fruit blenders and the surface of packaging machines are potential sources of yeast contamination [94]. The yeasts can grow relatively more easily at high acidic and low-temperature conditions than mesophilic and psychrotrophic bacteria. The growth of yeasts is rather limited in yogurt during cold storage, with an average generation time of 1 h. The sugar and fruit are utilized by the yeasts to meet their energy and nutritional requirements, making fruit yogurt and bioyogurt more perishable compared with the classical fermented milk products. Some metabolites (e.g., acetic acid) produced by yogurt starter bacteria can show inhibitive effect against yeasts [94]. Traditional concentrated yogurt is more readily subject to yeast contamination from the air as this product is produced by removing free water from the plain yogurt through gravity drainage at ambient temperature. To overcome this handicap, in some Middle Eastern countries, addition of potassium sorbate (>300 mg kg^{-1}) or sodium benzoate (up to 400 mg kg^{-1}) is a common practice [6,100,101].

The malt extract agar or broth, dichloran glycerol agar, and potato dextrose agar are among the growth media used in counting yeasts and molds. In recent years, ChemFlow (based on cytometric detection), the direct epifluorescent filter technique (DEFT), Petrifilm™ or the ISO-GRID technique are also gaining popularity for this purpose [6,102,103]. As with yeasts, the principal source of mold contamination is fruit itself. Heat treatment of fruit before incorporation into the product is the most effective way of preventing yeast and mold contamination. The molds can withstand very low temperature in fruit preparations (e.g., −23°C) [104].

Molds are aerobic organisms and require oxygen to secure their viability. Therefore, in set-type yogurts, the molds grow on the surface of the product, being recognized with the yellow filaments on the surface. The most common molds in yogurt and yogurt-type fermented milk products are *Mucor* spp., *Rhizopus* spp., *Aspergillus* spp., *Penicillum* spp., and *Alternia* spp. [17]. Since the aflatoxins produced by the molds carry risk for human health, the level of mold contamination in fermented milk products should not exceed 10 g^{-1} of the product. Aflatoxin can remain in yogurt throughout storage period. Hassanin [105], for example, demonstrated that Aflatoxin M1, which is present in yogurt bound to casein micelles, was found at detectable level in yogurt after 3 weeks of storage. Aflatoxin M1 may adversely affect the growth and acid-producing capacity of yogurt starter bacteria. Also, the cell morphology of the starter bacteria may be deformed by Aflatoxin M1 [106]. In contrast, Aflatoxin B1 has limited effect on the metabolic activities of yogurt starter bacteria and is largely degraded during fermentation [107]. Other aflatoxins produced by *Aspergillus flavus* and *Aspergillus parasiticus* (Aflatoxins B2, G1, and G2) can remain in yogurt and yogurt-type fermented milk products throughout storage period without being degraded [108,109]. The spores of *Aspergillus flavus* and *Aspergillus parasiticus* show great resistance against storage conditions of fermented milks [110,111].

To conclude, in order to prevent the growth of yeast and molds in yogurt and fermented milk products, the following measures should be taken:

- Hygienic conditions during and after production should be established efficiently
- The microbiological controls throughout the packaging line and in the fruit preparation tanks should be done routinely
- Storage temperature should be <4°C
- Incubation chambers and cold stores should be cleaned and sanitized routinely
- Fruits should be heat treated before adding into yogurt base [112]

8.5 SENSORY EVALUATION OF YOGURT AND FERMENTED MILKS

The chemical, physical, and microbiological qualities of yogurt and other fermented milk products are monitored routinely by means of advanced analytical testings. Although these testings provide us with scientific data on overall quality of the product in question, they cannot produce satisfactory data on the eating quality of the product. Two products with similar chemical and/or physical properties may be considered different by the consumers in terms of their eating qualities. Therefore, harmony between the overall quality properties and the organoleptic quality properties of a product is essential to ensure consumers' acceptability. In recent years, many kinds of yogurt and yogurt-type products have been introduced into the market and the sensory properties of yogurt and fermented milk products have become one of the principal factors that affect the consumers' choice. This has brought about the fact that sensory evaluation of foods has become a continuously developing and systematic scientific discipline that used to evoke measure, analyze, and interpret reactions to food and materials by the human senses [113].

In the past, in the organoleptic evaluation of yogurt and fermented milk products, nondescriptive hedonic tests based on texture, appearance, and color, and aroma and flavor of the product were used universally [114–117]. These tests were more appropriate for grading the consumer's preference on the product. A hedonic evaluation score card for yogurt is presented in Table 8.8. This evaluation method is simple but far from reflecting the actual sensory nature of the product in question. A similar approach was developed based on the relative importance of certain attributes by incorporating a multiplying factor (Table 8.9) [8]. Another organoleptic evaluation method of fermented milks is the Karl Ruher 9-point evaluation scheme (Table 8.10) [118]. According to this evaluation scheme, the samples are given points varying from 1 (very bad) to 9 (excellent) and divided into three intervals: I, II, and III. Each interval has three subclasses: upper, medium, and lower, and the samples taken in intervals I, II, and III are judged as no objection for consumption, still acceptable in commerce, and unsaleable, respectively. The American Dairy Science Association developed another sensory evaluation scheme for fermented dairy products in which

TABLE 8.8
Simplified Hedonic Evaluation Score Card

Property	Maximum Point	Defect	Product Code
Appearance and color	5		A
Body and texture	5		B
Aroma and flavor	10 (5 × 2)		C
Total score	20		D

1: Poor, 2: fair, 3: good, 4: very good, 5: excellent.

The overall score is obtained by multiplying the flavor score by 2 and then adding that score to the rest.

Defects:

Appearance and color: surface discolorization, fat separation on surface, wheying off, unnatural color, gassiness, and lack of uniformity.

Body and texture: too thin or too firm, dry, gelatinous, sticky, slimy, chalky, lumpy, or granular.

Aroma and flavor: buttery, lack of typical yogurt flavor, too sour, powdery, bitter/rancid, excess stabilizer, yeasty, unclean, and excess sugar.

Source: After Pearce, L.E. and Heap, H.A., *J. New Zeal. Milk Board*, 22, 18, 1974.

TABLE 8.9
Five-Point Scheme Proposed by Bergel in Germany

Characteristic	Maximum Point	Multiplying Factor	Total Points	Multiplying Factor
Flavor	5	5	25	50
Appearance	5	2	10	20
Consistency	5	2	10	20
Aroma	5	1	5	10
			50	**100**

Points	Description of property
5	Very good, ideal
4	Good
3	Satisfactory, few mistakes
2	Not very satisfactory, distinct mistakes
1	Not satisfactory
0	Bad, tainted

Source: Robinson, R.K. and Itsaranuwat, P., *Fermented Milks*, A.Y. Tamime, Ed., pp. 76–94, Blackwell Publishing, Oxford, 2006.

defects are described more clearly (Table 8.11). In this model, the evaluation is carried out based on the aroma/flavor, body/texture, and appearance/color defects of the product, and the samples are ranked according to their total scores [119].

In recent years, the quantitative descriptive analysis (QDA) has gained popularity in assessing the organoleptic properties of cultured dairy products. The quantitative descriptive analysis is based on a panelist's ability to verbalize perceptions of a

TABLE 8.10

Karl Ruher 9-Point Evaluation Scheme

Point	Decision	Quality	Aralık	Class	Overall judgment
9	Excellent	—		Upper	
8	Very good	Very good	I	Medium	No objection
7	Good	Good		Lower	
6	Satisfactory	Satisfactory		Upper	
5	Mediocre	Average	II	Medium	Still acceptable in commerce
4	Sufficient	Sufficient		Lower	
3	Imperfect	Bad		Upper	
2	Bad	Bad	III	Medium	Unsaleable
1	Very bad	Bad		Lower	

Source: Tamime, A.Y. and Robinson, R.K., *Yoghurt Science and Technology*, 3rd edition, p. 808, Woodhead Publishing, London, 2007.

TABLE 8.11

Sensory Evaluation Scheme Developed by American Dairy Science Association (ADSA)

Date: Panelist:

Aroma/Flavor Maximum 10 Points	Contestant Score →	1	2	3	Total Grades
	Score				
	Grade				
	Critisism				
No critisism: 10	Acetaldehyde (coarse)				
	Bitter				
	Cooked				
	Foreign				
	High acid				
	Lacks fine flavor				
	Lacks flavoring				
	Lacks freshness				
	Lacks sweetness				
	Low acid				
Normal range 1–10	Oxidized				
	Rancid				
	Too high flavoring				
	Too sweet				
	Unnatural flavoring				
	Unclean				

continued

TABLE 8.11 (continued)

Date: Panelist:

Body/Texture Maximum 5 Points	Contestant Score		Sample No.			Total Grades
		→	1	2	3	
	Score					
	Grade					
	Critisism					
No critisism: 5	Gel-like					
	Grainy					
	Ropy					
Normal range 1–5	Too firm					
	Weak					
Appearance Maximum 5 Points	**Contestant Score** →					
	Score					
	Grade					
	Critisism					
No critisism: 5	Atypical color					
	Color leaching					
	Excess fruit					
	Wheying off					
Normal range 1–5	Lumpy					
	Lacks fruit					
	Shrunken					
	Surface growth					
Total score	**Total score of each sample** →					
	Total grade per sample					
			Final grade			
			Rank			

Source: ADSA, American Dairy Science, Association, Committee on Evaluation of Dairy Products, Champaigne, IL, 1987.

product in a reliable manner. The method embodies a formal screening and training procedure, development and the scoring of products on repeated trials to obtain a complete, quantitative description. The panelists are given a training course for a period of 75–100 h and then they are asked to develop a terminology related to the product being evaluated. Table 8.12 shows a list of terminology developed by a group of panelists after 100 h of a training program. According to the alternative sensory evaluation method of fermented dairy products developed by the IDF, the defects of the products are divided into three groups and the panelists are asked to score the samples by taking these defects into account (Table 8.13).

TABLE 8.12

Terminology Developed for Organoleptic Evaluation of Yogurt and Fermented Milks

Odor	Taste	Aroma	Texture
Intensity	Intensity	Intensity	Firm
Sour	Sour/acidic	Bitter	Creamy
Fruity	Fruity	Sour/acidic	Viscous
Buttery	Buttery	Other	Ropy
Yeasty	Rancid		Lumpy
Creamy	Creamy		Mouth coating
Sweet	Salty		Chalky
Other	Bitter		Wheying off
	Lemon		
	Sweet		
	Chemical		

Source: Muir, D.D. and Hunter, E.A., *J. Soc. Dairy Technol.*, 45, 73–80, 1992.

For an objective evaluation of the product, the sample containers or lids should not contain any image associated with a brand. In general, the sensory evaluation of cultured dairy products is carried out at 4–6°C, and the order of presentation of samples is decided by using an appropriate statistical program [120,121]. For the estimation of treatment effects in experiments, the residual maximum likelihood (REML) method is widely used [122,123]. In order to simplify data obtained from REML analysis, the principal component analysis (PCA), which is a multiple variance analysis, is used [124,125]. PCA is a method that reduces data dimensionality by performing a covariance analysis between factors [126]. Figure 8.6 illustrates the simplified PCA pattern of a set of sensory data obtained from yogurt samples treated with microbial transglutaminase (m-TGase) ($n = 15$). The samples were analyzed according to the predeveloped terminology that consisted of 20 characteristics representing flavor, texture, and appearance of the products in question [127].

8.6 DETERMINATION OF THE SHELF LIFE OF YOGURT AND FERMENTED MILK PRODUCTS

Shelf life is that length of time that food, drink, medicine, and other perishable items are given before they are considered unsuitable for sale or consumption. For some dairy products including yogurt, shelf life is mandated by regulation at the state or even municipal level. However, in most cases, shelf life is determined by the manufacturer and is generally indicated to the consumer as a "sell by" or "best if used by" date [128]. Some instrumental analysis methods are also employed to determine the shelf life of foods. In the determination of shelf life of fermented milk products, the relationships between the quality parameters such as syneresis, flavor, pH, and appearance are

TABLE 8.13
Quality Terms for Fermented Milks

Appearance	Consistency	Taste
Overfilled	Setting	Watery
Underfilled	Lumps or flakes	Flat
Shrunken	Uneven	Bitter
Heterogeneous surface	Sticky	Cooked
Untypical color	Too thick	Burnt
Brown color	Too fluid	Smoked
Nonuniform color	Ropy/stringy	Oily
Marbled	Dried	Chemical
Air bubbles	Gelatinous	Feed flavor
Foreign matter	Brittle	Foreign flavor
Whey separation	Gritty	Oxide
Mold	Dripping	Defective aromatization
Yeast		Cheesy
Separation of phase		Malty
Sedimentation		Metallic
Lack of or poor distribution of ingredients		Musty
		Oxidized
		Acid
		Sharp
		Harsh
		Sour
		Tallowy
		Yeasty
		Rancid
		Astringent
		Unclean
		Stale/old
		Too sweet
		Too salty
		Soapy/alkaline

Source: IDF, *Sensory Evaluation of Dairy Products by Scoring: Reference Method*, Standard 99c, International Dairy Federation, Brussels, 1997.

evaluated by the panelists. In this evaluation, the product being analyzed is compared with its fresh counterpart in terms of the selected quality parameters. In the comparison of the samples, the 7-point difference-from-control category scale is usually used. In this scale, the numbers represent the following judgments: 0, no difference; 1, very slight difference; 2, slight difference; 3, moderate difference; 4, moderately big difference; 5, big difference; and 6, very big difference [131]. If the differences between the fresh control and the product being analyzed regarding the selected parameters exceed a threshold level, the shelf life of the product is decided to be ended. The threshold level

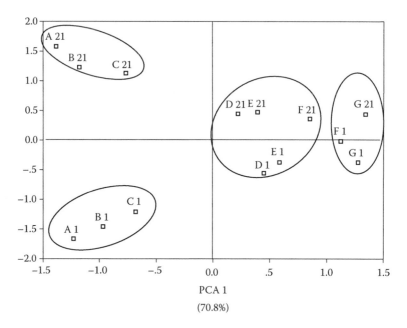

FIGURE 8.6   Simplified illustration of sensory evaluation data of yogurts added with TGase at various levels (g 100 g^{-1}). A: 0, B: 0.1, C: 0.2, D: 0.3, E: 0.4, F: 0.5, G: 0.5 (enzyme was deactivated before starter addition). 1 and 21 represent storage days.

for the differences between the quality parameters is determined by means of statistical models such as Weibull's hazard analysis [132–135].

Throughout storage period, the product in question is analyzed organoleptically by a group of panelists. At the storage time where the product is regarded as unsuitable for consumption by the majority of the panelists, the sensory evaluation data are processed to Weibull's hazard graphics and a probability factor (β) is calculated via the slope of the graphics (β = 1/slope). This probability factor is accepted as threshold level for the shelf life of the product.

8.7   DEFECTS OF YOGURT AND OTHER FERMENTED MILKS

Poor manufacturing practices often result in some sensory defects in yogurt and other fermented milk products. These defects may be divided into the following three groups: (i) defects of aroma and flavor, (ii) defects resulting in changes of appearance, and (iii) defects of body and texture.

8.7.1   AROMA/FLAVOR DEFECTS

Lack of the characteristic aroma/flavor profile is among the most common organoleptic defects in yogurt. The carbonyl compounds produced by the starter bacteria including acetaldehyde, acetone, acetoin, and diacetyl establish the characteristic yogurt aroma/flavor, acetaldehyde being the principal compound. Therefore, any factor interfering with the metabolic activity of the starter culture likely causes aroma/flavor defects in the end product. The major factors affecting starter culture activity are incubation temperature and period, presence of inhibitor substances in raw milk, and bacteriophage activity. *Lactobacillus delbrueckii* subsp. *bulgaricus* is principally responsible for the production of carbonyl compounds during yogurt fermentation, and insufficient growth or metabolic activity of this bacteria leads eventually to lack of characteristic aroma/flavor in yogurt. *Streptococcus thermophilus* is mainly responsible for the development of acidity during fermentation and any factor disturbing the growth or metabolic activity of this starter bacteria adversely affects the establishment of aroma/flavor balance in the final product. To obtain yogurt with a well-balanced aroma/flavor characteristics, the incubation temperature and inoculation level of starter culture should be selected properly. As the yogurt starter bacteria are thermophilic, the incubation temperature of fermenting milk should be set as 41–43°C. Too high or too low starter inoculation levels cause aroma/flavor defects in yogurt, and therefore, the level of inoculation should be designed as 2.5–3.0%. At higher inoculation levels, depending on the increased lactic acid concentration, the aroma/flavor compounds are masked. In contrast, at lower inoculation levels, characteristic aroma/flavor balance is established due to insufficient growth of starter bacteria. Too fast cooling after fermentation also results in aroma/flavor defects in fermented milks. Therefore, in order to avoid this problem, two-phase cooling is recommended, as discussed in Section 2.2.8. Excessive sourness is another major flavor problem in fermented milks. Although improper storage conditions (e.g., high storage temperature) and high starter inoculation level are the principal causes of sourness, other factors including too slow cooling after fermentation and low levels of fat and protein in yogurt also stimulate the development of excess sour taste in yogurt. Cooked flavor is developed in yogurt as a result of the heat treatment at high temperatures. In this respect, the heating temperature of yogurt milk should not be higher than 90–95°C for 5–10 min. Other factors causing aroma/flavor defects in yogurt and their remedies are presented in Table 8.14. Kefir and koumiss are among the popular fermented milks in the Eastern Europe and Central Asia. Kefir is characterized by having an acidic, milky taste and slight yeasty flavor, and the texture of the product should be uniform [136]. The common faults of kefir are attributed to taste and aroma [136]. Especially, *Saccharomyces cerevisiae* causes a vinegar-like or solvent-like aroma in kefir [137]. Similarly, *Acetobacter* spp. leads to development of acetic acid aroma. Molds (e.g., *Geotrichum candidum*) and some yeasts present in kefir can cause bitterness in the end product. In koumiss, the levels of acidity and alcohol influence the sensory quality of the final product. Table 8.15 shows the sensory properties of koumiss as affected by the levels of acidity and alcohol.

8.7.2 Appearance Defects

Appearance is one of the principal quality criteria for the acceptability of yogurt by consumers. The most widely encountered appearance problems in yogurt are dry surface and heterogeneous color distribution on the surface of the product. The first problem results from the evaporation of water from the yogurt pot during cold storage. This problem can be prevented by using a proper packaging material and/or

TABLE 8.14

Causes and Preventive Conditions of the Common Defects in Yogurt-Type Fermented Milk Products

Defects	Possible Causes	Preventive Measures
Aroma/Flavor Defects		
Insipid	– Insufficient incubation	– Ceasing incubation at pH <4.6
	– Presence of bacteriophages	– Evaluation of sanitation conditions and culture rotation
	– Insufficient growth of *Lactobacillus delbrueckii* subsp. *bulgaricus*	– Setting incubation temperatures at 42–43°C and monitoring the presence of inhibitor substances such as antibiotics
	– Insufficient inoculation	– Adding starter culture at the level of 2.0–2.5%
	– Too fast cooling after fermentation	– Applying two-phase cooling after incubation
Sour	– Too high starter culture inoculation level	– Adding starter culture at the level of 2.0–2.5%
	– High ratio of *Lactobacillus delbrueckii* subsp. *bulgaricus* in starter culture	– Inoculate milk with fresh culture
	– High incubation temperature	– Setting incubation temperatures at 42–43°C
	– Insufficient cooling after fermentation	– Applying two-phase cooling after incubation (1st phase at 20–22°C, 2nd phase at <7°C)
	– Too long incubation period	– Ceasing incubation at pH 4.6
	– Improper storage temperature	– Setting storage temperature at 4°C
Cooked flavor	– Reactivation of sulfhydryl groups as a result of high heat treatment	– Heat treatment at 80–85°C for 20–30 min or at 90–95°C for 5–10 min
Metallic flavor	– Metal contamination to yogurt or yogurt milk	– Using stainless steel equipment
Malty/yeasty flavor	– Contamination of yeasts and/or molds to yogurt	– Providing proper sanitation conditions throughout manufacturing
Feed flavor	– Feeding animals with rotten feeds	– Revision of silage production method and selection of right fermentation conditions for silage-making
	– Feeding animals with too aromatic feeds	– Removal of feeds with bad smell/odor from feeding program
Appearance Defects		
Color defects	– Heterogeneous color due to the growth of yeast/mold	– Establishing hygiene and sanitation protocols properly
	– Dirts coming from raw milk	– Cleaning of milk through mechanical separator
	– Heterogeneous distribution of fruits in fruit yogurt	– Blending fruit with yogurt base efficiently

continued

TABLE 8.14   (continued)

Defects	Possible Causes	Preventive Measures
	– Cooking milk at high temperature for longer period	– Heat treatment at 80–85°C for 20–30 min or at 90–95 °C for 5–10 min
Dry surface	– Surface evaporation during storage	– Proper packaging material, right storage temperature, and adjustment of relative humidity in cold store
Bubbles in coagulum	– Contamination with coliforms	– Establishing hygiene and sanitation protocols properly
	– Contamination with yeasts	
Crystal-like appearance	– Storage of yogurt at subzero temperatures	– Storage temperature at 2–4°C
Precipitated appearance	– Poor dissolving capacity of milk-based powder added into yogurt base	– Efficiently dissolving milk-based powders at 39–40°C, and filtering milk before fermentation to remove undissolved particles
Nodule	– Low incubation temperature	– Incubating milk at 42–43°C
	– Too low or too high inoculation level	– Adding starter culture at the level of 2.0–2.5%
	– Mechanical disturbance during fermentation	– Avoiding physical disturbance during fermentation
	– Seasonal variations in raw milk	

Body/Texture Defects

Defects	Possible Causes	Preventive Measures
Weak body	– Incomplete SS–SH interactions as a result of insufficient heat treatment	– Heat treatment at 80–85°C for 20–30 min or at 90–95°C for 5–10 min to provide whey protein denaturation at a ratio of >90%
	– Insufficient SNF and fat levels	– Increasing total solids content of yogurt milk to 15.5–16.0%. Avoiding to add caseinate at levels of higher than 4%
	– Presence of antibiotics in milk	– Discarding milk containing antibiotics
	– Presence of inhibitors such as alkaline, carbonate, H_2O_2	– Discarding milk containing inhibitors
	– Deformation as a result of physical disturbance during fermentation	– Avoiding mechanical disturbance during fermentation
	– Bacteriophage contamination	– Providing high hygienic and sanitation standards and culture rotation
	– Insufficient starter culture inoculation	– Adding starter culture at the level of 2.0–2.5%
	– Insufficient homogenization pressure	– Two-stage homogenization of milk (1st stage at 175 kg cm^2, 2nd stage at 125 kg cm^2, 65°C)
Wheying off	– Incomplete SS–SH interactions as a result of insufficient heat treatment	– Heat treatment at 80–85°C for 20–30 min or at 90–95°C for 5–10 min to provide whey protein denaturation at a ratio of >90%

continued

TABLE 8.14   (continued)

Defects	Possible Causes	Preventive Measures
	– Too low or too high starter culture activity	– Choosing medium acid-producing starter strains
	– Overacidification due to higher storage temperatures	– Keeping storage temperature at <4°C to control the development of acidity
	– Mechanical disturbances	– Avoiding mechanical disturbance and choosing correct type of pump and pressure

selecting correct storage temperature. Growth of yeasts and molds in yogurt likely causes heterogeneous color distribution on the surface of yogurt stored at higher temperatures. To avoid this problem, proper hygienic measures should be taken. Yogurt milk should be clarified before being converted to yogurt so that any solids materials coming from raw milk are removed completely. Otherwise, unclean appearance may develop in the end product. Bubbles in the coagulum may indicate the coliform contamination, and the products with bubbles should be destroyed and the sources of contamination should be eliminated effectively. Less likely, a crystal-like structure may be seen on yogurt surface resulting from keeping the product at subzero temperature. In this case, the temperature of the storage room should be adjusted to 2–4°C. Milk-based powders incorporated into yogurt milk to increase the total solids content is a common practice in yogurt-making. Poor-quality powders may not be dissolved properly and particulate at the bottom of the yogurt pots. Mixing the powder with milk at 39–40°C and passing the milk added with powder through a stainless steel mash can eliminate this handicap. For more information on the specifications of the milk-based powders used in yogurt production, readers may refer to Chapter 2.

TABLE 8.15

Classification of Koumiss Based on Acidity and Alcohol Contents

	Alcohol (g per 100 mL)	Acidity (mL per 100 mL)
Weak flavor Sweet-sour taste Yeasty odor	1.0	0.63–0.72
Medium flavor Boldly-sour taste Yeasty odor	1.5	0.73–0.90
Strong flavor Hardy-milk acid taste Yeasty odor	3.0	0.91–1.08

Source: Adapted from Lozovich, S., *Cult. Dairy Prod. J.*, 30, 18–20, 1991.

8.7.3 Body/Texture Defects

Major body/texture defects that can occur in yogurt are weak body and whey separation. The most important technological parameter determining the physical stability of yogurt gel network is total solids standardization. In some countries, the use of stabilizer to improve the textural quality of set-type yogurt is prohibited. Therefore, increasing the total solids level of yogurt milk to 15.5–16.0% prior to fermentation is a common practice. Insufficient total solids fortification leads often to a weak body and wheying off. On the contrary, addition of too much skim milk powder or caseinate powder into yogurt base results in a too firm body, with increased whey separation. The mechanism of this phenomenon is discussed in detail in Chapter 2. Homogenization affects the textural properties of yogurt-type set or stirred products positively. Similarly, heat treatment contributes to the establishment of desired textural structure in yogurt. Heat treatment of yogurt base at lower temperatures than usual heating norms (80–85°C for 20–30 min or 90–95°C for 5–15 min) causes textural defects due to incomplete denaturation of whey proteins.

The presence of nondispersible particles (nodules) suspended in the yogurt gel is considered as a textural defect. The terms "lumpy" or "granular" have also been used to describe this texture defect. Although the presence of these nodules does not affect the nutritional or the organoleptic qualities of yogurt, there is a detrimental influence on the appearance and hence the marketability of the product [139]. The exact mechanism of nodulation is yet to be established. High incubation temperatures, low starter activity, and high levels of starter inoculum (>3%) have long been known as possible causes of nodulation in yogurt. Fruit yogurt are usually subjected to mechanical agitation (i.e., pumping from cooling tank to packaging unit, fruit mixing). Therefore, low viscosity and/or wheying off are common problems in stirred yogurts. To overcome this problem, addition of stabilizers or incorporation of polysaccharide-producing starter culture strains are the common practices. Additionally, pretreatment to fruits and the type of fruit can stimulate the wheying off in fruit yogurt. To prevent the occurrence of textural defects in yogurt-type products, all processing parameters including incubation temperature, level of inoculum, type of starter culture, fortification of total solids, or cooling speed after fermentation should be established properly.

REFERENCES

1. Hoolasi, K., A HACCP study on yoghurt manufacture, MSc thesis, Deptartment of Operations & Quality Management, Durban Institute of Technology, p. 68, 2005.
2. Jones, M., Processing plants, in *Encyclopedia of Dairy Science*, H. Roginski, J. Fuquay and P. Fox, Eds., pp. 1288–1294, Elsevier Applied Science, London, 2002.
3. Byrne, R.D. and Bishop, J.R., Control of microorganisms in dairy processing: Dairy product safety systems, in *Applied Dairy Microbiology*, E.H. Marth and J.L. Steele, Eds., pp. 405–430, Marcel Dekker, New York, 1998.
4. Anonymous, EU 92/46/EEC Council Directive laying down the health rules for the production and placing on the market of raw milk, heat-treated milk and milk-based products. European Union, Commission Legislative Document, 1992.ec.europa.eu/food/fs/sfp/mr/mr03_en.pdf (accessed on 10.09.2008).

5. Kasimoglu, A., Sireli, U.T., and Akgun, S., Yogurt uretiminde kontaminasyon kaynak-larinin belirlenmesi, *Turkish J. Vet. Animal Sci.*, 28, 17–22, 2004.

6. Özer, B., *Yogurt Bilimi ve Teknolojisi*, Sidas Yayincilik, Izmir, 488, 2006.

7. Karaali, A., *Gida Isletmelerinde HACCP Uygulamalari ve Denetimi*, p. 196, Saglik Bakanligi Temel Saglik Hizmetleri Genel Mudurlugu Yayinlari, Ankara, 2003.

8. Robinson, R.K. and Itsaranuwat, P., Properties of yoghurt and their appraisal, in *Fermented Milks*, A.Y. Tamime, Ed., pp. 76–94, Blackwell Publishing, Oxford, 2006.

9. Varnam, A.H. and Sutherland, J.P., *Milk and Milk Products. Technology, Chemistry and Microbiology*, p. 451, Chapman & Hall, London, 1994.

10. Harrigan, W.F. and McCance, M.E., *Laboratory Methods in Food and Dairy Micro-biology*, p. 452, Academic Press, London, 1993.

11. Robinson, R.K. and Tamime, A.Y., Quality appraisal of yoghurt, *Soc. Dairy Technol.*, 29, 148–155, 1976.

12. Marquez, M.F., Ruiz, B.G.V., and Ruiz-Lopez, D., Determination of total solids in dairy products using the microwave-oven method, *Int. J. Food Sci. Technol.*, 30, 307–310, 1995.

13. Barrantes, E., Tamime, A.Y., Davies, G., and Barclay, M.N.I., Production of low calories yogurt using skim milk powder and fat-substitutes. 2. Compositional changes, *Milchwissenschaft*, 49, 135–139, 1994.

14. Dubert, A. and Robinson, R.K., Development of a low-fat yoghurt using Tapiocaline, *Dairy Ind. Int.*, 67, 18–20, 2002.

15. Monneuse, M.O., Bellisle, F., and de Antoni, G., Impact of sex and age on sensory evaluation of sugar and fat in dairy products, *Physiol. Behav.*, 59, 579–583, 2000.

16. Folkenberg, D.M. and Martens, M., Sensory properties of low-fat yohurts, *Milchwissenschaft*, 58, 48–51, 2003.

17. Tamime, A.Y. and Robinson, R.K., *Yoghurt Science and Technology*, 3rd edition, p. 808, Woodhead Publishing, London, 2007.

18. Anonymous, *Codex Standards for Fermented Milks*, Codex Stan 243, 2003.

19. Ellen, G. and Tudos, A.J., On-line measurement of product quality in dairy processing, in *Dairy Processing-Improving Quality*, G. Smit, Ed., pp. 263–288, Woodhead Publishing, Cambridge, UK, 2003.

20. I.D.F., *General Standard of Identity for Fermented Milks*, Standard 163, International Dairy Federation, Brussels, 1992.

21. Lin, M.Y. and Young, C.M., Folate levels in cultures of lactic acid bacteria, *Int. Dairy J.*, 10, 409–413, 2000.

22. Illic, D.B. and Ashoor, S.H., Stability of vitamins A and C in fortified yogurt, *J. Dairy Sci.*, 71, 1492–1498, 1988.

23. Kokini, J.L., Rheological properties of foods, in *Handbook of Food Engineering*, D.R. Heldman and D.B. Lund, Eds, pp. 1–38, Marcel Dekker, New York, 1992.

24. Barbosa-Canovas, G.V., Ibarz, A., and Peleg, M., Rheological properties of fluid foods: Review, *Alimentaria*, 241, 39–89, 1993.

25. Özer, B.H., Robinson, R.K., and Grandison, A.S., Effect of elevation of total solids by ultra-filtration and reverse osmosis on thiol groups in milk, *Milchwissenschaft*, 54, 609–611, 2002.

26. Vasbinder, A.J., Alting, A.C., Visscher, R.W., and de Kruif, G.G., Texture of acid milk gels: Formation of disulfide cross-links during acidification, *Int. Dairy J.*, 13, 29–38, 2003.

27. Bertrand-Harb, C., Ivanovai I.V., Dalgalarrondo, M., and Haetlle, T., Evolution of β-lactoglobulin and α-lactalbumin content during yoghurt fermentation, *Int. Dairy J.*, 13, 39–45, 2003.

28. Steventon, A.J., Parkinson, C.J., Fryer, P.J., and Bottomley, R.C., The rheology of yogurt, in *Rheology of Food, Pharmaceutical, and Biological Materials with General Rheology*, R.E. Carter, Ed., pp. 196–210, Elsevier Science, London, 1990.

29. Özer, B.H., Robinson, R.K., Grandison, A.S., and Bell, A.E., Comparison of techniques for measuring the rheological properties of labneh (concentrated yogurt), *Int. J. Dairy Technol.*, 50, 129–133, 1997.

30. Jaros, D. and Rohm, H., Controlling the texture of fermented dairy products: the case of yogurt, in *Dairy Processing*, G. Smit, Ed., pp. 155–184, Woodhead Publishing, Cambridge, UK, 2003.

31. Özer, B.H. and Atamer, M., Some properties of yoghurt produced from milk preserved by hydrogen peroxide, *Milchwissenschaft*, 54, 618–621, 1999.

32. Rohm, H., Viscosity determination of stirred yogurt, *Lebensm. Wiss. Technol.*, 25, 297–301, 1992.

33. Hassan, A.N., Frank, J.F., Schmidt, K.A., and Shalabi, S.I., Textural properties of yogurt made with encapsulated non-ropy lactic cultures, *J. Dairy Sci.*, 79, 2098–2103, 1996.

34. Rohm, H. and Kovac, A., Effect of starter cultures on linear viscoelastic and physical properties of yogurt gels, *J. Texture Stud.*, 25, 311–329, 1994.

35. Horne, D., Dynamic rheology in dairy research, in *Hannah Research Yearbook*, E. Taylor, Ed., p. 81, Hannah Research Institute, Ayr, UK, 1993.

36. Özer, B.H., Rheological properties of concentrated yoghurt (Labneh), PhD thesis, The University of Reading, Reading, UK, p. 275, 1997.

37. Clarke, A.H. and Ross-Murphy, S.B., Structural and mechanical properties of biopolymer gels, *Adv. Polym. Sci.*, 83, 57–92, 1987.

38. Lewis, M.J., *Physical Properties of Foods and Food Processing Systems*, p. 465, Woodhead Publishing Press, Cambridge, England, 1986.

39. Özer, B.H., Bell, A.E., Grandison, A.S., and Robinson, R.K., Rheological properties of concentrated yoghurt (labneh), *J. Texture Stud.*, 29, 67–79, 1998.

40. Özer, B.H., Robinson, R.K., Grandison, A.S., and Bell, A.E., Gelation profiles of milks concentrated by different techniques, *Int. Dairy J.*, 8, 793–799, 1998.

41. van Vliet, T., Rheological classification of foods and instrumental techniques for their study, in *Food Texture: Measurement and Perception*, A.J. Rosentahl, Ed., pp. 65–98, Aspen Publishers Inc., Gaithersburg, MD, 1999.

42. Dickinson, E. and McClement, D.J., *Advances in Food Colloids*, p. 333, Blackie Academic and Professionals Publ., Glasgow, UK, 1996.

43. Dickinson, E., Computer simulation of particle gel formation, *J. Chem. Soc. Faraday Trans.*, 90, 173–180, 1994.

44. Özer, B.H., Destructive effects of classical viscometers on the microstructure of yoghurt gel, *Turkish J. Agric. Forestry*, 28, 19–23, 2004.

45. Cayot, P., Fairise, J.F., Colas, B., Lorient, D., and Brule, G., Improvement of rheological properties of firm acid gels by skim milk heating is conserved after stirring, *J. Dairy Res.*, 70, 423–431, 2003.

46. Bianchi-Salvadori, B., Lactic acid bacteria: Biochemical characteristics affecting the texture of fermented milk products, in *Proceedings of IDF Symposium on Texture of Fermented Milk Products and Dairy Desserts*, 5–6 May, Vicenza, Italy, pp. 48–62, IDF Special Issue (no.: 9802), International Dairy Federation, Brussels, 1998.

47. Walstra, P., Relationship between structure and texture of cultured milk products, in *Proceedings of IDF Symposium on Texture of Fermented Milk Products and Dairy Desserts*, 5–6 May, Vicenza, Italy, pp. 9–15, IDF Special Issue (no.: 9802), International Dairy Federation, Brussels, 1998.

48. Beal, C., Louvet, P., and Corrieu, G., Influence of controlled pH and temperature on the growth and acidification of pure cultures of *Streptococcus thermophilus* 404 and *Lactobacillus bulgaricus* 398, *Appl. Microbiol. Biotechnol.*, 32, 148–154, 1999.

49. Harwalkar, V.R. and Kalab, M., Susceptibility of yoghurt to syneresis. Comparison of centrifugation and drainage methods, *Milchwissenschaft*, 38, 517–522, 1983.

50. Gohil, V.S., Ahmed, M.A., Davies, R., and Robinson, R.K., The incidence of *Listeria* in foods in the United Arab Emirates, *J. Food Protect.*, 5, 102–104, 1995.

51. Zuniga-Estrada, A., Lopez-Merino, A., and Mota de la Garza, L., Behaviour of *Listeria monocytogenes* in milk fermented with a yogurt starter culture. *Rev. Latinoamericana Microbiol.*, 37, 257–265, 1995.

52. Riberio, S.H.S. and Caminati, D., Survival of *Listeria monocytogenes* in fermented milk and yoghurt: effect of pH, lysozyme content and storage at 4°C, *Sci. Aliment.*, 16, 175–185, 1996.

53. Al-Haddad, K.S.H. and Robinson, R.K., Survival of salmonellae in bio-yoghurts, *Dairy Ind. Int.*, 69, 16–18, 2003.

54. Zuniga-Estrada, A., Sanchez-Mendoza, M., Mota de la Garza, L., and Ortigoza-Ferado, J., Behaviour of enterotoxigenic strains of *Staphylococcus aureus* in milk fermented with a yoghurt starter culture, *Rev. Latinoamericana Microbiol.*, 37, 257–265, 1999.

55. Halawa, M.A. and Abouzeid, A.M., Behaviour of enterohemorrhagic *Escherichia coli* and enterotoxigenic *Staphylococcus aureus* in yoghurt and acidified milk, *Vet. Medic. J. Giza*, 48, 319–326, 2000.

56. Gahan, G.C., O'Driscoll, B., and Hill, C., Acid adaptation of *Listeria monocytogenes* can enhance survival in acidic foods and during milk fermentation, *Appl. Environ. Microbiol.*, 62, 3128–3132, 1996.

57. Stanczak, B.J., Szczawinski, J., and Pocenek, J., Survival of *Listeria monocytogenes* in fermented milk products, *Medycyna Weterynaryjna*, 53, 592–595, 1997.

58. Aytac, S.A. and Ozbas, Z.Y., Survey of the growth and survival of *Yersinia enterocolitica* and *Aeromonas hydrophila* in yogurt, *Milchwissenschaft*, 49, 322–325, 1994.

59. Bodnaruk, P.W., Williams, R.C., and Golden, D.A., Survival of *Yersinia enterocolitica* during fermentation and storage of yogurt, *J. Food Sci.*, 63, 535–537, 1998.

60. Little, C.L., Adams, M.R., Anderson, W.A., and Cole, M.B., Application of a log-logistic model to describe the survival of *Yersinia enterocolitica* at sub-optimal pH and temperature, *Int. J. Food Microbiol.*, 22, 63–71, 1994.

61. Al-Haddad, A. and Khawla, S.H., Survival of salmonellae in bio-yoghurt, *Int. J. Dairy Technol.*, 56, 199–202, 2003.

62. Massa, S., Altieri, C., Quaranta, V., and Pace, R., Survival of *Escherichia coli* O157:H7 in yoghurt during preparation and storage at 4°C, *Lett. Appl. Microbiol.*, 24, 347–350, 1997.

63. Dineen, S.S., Takeuchi, K., Soudah, J.E., and Boor, K.J., Persistence of *Escherichia coli* O157:H7 in dairy fermentation system, *J. Food Protect.*, 61, 1602–1608, 1998.

64. Ghani, A.E., Sadek, Z.I., and Fathi, F.A., Reliability of coliform bacteria as an indicator of postprocessing contamination in yoghurt manufacture, *Dairy Food Environ. Sanit.*, 18, 494–498, 1998.

65. Elliker, P.R., Anderson A.E., and Hannesson, G., An agar culture medium for lactic acid streptococci and lactobacilli, *J. Dairy Sci.*, 39, 1611–1612, 1956.

66. Davis, J.G., Ashton, T.R., and McCaskill, M., Enumeration and viability of *L. bulgaricus* and *Str. thermophilus* in yoghurt, *Dairy Ind.*, 569–573, 1971.

67. Porubcan, R.S. and Sellars, R.L., Stabilized dry cultures of lactic acid-producing bacteria, US Patent no. 3 897 307, 1973.

68. Lee, S.Y., Vedamuthu, E.R., Washam, C.J., and Reingold, G.W., An agar medium for the differential enumeration of yogurt starter bacteria, *J. Milk Food Technol.*, 37, 272–276, 1974.

69. I.D.F., Yogurt: enumeration of characteristic microorganisms, Standard 117A, International Dairy Federation, Brussels, 1988.

70. Eloy, C. and Lacrosse, R., The composition of a culture medium intended for the enumeration of thermophilic microorganisms in yogurt, *Bull. Res. Agron. Gembloux*, 11, 83–86, 1976.

71. Bracquart, P., An agar medium for the differential enumeration of *Streptococcus thermophilus* and *Lactobacillus bulgaricus* in yoghurt, *J. Appl. Bacteriol.*, 51, 303–305, 1981.

72. Matalon, M.E. and Sandine, W.E., Improved media for differentiation of rods and cocci in yogurt, *J. Dairy Sci.*, 69, 2569–2576, 1986.
73. Millard, G.E., McKellar, R.C., and Holley, M.A., Counting yogurt starters, *Dairy Ind. Int.*, 54, 5, 1989.
74. Ghoddusi, H., Some aspects of the enumeration of bifidobacteria in white-brined cheese, PhD thesis, The Univeristy of Reading, Reading, UK, 1996.
75. Onggo, I. and Fleet, G.H., Media for the isolation and enumeration of lactic acid bacteria from yogurts, *Aus. J. Dairy Technol.*, 48, 89–92, 1993.
76. Kneifel, W. and Pacher, B., An X-Glu based agar medium for the selective enumeration of *Lactobacillus acidophilus* in yogurt-related milk products, *Int. Dairy J.*, 3, 277–291, 1993.
77. Lamoureux, L., Roy, D., and Gauthier, S.F., Production of oligosaccharides in yogurt containing bifidobacteria and yogurt cultures, *J. Dairy Sci.*, 85, 1058–1069, 2002.
78. Dave, R.I. and Shah, N.P., Ingredient supplementation effects of viability of probiotic bacteria in yogurt, *J. Dairy Sci.*, 81, 2804–2816, 1998.
79. Corbo, M.R., Albenzio, M., De Angelis, M., Sevi, A., and Gobbetti, M., Microbiological and biochemical properties of Canestrato Pugliese hard cheese supplemented with bifidobacteria, *J. Dairy Sci.*, 84, 551–561, 2001.
80. Breatry, S., Ross, R.P., Fitzgerald, G.F., Collins, K.J., Wallace, J.M., and Stanton, C., Influence of two commercially available bifidobacteria cultures on Cheddar cheese quality, *Int. Dairy J.*, 11, 599–610, 2001.
81. Crittenden, R.G., Morris, L.F., Harvey, M.L., Tran, L.T., Mitvhel, H.L., and Payne, M.J., Selection of a bifidobacterium strain to complement resistant starch in a synbiotic yoghurt, *J. Appl. Bacteriol.*, 90, 268–278, 2001.
82. Beerens, H., An elective and selective isolation medium for *Bifidobacterium* spp., *Lett. Appl. Microbiol.*, 11, 155–157, 1990.
83. Ghoddusi, H. and Robinson, R.K., Enumeration of starter cultures in fermented milks, *J. Dairy Res.*, 63, 151–158, 1996.
84. Kailasapathy, K. and Sureeta, B.S., Effect of storafe on shelf-life and viability of freze-dried and microencapsulated *Lactobacillus acidophilus* and *Bifidobacterium infantis* cultures, *Aus. J. Dairy Technol.*, 59, 204–208, 2004.
85. Picot, A. ve Lacroux, C., Encapsulation of bifidobacteria in whey protein-based microcapsules and survival in stimulated gastrointestinal conditions and in yoghurt. *Int. Dairy J.*, 14, 505–515, 2004.
86. Lankaputhra, W.E.V. and Shah, N.P., A simple method for selective enumeration of *Lactobacillus acidophilus* in yogurt supplemented with *L. acidophilus* and *Bifidobacterium* spp., *Milchwissenschaft*, 51, 446–450, 1996.
87. Dinakar, P. and Mistry, V.V., Growth and viability of *Bifidobacterium bifidum* in Cheddar cheese, *J. Dairy Sci.*, 77, 2854–2864, 1994.
88. Rybka, S. and Kailasapathy, K., Media for the enumeration of yoghurt bacteria, *Int. Dairy J.*, 6, 839–850, 1996.
89. Hudson, L.M., Chen, J., Hilla, R., and Griffiths, M.F., Bioluminescence; a rapid indicator of *Escherichia coli* O157:H7 in selected yogurt and cheese varieties, *J. Food Protect.*, 60, 891, 1997.
90. F.A.O., *Manual of Food Quality Control, 4 Rev.1. Microbiological Analysis*, FAO/WHO Publications, Rome, Italy, 1992.
91. FDA, *Bacterial Analytical Manual*, 8th edition, Revision A, AOAC International Publication, Washington, DC, 1998.
92. Bridson, E.Y., *The Oxoid Manual*, 8th edition, Oxoid Ltd., Hampshire, UK, 1998.
93. Vallone, L., Cantoni, C., Cocolin, L., and Comi, G., Yeasts and changes in fruit yoghurts, *Industrie Aliment.*, 40, 1001–1006, 2001.
94. Viljoen, B., Hattingh, A.L., Ikalafeng, B., and Peter, G., Temperature abuse initiating yeast growth in yoghurt, *Food Res. Int.*, 36, 193–197, 2003.

95. Fleet, G. and Mian, M.A., The occurence and growth of yeasts in dairy products, *Int. J. Food Microbiol.*, 4, 145–155, 1987.

96. Fleet, G., Yeast in dairy products, a review, *J. Appl. Bacteriol.*, 68, 199–211, 1990.

97. Giudici, P., Masin, G., and Caggia, C., The role of galactose fermenting yeast in plain yogurt spoilage, *Ann. Microbiol. Enzymol.*, 46, 11–19, 1996.

98. Canganella, F., Ovidi, M. Paganini, S., Vettraino, A., Bevilacqua, L., and Trovatelli, S., Survival of undesirable microorganisms in fruit yoghurt during storage at different temperatures, *J. Food Microbiol.*, 15, 71–77, 1998.

99. Hattingh, L.A. and Viljoen, B.C., Survival of dairy-associated yeasts in yoghurt and yoghurt related products, *Food Microbiol.*, 19, 597–604, 2002.

100. Mihyar, G.F., Yamani, M.I., and Al-Sa'ed, A.K., Resistance of yeast flora of labaneh to potassium sorbate and sodium benzoate, *J. Dairy Sci.*, 80, 2304–2309, 1997.

101. Yamani, M.I. and Abu-Jauber, M.M., Yeast flora of labaneh produced by in-bag straining of cow milk set yogurt, *J. Dairy Sci.*, 77, 3558–3564, 1994.

102. Entis, P. and Lerner, I., Two-day yeast and mold enumeration using the ISO-GRID(R) membrane filtration system in conjunction with YM-11 agar, *J. Food Protect.*, 59, 416–419, 1996.

103. Groote, J.M.F.H., Vroegop, L., and Brailsford, M., ChemFlow system: rapid detection and prediction of yeast contamination in fruit yoghurt, *Voedingsmidd.*, 28, 43–45, 1995.

104. Lopez, M.C., Medina, L., Toledano, A.M., Reiter, M.G., Dreyfuss, J., and Jordano, R., Fungal contamination of frozen yoghurt and its relationship with pH and titratable acidity, *Revisto do Instituto de Latinicios Candido Tostes*, 54, 58–64, 2000.

105. Hassanin, N.I., Stability of aflatoxin M1 during manufacture and storage of yoghurt, yoghurt cheese and acidified milk, *J. Sci. Food Agric.*, 65, 31–34, 1994.

106. El-Deeb, S.A., Interaction of aflatoxin M1 on the physiological and morphological properties of *Lactobacillus bulgaricus* and *Streptococcus thermophilus*, *Alexandria J. Agric. Res.*, 34, 61–72, 1989.

107. Rasic, J.L., Skrinjar, M., and Markov, S., Decrease of aflatoxin B1 in yoghurt and acidified milks, *Mycopathologia*, 113, 117–119, 1991.

108. Blanco, J.L., Dominguez, L., Gomez-Lucia, E., Garayzabal, J.F.F., Goyache, J., and Suarez, G., Experimental aflatoxin production in commerical yoghurt, *Zeitsch. Lebensmit. Unter. Forsch.*, 186, 218–222, 1988.

109. Blanco, J.L., Carrion, B.A., Liria, N., Diaz, S., Garcia, M.E., Dominguez, L., and Suarez, G., Behaviour of aflatoxins during manufacture and storage of yogurt, *Milchwissenschaft*, 48, 385–387, 1993.

110. Jordano, R. and Sameron, J., Growth and survival of *Aspergillus parasiticus* in commercial yoghurt, *Microbiol. Aliment Nutr.*, 8, 81–83, 1990.

111. Jordano, R., Jodrali M., Martinez, P., Salmeron, J., and Pozo, R., Aflatoxin-producing strains of *Aspergillus flavus* in yogurt, *J. Food Protect.*, 52, 823–824, 1989.

112. Pieckova, E., Valik, L., and Görner, F., Moulds in yoghurts, *Bull. Potrav. Vyskumu*, 41, 291–301, 2002.

113. Bodyfelt, F.W., Tobias, J., and Trout, G.M., *The Sensory Evaluation of Dairy Products*, p. 598, Van Nostrand Reinhold, New York, 1988.

114. Pearce, L.E. and Heap, H.A., Town milk, *J. New Zeal. Milk Board*, 22, 18, 1974.

115. McGill, A.E.J., Evaluation and prediction of the consumer acceptability of comercially manufactured yogurt, *South African J. Dairy Technol.*, 15, 139–141, 1983.

116. Tamime, A.Y., Davies, G., and Hamilton, M.P., The quality of yogurt on retail sale in Ayrshire. Part I. Chemical and microbiological evaluation, *Dairy Ind. Int.*, 52, 19–21, 1987.

117. Tamime, A.Y., Davies, G., and Hamilton, M.P., The quality of yogurt on retail sale in Ayrshire. Part II. Organoleptic evaluation, *Dairy Ind. Int.*, 52, 40–41, 1987.

118. Lawless, H.T. and Heymann, H., *Sensory Evaluation of Foods: Principles and Practices*, p. 891, Apsen Publishers Inc., Gaithersburg, MD, 1999.

119. ADSA, American Dairy Science Association, Committee on Evaluation of Dairy Products, Champaigne, IL, 1987.

120. Mac Fie, H.J., Bratchell, N., Greenhoff, N., and Vallis, L.V., Designs to balance the effect of order of presentation and first order carryover effects in hall tests. 2000, *J. Sens. Stud.*, 4, 129–148, 1989.

121. Muir, D.D. and Hunter, E.A., Sensory evaluation of Cheddar cheese: order of tasting and carryover effects, *Food Qual. Pref.*, 3, 141–145, 1991.

122. Patterson, H.D., Thompson, R., Hunter, A.E., and Kempton, R.A., *Analysis of Unbalanced Data Using REML*, University of Edinbrugh, Scottish Agricultural Service, 1990.

123. Muir, D.D., Hunter, A.E., and Dalaudier, C., Association of the sensory properties of commercial, strawberry flavoured fermented milks with product composition, *Int. J. Dairy Technol.*, 50, 28–34, 1997.

124. Piggott, J.R., *Sensory Analysis of Foods*, 2nd edition, p. 426, Elsevier Applied Science, Essex, UK, 1988.

125. Jollifee, I.T., Rotation of ill-defined principal components, *Appl. Stat.*, 38, 139–147, 1989.

126. Pereira, R.B., Singh, M, Munro, P.A., and Luckman, M.S., Sensory and instrumental textural characteritics of acid milk gels, *Int. Dairy J.*, 13, 655–667, 2003.

127. Özer, B.H., Kırmacı, H.A., Öztekin, Ş., Hayaloglu, A., and Atamer, M., Incorporation of microbial transglutaminase into non-fat yogurt production, *Int. Dairy J.*, 17, 199–207, 2007.

128. Roberts, B., Aspects of shelf life, *Dairy Foods*, 106, 68–70, 2005.

129. Muir, D.D. and Hunter, E.A., Sensory evaluation of fermented milks: Vocabulary development and the relations between sensory properties and composition and between acceptability and sensory properties, *J. Soc. Dairy Technol.*, 45, 73–80, 1992.

130. IDF, *Sensory Evaluation of Dairy Products by Scoring: Reference Method*, Standard 99C, International Dairy Federation, Brussels, 1997.

131. Meilgaard, M., Civille, G.V., and Carr, B.T., *Sensory Evaluation Techniques*, 3rd edition, p. 388, CRC Press, Boca Raton, FL, 1999.

132. Randell, R., Ahvenainen, R., Latva-kala, K., Hurme, E., Mattilasandhom, T., and Hyvonen, L., Modified atmosphere-packed marinated chicken breast and rainbow trout quality as affected by package leakage, *J. Food Sci.*, 60, 667–672, 1995.

133. Piga, A., D'Aquino, S., Agabbio, M., Emonti, G., and Farris, G.A., Influence of storage temperature on shelf-life of minimally processed cactus pear fruit, *Lebensm. Wiss. Technol.*, 33, 15–20, 2000.

134. Hough, L., Puglieso, M.L., Sanches, R., and Da Silva, O.M., Sensory and microbiological shelf-life of commercial ricotta cheese, *J. Dairy Sci.*, 82, 454–459, 1999.

135. Schmidt, K. and Bouma, J., Estimating shelf-life of cottage cheese using hazard analysis, *J. Dairy Sci.*, 75, 2922–2927, 1992.

136. Wszolek, M., Kupiec-Teahan, B., Skov-Guldager, and Tamime, A.Y., Production of kefir, koumiss and other related products, in *Fermented Milks*, A.Y. Tamime, Ed., pp. 174–216, Blackwell Publishing, Oxford, 2006.

137. Seiler, H., A review: yeasts in kefir and koumiss, *Milchwissenschaft*, 58, 392–396, 2003.

138. Lozovich, S., Medical uses of whole milk fermneted mare milk in Russia, *Cult. Dairy Prod. J.*, 30, 18–20, 1991.

139. Guirguis, N., Hickey, M.W., and Freeman, R., Some factors affecting nodulation in yoghurt, *Aus. J. Dairy Technol.*, 42, 45–47,1987.

9 Nutritional Aspects of Yogurt and Functional Dairy Products

Costas Chryssanthopoulos and Maria Maridaki

CONTENTS

9.1 INTRODUCTION

Milk, yogurt, and other dairy products have been recognized as important foods for centuries. Historically, the manufacturing of yogurt and fermented milks possibly started with the change of human life from food gathering and hunting to food producing. With the domestication of certain mammals such as the cow, sheep, goat, buffalo, and camel also emerged the need for milk preservation through processes such as lactic fermentation for yogurt production and curd formation for cheese-making [1].

Today, owing to major scientific advances in the dairy industry, consumers have the ability to choose from a vast variety of milks, yogurts, cheeses, and other dairy products in various forms and flavors with enhanced nutrition and product functionality for specific applications and population groups [2]. Food technology and instrumentation enable manufacturers to alter to a great extent milk composition, without compromising food safety [3], and to offer to the public dairy products that will contribute toward the development of an "optimum diet" [4]. Modern nutrition seems to be oriented to the concept of "optimum nutrition" or "optimized nutrition," which aims to maximize physiological functions of each individual to ensure both well-being and health, and simultaneously maintain a minimum risk of disease throughout the lifespan [4]. Within this framework seems to lie the development of functional foods and inevitably the development of functional dairy products.

This chapter will focus on the nutritional aspects of the four major dairy products, milk, yogurt, cheese, and butter; will outline their importance in maintaining a balanced healthy diet at all stages of life; and will briefly discuss the suggested health properties of these foods at "conventional" and "functional" levels since a detailed discussion concerning the health attributes of yogurt and functional dairy products will be presented in a different chapter of this book.

9.2 FACTORS AFFECTING NUTRIENT COMPOSITION OF DAIRY PRODUCTS

Nutrient composition of dairy products is influenced mainly by the factors that affect the basic raw material from which they are derived, that is, the milk. Factors affecting milk composition and its products may be categorized into four main categories, the ones concerning the animal from which the milk is taken, the methods of processing the milk, the fermentation procedure of the dairy product, and finally, the addition and fortification processes that take place before the product reaches the self.

Milk from different mammals differs in macronutrient as well as in micronutrient content. For instance, typical values for fat content in sheep's milk are higher than the average content observed in whole cow's milk (Table 9.1). Mare's raw milk possesses one of the lowest fat levels, which usually do not exceed 2 g/100 mL [5–8], and it also contains less amount of proteins than cow's milk [7]. However, when taken within the first 12 h postpartum, mare's colostrum contains almost 3% of fat and within 1 week postpartum drops below 2% [5]. Since fat content in sheep's milk is higher than that in cow's milk, yogurt made of sheep's milk (Greek-style yogurt) is more energy dense (92 kcal/100 g) than plain yogurt made of whole cow's milk (79 kcal/100 g) [8]. Differences in micronutrient composition of dairy products from different mammals also exist. For example, goat's raw milk has been reported to have more than twice the amount of iron (0.628 g/100 mL) found in cow's raw milk (0.284 g/100 mL) [9], whereas iron bioavailability of cow's milk has been found to be lower than that of goat's milk and human milk [10,11].

Different breeds may also produce milks with differences in composition. Holstein cows have been found to produce a higher concentration of conjugated linoleic acids (CLA), isomers of linoleic acid that may possess beneficial health properties [12], than Jersey cows [13,14], whereas Montbeliard cows seem to produce the highest concentrations of milk fat CLA [15].

TABLE 9.1
Macronutrient Composition of Various Types of Milk[a] (per 100 g Edible Portion)[b]

Type of Milk	Energy (kcal)	Water (g)	CHO[c] (g)	Fat (g)	FA (g)	Cholestrol (mg)	Protein (g)
Skimmed milk	34–36	90.8	4.8–5.1	0.1–0.3	0.2	4	3.5–3.6
Semiskimmed milk	46	89.4	4.7	1.7	1.6	6	3.5
Whole milk	65–66	87.3	4.4–4.9	3.5–3.9	3.7	14	3.3
Dried skimmed milk	348	3.0	52.9	0.6	0.6	12	36.1
Evaporated whole milk	151	69.1	8.5	9.4	8.9	34	8.4
Flavored milk (chocolate)	63	82.8	9.4	1.5	1.5	7	3.6
Cow milk children formula (with prebiotic—Friesland)	74	n.r.	8.5	2.8	n.r.	n.r.	3.4
Cow's milk with phytosterols (Becel)	48	n.r	4.8	1.8	n.r.	n.r.	3.2
Goat's milk	62	88.9	4.4	3.7	3.7	11	3.1
Sheep's milk	93	83.0	5.1	5.8	5.8	12	5.4
Mare's milk	47	n.r.	5.8–7.5	0.5–2.0	n.r.	n.r.	1.9
Human Milk	69	87.1	6.3–7.2	3.5–4.1	3.9	16	1.3

CHO, carbohydrate; FA, fatty acids; n.r., not reported; Tr, trace.

[a] Pasteurized.

[b] Data from references [5–8,203] and food labels.

[c] The main type of CHO is in the form of lactose in the vast majority of different types of milk.

It has been recognized for decades that dietary manipulation alters the milk composition of the animal [12], and different mammals have a diverse response to the same diet or dietary supplement. For instance, goats seem to increase the fat content of their milk with the majority of fat supplements, something that is not observed in cows [16]. Other than diet, other factors such as feeding-production (conventional farming–whole year indoor feeding versus conventional farming–summer grazing versus ecological farming–summer grazing) and farming systems (organic versus conventional dairy farms) may influence the content of milk too [13,14,17,18]. The highest level of CLA was observed in the ecologically fed animals, whereas the lowest was found in the most intensive production farm system [17]. Furthermore, organic dairy farms in the United Kingdom have been reported to produce milk having a higher level of polyunsaturated fatty acids (PUFA) and, in particular, Omega-3 fatty acids [18] that seem to play a protective role against coronary heart disease [19,20] and against some forms of cancer [21,22].

Environmental factors may also affect the animal and consequently its milk composition. Thorsdottir et al. in 2004 reported that CLA content of cow milk was higher during summer (0.68 g/100 g) than during winter (0.48 g/100 g) in samples taken from all five different Nordic countries [23]. Furthermore, the authors observed that CLA concentration in milk from Nordic countries was lower than that in milk from other

European countries possibly due to shorter summers and longer winters in the Nordic countries [23]. The altitude has also been reported to affect milk fatty acid content and composition [24]. Milk fat from the highlands (1275–2120 m) possessed a higher PUFA content and a lower saturated fatty acid level than the milk fat content from the low-lands (600–650 m) [24]. Finally, factors such as milking frequency [25,26], stage of lactation [26,27] and certainly the age of the animal, a factor that has been observed more than 80 years ago [28], have been reported to affect milk composition.

Safety of raw milk is of ultimate importance for public health. Therefore, milk pathogenic bacteria should be almost eliminated or at least be kept to a low concentration that makes the product safe for human consumption till the end of its shelf life. Various methods have been employed for achieving this such as milk thermization, pasteurization, microfiltration, and addition of lactic acid starter cultures, carbon dioxide, or niacin [29]. The most common procedure, however, is pasteurization, which when properly applied eliminates not only all common pathogenic organisms in milk but also kills the Gram-negative psychrotrophs, which spoil raw and thermized milk [29]. Unfortunately, during the pasteurization process where the milk may reach or exceed an ultrahigh temperature (UHT) of 135°C, several nutrients are lost. Hansen and Melo in 1977 heated skim milk to an average UHT of 143°C for 8–10 s and reported a decrease in concentration of Ca [30]. A significant loss of vitamin C (32.5%) was also reported by Oamen et al. in 1989 [31] after heating raw milk at 149°C for 3.4 s and at 138°C for 20.3 s and by Haddad and Loewenstein in 1983 [32] during heating raw milk at 72–80°C for 16 s and at 110–140°C for 3.5 s. The authors reported that vitamins from B group such as B_{12}, B_6, B_2, folic acid, and riboflavin were less susceptible to heat treatment and were lost by 17.9%, 3.4%, 2.6%, 12.5%, and 2.7%, respectively. Nevertheless, after the UHT treatment, prolonged storage of the milk to room temperature resulted in major vitamin losses except for vitamin B_2 that was very little affected [31]. However, not all vitamins are susceptible to UHT processing. Vitamin A has demonstrated a good stability after UHT treatment of raw milk, skimmed milk, or 2% chocolate milk at 140–144°C for 3–4 s [32,33]. Despite certain nutrient losses during pasteurization, this procedure is worth applying due to its value in food safety and public health.

A vast number of dairy products are milk-based products that have undergone the process of fermentation. One of the most popular is yogurt that is made by introducing specific bacteria strains into milk, which is subsequently fermented under controlled temperatures and environmental conditions. These bacteria will metabolize lactose, which is the dominant form of milk carbohydrate (see Table 9.1). Factors such as the type of yogurt cultures, the use of other bacteria such as bifidobacteria, the application of enzyme preparations for inoculation, and the time of fermentation may alter the amount and composition of carbohydrates in the final product. For instance, yogurt prepared using *Lactobacillus bulgaricus* and *Streptococcus thermophilus* reduced lactose content from 6.53% to 4.22%, increased galactose content from 0.04% to 1.46%, and elevated the content of oligosaccharides, a type of carbohydrate that may help in intestinal infections or constipation [34,35], from undetected levels to 0.08% after 10 h of fermentation [36]. The simultaneous inoculation with β-galactosidase enzyme further reduced the lactose content of yogurt to about 2.5% from an initial value of 6.5% when 4.7 units/100 mL of the enzyme preparation was used; when 93 units/100 mL of the enzyme was used, lactose was completely hydrolyzed [37], whereas the addition of bifidobacteria in yogurt cultures further increased the content of oligosaccharides in the final product [38]. The time of fermentation, to a significant degree, and the storage time after fermentation even at refrigeration temperatures, to a lower degree, may also change the composition of carbohydrates in yogurt [36–38]. In addition, the alteration of milk protein composition during the process of cheese ripening is well recognized [39].

Fermentation and storage may influence not only the macronutrient composition but also the micronutrient concentration in milk products. During the manufacturing process of cottage cheese, considerable amounts of vitamin B_{12} and folic acid were synthesized by cottage cheese starter culture during a 16-h incubation period and resulted in higher concentrations of these vitamins in the cheese curd [40]. Also, the authors reported that the storage of creamed cottage cheese for a period of 2 weeks did not affect the content of these vitamins [40], whereas other investigators have reported that the level of vitamin B_{12} and folic acid in cultured and acidified yogurt may be affected [41]. Reddy et al. observed that during yogurt fermentation at 42°C for 3 h, folic acid and niacin were synthesized, and from an initial value of 0.371 and 120 µg/100 g, these vitamins peaked to 4.317 and 142 µg/100 g, respectively [41]. The changes in vitamin content during milk fermentation also depend on the lactic culture bacteria used [42,43]. Skim milk fermentation by *Streptococcus thermophilus* and *Lactobacillus acidophilus* increased the folate concentration by twofold, whereas the application of *L. bulgaricus* reduced folate to negligible amounts [43]. In addition to affecting milk protein composition, cheese ripening also exerts an effect on vitamin content too. A wide variation in B-complex vitamin content among cheese samples of the same variety has been observed [44]. The investigators analyzed a large number of samples from about 31 cheese varieties and reported that about 9–55% of the vitamin content of milk remained in cheese at the time of analysis [44].

The fact that dairy products may be poor sources of some vitamins or minerals such as vitamin C and iron and that public demand for fortified foods has increased has led manufacturers and scientists to fortify dairy products with almost all major vitamins and minerals, altering in this way the dairy product micronutrient content [8,39,45–53]. This fortification not only helps people avoid hypovitaminosis but also helps special populations such as infants and children to reduce the burden of common morbidities and avoid certain dietary disorders such as iron deficiency [54,55]. Finally, the addition of fruits, cereals, nuts, chocolate, marmalade, honey, and various other substances by manufacturers in an attempt to provide greater food variety may further modify the final composition of yogurt, cheese, and other dairy products. Bearing in mind all the above factors that alter dairy product composition, the nutritional composition of dairy foods presented in Tables 9.1 through 9.6 should only be considered as typical.

9.3   NUTRITIONAL ASPECTS OF MILK AND YOGURT

Worldwide, milk, yogurt, and dairy products contribute ~5% of total energy. However, in traditional pastoral regions such as China, India, Africa, and Northern Europe, dairy and milk products supply about 10% total energy and 15–25% dietary protein and fat intake [56]. Dairy products are foods of high nutrient density and that means that they have a high concentration of major nutrients in relation to their energy value. Milk is the base for all dairy products, whereas yogurt is possibly the most commonly found fermented milk product around the world. Traditionally, yogurt is made of milk fermented with *Streptococcus thermophilus* and *Lactobacillus delbrueckii* subsp. *bulgaricus*, which grow in synergy in milk [57]. The fermentation process is carried out at 30–43°C for a period of 2.5–20 h [58]. Using different types of bacteria other products can be made such as viili, which is popular in Finland, or koumiss and kefir made by combining lactic acid and alcohol fermentation [59]. Today, there is a large variety of milks and yogurts of different flavors that have been fortified with vitamins and minerals and may contain fruits, nuts, or cereals, and different forms of live bacteria. Tamime in 2002 reported that about 400 generic names were applied to traditional and industrialized products concerning only fermented milks [1]. Therefore, the composition of milk and yogurt may be as variable as the product diversity of these foods. Some typical values of milk regarding macronutrient and micronutrient composition are presented in Tables 9.1 and 9.2, respectively, whereas the composition of various types of yogurt, milk beverages, and ice creams is presented in Tables 9.3 and 9.4.

9.3.1 CARBOHYDRATES

The main type of carbohydrate in milk is in the form of lactose [8]. It is a disaccharide formed from galactose and glucose and forms about 54% of the total nonfat milk solids [58]. Lactose content is about 4.5–6% although higher values have been reported for mare's milk [6]. In the human intestine lactose is hydrolyzed by lactase (β-galactosidase) developed in the intestinal brush border into its constituents glucose and galactose, which in turn are absorbed and used as energy sources [60]. If an individual has a lactase deficiency, lactose intake may cause intestinal discomfort and other symptoms, a condition known as lactose intolerance or lactose maldigestion [58,60]. The consumption of yogurt, however, is tolerated better than milk by people with lactose deficiency even if the content of lactose is similar in both foods [61–64]. The enhanced absorption of lactose in yogurt might be due to intraintestinal digestion of lactose by lactase released from the yogurt organisms [61]. Some lactic acid bacteria (LAB) used as starter cultures in milk and fermentation and probiotic bacteria such as *L. acidophilus* and *Bifidobacterium bifidum* produce β-galactosidase [65]. The addition of 2.5×10^8 *L. acidophilus*/mL in milk consumed for 1 week improved lactose digestion [66]. The authors reported that the improved digestion of lactose was not due to hydrolysis prior to consumption but the beneficial effect took place in the digestive tract after consumption of the milk containing *L. acidophilus* [66]. Industry offers milk with low lactose content where lactose has been hydrolyzed enzymatically. In long-life milks, the enzyme is added to the milk after sterilization, and the product is released for sale after a certain period, when the lactose level has decreased. In fermented milks the enzyme is added before fermentation or at the same time as the culture [58].

Milk contains not only lactose but also some other forms of carbohydrates such as glucose, galactose, and oligosaccharides that possess a degree of polymerization

TABLE 9.2
Selected Micronutrients of Various Types of Milk[a] (per 100 g Edible Portion)[b]

Type of Food	Ca (mg)	Na (mg)	K (mg)	Fe (mg)	Cl (mg)	Vit. A (RE) (µg)	Vit. E (mg)	Vit. C (mg)	Vit. D (µg)	Vit. B$_2$ (mg)	Vit. B$_5$ (mg)
Skimmed milk	121–125	44–52	145–162	0.03	87	1	Tr	1	Tr	0.18–0.22	0.37–0.50
Semiskimmed milk	118–143	43–50	129–156	0.02–0.28	87–107	19	0.04–0.11	1.5–2	Tr	0.17–0.24	0.46–0.68
Whole milk	118	43–50	144–155	0.03	89	30	0.08	1–2	Tr	0.17–0.23	0.30–0.58
Dried skimmed milk	1280	550	1590	0.27	1070	350	0.27	13	2.1	1.63	3.28
Evaporated whole milk	290	180	360	0.26	250	105	0.19	1	4.0	0.42	0.75
Flavored milk (chocolate)	115	45	206	0.62	110	20	0.03	Tr	0	0.17	0.30
Cow milk children formula (with prebiotic—Friesland)	120	49	164	1.30	104	39	0.96	13	0.9	0.14	0.70
Cow's milk with phytosterols (Becel)	120	55	n.r.	n.r.	n.r.	n.r.	n.r.	n.r.	n.r.	n.r.	n.r.
Goat's milk	100–134	42	170	0.12–0.56	113–150	44	0.03	1	0.1	0.04–0.08	0.41
Sheep's milk	170	44	120	0.03	82	83	0.11	5	0.2	0.32	0.45–0.46
Mare's milk	80–82	15–17	52–59	0.12	n.r.	6	0.01–0.11	1–1.7	n.r.	0.0	n.r.
Human milk	34	15	58	0.07	42	58	0.34	4	Tr	0.03	0.25

Vit., vitamin; RE, retinol equivalent; Tr, Trace; n.r., not reported.
[a] Pasteurized.
[b] Data from references [5,6,9,203,204] and food labels.

TABLE 9.3

Macronutrients of Various Types of Yogurt, Fermented Milk Beverages, and Ice Creams (per 100 g Edible Portion)[a]

Type of Food	Energy (kcal)	Water (g)	CHO (g)	Fat (g)	FA (g)	Cholesterol (mg)	Protein (g)
Whole milk yogurt plain	79	81.9	7.8	3.0	2.8	11	5.7
Low-fat yogurt plain	56–63	87.2	7.0–7.4	1.0–1.6	0.9	1	3.0–4.8
Fat-free yogurt plain	54	86.9	8.2	0.2	0.2	n.r.	5.4
Fat-free yogurt plain with fruit[b]	47	85.4	7.0	0.2	0.2	n.r.	4.8
Cow milk yogurt with phytosterols and strawberries (Becel)	62	n.r.	7.0	0.9	n.r.	n.r.	6.5
Cow milk yogurt with cereals for children with prebiotics and probiotics (Fage)	122	n.r.	17.0	3.8	n.r.	n.r.	4.9
Cow milk yogurt with plums and probiotics (Danone)	102	n.r.	15.1	2.6	n.r.	n.r.	4.6
Drinking yogurt	62	84.4	13.1	Tr	Tr	Tr	3.1
Sheep milk yogurt	92	80.9	5.0	6.0	6.0	14	4.8
Lassi (sweetened)	62	83.3	11.6	0.9	0.8	n.r.	2.6
Kefir	65	87.5	4	3.5	n.r.	13	3.3
Cornetto-type ice cream (chocolate and nuts)	284	42.5	28.8	17.8	17.7	15	4.0
Ice-cream bar (chocolate coated)	311	33.1	21.8	23.3	22.3	n.r.	5.0
Ice-cream dairy vanilla	177	62.5	19.8	9.8	9.8	24	3.6

CHO, carbohydrate; FA, fatty acids; n.r., not reported; Tr, trace.

[a] Data from references [8,203,205] and food labels.

[b] Ten different brands including bio-varieties and different flavors.

from 2 to 20 [34]. Human milk is particularly rich in oligosaccharides, whereas the concentration of this type of carbohydrate is much lower in most domestic mammals [34]. Human milk oligosaccharides are high in complexity because of the variable combination of glucose, sialic acid, galactose, fructose, and N-acetylglucosamine [67].

TABLE 9.4
Selected Micronutrients of Various Types of Yogurt, Fermented Milk Beverages, and Ice Creams (per 100 g Edible Portion)[a]

Type of Food	Ca (mg)	Na (mg)	K (mg)	Fe (mg)	Cl (mg)	Vit. A (RE) (μg)	Vit. E (mg)	Vit. C (mg)	Vit. D (μg)	Vit. B₂ (mg)	Vit. B₅ (mg)
Whole milk yogurt plain	200	80	280	0.1	170	28	0.05	1	0	0.27	0.50
Low-fat yogurt plain	162–183	63–70	228–234	0.1–0.08	235	8	Tr	1–0.8	0.1	0.22–0.21	0.56–0.59
Fat-free yogurt plain	160	71	247	0.1	252	Tr	Tr	1	Tr	0.29	n.r.
Fat-free yogurt plain with fruit (average)[b]	130	73	180	0.1	120	Tr	0.03	1	Tr	0.29	n.r.
Cow milk yogurt with phytosterols and strawberries (Becel)	110	50	n.r.	n.r.	n.r.	n.r.	n.r.	n.r.	n.r.	n.r.	n.r.
Cow milk yogurt with cereals for children with prebiotics and probiotics (Fage)	100	n.r.	n.r.	1.2	n.r.	n.r.	n.r.	n.r.	n.r.	n.r.	n.r.
Cow milk yogurt with plums and probiotics (Danone)	n.r.	60	n.r.	n.r.	n.r.	n.r.	n.r.	n.r.	n.r.	n.r.	n.r.
Drinking yogurt	100	47	130	0.1	75	Tr	Tr	0	Tr	0.16	0.19
Sheep milk yogurt	150	150	190	Tr	220	86	0.73	Tr	0.2	0.33	n.r.
Lassi (sweetened)	92	45	109	Tr	85	9	n.r.	n.r.	Tr	0.21	n.r.
Kefir	120	50	150	0.05	100	60	0.11	1	0.8	0.13–0.17	0.45
Ice-cream cone (chocolate and nuts)	84	69	181	0.7	209	27	0.06	n.r.	1.2	0.18	0.47
Ice-cream bar (chocolate coated)	140	91	250	0.7	175	78	1.10	0	0.2	0.29	0.50
Ice-cream dairy vanilla	100	60	174	Tr	110	91	0.49	1	0.5	0.28	1.05

Vit., vitamin; RE, retinol equivalent; Tr, trace; n.r., not reported.
[a] Data from references [8,98,203,205] and food labels.
[b] Ten different brands including bio-varieties and different flavors.

Because breast milk oligosaccharides are partially digested in the small intestine, they reach the colon and stimulate the development of a bifidogenic microbiota acting in this way as the first prebiotic for the infant [68]. Furthermore, certain types of oligosaccharides can inhibit pathogens such as *Streptococcus pneumoniae*, *Hemophilus influenzae*, *Escherichia coli*, and *Campylobacter jejuni* from binding to their receptors [69]. Therefore, oligosaccharides are included in infant milk formulas in an attempt to improve gut microflora of bottle-fed infants. A prebiotic mixture added to an infant milk formula containing 90% short-chain galacto-oligosaccharides and 10% long-chain fructo-oligosaccharides stimulates the growth of lactobacilli and bifidobacteria, decreases the fecal pH, and reduces the presence of pathogens to levels similar to those of breast-fed infants [70]. Also, the inclusion of mixed cultures of bifidobacteria (*Bifidobacterium animalis*, *B. bifidum*, *Bifidobacterium breve*, *Bifidobacterium infantis*, and *Bifidobacterium longum*) increases the oligosaccharide content of yogurt [38].

9.3.2 Proteins

The protein content of milk does not differ substantially from that of yogurt although commercial yogurts may have higher protein levels because of the addition of nonfat dry milk during processing, which increases the protein content of the final product [60]. Cow's milk is a rather heterogeneous mixture of proteins. About 80% of the total bovine milk protein is casein and 20% is whey protein. There are also traces of nonprotein nitrogenous compounds such as ammonia, urea, creatinine, creatine, and uric acid [71]. Casein can be fractionated electrophoretically into four major components: α, β, γ, and κ. α-caseins are present in two forms: α_{S1}-casein and α_{S2}-casein. α_{S1}-casein with the β-casein form more than 70% of bovine milk caseins [72]. Whey protein consists predominantly of α- and β-lactalbumins that form about 80% of the total whey proteins, whereas the remainder is serum albumin, immunoglobulins, glycomacropeptide, lactoferrin, and various enzymes [72]. α-lactalbumin has a high content of the amino acid tryptophan, a precursor of niacin. Because of milk's tryptophan content, this food is an excellent source of niacin equivalents (1 niacin equivalent = 1 mg niacin = 60 mg of tryptophan) [71]. Bovine milk is an excellent source of high-quality protein that provides significant amounts of all of the essential amino acids that humans cannot synthesize. A cup (about 250 mL) of semiskimmed (2%) cow's milk provides about 25–80% of a male adult's estimated daily requirements of the essential amino acids [71]. However, the quantity and composition of human milk and cow's milk are different. Protein quantity in human milk is about threefold lower than that in cow's milk (Table 9.1; reference [73]). In addition, β-lactalbumin does not exist in human milk where α-lactalbumin and lactoferrin are the major whey proteins. Moreover, caseins predominate in cow's milk, whereas whey predominates in human milk. The ratio of caseins to whey proteins is generally stated to be 40:60 in human milk and 82:18 in cow's milk [73]. β-casein forms nearly all of the casein protein in human milk, whereas although β-casein is a major protein in cow's milk, α_{S1}-casein and α_{S2}-casein account for more than half of the caseins in bovine milk [73].

Apart from the nutritional value, milk proteins have various physiological roles such as ion carriers, lactose synthesis in mammary glands, immunomodulation, and immune protection, and can also act as anticarcinogenic, antimicrobial, antiviral, and antioxidative agents [58]. In addition, dairy proteins may help maintain a feeling of satiety, which in turn facilitates weight control [74]. Furthermore, milk proteins are a rich source of precursors of biologically active peptides. Bioactive peptides are formed *in vivo* by the enzymatic hydrolysis of the digestive enzymes, in food processing with heat and/or alkali treatment as for example during manufacturing of hypoallergic infant formulae, or by the proteolytic activity of LAB in microbial fermentations [75]. Lactorphins, casoxins, casokinins, casoplatelins, casecidin, immunopeptides, and lactoferricin are some of the bioactive peptides derived from bovine milk that possess antihypertensive, antimicrobial, and antithrombotic properties or may act as immunostimulants or as opioid agonists and antagonists [75,76].

In yogurt production, the process of fermentation or the addition of bacterial cultures may increase the amount of free amino acids. Actually, bacterial strains may have higher proteolytic activity than others. The application of *L. bulgaricus* showed higher proteolytic activity compared with *Streptococcus thermophilus* and resulted in higher individual amino acid concentrations [77]. Also, the activity of proteolytic enzymes is maintained throughout the shelf life of yogurt. As a consequence, the concentration of free amino groups increases to twofold during the first 24 h and then doubles again during the next 3 weeks of storage at 7°C [60]. Therefore, it has been argued that the bacterial predigestion of milk proteins in yogurt makes this product's proteins more easily digested than the milk proteins. Furthermore, yogurt provided higher feed efficiency and yielded a better growth rate than did milk or other fermented milk products in rats [78]. However, in 16 healthy humans it has been reported that proteins from both milk and yogurt were rapidly hydrolyzed and were digested well and that only the gastric emptying rate of yogurt was slower than that of the milk [79].

9.3.3 LIPIDS

Milk fat is a natural fat with unique physical, chemical, and biological properties that contributes to the appearance, texture, flavor, and stability of dairy foods. Milk fat is a source of energy, essential fatty acids, fat-soluble vitamins, and several other potential health-promoting components. Fat in the milk is a complex of lipids and exists in microscopic globules in an oil-in-water emulsion in milk. Triglycerides form the majority of milk lipids (97–98%), and the minority are phospholipids (0.2–1%), free sterols such as cholesterol, waxes, and squalence (0.2–0.4%), and traces of free fatty acids [58]. About 62% of milk fat is saturated, 30% is monounsaturated (oleic acid), 4% is polyunsaturated and 4% is minor types of fatty acids [58]. More than 400 different fatty acids and fatty acid derivatives are found in milk, ranging from butyric acid with four carbon atoms to fatty acids with 26 carbon atoms [71]. Milk fat contains about 7% short-chain fatty acids (C4–C8), 15–20% medium-chain fatty acids (C10–C14), and 73–78% long-chain fatty acids (>C16) [71]. The major saturated fatty acids present in milk fat are myristic (14 : 0), palmitic (16 : 0), and stearic (18 : 0) acids, whereas the major unsaturated fatty acids are oleic (18 : 1), linoleic (18 : 2), and linolenic (18 : 3) acids [71].

Omega-3 linoleic acid, which may play a protective role against coronary heart disease and some forms of cancer [20–22], and its products eicosapentaenoic acid and docosahexaenoic acid are also found in small but significant amounts in milk fat [71].

Furthermore, milk fat components such as sphingomyelin and butyric acid are under investigation for their effect in reducing the risk of colon cancer [80,81]. The greatest interest, however, exists regarding the health benefits attributed to CLA that naturally exist in milk and dairy products [12,82]. Actually, CLA is a generic term to describe positional and geometric isomers of linoleic acid. Ruminant meat, milk, and dairy products are the predominant sources of CLA in the human diet. There are two major CLA isomers that have physiological significance: rumenic acid (*cis-9,trans-*11) isomer and *trans-*10,*cis-*12 isomer. It has been reported that these CLA isomers may act as anticarcinogens and reduce the risk of atherogenesis, adipogenesis, diabetogenesis, inflammation, bone density loss, and immune dysfunction [12]. The CLA content in milk is affected by several factors such as the animal's breed, age, and diet, seasonal and regional variation, milk processing, and also management factors related to feed supplements affecting the diet [15,23,83]. Of all these factors, animal diet is the primary one and could be manipulated to a great extent for enhancing the concentration of CLA in food products, both from ruminants and nonruminants [83]. CLA in milk has been shown to be a stable compound under normal cooking and storage conditions and its total content has been reported to vary from 0.32% to 3.3% in Holstein cows under pasture diet supplemented with fish oil [15,83]. About 82–97% of CLA in milk is in the form of rumenic acid (*cis-9,trans-*11); *trans-*10,*cis-*12 constitutes 3–5%; another isomer of quantitative importance is the *trans-*7,*cis-*9 (18:2) isomer that has been reported to constitute 3–16% of the total CLA [83,84]. For milks that have not been enriched with CLA, a low milk fat content usually results in a low CLA level. Skim milk (<0.5% fat) has a CLA concentration of about 1.8 mg/g of fat, whereas CLA in a 2% milk may exceed the value of 5 mg/g of fat [85,86]. CLA content in yogurt is usually 4–5 mg/g of lipid, although concentrations as high as 9.01 mg/g of fat for 1% yogurt and as low as 1.7 mg/g of fat for nonfat yogurt have been reported [12,82,85,86]. Due to the health attributes of CLA, many attempts are made to increase the CLA levels of milk and yogurt either by manipulating the animal's milk CLA content or through the use of various starter cultures and strains that have the ability to biosynthesize CLA. Such strains are lactococci, streptococci, enterococci, propionibacteria, lactobacilli, and bifidobacteria [12]. Furthermore, the application of UHT on milk has been used successfully and increases total CLA content from 0.54 g/100 g of fatty acids in the control milk to 4.68 g/100 g of fatty acids in the CLA-enriched milk [87]. Also, another factor that may elevate CLA content is storage. Although the combination of yogurt cultures and propionibacteria resulted in a stable CLA level during refrigerated storage, the use of LAB either alone or in coculture with yogurt cultures significantly elevated CLA content of the fermented product after 2 weeks of storage [88]. Despite the variety of milk, yogurt, and dairy products enriched with CLA, it has been estimated that the average adult consumes only one-third to one-half of the amount of CLA that has been shown to reduce cancer in animal studies [15].

9.3.4 VITAMINS AND MINERALS

Vitamins and minerals play an important role in many metabolic functions, growth, repair, and development of tissues, fluid and electrolyte balance, maintenance of bone health, adequate immune function, or even genetic regulation [89]. Milk and consequently yogurt contain most of the major vitamins and minerals necessary for the normal function of the human body. Water-soluble vitamins such as thiamine (vitamin B_1), riboflavin (vitamin B_2), niacin (vitamin B_3), pantothenic acid (vitamin B_5), vitamin B_6, biotin, folate, vitamin B_{12}, and ascorbic acid (vitamin C), fat-soluble vitamins such as vitamins A, D, E, and K, and minerals such as calcium, phosphorus, magnesium, iron, zinc, iodine, copper, manganese, selenium, chloride, potassium, and sodium are detected in milk, some in small and others in large quantities [71]. However, the most important single nutrient that has made milk and dairy products famous is calcium. It contributes to the electrical potential of cell membranes and is involved in many fundamental processes including DNA synthesis, enzyme activity, neurotransmitter release, membrane permeability, intracellular communication, and of course bone metabolism [90]. Taking into account all these important functions, it is not surprising that disturbances in calcium metabolism have been implicated in many chronic diseases including osteoporosis, kidney disease, obesity, heart disease, and hypertension [90]. Despite the importance of calcium in human diet, modern societies such as the USA population do not receive the recommended calcium intakes [90,91]. Milk and yogurt are excellent sources of calcium. It has been shown to have beneficial effects on bone mass at all ages, although the results are not always consistent [92]. In growing children, however, long-term avoidance of cow's milk was reported to be associated with small stature and poor bone health [93]. The recommended dietary reference intakes for calcium vary from 800 mg/day for 3–8 year olds to 1300 mg/day for ages 9–17 years, whereas for people over 50 years the value is 1200 mg/day [94]. Three cups of cow's milk can cover about 75–90% of the adult requirements [71]. In terms of absorption, about 20–30% of dietary calcium is absorbed, although the bioavailability of calcium can vary considerably depending on the dietary source of calcium [91]. The fact that high dietary fiber reduces the bioavailability of dietary calcium and that vegetables possess a low calcium density (calcium per serving) makes impractical for someone to meet calcium needs from nondairy food sources alone [91]. Furthermore, special populations such as lactase-deficient people may run the risk of osteoporosis since they avoid consuming milk due to its lactose content, and also even when they consume lactose, calcium absorption is reduced [95]. Under these circumstances, yogurt with its auto-digesting lactose properties [61] may seem to be the ideal solution for these individuals. In fact, yogurt is also a rich source of calcium and can become even richer than milk if the amount of proteins in the product is elevated [96]. Nevertheless, Smith et al. reported that lactase-deficient subjects and controls absorbed calcium (270 mg Ca in 250 g milk or in 147 g yogurt) equally well from yogurt and milk, and that there was no difference in calcium absorption between the two groups [97].

On the other hand, milk is not a very good source of fat-soluble vitamins, ascorbic acid, folate, and iron (Tables 9.2 and 9.4; reference [71]), although the level of vitamin A varies upon milk fat content. Because the vitamin A in milk exists in the fat portion, much of the vitamin A activity is removed during the manufacture of low-fat and nonfat milks. Also, considerable variation exists among different mammals' milk regarding vitamin levels. For example, when kefir, a cultured milk beverage, was made by cow's milk, biotin content was about 13.5 μg/kg, whereas when ewe's milk was used the biotin level was only 5.9 μg/kg [98]. Furthermore, heat and storage may also affect the labile water-soluble vitamins C, B_2, B_6, B_{12}, and folic acid [31,32]. Heat has been reported to decrease the concentration of free Ca^{++} too [30], whereas although vitamin A is affected by storage it seems to be more stable with UHT treatment [32,33].

However, there are factors that increase vitamin and mineral levels of milk, yogurt, and dairy products improving in this way their nutritional value. These factors are fermentation and in particular the use of various LAB and bifidobacteria and also the process of fortification. It has been demonstrated that a large number of bifidobacteria and LAB strains increase the concentration of folate, vitamin K, cobalamin (vitamin B_{12}), riboflavin, and thiamine when used in yogurt and fermented milks [99]. On the other hand, through the fortification process, manufacturers can overcome the possible losses of vitamins and minerals due to heat, storage, and processing or due to inherent low levels of some micronutrients in milk. Actually, in some countries fortification is compulsory as it happens in United States and Canada where milk is fortified with vitamins A and D [51]. Fortification of milk and yogurt with iron, vitamin C, vitamin A, and vitamin D, that facilitates calcium absorption, is a common practice that does not alter the properties of the product and improves its nutritional value [8,39,45,48,51,71,100]. This approach helps the consumer to reduce the risk of certain health problems such as osteoporosis [101], and to overcome iron deficiency [54], and common morbidities among preschool children [55].

9.4 NUTRITIONAL ASPECTS OF CHEESE AND BUTTER

Cheese is made mainly from bovine milk although goat and sheep milks may be used. It can be fresh or matured and is obtained by draining the whey, the moisture of the original milk, after coagulation of casein that is the milk's major protein. Casein coagulation is achieved by acid produced by microorganisms and/or by coagulating enzymes resulting in curd formation. Milk may also be acidified by adding food-grade acidulants in manufacture of certain varieties of cheese (e.g., cottage cheese). Cheese can also be natural or blended (processed). Natural cheese such as cheddar is produced directly from milk, whereas blended cheeses (e.g., pasteurized blended cheese, cheese spreads, and cold-pack cheeses) are made by blending one or more natural cheeses of the same or different varieties into a homogeneous mass with the aid of heat and emulsifying agent (e.g., sodium salts of phosphoric acid) [71]. After curd is formed, it is broken or cut to speed up whey expulsion and then the curd is cooked. Then the whey is drained off, followed by "knitting" of the curd to provide the cheese its characteristic texture. Afterwards the curd is salted, pressed, and exposed to a temperature- and humidity-controlled environment for a specified length of time, which depends on the type of cheese, for ripening or curing [71]. Of course, this simplistic description of the manufacturing process for cheese-making may vary substantially according to the type and variety of cheese someone wishes to produce. As one can appreciate, the composition of milk used in cheese-making changes as a result of separation of the curd from the whey, and also during ripening or curing of cheese. The separation of the curd from the whey causes a significant partition of nutrients and considerable change in the nutrient content of cheese compared with that of original milk. Since about 10 parts of milk are needed to make 1 part of cheese [102], the water-insoluble components of milk (e.g., fat, fat-soluble vitamins, and caseins) are retained in the curd and may appear in about 10 times the amount of water-insoluble components of milk (Tables 9.1 and 9.5). For instance, the 3–3.5% fat in milk used to make ripened cheeses such as Cheddar and Edam is increased to about 30–35% in cheese. On the other hand, the water-soluble constituents such as lactose, dissolved salts, lactalbumin, and lactoglobulin, which remain in the whey, are lower in cheese than in milk. However, the amount of whey retained in the curd, the type of milk used (whole, low fat, and nonfat), the manner of coagulation (enzyme or acid coagulation), and of course the type of cheese being manufactured largely affect the concentration of these nutrients in the final product. Ripening also influences the nutrient content of cheese affecting all three major macronutrients (carbohydrate, protein, and fat) and gives to the finished products its characteristic odor and flavor [71].

In terms of carbohydrate content, cheese usually contains insignificant amounts since lactose, milk's main type of carbohydrate, is largely removed in the whey

TABLE 9.5
Macronutrients of Various Types of Cheese, Butter, and Cream (per 100 g Edible Portion)[a]

Type of Food	Energy (kcal)	Water (g)	CHO (g)	Fat (g)	FA (g)	Cholestrol (mg)	Protein (g)
Camembert	290	54.4	Tr	22.7	21.5	72	21.5
Cheddar cheese	416	36.6	0.1	34.9	33.6	97	25.4
Cottage cheese plain	101	78.6	3.1	4.3	3.9	16	12.6
Danish Blue	342	46.3	Tr	28.9	28.7	75	20.5
Edam	341	43.8	Tr	26.0	22.1	71	26.7
Feta	250	56.5	1.5	20.2	18.4	70	15.6
Goat milk cheese (soft, full fat)	320	50.8	1.0	25.8	24.8	93	21.1
Gouda	377	40.4	Tr	30.6	29.7	85	25.3
Parmesan	415	27.6	0.9	29.7	29.2	93	36.2
Spreadable cheese (soft white, low fat)	132	72.5	3.5	8.0	7.8	24	14.9
Spreadable cheese (soft white, full fat)	312	58.6	Tr	31.3	30.5	92	7.5
Butter (>70% fat)	744	14.9	0.6	82.2	78.7	213	0.6
Spreadable butter (40% fat)	390	51.4	0.4	40.3	38.8	46	6.5
Dairy spread (40% fat)	388	52.9	0.1	40.0	38.0	n.r.	7.0
Single cream	193–211	77.0	2.2–4.3	19.1–20.6	18.6	55	3.0–3.3
Double cream	496	46.9	1.7	53.7	50.9	137	1.6

CHO, carbohydrate; FA, fatty acids; Tr, trace; n.r., not reported.

[a] Data from references [8,203] and food labels.

during cheese-making. In some fresh cheeses, however, made of goat's or sheep's milk, lactose is about 1–1.5 g/100 g, or even greater than 3 g/100 g for cottage cheeses where lactose may be added as an optional ingredient to the creaming mixture [8,102]. Ripening process further decreases lactose because the remaining lactose entrapped in the curd is converted to lactic and other acids. The low lactose content of most cheeses, particularly aged cheeses, makes this food well tolerated by individuals who have difficulty digesting lactose [102].

Protein levels in cheese are particularly high and cheese is the largest contributor among dairy foods to the total amount of protein intake. Protein content in milk and yogurt usually do not exceed 3–6 g/100 g. In cheese, protein levels are higher than 20 g/100 g, although some varieties with higher moisture such as cottage and feta cheeses may have lower protein concentration than 15 g/100 g (Tables 9.1, 9.3, and 9.5). The main cheese protein components are in casein, although water-soluble milk proteins such as lactalbumin and lactalglobulin may be present depending on the amount of whey entrapped in cheese [102]. Furthermore, the method of coagulation and the degree of ripening influence the protein in cheese. In enzyme-coagulated cheese (e.g., Cheddar), protein is present as di- and monocalcium paracasein. During curing, paracasein is hydrolyzed resulting in a more pliable and easier to digest food. In hard cheeses, however, less hydrolysis occurs compared with soft cheeses that possess this soft nature due to higher moisture and also due to extensive solubilization of their proteins [71]. On the other hand, in acid-coagulated cheeses (e.g., cottage cheese) proteins are not greatly hydrolyzed or digested before use. Nevertheless, cheese protein is of high quality and provides all the essential amino acids in significant amounts for the human body. For instance, 100 g of cottage cheese, which is not a nutrient dense type of cheese due to its high moisture levels (about 80% water), provides about 45–140% of the daily adult requirements in essential amino acids [102].

The fat content of cheese is mainly responsible for its texture and flavor. High-fat cheeses (>30% of fat) are described as "creamy" and "buttery" compared with both reduced-fat and low-fat cheeses [103]. Cheeses vary widely in fat, saturated fat, and cholesterol, mainly due to the type of milk (whole, semiskimmed, and skimmed) and milk product (e.g., cream) used to make cheese. Cottage cheese of reduced fat may contain only 1.5 g fat/100 g, 1 g saturated fatty acids/100 g, and 5 mg cholesterol/100 g. On the other hand, cream cheese contains 95 mg cholesterol/100 g and more than 47 g fat/100 g of which about 30 g are from saturated fatty acids [8]. However, dietary guidelines recommend a fat intake of no more than 30%–35% of the total energy intake and the saturated fat intake should be less than 10% of the total caloric intake [104]. Also, the association of high dietary fat intake with a high risk of cardiovascular diseases has led the American Heart Association to recommend low-fat or nonfat dairy products for reducing the risk of cardiovascular disease [105]. Therefore, industry using new technologies has offered the consumers cheeses with low fat content that does not exceed 3 g per serving [71]. Furthermore, cheese fat may contain beneficial health fats such as CLA that may help to reduce the risk of heart disease and certain types of cancer [12]. As it happens with milk and yogurt, the CLA content of cheese can also be increased through manipulation of animal diet [87,106]. In fact, cheese may be the richest source of CLA among dairy products. In a recent study, Prandini et al. analyzed more than 100 different types of dairy products from Italy including milks, yogurts, fermented milks, and cheeses and reported that the highest amount of CLA, exceeding 7 mg/g fat, was in three cheeses (Fontina Valdostana, Pecorino, and Swiss Emmental) followed by sheep yogurt [107]. Also, cheese fat can be partially substituted by vegetable oils resulting in favorable changes in the cholesterol profile of both animals and humans [108,109]. In addition, cheese's nutritional profile can further be enhanced by including various types of LAB in the fermentation and maturation processes giving cheese probiotic qualities [57].

The vitamin content of cheeses varies widely as a result of the vitamins' level in the milk used, the manufacturing of cheese, the cultures and microorganisms used, the fortification process, and the conditions and time of ripening. Since most of the fat in milk is retained in the curd, cheese contains the fat-soluble vitamins of the milk used in cheese-making. However, the amount of milk fat has a major influence. For instance, Cheddar cheese and goat cheeses made with full-fat milk may have more than 300 µg retinol equivalents of vitamin A per 100 g, whereas cottage cheese made with skimmed milk may contain less than 50 µg retinol equivalents per 100 g (Table 9.6). The level of water-soluble vitamins depends on the amount of whey retained in the cheese. For instance, in cottage cheese, considerable quantities of B-complex vitamins were lost in the whey and about 16–64% of niacin, vitamin B_6, and vitamin B_{12} were retained in the cheese [40]. On the other hand, cottage cheese starter culture synthesized considerable amounts of vitamin B_{12} and folic acid during the setting period resulting in higher concentrations of these vitamins in the cheese curd [40]. The bacterial surface-ripened and mold-ripened cheeses (e.g., Camembert, blue, and Roquefort) may contain a higher concentration of the B-complex vitamins than the hard and semihard types of cheeses (e.g., Cheddar, Swiss, and Mozzarella) [71]. In general, there is a great variation in vitamin content among cheese samples even of the same variety. Shahani et al. analyzed 2122 cheese samples from 23 varieties and found that the cheeses contained 9–55% of the B-complex vitamin content of milk [44]. The authors reported that the cheeses contained on average 277 µg niacin, 94 µg of vitamin B_6, 691 µg of pantothenic acid, 1.79 µg of biotin, and 22.3 µg of folic acid per 100 g [44].

Cheese is also a good source of several minerals, although the amounts of specific minerals in different cheese types are influenced by factors such as addition of salt, the method of coagulation, the treatment of the curd, and the acidity levels. As in milk and yogurt, cheese's most important mineral is calcium. In some low-moisture hard cheeses such as Parmesan, calcium content may exceed 1 g/100 g, while in high-moisture low-fat cheeses such as cottage cheese, calcium may not exceed 150 mg/100 g (Table 9.6). Calcium content is also affected by the coagulation process. In ripened whole milk cheeses made with a coagulating enzyme (e.g., Cheddar and Swiss), the calcium largely remains in the curd, whereas cheese coagulated by lactic acid alone (e.g., Cottage) retains less calcium because the calcium salts are removed from the casein [71]. The absorbability of calcium from cheese sources, however, is as good as from other dairy foods such as whole milk and yogurt [110]. Sodium content is also at significant levels but it varies depending on the amount of salt (sodium chloride) added. Some varieties such as Fata cheese (made of sheep's and/or goat's milk) and Danish Blue that have a particularly salty flavor may contain sodium in excess of 1 g/100 g (Table 9.6). Due to the negative effects of dietary sodium on blood pressure

TABLE 9.6

Selected Micronutrients of Various Types of Cheese, Butter, and Cream (per 100 g Edible Portion)[a]

Type of Food	Ca (mg)	Na (mg)	K (mg)	Fe (mg)	Cl (mg)	Vit. A (RE) (µg)	Vit. E (mg)	Vit. C (mg)	Vit. D (µg)	Vit. B$_2$ (mg)	Vit. B$_5$ (mg)
Camembert	235	605	104	Tr	1120	230	0.65	Tr	0.1	0.52	0.46–0.80
Cheddar cheese	739	723	75	0.3	1040	364	0.52	Tr	0.3	0.39	0.11–0.71
Cottage cheese plain	127	300	161	Tr	490	46	0.10	Tr	0	0.24	0.02–0.87
Danish Blue	488	1220	88	Tr	1950	244	0.71	Tr	0.2	0.41	0.53–2.62
Edam	795	996	89	0.3	1570	188	0.80	Tr	0.2	0.35	0.10–1.26
Feta	360	1440	95	0.2	2350	220	0.37	Tr	0.5	0.21	0.36
Goat milk cheese (soft, full fat)	133	601	132	Tr	1060	333	0.63	Tr	0.5	0.39	0.40
Gouda	773	925	82	0.3	1440	258	0.57	Tr	0.2	0.30	0.32–0.74
Parmesan	1025	756	152	0.8	1260	371	0.76	Tr	0.3	0.32	0.43
Spreadable cheese (soft white, low fat)	116	438	135	Tr	745	86	0.42	Tr	n.r.	0.52	0.40
Spreadable cheese (soft white, full fat)	76	288	89	Tr	490	260	0.24	Tr	0.1	0.26	0.20
Butter (>70% fat)	18	606[b]	27	Tr	994[b]	958	1.85	Tr	0.9	0.07	0.05
Spreadable butter (40% fat)	n.r.	510	n.r.	n.r.	780	160	3.88	0	0.2	Tr	Tr
Dairy spread (40% fat)	n.r	600	n.r.	n.r.	930	n.r.	n.r.	0	n.r.	Tr	Tr
Single cream	89–102	29–43	104–122	Tr	80	291	0.47	1	0.3	0.15–0.19	0.26–0.34
Double cream	49	22	65	0.1	36	779	1.64	1	0.3	0.19	0.23

Vit., vitamin; RE, retinol equivalents; Tr, trace; n.r., not reported.

[a] Data from references [8,44,203] and food labels.

[b] Average of salted and unsalted. Unsalted butter may contain 9 mg Na and 19 mg Cl per 100 g, whereas salted varieties may contain up to 1500 mg Na.

and hypertension [111], however, low-sodium (<140 mg per serving) or even sodium-free cheeses (<5 mg per serving) are available to the consumers [71].

Finally, the micronutrient content of cheeses can be improved through fortification procedures that elevate the content of certain vitamins and minerals, such as iron and vitamin D that are particularly low in cheese (Table 9.6). Cheese fortification with iron, vitamins D, C, and A, or even with microelements such as zinc and selenium has been carried out successfully resulting in good recovery levels and without substantial problems concerning flavor, stability, or chemical oxidation [46,47,49,50,52,53].

Butter is a concentrated milk fat made from milk or cream, or a mixture of both, that usually contain a minimum of 80% fat with some water and nonfat solids such as casein, lactose, and minerals. Various types of butter are available on the market, such as sweet cream (which can be salted or unsalted), cultured, whipped, and whey butter [71,112]. Sweet cream butter is made from pasteurized sweet cream to which no starter has been added, whereas cultured cream butter is cultured with lactic bacteria. Whey butter is produced using whey cream that is removed from whey after cheese-making and before whey is processed for spray-drying or protein concentration [112]. Butter is an energy-dense food rich in saturated fat and cholesterol. It contains about 40 kcal of energy and 10 mg of cholesterol per serving (5 g) (Table 9.6). Also, butter contains about 66% saturated fat, 30% monounsaturated fat, and only 4% polyunsaturated fat [71]. However, there is butter with reduced fat content that does not exceed 40% of milk fat and offers about 20 kcal of energy and 2 mg of cholesterol per serving (Table 9.6). Although calcium content of butter is lower than that of cheese, it contains higher amounts of fat-soluble vitamins A and E. Also, the amounts of Na and Cl in butter may vary tremendously depending on the amount of salt (sodium chloride) added to the product. Unsalted butter may contain only 9 mg Na and 19 mg Cl/100 g, while salted butter may have more than 1 g/100 g of Na and Cl (Table 9.6). Despite its high levels of saturated fat, butter contains some acids that may be beneficial to health such as CLA and especially rumenic acid (*cis*-9,*trans*-11). The CLA content of butter may even be higher than that of milk, yogurt, or cheese and exceeds 2 g/100 g of total fatty acids [85,113]. In fact, butter can be enriched in rumenic acid through the use of rumenic acid-enriched milk that is obtained from animals fed with animal or plant oils such as fish oil, sunflower oil, or extruded soyabeans [87,114,115]. Finally, butter and especially whey butter contain sphingomyelin [112] that may prevent the onset of cancer and control the growth of cancerous cells [81].

9.5 MILK, YOGURT, AND OTHER DAIRY PRODUCTS THROUGHOUT LIFE

Milk, yogurt, and dairy products are important food components of the human diet. In fact, humans are possibly the only mammals that consume milk not only during infancy but throughout their entire life. In terms of infant nutrition, it is well recognized that breastfeeding is associated with several benefits. According to the American Dietetic Association, exclusive breastfeeding provides optimal nutrition and health protection for the first 6 months of life and the combination of breastfeeding with complementary foods for at least 12 months is the ideal feeding pattern for infants [116]. Other health organizations such as the American Academy of Pediatrics also firmly support the position that human milk ensures the best possible health as well as the best developmental and psychological outcomes for the infant [117]. In addition, the World Cancer Research Fund and the American Institute for Cancer Research in their recent joint project recommend mothers to breastfeed and children to be breastfed exclusively up to 6 months, an approach that may prevent breast cancer in mothers and overweight and obesity in children [118]. Benefits of breastfeeding for the infant also include protection against infectious and noninfectious diseases, allergies and intolerances, reduced risk of diarrhea, heart disease, promotion of correct development of jaws, teeth, and speech patterns, and a guarantee of safe and fresh milk. Health benefits for the lactating mother are the promotion of faster shrinking of the uterus, reduced postpartum bleeding, improved bone density and glucose profile in gestational diabetes, and decreased risk for hip fracture, breast cancer, and ovarian cancer [116]. The neonatal immunodeficiency is limited by the introduction of protective and immunological components of human milk in the infant. This protection may be ensured either passively by factors with anti-infective, hormonal, enzymatic, trophic, and bioactive activity present in breast milk, or through a modulator effect on the neonatal immune system exerted by cells, cytokines, and other immune agents in human milk [119]. It seems that the immunological memory of the mother is passed to the infant through breast milk that contains a variety of immune-modulating compounds causing immunological imprinting and programming [120]. Furthermore, human milk is rich in oligosaccharides and because these carbohydrates are partially digested in the small intestine, they reach the colon and stimulate the development of bifidogenic microbiota acting in this way as the first prebiotic for the infant [68,121]. It has been reported that breastfed infants develop an intestinal flora dominated by bifidobacteria and lactobacilli with less pathogenic bacteria compared with formula-fed babies [122]. Therefore, attempts have been made to influence the intestinal flora of infants who are not breastfed. The addition of milk formulas with nonmilk oligosaccharides and especially with a mixture of short-chain galacto-oligosaccharides and long-chain fructo-oligosaccharides stimulates the growth of lactobacilli and bifidobacteria, reduces the presence of pathogens, and reduces the number of infections [70,121,123]. Also, although predominant breastfeeding for the first 6 months reduces the risk for gastrointestinal infections, it may increase the risk for iron deficiency in infants living in disadvantaged environments [124]. Iron deficiency, however, can be overcome using a milk formula fortified with iron [102]. In terms of other dairy products, cheese may be introduced at about 4–6 months of age when solid foods begin to complement the infant's liquid diet. Yogurt can also be introduced to infants at about 8–10 months of age [71].

Milk and dairy products and their high calcium content are also important for children and adolescents. In toddlers, calcium retention is relatively low and slowly increases as puberty approaches [125]. For children up to 8 years old, a calcium intake of about 800 mg/day is adequate, whereas for adolescents 1200–1500 mg/day are recommended [94,125]. Possibly, the most important issue during childhood is the development of eating patterns that will be associated with adequate calcium intake later in life [125]. During adolescence there is a great opportunity to influence lifelong bone mass especially in women since 86% of the adult bone mass of the spine is acquired before the skeletal age of 14 or the second year after menarche [126]. Despite the recommended or dietary reference intakes by certain associations [94,125], calcium absorption and metabolism is influenced by several factors such as diet, genetics, or activity level and therefore the question of what type of diet constitutes the best support for optimal bone growth and development remains open [127]. Also, some authors have concluded that there is scant evidence to support increased milk or other dairy product intake for promoting child and adolescent bone mineralization [128], whereas others restrict the possible beneficial effects of dairy food intake on bone health to milk and yogurt and to white women below the age of 30 [129]. However, data from studies examining children aged 3–13 years who avoid drinking milk have reported associations with small stature, poor bone health, and a high risk of bone fractures [93,130]. A recent controlled trial on ninety-six 12-year-old girls with low calcium intakes reported that calcium supplementation enhanced bone mineral accrual, but this benefit was no longer present 2 years after supplemental withdrawal [131]. Furthermore, a recent meta-analysis study has shown that increased dietary calcium/dairy products significantly increases total body and lumbar spine bone mineral content in children with low baseline calcium intake levels [132]. In addition, adolescents aged 9–18 years could not meet an adequate calcium intake with a dairy-free diet [133]. Under these circumstances, it may not be wise to leave children and adolescents to run the risk of suboptimal calcium intake and bone mass but adopt dietary habits such as consumption of 3–4 servings per day of milk and dairy products [71], since there is greater chance for this strategy to help rather than to harm these young individuals.

Adults and especially postmenopausal women and elderly people also benefit from dairy food intake. Although there is a high dietary calcium need in older people [94], consumption of dairy foods in some Western societies such as the USA population decreases as people age [91]. In a recent study, calcium supplementation reduced the risk of all fractures and of minimal trauma fractures in 61-year-old healthy individuals, but this benefit appeared to dissipate after treatment was stopped [134]. However, other authors have reported that the supplementation with calcium and vitamin D_3 fortified milk for 2 years provided some sustained benefits for bone mineral density in older men after withdrawal of supplementation [135]. Furthermore, postmenopausal women aged 55–65 years significantly reduced the rate of bone loss at lumbar spine and hip sites with the ingestion of high-calcium skimmed milk for 24 months [136]. The addition of 3 servings of yogurt to the daily diet of older women with habitually low calcium intakes has also been found to reduce urinary excretion of N-telepeptide, a marker for bone resorption [137].

9.6 HEALTH PROPERTIES OF YOGURT AND FUNCTIONAL DAIRY PRODUCTS

Conventional as well as functional milk, yogurt, and dairy products are supposed to possess health properties that may benefit humans who suffer from certain health problems or exert a protective role against certain diseases. Except for their role in bone health and osteoporosis that was mentioned earlier, dairy products and some of their components may reduce the risk of certain types of cancer, help people with lactose intolerance, have a hypocholesterolemic effect, and help in gastrointestinal infections, dental health, hypertension, and in weight management and obesity. In this section, a brief outline of the health properties of the dairy products will be presented since a detailed description of health attributes of yogurt and dairy foods will be presented in a different chapter of this book.

9.6.1 CANCER RISK

The World Cancer Research Fund and the American Institute for Cancer Research in their recent joint report have stated that "the evidence on milk and dairy products shows that their impact on the risk of cancer varies in different tissues" [118]. There is reasonably consistent evidence from cohort studies that milk probably protects against colorectal cancer [118]. In a pooled analysis from 10 cohort studies that included 4992 colorectal cancer cases from a population of 534,536 individuals, the authors concluded that higher consumption of milk is associated with a lower risk of colorectal cancer [138]. This outcome is supported further by data from experimental studies in animals and humans that more regularly report a beneficial role of calcium in colon cancer [56,138]. Also, despite the high fat content of cheese there is limited evidence to suggest that cheese is a cause of colorectal cancer [118]. Despite the protective role of milk in colon cancer, a recent pooled analysis from 12 cohort studies that included 2132 epithelial ovarian cancer cases from 553,217 women showed no significant associations between intakes of milk, yogurt, cheese, ice cream, and dietary calcium and risk of ovarian cancer [139]. Also, the evidence from cohort and case-control studies is inconsistent regarding the protective role of milk against bladder cancer or that milk and dairy products are a cause of prostate cancer [118].

Despite the inconsistent epidemiological evidence concerning the effect of dairy products on certain types of cancer, several individual ingredients of dairy foods such as calcium, casein, whey, CLA, and sphingolipids may possess anticancer properties and contribute in this way to the potential anticancer effect of dairy products and especially to the effect against colorectal cancer [56]. Furthermore, functional dairy products containing lactobacilli and bifidobacteria exert antimutagenic and anticarcinogenic effects possibly through microbial binding of mutagens to the cell surface, producing metabolic products such as butyrate that promote apoptosis, alteration of intestinal microecology and intestinal metabolic activity, normalization of intestinal permeability, and suppression of the growth of bacteria that convert pro-carcinogens into carcinogens or enhanced intestinal immunity [140,141].

9.6.2 LACTOSE INTOLERANCE

The inability to digest lactose that is the main type of carbohydrate in milk is quite common worldwide and exceeds 50% of adults with the exception of people from northern and central Europe and Caucasians in North America and Australia [60,141]. People suffering from lactose intolerance have low levels or even absence of the enzyme β-galactosidase in the human intestine that is responsible for the hydrolysis of lactose. The undigested lactose remains in the intestinal lumen and, when it reaches the colon, is fermented by colonic bacteria. By-products of this process include short-chain fatty acids, which associate with electrolytes leading to an osmotic load that can induce diarrhea [60]. Other clinical symptoms include bloating, flatulence, and abdominal pain [142]. Several studies have shown that the consumption of fermented milk products such as yogurt is tolerated better than milk by individuals with lactose deficiency [61–64]. One reason for the enhanced absorption of lactose might be the fact that the traditional cultures used in dairy fermentations utilize lactose as an energy source during growth, reducing in this way the lactose content in fermented products [141]. In yogurt, for instance, there might be some degree of intraintestinal digestion of lactose by lactase released from yogurt organisms [61]. However, Kim and Gilliland [66] who added *L. acidophilus* in milk to improve lactose digestion found that the improved digestion of lactose was not caused by hydrolysis of the lactose prior to consumption, indicating that the beneficial effect must have occurred in the digestive tract after consumption of milk containing *L. acidophilus*. Also, Vesa et al. [143] found no difference in digestion and tolerance to lactose in several fermented dairy products with substantially different lactase activities and suggested that possibly fermented milks slowed gastric emptying and consequently prolonged transit time through the gastrointestinal tract, improving absorption and lactose tolerance.

Besides yogurt, cheese is another alternative dairy food to milk for lactose maldigesters, since cheese and particularly aged cheese contains negligible amounts of lactose (Table 9.5). Actually, it has been reported that women suffering from lactose maldigestion could receive about 1500 mg calcium from dairy products without a major impediment when cheese, yogurt, and milk were combined in their diet [144]. Finally, the American Academy of Pediatrics recommends that children with lactose intolerance should include cheese in their diet so that the appropriate amount of calcium is consumed [125].

9.6.3 Hypocholesterolemic Effect

High serum cholesterol has been increasingly acknowledged as being a major risk factor for coronary heart disease [145]. Therefore, scientists have attempted to develop food products that lower cholesterol. Mann and Spoerry were probably the first to report a hypocholesterolemic effect of milk fermented by wild types of starters including *Lactobacillus* in Maasai tribesmen [146]. The authors attributed this finding to the production of hydroxymethylglutarate by probiotic bacteria, which inhibited hydroxymethylglutaryl-CoA reductases required for the synthesis of cholesterol. There are claims that *L. acidophilus* strains are able to lower cholesterol levels within the intestine. Cholesterol coprecipitates with deconjugated bile salts as the pH declines as a result of lactic acid production by the LAB [65]. Another mechanism might be that *L. acidophilus* deconjugates bile acids. The deconjugated bile acids do not absorb lipid as readily as their conjugated counterparts leading to a reduction in cholesterol level [147]. Also, in an *in vitro* culture *L. acidophilus* was reported to take up cholesterol during growth as a result of its bile salt-deconjugating activity [148]. However, *in vivo* human studies have produced somehow contradictory results. The consumption of 125 mL of yogurt with *L. acidophilus* and 2.5% fructo-oligosaccharides three times daily for 3 weeks reduced serum total cholesterol, LDL (low-density lipoprotein) cholesterol, and the LDL/HDL (high-density lipoprotein) ratio in normal healthy males with borderline elevated levels of serum total cholesterol [149]. Similarly, the administration of 450 mL of yogurt that contained strains of *Enterococcus faecium* and *Streptococcus thermophilus* for 8 weeks reduced LDL cholesterol in overweight individuals [150]. On the other hand, when subjects with normal to borderline high cholesterol levels ingested yogurt enriched with *L. acidophilus* for 6 weeks, no change in serum total cholesterol or LDL cholesterol was observed [151]. Neither there was a change in cholesterol levels in humans who received *L. acidophilus* in the form of capsules for 6 weeks despite the fact that this strain reduced cholesterol *in vitro* [152]. Therefore, some authors believe that the reduction in serum cholesterol by probiotic bacteria is still not considered an established effect and more double-blind placebo-controlled human clinical studies are needed to substantiate this claim [141].

Apart from probiotic bacteria, dairy products can be enriched with plant sterols and plant stanols, substances that have been known to reduce the assimilation of dietary cholesterol. Yogurt and low-fat milk enriched with plant sterol esters and plant stanol esters when taken for a period of 3 weeks lowered total and LDL cholesterol in modestly hypercholesterolemic humans [153]. Similarly, the addition of plant stanols in yogurt, yogurt drink, and milk resulted in lower serum total cholesterol and LDL cholesterol levels compared with the dairy products without the plant stanol enrichment in subjects with mild or moderate hypercholesterolemia [154]. Similar results have been reported by other investigators who reported a more than 10% reduction in LDL cholesterol as a result of consuming phytosterol-enriched drinkable yogurt for 42 days [155]. The hypocholesterolemic effect of phytosterols seems to be enhanced if the plant-sterol dairy product is consumed with a meal rather than without a meal [156].

9.6.4 Gastrointestinal Infections and Dysfunction

There is significant research to date supporting the role of functional fermented milk products containing probiotics in reducing the risk and alleviate the symptoms of gastrointestinal diseases and dysfunctions such as *Helicobacter pylori* infection, diarrhea, irritable bowel syndrome (IBS), and constipation [157,158]. Also, the role of probiotics, mainly from the genera *Lactobacillus* and *Bifidobacterium*, in the prevention and treatment of gastrointestinal infections is increasingly documented as a complement or an alternative to antibiotics, with the potential to decrease the use of antibiotics [158].

H. pylori infection that produces local inflammatory responses and mucosal injury is an area where probiotics have shown their beneficial role. Sheu et al. [159] reported that patients in whom triple therapy had failed had a higher *H. pylori* eradication rate as a result of supplementing the quadruple therapy with yogurt containing *L. acidophilus* La5 and *Bifidobacterium lactis* Bb12 compared with the patients who only received the quadruple therapy. Also, the probiotic yogurt reduced the number of patients who reported side effects such as constipation, diarrhea, nausea, or vomiting. Similar results were reported by Wang et al. [160] in 59 adults infected with *H. pylori*. The consumption of yogurt that contained the same bacteria as in the previous study [159] twice daily after a meal for 6 weeks suppressed *H. pylori* [160]. Furthermore, yogurt containing *Lactobacillus gasseri* OLL 2716 (LG21) when consumed for 8 weeks (90 g twice daily) suppressed *H. pylori* and reduced gastric mucosal inflammation in 31 patients [161]. In addition, the supplementation of triple therapy with a fermented milk product containing *Lactobacillus casei* DN-114 001 elevated eradication rate in infected children with gastritis [162]. The mechanism of probiotics on *H. pylori* infection is unclear, but some *Lactobacillus* and *Bifidobacterium* strains may produce antimicrobial substances such as organic acids and hydrogen peroxide, compete with pathogens for nutrients and ecological sites, or stimulate nonspecific and specific immune responses [158].

Another common gastrointestinal infection is diarrhea. In industrialized countries diarrhea is mainly a problem of morbidity, whereas in developing countries it is a major cause of mortality in children [163]. As in *H. pylori* certain probiotic bacteria can help in the relief of acute diarrhea in children. In a meta-analysis study, Van Niel et al. [164] reported that *Lactobacillus* reduced the duration of diarrhea in children by about 1 day, whereas other authors have reported a more pronounced effect in nonhospitalized children with mild diarrhea who received early treatment containing *Lactobacillus rhamnosus* and *Lactobacillus reuteri* [165]. However, the consumption of yogurt containing *L. casei* was not effective in reducing the incidence and the duration of diarrhea among young adults [166].

Also, probiotics have been used for the treatment and prevention of antibiotic-associated diarrhea. In a recent meta-analysis report, *Saccharomyces boulardii*, *L. rhamnosus* GG, and other probiotic mixtures were found to significantly reduce the development of antibiotic-associated diarrhea [167]. Similar to antibiotic- and rotavirus-associated diarrhea, probiotics may prevent and alleviate symptoms of traveler's diarrhea, which is caused by bacteria, particularly *E. coli* [141].

A possible mechanism by which probiotics reduce the duration of diarrhea might be the competitive inhibition of the mucosal adherence of pathogens. Furthermore, lactobacilli and bifidobacteria may also demonstrate antimicrobial activity against pathogens by producing various antimicrobial substances [158].

The IBS is a common functional gastrointestinal disorder characterized by symptoms of abdominal pain or discomfort that is associated with disturbed defecation, bloating, and flatulence [158,168]. The disorder can also be associated with significant emotional distress, impaired health-related quality of life, disability, and high health care costs [168,169]. Results from intervention studies on the use of probiotics in IBS have produced contradictory results. The administration of *Lactobacillus plantarum* for a period of 4 weeks decreased pain and flatulence in the experimental group compared with the control group [170], whereas other authors using the same probiotic strain found no improvement in the symptoms of patients with IBS [171]. Furthermore, the use of *Lactobacillus* GG for 6 weeks was not superior to placebo in the treatment of abdominal pain in children with IBS, although a lower incidence of perceived abdominal distention was reported in the experimental group [172]. However, a probiotic mixture containing four different strains for a period of 6 months was effective in alleviating IBS symptoms [173]. It seems that the effects of probiotics on IBS are strain-specific and therefore all strains or combination of strains should be studied for long periods in double-blind human interventions in order to clarify whether and which probiotics are beneficial to IBS patients [158].

Besides IBS, constipation is another gastrointestinal disorder that reduces the quality of life and places a financial load on patients and on the health care system [169].

Constipated patients seem to possess a colonic flora associated with low levels of lactobacilli and bifidobacteria and an increased number of pathogenic bacteria and/ or fungi [171]. Also, the relief of constipation tends to normalize these findings [174]. Therefore, the use of probiotics and prebiotics might be beneficial in relieving constipation and normalizing gut microflora of constipated individuals. For instance, *L. casei* Shirota in a 65-mL beverage given daily for 4 weeks improved gastrointestinal symptoms in patients with chronic constipation [175]. In another study, the use of a commercial fermented milk with *B. animalis* DN-173 010 for 2 weeks reduced gut transit time in elderly subjects, a beneficial effect that lasted 4–6 weeks after intervention was stopped [176]. Finally, prebiotics such as galacto-oligosaccharides and inulin have also demonstrated laxative effects in elderly people suffering from constipation [35,177].

9.6.5   HYPERTENSION

Substantial scientific evidence from animal, observational, and interventional studies indicates that dairy products and more specifically calcium and certain bioactive milk peptides have antihypertensive properties. In the Dietary Approaches to Stop Hypertension study (DASH), the so-called combination diet that was rich in fruits, vegetables, and low-fat dairy products reduced systolic and diastolic blood pressure more than the control diet [178]. In another epidemiological study (CARDIA study), increased dairy consumption had a strong inverse association with the insulin resistance syndrome and with the incidence of hypertension in overweight young adults [179]. Similar results were presented by Ruidavets et al. [180] who reported that dairy products and dairy calcium are both significantly and independently associated with low levels of systolic blood pressure. Also, in a meta-analysis study including 2492 subjects who were supplemented with calcium, a larger blood pressure reduction estimate was observed in people who had relatively low (<800 mg/day) calcium intake in their diet [181].

Both casein and whey milk proteins are rich sources of bioactive peptides that have been shown to inhibit the activity of the angiotensin converting enzyme (ACE). ACE converts angiotensin I to angiotensin II, increasing blood pressure and aldosterone, and inactivating the depressor action of bradykinin [76]. Inhibition of ACE results in lowering blood pressure and therefore is a main target for blood pressure control. Several studies in spontaneously hypertensive rats as well as in humans show that ACE inhibitory peptides found in milk proteins can significantly reduce blood pressure [182]. For instance, fermented milks with *Lactobacillus helveticus* LBK-16H, *L. helveticus* CM4, and *Saccharomyces cerevisiae* have lowered blood pressure in individuals with moderate and mild hypertension [183–185]. However, other authors have found no or modest hypotensive effects with fermented milks containing lactotripeptides that inhibit ACE [186,187].

9.6.6   DENTAL HEALTH

Dental health is essential to an individual's overall well-being. Despite efforts with fluoride-enriched water and personal hygiene products, dental caries remains a major public health problem that economically burdens the health care system to an extent greater than many widespread diseases such as heart disease, cancer, and hypertension [188]. Caries lesions result from interactions of odontopathogenic bacteria that colonize the tooth surface. These bacteria utilize dietary sugars to produce mutans and organic acids, which in turn demineralize calcium and other cations from the tooth's enamel. The body, however, counteracts demineralization by the salivary protein statherin binding calcium to remineralize the tooth's surface. Simply, dental caries worsen if odontopathogenic bacteria overcome the body's ability to remineralize the tooth [189].

There is considerable evidence from laboratory animal, human, *in situ*, and *in vitro* studies to suggest that dairy products and especially milk and cheese possess anticariogenic and tooth protecting properties [189–191]. Papas et al. [192] conducted an epidemiological study on 275 humans aged 44–64 years and reported that high intake of cheese was negatively associated with root caries. Another epidemiological study found that in 6–11-year-old children, who did not use fluoride and had a high daily sucrose-consuming frequency, milk had a caries preventive effect [193]. It seems that there are several mechanisms by which milk and cheese exert their protective role. Such mechanisms may involve buffering, salivary stimulation, reduction of bacterial adhesion, reduction of enamel demineralization, and/or promotion of remineralization by casein and calcium and phosphate ions [191]. Also, milk bioactive peptides such as caseinophosphopeptides and glycomacropeptides have shown to exert an inhibitory effect on cariogenic bacteria such as *Streptococcus mutans* and other species and are used in common personal hygiene products to prevent dental caries [188]. In addition, probiotic milk containing *L. rhamnosus* has been shown to lower mutans streptococcus counts and to reduce dental caries after 7 months of intake in children aged 1–6 years [194]. However, extra attention should be paid in the selection of strain if a prebiotic product should be administered since some strains such as *Lactobacillus salivarius* may have cariogenic properties [195].

9.6.7 WEIGHT MANAGEMENT AND OBESITY

A variety of epidemiological, clinical, animal, and *in vitro* investigations provide evidence that dairy products play a role in controlling body weight and enhancing fat loss [157]. This beneficial effect is mainly observed with the consumption of low-fat dairy products such as milk and yogurt and is specifically attributed to their calcium content. In a well-designed randomized, placebo-controlled study, 32 obese adults were instructed to consume a nutritionally balanced weight loss diet reduced in energy intake by 500 kcal/day for 24 weeks and randomized to a standard diet (400–500 mg of dietary calcium/day supplemented with placebo), a high-calcium diet (standard diet + 800 mg of calcium supplement/day), or a high-dairy diet (1200–1300 mg of dietary calcium/day supplemented with placebo) [196]. Subjects in the high-dairy diet lost significantly more body weight and body fat compared with the other two treatments. Furthermore, the authors reported that the patients in the high-dairy diet group lost more fat from the trunk region than it was lost from the same body region by the other two experimental groups. This is particularly important because abdominal obesity is associated with metabolic syndrome. Other findings from epidemiological studies also support the beneficial role of calcium in weight control. A significant inverse relationship between dietary calcium and body fat was reported in a 5-year longitudinal study of preschool children [197]. In a reanalysis of data from five studies that involved 780 women, the authors reported a significant negative association between calcium intake and body weight for all age groups and an odds ratio for being overweight of 2.25 for young women in the lower half compared with the upper half of calcium intake [198].

There are two mechanisms by which calcium facilitates weight and fat loss. The calcitrophic hormone 1,25 dihydroxy-vitamin D is increased when dietary calcium is low. The elevated levels of 1,25 dihydroxy-vitamin D favor the entrance of calcium in adipocytes, and this increases lipogenesis, reduces lipolysis, and promotes fat storage. Conversely, when dietary calcium is high, calcium levels in adipocytes decline, lipogenesis is reduced, lipolysis is facilitated, and fat loss is promoted [199]. Another mechanism whereby dietary calcium intake may reduce body adiposity is by inhibiting fat absorption from the gastrointestinal tract and increasing fecal loss of fatty acids and energy through the formation and excretion of calcium–fatty acid soaps [200]. A high calcium/normal protein diet was reported to produce a 2.5-fold increase in fecal fat excretion compared with a low-calcium/normal-protein diet and a high-calcium/high-protein diet [200]. On the other hand, some authors believe that this mechanism seems to appear insufficient to fully explain the great weight and fat losses found in the human studies of high-calcium and high-dairy food diets [101,199].

However, it should be pointed out that there are studies that have found no association between high-dairy consumption and low body weight [201–203]. Nevertheless, low-fat dairy products seem to provide a nutritional base for losing weight and high dietary calcium influences adipocyte metabolism indirectly, possibly through calcitrophic hormone levels [74,204,205].

REFERENCES

1. Tamime, A.Y. Fermented milks: A historical food with modern applications—a review, *Eur. J. Clin. Nutr.*, 56 (Suppl. 4), S2–S15, 2002.
2. Henning, D.R., Baer, R.J., Hassan, A.N., and Dave, R., Major advances in concentrated and dry milk products, cheese, and milk fat-based spreads, *J. Dairy Sci.*, 89, 1179–1188, 2006.
3. Jenkins, T.C. and McGuire, M.A., Major advances in nutrition: Impact on milk composition, *J. Dairy Sci.*, 89, 1302–1310, 2006.
4. Robertfroid, M.B., A European consensus of scientific concepts of functional foods, *Nutrition*, 16, 689–691, 2000.
5. Csapo, J., Stefler, J., Martin, T.G., Makray, S., and Csapo-Kiss, Z.S., Composition of mares' colostrum and milk. Fat content, fatty acid composition and vitamin content, *Int. Dairy J.*, 5, 393–402, 1995.
6. Marconi, E. and Panfili, G., Chemical composition and nutritional properties of commercial products of mare milk powder, *J. Food Comp. Anal.*, 11, 178–187, 1998.
7. Malacarne, M., Martuzzi, F., Summer, A., and Mariani, P., Protein and fat composition of mare's milk: Some nutritional remarks with reference to human and cow's milk, *Int. Dairy J.*, 12, 869–877, 2002.
8. Food Standards Agency, *McCance and Widdowson's the Composition of Foods*, Royal Society of Chemistry, Cambridge, 2002.

9. Lopez, A., Collins, W.F., and Williams, H.L., Essential elements, cadmium, and lead in raw and pasteurized cow and goat milk, *J. Dairy Sci.*, 68, 1878–1886, 1985.

10. Saarinen, U.M. and Siimes, M.A., Iron absorption from breast milk, cow's milk, and iron-supplemented formula: An opportunistic use of changes in total body iron determined by haemoglobin, ferritin, and body weight in 132 infants, *Pediatr. Res.*, 13, 143–147, 1979.

11. Park, Y.W., Mahoney, A.W., and Hendricks, D.G., Bioavailability of iron in goat milk compared with cow milk fed to anemic rats, *J. Dairy Sci.*, 69, 2608–2615, 1986.

12. Hennessy, A.A., Ross, R.P., and Stanton, C., Development of dairy based functional foods enriched in conjugated linoleic acid with special reference to rumenic acid, in *Functional Dairy Products*, M. Saarela, Ed., Vol. 2, pp. 443–495, CRC Press, Boca Raton and Woodhead Publishing Limited, England, 2007.

13. Morales, M.S., Palmquist, D.L., and Weiss, W.P., Milk fat composition of Holstein and Jersey cows with control or depleted copper status and fed whole soybeans or tallow, *J. Dairy Sci.*, 83, 2112–2119, 2000.

14. White, S.L., Bertrand, J.A., Wade, M.R., Washburn, S.P., Green, J.T., Jr., and Jenkins, T.C., Comparison of fatty acid content of milk from Jersey and Holstein cows consuming pasture or a total mixed ration, *J. Dairy Sci.*, 84, 2295–2301, 2001.

15. Dhiman, T., Nam, S.-H., and Ure, A.L., Factors affecting conjugated linoleic acid content in milk and meat, *Crit. Rev. Food Sci. Nutr.*, 45, 463–482, 2005.

16. Chilliard, Y., Ferlay, A., Rouel, J., and Lamberet, G., A review of nutritional and physiological factors affecting goat milk lipid synthesis and lipolysis, *J. Dairy Sci.*, 86, 1751–1770, 2003.

17. Jahreis, G., Fritsche, J., and Steinhart, H., Conjugated linoleic acid in milk fat: High variation depending on production system, *Nutr. Res.*, 17, 1479–1484, 1997.

18. Ellis, K.A., Innocent, G., Grove-White, D., Cripps, P., McLean, W.G., Howard, C.V., and Mihm, M., Comparing the fatty acid composition of organic and conventional milk, *J. Dairy Sci.*, 89, 1938–1950, 2006.

19. Bucher, H.C., Hengstler, P., Schindler, C., and Meier, G., N-3 polyunsaturated fatty acids in coronary heart disease: A meta-analysis of randomized controlled trials, *Am. J. Med.*, 112, 298–304, 2002.

20. Harris, W.S., Park, Y., and Isley, W.L., Cardiovascular disease and long-chain omega-3 fatty acids, *Curr. Opin. Lipidol.*, 14, 9–14, 2003.

21. Roynette, C.E., Calder, P.C., Dupertuis, Y.M., and Pichard, C., n-3 Polyunsaturated fatty acids and colon cancer prevention, *Clin. Nutr.*, 23, 139–151, 2004.

22. Saadatian-Elahi, M., Norat, T., Goudable, J., and Riboli, E., Biomarkers of dietary fatty acid intake and the risk of breast cancer: A meta-analysis, *Int. J. Cancer*, 111, 584–591, 2004.

23. Thorsdottir, I., Hill, J., and Ramel, A., Short communication: Seasonal variation in cis-9, trans-11 conjugated linoleic acid content in milk fat from Nordic countries, *J. Dairy Sci.*, 87, 2800–2802, 2004.

24. Collomb, M., Butikofer, U., Sieber, R., Jeangros, B., and Bosset, J.-O., Composition of fatty acids in cow's milk fat produced in the lowlands, mountains and highlands of Switzerland using high-resolution gas chromatography, *Int. Dairy J.*, 12, 649–659, 2002.

25. Klei, L.R., Lynch, J.M., Barbano, D.M., Oltenacu, P.A., Lednor, A.J., and Bandler, D.K., Influence of milking three times a day on milk quality, *J. Dairy Sci.*, 80, 427–436, 1997.

26. Sapru, A., Barbano, D.M., Yun, J.J., Klei, L.R., Oltenacu, P.A., and Bandler, D.K., Cheddar cheese: Influence of milking frequency and stage of lactation on composition and yield, *J. Dairy Sci.*, 80, 437–446, 1997.

27. Lynch, J.M., Barbano, D.M., Bauman, D.E., Hartnell, G.F., and Nemeth, M.A., Effect of a prolonged-release formulation of *n*-methionyl bovine somatotropin (Sometribove) on milk fat, *J. Dairy Sci.*, 75, 1794–1809, 1992.

28. Ragsdale, A.C., Turner, C.W., and Brody, S., The relation between age and fat production in dairy cows, *J. Dairy Sci.*, 7, 189–196, 1924.

29. Muir, D.D., The shelf-life of dairy products: 1. Factors influencing raw milk and fresh products, *J. Soc. Dairy Technol.*, 49, 24–32, 1996.

30. Hansen, A.P. and Melo, T.S., Effect of ultra-high-temperature steam injection upon constituents of skim milk, *J. Dairy Sci.*, 60, 1368–1373, 1977.

31. Oamen, E.E., Hansen, A.P., and Swartzel, K.R., Effect of ultra-high temperature steam injection processing and aseptic storage on labile water-soluble vitamins in milk, *J. f Dairy Sci.*, 72, 614–619, 1989.

32. Haddad, G.S. and Loewenstein, M., Effect of several heat treatments and frozen storage on thiamine, riboflavin, and ascorbic acid content of milk, *J. f Dairy Sci.*, 66, 1601–1606, 1983.

33. Maguer, I.L. and Jackson, H., Stability of vitamin A in pasteurized and ultra-high temperature processed milks, *J. Dairy Sci.*, 66, 2452–2458, 1983.

34. Boehm, G. and Stahl, B., Oligosaccharides, in *Functional Dairy Products*, T. Mattila-Sandholm and M. Saarela, Eds, pp. 203–243, CRC Press, Boca Raton and Woodhead Publishing Limited, England, 2003.

35. Teuri, U. and Korpela, R., Galacto-oligosaccharides relieve constipation in elderly people, *Ann. Nutr. Metab.*, 42, 319–327, 1998.

36. Toba, T., Watanabe, A., and Adachi, S., Quantitative changes in sugars, especially oligo-saccharides, during fermentation and storage of yogurt, *J. Dairy Sci.*, 66, 17–20, 1983.

37. Toba, T., Arihara, K., and Adachi, S., Quantitative changes in oligosaccharides during fermentation and storage of yogurt inoculated simultaneously with starter culture and β-galactosidase preparation, *J. Dairy Sci.*, 69, 1241–1245, 1986.

38. Lamoureux, L., Roy, D., and Gauthier, S.F., Production of oligosaccharides in yogurt containing bifidobacteria and yogurt cultures, *J. Dairy Sci.*, 85, 1058–1069, 2002.

39. Graham, D.M., Alteration of nutritive value resulting from processing and fortification of milk and milk products, *J. Dairy Sci.*, 57, 738–745, 1974.

40. Reif, G.D., Shahani, K.M., Vakil, J.R., and Crowe, L.K., Factors affecting B-complex vitamin content of cottage cheese, *J. Dairy Sci.*, 59, 410–415, 1976.

41. Reddy, K.P., Shahani, K.M., and Kulkarni S.M., B-complex vitamins in cultured and acidified yogurt, *J. Dairy Sci.*, 59, 191–195, 1976.

42. Alm, L., Effect of fermentation on B-vitamin content of milk in Sweden, *J. Dairy Sci.*, 65, 353–359, 1982.

43. Rao, D.R., Reddy, A.V., Pulusani, S.R., and Cornwell, P.E., Biosynthesis and utilization of folic acid and vitamin B_{12} by lactic cultures in skim milk, *J. Dairy Sci.*, 67, 1169–1196, 1984.

44. Shahani, K.M., Hathaway, I.L., and Kelly, P.L., B-complex vitamin content of cheese II. Niacin, pantothenic acid, pyridoxine, biotin and folic acid, *J. Dairy Sci.*, 45, 833–841, 1962.

45. Ilic, D.B. and Ashoor, S.H., Stability of vitamins A and C in fortified yogurt, *J. Dairy Sci.*, 71, 1492–1498, 1988.

46. Sweeney, M.A. and Ashoor, S.H., Fortification of cottage cheese with vitamins A and C, *J. Dairy Sci.*, 72, 587–590, 1989.

47. Zhang, D. and Mahoney, A.W., Iron fortification of process cheddar cheese, *J. Dairy Sci.*, 74, 353–358, 1991.

48. Hekmat, S. and McMahon, D.J., Manufacture and quality of iron-fortified yogurt, *J. Dairy Sci.*, 80, 3114–3122, 1997.

49. Rice, W.H. and McMahon, D.J., Chemical physical, and sensory characteristics of mozzarella cheese fortified using protein-chelated iron or ferric chloride, *J. Dairy Sci.*, 81, 318–326, 1998.

50. Upreti, P., Mistry, V.V., and Warthesen, J.J., Estimation and fortification of vitamin D_3 in pasteurized process cheese, *J. Dairy Sci.*, 85, 3173–3181, 2002.

51. Calvo, M.S., Whiting, S.J., and Barton, C.N., Vitamin D fortification in the United Status and Canada: Current status and data needs, *Am. J. Clin. Nutr.*, 80 (Suppl.), 1710S–1716, 2004.

52. Gulbas, S.Y. and Saldamli, I., The effect of selenium and zinc fortification on the quality of Turkish white cheese, *Int. J. Food Sci. Nutr.*, 56, 141–146, 2005.

53. Wagner, D., Rousseau, D., Sidhom, G., Pouliot, M., Audet, P., and Vieth, R., Vitamin D_3 fortification, quantification, and long-term stability in cheddar and low-fat cheeses, *J. Agric. Food Chem.*, 56, 7964–7969, 2008.

54. Stekel, A., Olivares, M., Cayazzo, M., Chadud, P., Llaguno, S., and Pizarro, F., Prevention of iron deficiency by milk fortification. II A field trial with a full-fat acidified milk, *Am. J. Clin. Nutr.*, 47, 265–269, 1988.

55. Sazawal, S., Dhingra, U., Hiremath, G., Kumar, J., Dhingra, P., Sarkar, A., Menon, V.P., and Black, R.E., Effects of fortified milk on morbidity in young children in north India: Community based, randomized, double masked placebo controlled trial, *Br. Med. J.*, 334, 140, 2007.

56. Gill, C. and Rowland, I., Cancer, in *Functional Dairy Products*, T. Mattila-Sandholm and M. Saarela, Eds, pp. 19–53, CRC Press, Boca Raton and Woodhead Publishing Limited, England, 2003.

57. Fonden, R., Saarela, M., Matto, J., and Mattila-Sandholm, T., Lactic acid bacteria (LAB) in functional dairy products, in *Functional Dairy Products*, T. Mattila-Sandholm and M. Saarela, Eds, pp. 244–262, CRC Press, Boca Raton and Woodhead Publishing Limited, England, 2003.

58. Saxelin, M., Korpela, A., and Mayra-Makinen, A., Introduction: Classifying functional dairy products, *Functional Dairy Products*, in T. Mattila-Sandholm and M. Saarela, Eds, pp. 1–16, CRC Press, Boca Raton and Woodhead Publishing Limited, England, 2003.

59. Buttriss, J., Nutritional properties of fermented milk products, *Int. J. Dairy Technol.*, 50, 21–27, 1997.

60. Adolfson, O., Meydani, S.N., and Russel, R.M., Yogurt and gut function, *Am. J. Clin. Nutr.*, 80, 245–256, 2004.

61. Kolars, J.C., Levitt, M.D., Aouji, M., and Savaiano, D.A., Yogurt-an autodigesting source of lactose, *New Engl. J. Med.*, 310, 1–3, 1984.

62. Savaiano, D.A., AbouElAnouar, A., Smith, D.E., and Levitt, M.D., Lactose malabsorption from yogurt, pasteurized yogurt, sweet acidophilus milk, and cultured milk in lactase-deficient individuals, *Am. J. Clin. Nutr.*, 40, 1219–1223, 1984.

63. Martini, M.C., Lerebours, E., Lin, W.-J., Harlander, S.K., Berrada, N.M., Antoine, J.M., and Savaiano, D.A., Strains and species of lactic acid bacteria in fermented milks (yogurts): Effect on in vivo lactose digestion, *Am. J. Clin. Nutr.*, 54, 1041–1046, 1991.

64. Rosado, J.L., Solomons, N.W., and Allen, L.H., Lactose digestion from unmodified, low-fat and lactose-hydrolyzed yogurt in adult lactose-maldigesters, *Eur. J. Clin. Nutr.*, 46, 61–67, 1992.

65. Lourens-Hattingh, A. and Viljoen, B.C., Yogurt as probiotic carrier food, *Int. Dairy J.*, 11, 1–17, 2001.

66. Kim, H.S. and Gilliland, S.E., Lactobacillus acidophilus as a dietary adjunct for milk to aid lactose digestion in humans, *J. Dairy Sci.*, 66, 959–966, 1983.

67. Lukewille, U. and Uhlig, H.H., Dairy products, probiotics and the health of infants and children, in *Functional Dairy Products*, M. Saarela, Ed., Vol. 2, pp. 46–62, CRC Press, Boca Raton and Woodhead Publishing Limited, England, 2007.

68. Coppa, G.V., Bruni, S., Morelli, L., Soldi, S., and Gabrielli, O., The first prebiotics in humans. Human milk oligosaccharides, *J. Clin. Gastroenterol.*, 38 (Supp. 2), S80–S83, 2004.

69. Koletzko, B., Aggett, P.J., Bindels, J.G., Bung, P., Ferre, P., Gil, A., Lentze, M.J., Roberfroid, M., and Strobel, S., Growth, development and differentiation: A functional food science approach, *Br. J. Nutr.*, 80 (Suppl. 1), S5–S45, 1998.

70. Boehm, G., Stahl, B., Jelinek, J., Knol, J., Miniello, V., and Moro, G. Prebiotic carbohydrates in human milk and formulas, *Acta Pediatr.*, 94 (S449), 18–21, 2005.

71. National Dairy Council, *Newer Knowledge of Dairy Foods*, 2000, Available at www.nationaldairycouncil.org.

72. Jensen, G., *Handbook of Milk Composition*, Academic Press, New York, 1995.

73. Nasirpour, A., Scher, J., and Desobry, S. Baby foods: Formulations and interactions (A review), *Clin. Rev. Food Sci. Nutr.*, 46, 665–681, 2006.

74. Ward, L.S. and Bastian, E.D., Dairy components in weight management: A broad perspective, in *Functional Dairy Products*, M. Saarela, Ed., Vol. 2, pp. 3–18, CRC Press, Boca Raton and Woodhead Publishing Limited, England, 2007.

75. Haque, E. and Rattan, C., *Milk Protein Derived Bioactive Peptides*, 2006, Available at www.dairyscience.info/bio-peptides.htm.

76. Clare, D.A. and Swaisgood, H.E., Bioactive milk peptides: A prospectus, *J. Dairy Sci.*, 83, 1187–1195, 2000.

77. Beshkova, D.M., Simova, E.D., Frengova, G.I., Simov, Z.I., and Adilov, E.F., Production of amino acids by yogurt bacteria, *Biotechnol. Progr.*, 14, 963–965, 1998.

78. Hargrove, R.E. and Alford, J.A. Growth rate and feed efficiency of rats fed yogurt and other fermented milks, *J. Dairy Sci.*, 61, 11–19, 1978.

79. Gaudichon, C., Mahe, S., Roos, N., Benamouzig, R., Luengo, C., Huneau, J.-F., Sick, H., Bouley, C., Rautureau, J., and Tome, D. Exogenous and endogenous nitrogen flow rates and level of protein hydrolysis in the human jejunum after [^{15}N]milk and [^{15}N] yoghurt ingestion, *Br. J. Nutr.*, 74, 251–260, 1995.

80. Dillehay, D.L., Webb, S.K., Schmelz, E.-M., and Merrill, A.H., Jr., Dietary sphingomyelin inhibits 1,2-dimethylhydrazine-induced colon cancer in CF1 mice, *J. Nutr.*, 124, 615–620, 1994.

81. Parodi, P.W. Cow's milk fat components as potential anticarcinogenic agents, *J. Nutr.*, 127, 1055–1060, 1997.

82. Lin, H., Boylston, T.D., Chang, M.J., Luedecke, L.O., and Shultz, T.D., Survey of the conjugated linoleic acid contents of dairy products, *J. Dairy Sci.*, 78, 2358–2365, 1995.

83. Khanal, R.C. and Olson, K.C., Factors affecting conjugated linoleic acid (CLA) content in milk, meat, and egg: A review, *Pakistan J. Nutr.*, 3, 82–98, 2004.

84. Yurawecz, M.P., Roach, J.A., Sehat, N., Mossoba, M.M., Kramer, J.K., Fritsche, J., Steinhart, H., and Ku, Y., A new conjugated linoleic acid isomer, 7 trans, 9 cis-octadecadienoic acid, in cow milk, cheese, beef and human milk and adipose tissue, *Lipids*, 33, 803–809, 1998.

85. Chin, S.F., Liu, W., Storkson, J.M., Ha, Y.L., and Pariza, M.W., Dietary sources of conjugated dienoic isomers of linoleic acid, a newly recognized class of anticarcinogens, *J. Food Comp. Anal.*, 5, 185–197, 1992.

86. Ma, D.W.L., Wierzbicki, A.A., Field, C.J., and Clandinin, M.T., Conjugated linoleic acid in Canadian dairy and beef products, *J. Agric. Food Chem.*, 47, 1956–1960, 1999.

87. Jones, E.L., Shingfield, K.J., Kohen, C., Jones, A.K., Lupoli, B., Grandison, A.S., Beever, D.E., Williams, C.M., Calder, P.C., and Yaqoob, P., Chemical, physical, and sensory properties of dairy products enriched with conjugated linoleic acid, *J. Dairy Sci.*, 88, 2923–2937, 2005.

88. Xu, S., Boylston, T.D., and Glatz, B.A., Conjugated linoleic acid and organoleptic attributes of fermented milk products produced with probiotic bacteria, *J. Agric. Food Chem.*, 53, 9064–9072, 2005.

89. Olson, J.A., Vitamins: The tortuous path from needs to fantasies, *J. Nutr.*, 124, 1771S-1776S, 1994.

90. Tordoff, M.G., Calcium: Taste, intake, and appetite, *Physiol. Rev.*, 81, 1567–1597, 2001.

91. Wood, R., Osteoporosis, in *Functional Dairy Products*, T. Mattila-Sandholm and M. Saarela, Eds, pp. 94–107, CRC Press, Boca Raton and Woodhead Publishing Limited, England, 2003.

92. Nieves, J.W., Osteoporosis: The role of micronutrients, *Am. J. Clin. Nutr.*, 81(Suppl.), 1232S–1239S, 2005.

93. Black, R.E., Williams, S.M., Jones, I.E., and Goulding, A., Children who avoid drinking cow milk have low dietary calcium intakes and poor bone health, *Am. J. Clin. Nutr.*, 76, 675–680, 2002.

94. Institute of Medicine of the National Academies of Science, *Dietary Reference Intakes for Calcium, Phosphorus, Magnesium, Vitamin D, and Fluoride*, National Academy Press, Washington, DC, 1997.

95. Cochet, B.A., Jung, M., Griessen, P., Bartholdi, P., Schaller, P., and Donath, A., Effects of lactose on intestinal calcium absorption in normal and lactase-deficient subjects, *Gastroenterology*, 84, 935–940, 1983.

96. Tunick, M.H., Calcium in dairy products, *J. Dairy Sci.*, 70, 2429–2438, 1987.

97. Smith, T.M., Kolars, J.C., Savaiano, D.A., and Levitt, M.D., Absorption of calcium from milk and yogurt, *Am. J. Clin. Nutr.*, 42, 1197–1200, 1985.

98. Kneifel, W. and Mayer, H.K., Vitamin profiles of kefirs made from milks of different species, *Int. J. Food Sci. Technol.*, 26, 423–428, 1991.

99. O'Connor, E.B., Barrett, E., Fitzgerald, G., Hill, C., Stanton, C., and Ross, R.P., Production of vitamins, exopolysaccharides and bacteriocins by probiotic bacteria, in *Probiotic Dairy Products*, A.Y. Tamime, Ed., pp. 167–194, Blackwell Publishing Ltd, Iowa, 2005.

100. Piirainen, T., Laitinen, K., and Isolauri, E., Impact of national fortification of fluid milks and margarines with vitamin D on dietary intake and serum 25-hydroxyvitamin D concentration in 4-year-old children, *Eur. J. Clin. Nutr.*, 61, 123–128, 2007.

101. Huth, P.J., DiRienzo, D.B., and Miller, G.D., Major scientific advances with dairy foods in nutrition and health, *J. Dairy Sci.*, 89, 1207–1221, 2006.

102. Dairy Council Digest, *Health Benefits of Cheese*, 73, 25–30, 2002, Available at www.nationaldairycouncil.org.

103. Fenelon, M.A., Guinec, T.P., Delahunty, C., Murray, J., and Crowe, F., Composition and sensory attributes of retail cheddar cheese with different fat contents, *J. Food Comp. Anal.*, 13, 13–26, 2000.

104. Institute of Medicine of the National Academies of Science, *Dietary Reference Intakes for Energy, Carbohydrates, Fiber, Fat, Fatty Acids, Cholesterol, Protein, and Amino Acids*, National Academy Press, Washington, DC, 2002.

105. Krauss, R.M., Eckel, R.H., Howard, B., Appel, L.J., Daniels, S.R., Deckelbaum, R.J., Erdman, J.W., Jr., Kris-Etherton, P., Goldberg, I.J., Kotchen, T.A., Lichtenstein, A.H., Mitch, W.E., Mullis, R., Robinson, K., Wylie-Rosett, J., Jeor, S.S., Suttie, J., Tribble, D.L., and Bazzarre, T.L., AHA scientific statement: AHA dietary guidelines. Revision 2000: A statement for healthcare professionals from the nutrition committee of the American Heart Association, *J. Nutr.*, 131, 132–146, 2001.

106. Coakley, M., Barrett, E., Murphy, J.J., Ross, R.P., Devery, R., and Stanton, C., Cheese manufacture with elevated conjugated linoleic acid levels caused by dietary manipulation, *J. Dairy Sci,*, 90, 2919–2927, 2007.

107. Prandini, A., Sigolo, S., Tansini, G., Brogna, N., and Piva, G., Different level of conjugated linoleic acid (CLA) in dairy products from Italy, *J. Food Comp. Anal.*, 20, 472–479, 2007.

108. Davis, P.A., Platon, J.-F., Gershwin, M.E., Halpern, G.M., Keen, C.L., DiPaolo, D., Alexander, J., and Ziboh, V.A., A linoleate-enriched cheese product reduces low-density

lipoprotein in moderately hypercholesterolemic adults, *Ann. Int. Med.*, 119, 555–559, 1993.

109. During, A., Combe, N., Mazette, S., and Entressangles, B., Effects on cholesterol balance and LDL cholesterol in the rat of a soft-ripened cheese containing vegetable oils, *J. Am. College Nutr.*, 19, 458–466, 2000.

110. Recker, R.R., Bammi, A., Barger-Lux, M.J., and Heaney, R.P., Calcium absorbability from milk products, an imitation milk, and calcium carbonate, *Am. J. Clin. Nutr.*, 47, 93–95, 1988.

111. Appel, L.J., Brands, M.W., Daniels, S.R., Karanja, N., Elmer, P.J., and Sacks, F.M., Dietary approaches to prevent and treat hypertension. A scientific statement from the American Heart Association, *Hypertension*, 47, 296–308, 2006.

112. Jinjarak, S., Olabi, A., Jimenez-Flores, R., and Walker, J.H., Sensory, functional, and analytical comparisons of whey butter with other butters, *J. Dairy Sci.*, 89, 2428–2440, 2006.

113. Gnadig, S., Xue, Y., Berdeaux, O., Chardigny, J.M., and Sebedio, J.-L., Conjugated linoleic acid (CLA) as a functional ingredient, in *Functional Dairy Products*, T. Mattila-Sandholm and M. Saarela, Eds, pp. 263–298, CRC Press, Boca Raton, Woodhead Publishing Limited, England, 2003.

114. Bauman, D.E., Barbano, D.M., Dwyer, D.A., and Griinari, J.M., Technical note: Production of butter with enhanced conjugated linoleic acid for use in biomedical studies with animal models, *J. Dairy Sci.*, 83, 2422–2425, 2000.

115. Ramaswamy, N., Baer, R.J., Schingoethe, D.J., Hippen, A.R., Kasperson, K.M., and Whitlock, L.A., Composition and flavour of milk and butter from cows fed fish oil, extruded soybeans, or their combination, *J. Dairy Sci.*, 84, 2144–2151, 2001.

116. ADA Reports Position of the American Dietetic Association: Promoting and supporting breastfeeding, *J. Am. Diet. Assoc.*, 105, 810–818, 2005.

117. American Academy of Pediatrics Work group on breastfeeding. Breastfeeding and the use of human milk, *Pediatrics*, 100, 1035–1039, 1997.

118. World Cancer Research Fund/American Institute for Cancer Research Food, *Nutrition, Physical Activity, and the Prevention of Cancer: A Global Perspective*, American Institute for Cancer Research Food, Washington, DC, 2007.

119. Chirico, G., Marzollo, R., Cortinovis, S., Fonte, C., and Gasparoni, A., Antiinfective properties of human milk, *J. Nutr.*, 138, 1801S–1806S, 2008.

120. M'Rabet, L., Vos, A.P., Boehm, G., and Garssen, J., Breast-feeding and its role in early development of the immune system in infants: Consequences for health later in life, *J. Nutr.*, 138, 1782S–1790S, 2008.

121. Boehm, G. and Moro, G., Structural and functional aspects of probiotics used in infant nutrition, *J. Nutr.*, 138, 1818S–1828S, 2008.

122. Mackie, R.I., Sghir, A., and Gaskins, H.R., Developmental microbial ecology of the neonatal gastrointestinal tract, *Am. J. Clin. Nutr.*, 69 (Suppl.), 1035S–1045S, 1999.

123. Arslanoglu, S., Moro, G.E., and Boehm, G., Early supplementation of prebiotic oligosaccharides protects formula-fed infants against infections during the first 6 months of life, *J. Nutr.*, 137, 2420–2424, 2007.

124. Monterrosa, E.C., Frongillo, E.A., Vasquez-Garibay, E.M., Romero-Velarde, E., Casey, L.M., and Willows, N.D., Predominant breast-feeding from birth to six months is associated with fewer gastrointestinal infections and increased risk for iron deficiency among infants, *J. Nutr.*, 138, 1499–1504, 2008.

125. American Academy of Pediatrics Committee on nutrition, Calcium requirements of infants, children, and adolescents, *Pediatrics*, 104, 1152–1157,1999.

126. Sabatier, J.P., Guaydier-Souquieres, G., Laroche, D., Benmalek, A., Fournier, L., Guillon-Metz, F., Delavenne, J., and Denis, A.Y., Bone mineral acquisition during adolescence and early adulthood: A study in 574 healthy females 10–24 years of age, *Osteoporos. Int.*, 6, 141–148, 1996.

127. Prentice, A., Schoenmakers, I., Laskey, M.A., de Bono, S., Ginty, F., and Goldberg, G.R., Symposium on 'Nutrition and health in children and adolescents.' Session 1: Nutrition in growth and development: Nutrition and bone growth and development, *Proc. Nutr. Soc.*, 65, 348–360, 2006.
128. Lanou, A.J., Berkow, S.E., and Barnard, N.D., Calcium, dairy products, and bone health in children and young adults: A reevaluation of the evidence, *Pediatrics*, 115, 736–743, 2005.
129. Weinsier, R.L. and Krumdieck, C.L., Dairy foods and bone health: Examination of the evidence, *Am. J. Clin. Nutr.*, 72, 681–689, 2000.
130. Goulding, A., Rockell, J.E.P., Black, R.E., Grant, A.M., Jones, I.E., and Williams, S.M., Children who avoid drinking cow's milk are at increased risk for prepubertal bone fractures, *J. Am. Diet. Assoc.*, 104, 250–253, 2004.
131. Lambert, H.L., Eastell, R., Karnik, K., Russell, J.M., and Barker, M.E., Calcium supplementation and bone mineral accretion in adolescent girls: An 18-mo randomized controlled trial with 2-y follow-up, *Am. J. Clin. Nutr.*, 87, 455–462, 2008.
132. Huncharek, M., Muscat, J., and Kupelnick, B., Impact of dairy products and dietary calcium on bone-mineral content in children: Results of meta-analysis, *Bone*, 43, 312–321, 2008.
133. Gao, X., Wilde, P.E., Lichtenstein, A.H., and Tucker, K.L., Meeting adequate intake for dietary calcium without dairy foods in adolescents aged 9 to 18 years (National Health and Nutrition Examination Survey 2001–2002), *J. Am. Diet. Assoc.*, 106, 1759–1765, 2006.
134. Bischoff-Ferrari, H.A., Rees, J.R., Grau, M.V., Barry, E., Gui, J., and Baron, J.A., Effect of calcium supplementation on fracture risk: A double-blind randomized controlled trial, *Am. J. Clin. Nutr.*, 87, 1945–1951, 2008.
135. Daly, R.M., Petrass, N., Bass, S., and Nowson, C.A., The skeletal benefits of calcium- and vitamin D_3-fortified milk are sustained in older men after withdrawal of supplementation: An 18-mo follow-up study, *Am. J. Clin. Nutr.*, 87, 771–777, 2008.
136. Chee, W.S.S., Suriah, A.R., Chan, S.P., Zaitum, Y., and Chan, Y.M., The effect of milk supplementation on bone mineral density in postmenopausal Chinese women in Malaysia, *Osteoporos. Int.*, 14, 828–834, 2003.
137. Heaney, R.P., Rafferty, K., and Dowell, M.S., Effect of yogurt on a urinary marker of bone resorption in postmenopausal women, *J. Am. Diet. Assoc.*, 102, 1672–1674, 2002.
138. Cho, E., Smith-Warner, S.A., Spiegelman, D., Beeson, L.W., van den Brandt, P.A., Colditz, G.A., Folsom, A.R., Fraser, G.E., Freudenheim, J.L., Giovannucci, E., Goldbohm, R.A., Graham, S., Miller, A.B., Pietinen, P., Potter, J.D., Rohan, T.E., Terry, P., Toniolo, P., Virtanen, M.J., Willett, W.C., Wolk, A., Wu, K., Yaun, S.-S., Zeleniuch-Jacquotte, A., and Hunter, D.J., Dairy foods, calcium, and colorectal cancer: A pooled analysis of 10 cohort studies, *J. Nat. Cancer Inst.*, 96, 1015–1022, 2004.
139. Genkinger, J.M., Hunter, D.J., Spiegelman, D., Anderson, K.E., Arslan, A., Beeson, L.W., Buring, J.E., Fraser, G.E., Freudenheim Jo, L., Goldbohm, R.A., Hankinson, S.E., Jacobs, D.R., Jr., Koushik, A., Lacey, J.V., Jr., Larsson, S.C., Leitzmann, M., McCullough, M.L., Miller, A.B., Rodriguez, C., Rohan, T.E., Schouten, L.J., Shore, R., Smit, E., Wolk, A., Zhang, S.M., and Smith-Warner, S.A., Dairy products and ovarian cancer: A pooled analysis of 12 cohort studies, *Cancer Epidemiol., Biomarkers Prev.*, 15, 364–372, 2006.
140. Parvez, S., Malik, K.A., Ah Kang, S., and Kim, H.-Y., Probiotics and their fermented food products are beneficial for health, *J. Appl. Microbiol.*, 100, 1171–1185, 2006.
141. Vasiljevic, T., Shah, N.P., Probiotics—from Metchnikoff to bioactives, *Int. Dairy J.*, 18, 714–728, 2008.
142. Suarez, F.L., Savaiano, D.A., and Levitt, M.D., A comparison of symptoms after the consumption of milk or lactose-hydrolyzed milk by people with self-reported severe lactose intolerance, *New Engl. J. Med.*, 333, 1–4, 1995.

143. Vesa, T.H., Marteau, P., Zidi, S., Briet, F., Pochart, P., and Rambaud, J.C., Digestion and tolerance of lactose from yogurt and different semi-solid fermented dairy products containing Lactobacillus acidophilus and bifidobacteria in lactose maldigesters- is bacterial lactase important? *Eur. J. Clin. Nutr.*, 50, 730–733, 1996.
144. Suarez, F.L., Adshead, J., Furne, J.K., and Levitt, M.D., Lactose maldigestion is not an impediment to the intake of 1500 mg calcium daily as daily products, *Am. J. Clin. Nutr.*, 68, 1118–1122, 1998.
145. Grundy, S.M., Small LDL, atherogenic dyslipidemia, and the metabolic syndrome, *Circulation*, 95, 1–4, 1997.
146. Mann, G.V. and Spoerry, A., Studies of a surfactant and cholesteremia in Maasai, *Am. J. Clin. Nutr.*, 27, 464–469, 1974.
147. Shah, N.P., Functional cultures and health benefits, *Int. Dairy J.*, 17, 1262–1277, 2007.
148. Klaver, F.A.M. and Van Der Meer, The assumed assimilation of cholesterol by Lactobacilli and Bifidobacterium bifidum is due to their bile salt-deconjugating activity, *Appl. Environ. Microbiol.*, 59, 1120–1124, 1993.
149. Schaafsma, G., Meuling, W.J.A., Van Dokkum, W., and Bouley, C., Effects of a milk product, fermented by Lactobacillus acidophilus and with fructo-oligosaccharides added, on blood lipids in male volunteers, *Eur. J. Clin. Nutr.*, 52, 436–440, 1998.
150. Agerholm-Larsen, L., Raben, A., Haulrik, N., Hansen, A.S., Manders, M., and Astrup, A., Effect of 8 week intake of probiotic milk products on risk factors for cardiovascular diseases, *Eur. J. Clin. Nutr.*, 54, 288–297, 2000.
151. De Ross, N.M., Schouten, G., and Katan, M.B., Yogurt enriched with Lactobacillus acidophilus does not lower blood lipids in healthy men and women with normal to borderline high serum cholesterol levels, *Eur. J. Clin. Nutr.*, 53, 277–280, 1999.
152. Lewis, S.J. and Burmeister, S., A double-blind placebo-controlled study of the effects of Lactobacillus acidophilus on plasma lipids, *Eur. J. Clin. Nutr.*, 59, 776–780, 2005.
153. Noakes, M., Clifton, P.M., Doornbos, A.M.E., and Trautwein, E.A., Plant sterol ester-enriched milk and yoghurt effectively reduce serum cholesterol in modesty hyper-cholesterolemic subjects, *Eur. J. Nutr.*, 44, 214–222, 2005.
154. Seppo, L., Jauhiainen, T., Nevala, R., Poussa, T., Korpela, R., Plant stanol esters in low-fat milk products lower serum total and LDL cholesterol, *Eur. J. Nutr.*, 46, 111–117, 2007.
155. Plana, N., Nicolle, C., Ferre, R., Camps, J., Cos, R., Villoria, J., and Masana, L., Plant sterol-enriched fermented milk enhances the attainment of LDL-cholesterol goal in hypercholesterolemic subjects, *Eur. J. Nutr.*, 47, 32–39, 2008.
156. Doornbos, A.M.E., Meynen, E.M., Duchateau, G.S.M.J.E., Van Der Knaap, H.C.M., and Trautwein, E.A., Intake occasion affects the serum cholesterol lowering of a plant sterol-enriched single-dose yogurt drink in mildly hypercholesterolaemic subjects, *Eur. J. Clin. Nutr.*, 60, 325–333, 2006.
157. Hoolihan, L., Beyond calcium. The protective attributes of dairy products and their constituents, *Nutr. Today*, 39, 69–77, 2004.
158. Myllyluoma, E., Kajander, K., and Saxelin, M., Functional dairy products for gastrointestinal infections and dysfunction, in *Functional Dairy Products*, M. Saarela, Ed., Vol. 2, pp. 63–89, CRC Press, Boca Raton and Woodhead Publishing Limited, England, 2007.
159. Sheu, B.S., Cheng, H.C., Kao, A.W., Wang, S.T., Yang, Y.J., Yang, H.B., and Wu, J.J., Pretreatment with Lactobacillus- and Bifidobacterium-containing yogurt can improve the efficacy of quadruple therapy in eradicating residual Helicobacter pylori infection after failed triple therapy, *Am. J. Clin. Nutr.*, 83, 864–869, 2006.
160. Wang, K.Y., Li, S.N., Liu, C.S., Perng, D.S., Su, Y.C., Wu, D.C., Jan, C.M., Lai, C.H., Wang, T.N., and Wang, W.M., Effects of ingesting Lactobacillus- and bifidobacterium-containing yogurt in subjects with colonized Helicobacter pylori, *Am. J. Clin. Nutr.*, 80, 737–741, 2004.

161. Sakamoto, I., Igarashi, M., Kimura, K., Takagi, A., Miwa, T., and Koga, Y., Suppressive effect of Lactobacillus gasseri OLL 2716 (LG21) on Helicobacter pylori infection in humans, *J. Antimicrob. Chemother.*, 47, 709–710, 2001.

162. Sykora, J., Valeckova, K., Amlerova, J., Siala, K., Dedek, P., Watkins, S., Varvarovska, J., Stozicky, F., Pazdiora, P., and Schwarz, J., Effects of a specially designed fermented milk product containing probiotic Lactobacillus casei DN-114 001 and the eradication of H., pylori in children, *J. Clin. Gastroenterol.*, 39, 692–698, 2005.

163. Cheng, A.C., McDonald, J.R., and Thielman, N.M., Infectious diarrhea in developed and developing countries, *J. Clin. Gastroenterol.*, 39, 757–773, 2005.

164. Van Niel, C.W., Feudtner, C., Garrison, M.M., and Christakis, D.A., Lactobacillus therapy for acute infectious diarrhoea in children: A meta-analysis,. *Pediatrics*, 109, 678–684, 2002.

165. Rosenfeldt, V., Michaelsen, K.F., Jakobsen, M., Larsen, C.N., Moller, P.L., Tvede, M., Weyrehter, H., Valerius, N.H., and Paerregaard, A., Effect of probiotic Lactobacillus strains on acute diarrhea in a cohort of nonhospitalized children attending day-care centres, *Pediatr. Infect. Dis. J.*, 21, 417–419, 2002.

166. Pereg, D., Kimhi, O., Tirosh, A., Orr, N., Kayouf, and R., Lishner, M., The effect of fermented yogurt on the prevention of diarrhea in a healthy adult, *Am. J. Infect. Control*, 33, 122–125, 2005.

167. McFarland, L.V., Meta-analysis of probiotics for the prevention of antibiotic associated diarrhea and the treatment of *Clostridium difficile* disease, *Am. J. Gastroenterol.*, 101, 812–822, 2006.

168. Drossman, D.A., Camilleri, M., Mayer, E.A., and Whitehead, W.E., AGA technical review on Irritable Bowel Syndrome, *Gastroenterology*, 123, 2108–2131, 2002.

169. Chang, L., Review article: Epidemiology and quality of life in functional gastrointestinal disorders, *Aliment. Pharmacol. Therapeut.*, 20 (Suppl. 7), 31–39, 2004.

170. Nobaek, S., Johansson, M.-L., Molin, G., Ahrne, S., and Jeppsson, B., Alteration of intestinal microflora is associated with reduction in abdominal bloating and pain in patients with Irritable Bowel Syndrome, *Am. J. Gastroenterol.*, 95, 1231–1238, 2000.

171. Sen, S., Mullan, M.M., Parker, T.J., Woolner, J.T., Tarry, S.A., and Hunter, J.O., Effect of Lactobacillus plantarum 299v on colonic fermentation and symptoms of Irritable Bowel Syndrome, *Digest. Dis. Sci.*, 47, 2615–2620, 2002.

172. Bausserman, M. and Michail, S., The use of Lactobacillus GG in irritable bowel syndrome in children: A double-blind randomized control trial, *J. Pediatr.*, 147, 197–201, 2005.

173. Kajander, K., Hatakka, K., Poussa, T., Farkkila, M., and Korpela, R., A probiotic mixture alleviates symptoms in irritable bowel syndrome patients: A controlled 6-month intervention, *Aliment. Pharmacol. Therapeut.*, 22, 387–394, 2005.

174. Khalif, I.L., Quigley, E.M.M., Konovitch, E.A., and Maximova, I.D., Alterations in the colonic flora and intestinal permeability and evidence of immune activation in chronic constipation, *Digest. Liver Dis.*, 37, 838–849, 2005.

175. Koebnick, C., Wagner, I., Leitzmann, P., Stern, U., and Zunft, H.J., Probiotic beverage containing Lactobacillus casei Shirota improves gastrointestinal symptoms in patients with chronic constipation, *Can. J. Gastroenterol.*, 17, 655–659, 2003.

176. Meance, S., Cayuela, C., Raimondi, A., Turchet, P., Lucas, C., and Antoine, J.-M., Recent advances in the use of functional foods: Effects of the commercial fermented milk with Bifidobacterium animalis strain DN-173 010 and yoghurt strains on gut transit time in the elderly, *Microbial Ecol. Health Dis.*, 15, 15–22, 2003.

177. Kleessen, B., Sykura, B., Zunft, H.-J., and Blaut, M., Effects of inulin and lactose on fecal microflora, microbial activity, and bowel habit in elderly constipated persons, *Am. J. Clin. Nutr.*, 65, 1397–1402, 1997.

178. Appel, L.J., Moore, T.J., Obarzanek, E., Vollmer, W.M., Svetkey, L.P., Sacks, F.M., Bray, G.A., Vogt, T.M., Cutler, J.A., Windhauser, M.M., Lin, P.-H., and Karanja, N., for the DASH Collaborative Research Group A clinical trial of the effects of dietary patterns on blood pressure, *New Engl. J. Med.*, 336, 1117–1124, 1997.
179. Pereira, M.A., Jacobs, D.R., Van Horn, L., Slattery, M.L., Kartashov, A.I., and Ludwig, D.S., Dairy consumption, obesity, and the insulin resistance syndrome in young adults. The CARDIA study, *J. Am. Med. Assoc.*, 287, 2081–2089, 2002.
180. Ruidavets, J.-B., Bongard, V., Simon, C., Dallongeville, J., Ducimetiere, P., Arveiler, D., Amouyel, P., Bingham, A., and Ferrieres, J., Independent contribution of dairy products and calcium intake to blood pressure variations at a population level, *J. Hypertens.*, 24, 671–681, 2006.
181. Van Mierlo, L.A., Arends, L.R., Streppel, M.T., Zeegers, M.P.A., Kok, F.J., Grobbee, D.E. and Geleijnse, J.M., Blood pressure response to calcium supplementation: A meta-analysis of randomized controlled trials, *J. Human Hypertens.*, 20, 571–580, 2006.
182. FitzGerald, R.J., Murray, B.A., and Walsh, D.J., Hypotensive peptides from milk proteins, *J. Nutr.*, 134, 980S–988S, 2004.
183. Hata, Y., Yamamoto, M., Ohni, M., Nakajima, Y., and Takano, T., A placebo-controlled study of the effect of sour milk on blood pressure in hypertensive subjects, *Am. J. Clin. Nutr.*, 64, 767–771, 1966.
184. Seppo, L., Jauhiainen, T., Poussa, T., and Korpela, R., A fermented milk high in bioactive peptides has a blood pressure-lowering effect in hypertensive subjects, *Am. J. Clin. Nutr.*, 77, 326–330, 2003.
185. Aihara, K., Kajimoto, O., Hirata, H., Takahashi, R., and Nakamura, Y., Effect of powdered fermented milk with *Lactobacillus helveticus* on subjects with high-normal blood pressure or mild hypertension, *J. Am. College Nutr.*, 24, 257–265, 2005.
186. Tuomilehto, J., Lindstrom, J., Hyyrynen, J., Korpela, R., Karhunen, M.-L., Mikkola, L., Jauhiainen, T., Seppo, L., and Nissinen, A., Effect of ingesting sour milk fermented using *Lactobacillus helveticus* bacteria producing tripeptides on blood pressure in subjects with mild hypertension, *J. Human Hypertens.*, 18, 795–802, 2004.
187. Engberink, M.F., Schouten, E.G., Kok, F.J., van Mierlo, L.A.J., Brouwer, I.A., Geleijnse, J.M., Lactotripeptides show no effect on human blood pressure. Results from a double-blind randomized controlled trial, *Hypertension*, 51, 399–405, 2008.
188. Aimutis, W.R., Bioactive properties of milk proteins with particular focus on anticariogenesis, *J. Nutr.*, 134, 989S–995S, 2004.
189. Aimutis, W.R., Dairy products and oral health, in *Functional Dairy Products*, M. Saarela, Ed., Vol. 2, pp. 134–162, CRC Press, Boca Raton and Woodhead Publishing Limited, England, 2007.
190. Herod, E.L., The effect of cheese on dental caries: A review of the literature, *Aus. Dent. J.*, 36, 120–125, 1991.
191. Kashket, S. and DePaola, D.P., Cheese consumption and the development and progression of dental caries, *Nutr. Rev.*, 60, 97–103, 2002.
192. Papas, A.S., Joshi, A., Belanger, A.J., Kent, R.L., Jr., Palmer, C.A., and DePaola, P.F., Dietary models for root caries, *Am. J. Clin. Nutr.*, 61, 417S–422S, 1995.
193. Petti, S., Simonetti, R., and D'Arca, S., The effect of milk and sucrose consumption on caries in 6-to-11-year-old Italian schoolchildren, *Eur. J. Epidemiol.*, 13, 659–664, 1997.
194. Nase, L., Hatakka, K., Savilahti, E., Saxelin, M., Ponka, A., Poussa, T., Korpela, R., and Meurman, J.H., Effect of long-term consumption of a probiotic bacterium, *Lactobacillus rhamnosus* GG, in milk on dental caries and caries risk in children, *Caries Res.*, 35, 412–420, 2001.
195. Matsumoto, M., Tsuji, M., Sasaki, H., Fujita, K., Nomura, R., Nakano, K., Shintani, S., and Ooshima, T., Cariogenicity of the probiotic bacterium Lactobacillus salivarius in rats, *Caries Res.*, 39, 479–483, 2005.

196. Zemel, M.B., Thompson, W., Milstead, A., Morris, K., and Campbell, P., Calcium and dairy acceleration of weight and fat loss during energy restriction in obese adults, *Obesity Res.*, 12, 582–590, 2004.
197. Carruth, B.R. and Skinner, J.D., The role of dietary calcium and other nutrients in moderating body fat in preschool children, *Int. J. Obesity*, 25, 559–566, 2001.
198. Davies, K.M., Heaney, R.P., Recker, R.R., Lappe, J.M., Barger-Lux, M.J., Rafferty, K., and Hinders, S., Calcium intake and body weight, *J. Clin. Endocrinol. Metab.*, 85, 4635–4638, 2000.
199. Zemel, M.B., Regulation of adiposity and obesity risk by dietary calcium: Mechanisms and implications, *J. Am. College Nutr.*, 21, 146S–151S, 2002.
200. Jacobsen, R., Lorenzen, J.K., Toubro, S., Krog-Mikkelsen, I., and Astrup, A., Effect of short-term high dietary calcium intake on 24-h energy expenditure, fat oxidation, and fecal fat excretion, *Int. J. Obesity*, 29, 292–301, 2005.
201. Rajpathak, S.N., Rimm, E.B., Rosner, B., Willett, W.C., and Hu, F.B., Calcium and dairy intakes in relation to long-term weight gain in US men, *Am. J. Clin. Nutr.*, 83, 559–566, 2006.
202. Snijder, M.B., Van der Heijden AWA, Van Dam, R.M., Stehouwer, C.D.A., Hiddink, G.J., Nijpels, G., Heine, R.J., Bouter, L.M., and Dekker, J.M. Is higher dairy consumption associated with body weight and fewer metabolic disturbances? The Hoorn study, *Am. J. Clin. Nutr.*, 85, 989–995, 2007.
203. Shahani, K.M. and Chandan, R.C., Nutritional and healthful aspects of cultured and culture-containing dairy foods, *J. Dairy Sci.*, 62, 1658–1694, 1979.
204. Csapo-Kiss Zs, Stefler, J., Martin, T.G., Makray, S., and Csapo J., Composition of Mares' colostrums and milk. Protein content, amino acid composition and contents of macro- and micro-elements, *Int. Dairy J.*, 5, 403–415, 1995.
205. Otles, S. and Cagindi, O., Kefir: A probiotic dairy-composition, nutritional and therapeutic aspects, *Pakistan J. Nutr.*, 2, 54–59, 2003.

10 Health Attributes of Yogurt and Functional Dairy Products

Yonca Karagül-Yüceer and Yahya Kemal Avşar

CONTENTS

10.1 INTRODUCTION

Functional foods are popular food products that meet the healthy lifestyle of consumers' demands. They contain some components that have health-promoting functions beyond traditional nutrients. Designer foods, medicinal foods, nutraceuticals, therapeutic foods, super foods, foodiceuticals, and medifoods are known as functional foods.[1]

Dairy foods and their components have a large number of functions, including a positive role in bone health, improving blood pressure, reducing risks of certain types of cancer, enhancing immunity and preventing some diseases, improving intestinal health, preventing the formation of kidney stones, enhancing nutrient absorption, and regulating body weight.[2] Fermentation adds additional functional properties to dairy products. As a result of fermentation, milk components undergo some changes and some new compounds such as organic acids and intermediates are produced. This makes fermented dairy products even more nutritious and healthier compared to milk.

One way to modify a food to make it functional is to add probiotic microorganisms, and dairy products are no exception. A probiotic is defined as a food/supplement containing concentrates of certain types of microorganisms that provide health benefits when it is consumed.[3] *Lactobacillus acidophilus*, *Bifidobacterium* spp., and *Lactobacillus casei* are the most popular probiotic cultures used in the food industry.[4] Also, *Enterococcus faecium*, *Saccharomyces cerevisiae* Boulardii, and *Propionibacterium* have the potential to be used as probiotic cultures because of several health benefits. Yogurt is the most common vehicle to deliver probiotic microorganisms. Other than yogurt, cheese, dips, and spreads are gaining popularity for incorporation of probiotic cultures.

In today's world, consumers are aware of the physiological and therapeutic properties of fermented dairy products. In response, dairy companies are exploiting this demand by producing new dairy (fermented) products with additional functional properties. Therapeutic properties of fermented milk were well reviewed in a book edited by Robinson.[5] In this chapter, the recent findings related to different health aspects of fermented dairy products will be reviewed.

10.2   HEALTH BENEFITS OF YOGURT AND FUNCTIONAL DAIRY PRODUCTS

The health benefits of fermented dairy foods are divided into two groups: nutritional function and physiological function.[3,6] The nutritional effect is explained as the function of supplying sufficient nutrition. Dairy foods are good sources of macronutrients (including carbohydrates, fats, and proteins) and micronutrients (including calcium, phosphorus, magnesium, and zinc). The physiological function is prophylactic and therapeutic functions.[6] Figure 10.1 shows the potential mode of health attributes of yogurt and fermented dairy products.

10.2.1   Nutritional Function

Milk components have many health benefits. Table 10.1 shows some of the potential benefits of milk components. Among the milk components, bioactive peptides deserve a special mention. They are specific fragments of proteins, which have a positive effect on health.[7] Proteolytic strains of probiotic microorganisms release bioactive peptides such as angiotensin I-converting engyme (ACE)-inhibitor peptides.[4] Consumption of bioactive peptides influences the cardiovascular, digestive, immune, and nervous systems. These peptides are not active in the parent protein and can be liberated by the following ways: (a) hydrolysis by digestive enzymes, (b) fermentation of milk by proteolytic starter cultures, and (c) effect of proteolytic enzymes produced by microorganisms or plants.[8,9]

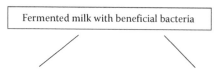

FIGURE 10.1   Health attributes of yogurt and fermented milks. (Adapted from Chandan, R.C. and Shah, N.P., in *Manufacturing Yogurt and Fermented Milks*, R.C. Chandan et al., Eds, pp. 311–325, Blackwell Publishing, Iowa, 2006.)

TABLE 10.1
Health Benefits of Milk Constituents

Component	Health Effect
Bioactive peptides	Immune system modulation
β-CN[a]	Immunoglobulin enhancement
Glycomacropeptides	Prevention of dental caries, gingivitis
Immunoglobulins	Antibodies against diarrhea and gastrointestinal track disturbances
Lactoferrin	Antibacterial
Lactoperoxide	Antimicrobial
Lysozyme	Antimicrobial
Lactose	Calcium absorption
Calcium	Prevention of osteoporosis and cancer, control of hypertension, reduces risk of colon cancer, and kidney stones
Butyric acid	Reduces risk of colon cancer
Conjugated linoleic acid	Modulates immune function, reduces risk of cancer
Sphingolipids	Reduces risk of colon cancer
Stearic acid	Modulates blood lipids to reduce risk of cardiovascular and heart disease
Triglycerides	Enhances long-chain fatty acids and calcium absorption
Whey proteins	Modulates immune system, reduce risk of heart disease and cancer, and lower blood pressure

Sources: Adapted from Chandan, R.C., *J. Dairy Sci.*, 82, 2245–2256, 1999; Hoolihan, L., *Nutr. Today*, 39 (2), 69, 2004.

[a] β-CN: β-casein.

TABLE 10.2
Health Benefits of Fermented Foods and Possible Mechanisms

Beneficial Effect	Possible Mechanisms
Improved digestibility	Breakdown of proteins, fats, and carbohydrates
Improved nutritional value	Higher levels of B vitamins and certain amino acids (methionine, lysine, and tryptophan)
Improved lactose utilization	Reduced lactose in product
Antimicrobial effect against pathogens	Reduction of carcinogen-promoting enzymes, degradation of precarcinogens; modulation of the immune system
Hypocholesterolemic action	Inhibition of cholesterol synthesis; use of cholesterol by assimilation and precipitation with deconjugated bile salts
Immune system modulation	Enhancement of macrophage formation and production of suppressor cells and γ-interferon

Source: Gomes, A.M.P. and Malcata, F.X. *Trend Food Sci. Technol.*, 10, 139–157, 1999.

10.2.2 Physiological Functions

Shah[10] stated that bacteria and yeasts are used as probiotics such as *Lactobacillus*, *Streptococcus*, *Leuconostoc*, *Pediococcus*, *Bifidobacterium*, and *Enterococcus* in general. However, *Lactobacillus acidophilus*, *Bifidobacterium* spp., and *Lactobacillus casei* are believed to be the main species that have probiotic properties. Some of the health benefits of probiotic microorganisms include improvement of lactose metabolism, antimutagenic and anticarcinogenic properties, production of antimicrobial substances that inhibit the growth of undesirable microorganisms, stimulation of the host immune system, reduction of serum cholesterol, and treatment/prevention of some diseases.[4,11,12] Health benefits of fermented dairy foods and possible mechanisms are summarized in Table 10.2.

10.2.2.1 Antimicrobial Activity and Gastrointestinal Infections

Probiotic cultures produce organic acids, hydrogen peroxide, and bacteriocins as antimicrobial substances that inhibit the growth of some pathogenic and putrefying microorganisms. Low pH due to the production of lactic or acetic acids in the intestine has a bacteriocidal or bacteriostatic effects. For example, bifidobacteria and *Lactobacillus acidophilus* show antagonistic effects on enteropathogenic *Escherichia coli*, *Salmonella typhimurium*, *Staphylococcus aureus*, and *Clostridium perfringensis*. In addition, various bacteriocins and antibacterial substances are produced by *Lactobacillus acidophilus* (e.g., lactocidin, acidolin, acidophilin, and lactacium-B) and *Bifidobacterium* spp. (e.g., bifidolin and bifilong).[13]

Using probiotic cultures, *Lactobacillus acidophilus* and bifidobacteria inhibit the growth of some enteropathogenic microorganisms including *Escherichia coli*, *Salmonella typhi*, and *Staphylococcus aureus*.[14,15]

Helicobacter pylori is a pathogenic bacterium that causes pectic ulcers, type B gastritis, and chronic gastritis.[16] Probiotic organisms do not eradicate *H. pylori*, but they reduce the number of bacteria. For example, *Lactobacillus johnsonii* La1 and

Lactobacillus gasseri OLL2716 reduce colonization and inflammation of *H. pylori.*[17] Also, *Lactobacillus casei* Shirota and *Lactobacillus acidophilus* inhibit the growth of *H. pylori.*[18]

The antimicrobial activities of some commercial and noncommercial probiotic bacteria was investigated.[19] The results showed that the antimicrobial compound was a proteinaceous substance. *Enterococcus faecium* B20, *Pediococcus acidilactis* S1, *Lactobacillus helveticus* S57, and *Lactobacillus reuteri* T17 (noncommercial sources) and *Lactobacillus plantarum* AS2, *Lactobacillus acidophilus* DC1, *Lactobacillus pontis* H3, and *Lactobacillus reuteri* PBC2 (commercial sources) showed antimicrobial activities against some indicator pathogens including *Listeria monocytogenes*, *Escherichia coli* O157:H7, and *Salmonella* spp.

Inflammatory bowel disease (ulcerative colits and Crohn's disease) is related to the microflora of the intestine. Disturbance in bowel habits and mucosal inflammation are some of the symptoms of this disease. Individuals with inflammatory bowel disease have a higher number of coccoids and anaerobes than *Lactobacillus* and *Bifidobacterium* in the intestine.[4] Probiotic bacteria do not cure the disease, but they can prolong the remission period to reduce the incidence of relapse and the use of corticosteroids. Specifically, *Lactobacillus plantarum* is effective in reducing inflammation in this disease.[20]

10.2.2.2   Effectiveness against Diarrhea

Clostridium difficile is found in small numbers in the healthy intestine, but antibiotic treatment may cause an increase in their number and toxin production. Development of these microorganisms in the intestine causes diarrhea. It was found that probiotics are useful for treating diarrhea. For example, a daily intake of *Lactobacillus* GG is effective in the termination of diarrhea. In addition, *Saccharomyces cerevisiae* Boulardii can be used to treat *C. difficile*–related colitis.[10]

Rotavirus is also a common diarrhea in children. Certain strains of probiotics, such as *Lactobacillus rhamnosus* GG and *Bifidobacterium animalis* Bb-12, have a beneficial effect on the treatment of rotaviruses.[10] In addition, a mix of pediatric beverage having *B. animalis*, *Lactobacillus acidophilus*, and *Lactobacillus reuteri* showed a preventive effect on diarrhea caused by rotavirus.[21] Probiotics can also prevent traveler's diarrhea, caused by enterotoxigenic *Escherichia coli*.

10.2.2.3   Improvement in Lactose Metabolism

Lactose malabsorption is a disturbance in which lactose is not hydrolyzed into its monosaccharides, glucose and galactose, because of a deficiency of the β-D-galactosidase enzyme. Individuals with a deficiency of this enzyme may have gastric distress after consuming unfermented milk or milk products due to the formation of hydrogen gas by microbial activity in the intestine.[22] Probiotic cultures have a positive effect on relief of lactose malabsorption. Specifically, yogurt is very good for lactose malabsorbers. Lactose tolerance of yogurt is better than that of some other fermented dairy foods. The factors responsible for better tolerance of lactose by consuming yogurt include (a) yogurt bacteria, (b) lactase enzyme elaborated by yogurt bacteria, and (c) orocoecal transit time.[6] Yogurt starter bacteria (*Lactobacillus delbrueckii* ssp. *bulgaricus* and *Streptococcus thermophilus*) contain high levels of lactase enzyme, which autodigest lactose intracellularly before reaching the intestine.[23] In addition, products having *Lactobacillus acidophilus* and bifidobacteria can easily be consumed by individuals who are lactose intolerant.[24,25]

Slower gastric emptying of semisolid fermented milks is another factor responsible for better digestion of lactose. Lactose is hydrolyzed by indigenous lactase enzyme located in the sides and tips of the viili of the jejunum and by bacterial lactase when gastric emptying is delayed. Yogurt-like viscous foods delay gastric emptying and decrease the symptoms of lactose intolerance.[26]

10.2.2.4   Anticarcinogenic Properties

Certain types of cancer are related to diet. Some bacteria and metabolic products including nitrosamine, heterocyclic amines, phenolic compounds, and ammonia may cause colorectal cancer. Specifically, consumption of barbequed red meat and not enough fiber in the diet play a major role in colorectal cancer. In addition, colonic microflora cause carcinogenesis mediated by enzymes produced by microorganisms such as β-glucuronidase, azoreductase, and nitroreductase. These enzymes convert procarcinogens into carcinogens.[4] Certain strains of *Lactobacillus acidophilus* and *Bifidobacterium* spp. decrease the amount of these enzymes. Therefore, the risk of tumor development is reduced.[27]

Singh et al.[28] reported the mechanisms of the anticarcinogenic effect of probiotic bacteria. These effects may be due to the removal of procarcinogen sources, improving the balance of intestinal microflora, preventing/delaying toxin production, strengthening of intestinal barrier mechanisms, and activation of nonspecific cellular factors (such as macrophages and natural killer cells) via the regulation of γ-interferon production.

Fermented milks, including yogurt, milk fermented with *Lactobacillus delbrueckii* spp. *bulgaricus*, *Streptococcus thermophilus*, and *Lactobacillus acidophilus*, or milk fermented with *Lactobacillus helveticus*, are reported to inhibit the growth of cancer cells. Also exopolysaccharides in kefir inhibit cancer cell growth.[6] Yogurt bacteria also have antitumor actions due to the stimulation of the immune function and the detoxification of genotoxins.[6,29] Yogurt reduces the level of bacterial enzymes such as β-glucuronidase, azoreductase, and nitroreductase. These enzymes may contribute to the formation of bowel cancer.[30,31] Salminen et al.[32] stated that the following mechanisms are related to the consumption of lactic acid bacteria and cancer:

1. Modulation of intestinal microecology
2. Alteration of metabolic activity (decrease in conversion of precarcinogens to carcinogens)
3. Prevention or delay of toxin absorption
4. Enhancement of intestinal immunity
5. Strengthening intestinal barrier mechanisms
6. Butyrate supply to villi
7. Folate supply in regulation of intestinal cell division

10.2.2.5   Reduction in Serum Cholesterol

Cholesterol is an essential component of the cell membrane and is synthesized by the liver and absorbed from foods. Cholesterol is required to produce some hormones and bile acids. Controlling blood cholesterol level has a complex mechanism. Hydroxymethylglutaryl-CoA is a required enzyme for the synthesis of cholesterol in the body. However, hydroxymethylglutarate produced by the metabolites of starter cultures in fermented milks inhibits this enzyme.[6]

Dietary saturated fat intake and serum cholesterol levels are highly correlated. A high level of cholesterol, specifically low-density lipoprotein (LDL), is a risk factor for cardiovascular disease.[33] Probiotics deconjugate bile salts. Deconjugated bile acid cannot absorb lipids as its conjugated counterpart. Therefore, the cholesterol level is decreased. *Lactobacillus acidophilus* can also take up cholesterol during growth. For this reason, cholesterol will be unavailable for absorption into the bloodstream.[34] *Lactobacillus reuteri*[35] and *Bifidobacterium longum*[36] showed the reducing effect in triglycerides and LDL cholesterol.

10.2.2.6 Stimulation of the Immune System

Starter bacteria used in fermented milks have the ability to survive in the gastrointestinal tract. The intestinal system is important to defend the body against bacterial and viral infections, cancer, and allergies. Therefore, the health benefits of fermented milk products are affected by intestinal microflora.[6] The major mechanism by which lactobacilli and bifidobacteria affect the immune system is related to their ability to differentially modulate the expression of cytokines and costimulatory molecules.[37,38] Another mechanism of probiotic therapy is enhanced IgA response because of the administration of probiotics. Tejada-Simon et al.[39] showed that ingestion of yogurt with *Lactobacillus acidophilus* and *Bifidobacterium* by mice potentiated IgA response to cholera toxin. Probiotics produce γ-interferon by T-cells and stimulate cytokines.[4]

10.2.2.7 Others

The effect of *Lactobacillus helveticus* fermented milk on acute changes in calcium metabolism in postmenopausal women was investigated.[40] The result showed that the fermentation of milk with *Lactobacillus helveticus* positively affected calcium metabolism by suppressing serum parathyroid hormone (PTH) and increasing serum calcium concentration.

10.3 FINAL REMARKS

The scientific findings up until today have justified Ilya Methcnikoff's (1908) theory about auto-intoxication. His theory claims that "the human body is slowly being poisoned and its resistance weakened by the action of the wrong type of intestinal flora." Today it is well agreed that a well-functioning intestinal flora is a key element for a healthy life. Therefore, it has become important to consume fermented milk products containing probiotic bacteria for several reasons, such as

- Fighting against several types of infections and cancer
- Reducing the side effects of drugs and x-ray treatments, lactose-intolerant symptoms, and gastrointestinal secretions
- Reducing the number of potentially pathogenic microorganisms in the gut
- Improving the bioavailability of nutrients

REFERENCES

1. Shah, N.P., Functional foods, probiotics and prebiotics, *Food Technol.*, 55, 46, 2001.
2. Hoolihan, L., Beyond calcium. The protective attributes of dairy products and their constituents, *Nutr. Today*, 39 (2), 69, 2004.
3. Chandan, R.C. and Shah, N.P., Functional foods and disease prevention, in *Manufacturing Yogurt and Fermented Milks*, R.C. Chandan, C.H. White, A. Kilara, and Y.H. Hui, Eds, pp. 311–325, Blackwell Publishing, Iowa, 2006.
4. Shah, N.P., Functional cultures and health benefits, *Int. Dairy J.*, 17, 1262, 2007.
5. Robinson, R.K., *Therapeutic Properties of Fermented Milks*, p. 185, Elsevier Science Publishers Ltd., Essex, England, 1991.
6. Shah, N.P., Health benefits of yogurt and fermented milks, in *Manufacturing Yogurt and Fermented Milks*, R.C. Chandan, C.H. White, A. Kilara, and Y.H. Hui, Eds, pp. 327–254, Blackwell Publishing, Iowa, USA, 2006.
7. Kitts, D.D. and Weiler, K., Bioactive proteins and peptides from food sources. Applications of bioprocesses used in isolation and recovery, *Curr. Phar. Des.*, 9, 1309, 2003.
8. FitzGerald, R.J. and Meisel, H., Milk protein hydrolysates and bioactive peptides, in *Advanced Dairy Chemistry, Vol. 1: Proteins*, 3rd edition, P.F. Fox and P.L.H. McSweeney, Eds,. pp. 675–698, Elsevier Science Publishers Ltd., England, 2003.
9. Korhonen, H. and Pihlanto, A., Food-derived bioactive peptides-opportunities for designing future foods, *Curr. Phar. Des.*, 9, 1297, 2003.
10. Shah, N.P., Probiotics and fermented milks, in *Manufacturing Yogurt and Fermented Milks*, R.C. Chandan, C.H. White, A. Kilara, and Y.H. Hui, Eds, pp. 341–354, Blackwell Publishing, Iowa, USA, 2006.
11. Roberfroid, M.B., Prebiotics and probiotics: Are they functional foods? *Am. J. Clin. Nutr.*, 71 (Suppl.), 1682S–1687S, 2000.
12. Varnam, A.H. and Sutherland, J.P., Fermented milks, in *Milk and Milk Products. Technology, Chemistry and Microbiology*, pp. 346–386, Chapman & Hall, London, 1996.
13. Shah, N.P., Probiotic bacteria: Antimicrobial and antimutagenic properties, *Probiotica*, 6, 1, 1999.
14. Hekmat, S. and McMahon, D.J., Survival of *Lactobacillus* and *Bifidobacterium bifidum* in ice cream for use as a probiotic food, *J. Dairy Sci.*, 75, 1415, 1992.
15. Klupsch, H.J., Man and microflora-bioghurt-biogarde, *S. Afr. J. Dairy Technol.*, 17, 153, 1985.
16. Armuzzi, A., et. al., The effect of oral administration of *Lactobacillus* GG on antibiotic-associated gastrointestinal side-effects during *Helicobacter pylori* eradication therapy, *Aliment. Phar. Therap.*, 15, 163, 2001.
17. Felley, C.P., et al., Favourable effect of an acidified milk (LC-1) on *Helicobacter pylori* gastritis in man, *Eur. J. Gastroenterol. Hepatol.*, 13, 25, 2001.
18. Cats, A., et al., Effect of frequent consumption of *Lactobacillus casei*-containing milk drink in *Helicobacter pylori*-colonised subjects, *Aliment. Phar. Therap.*, 17, 429, 2003.
19. Çakır, İ. and Çakmakçı, M.L., Antimicrobial activities of some commercial and non-commercial probiotic bacteria, in *Proc. Int. Dairy Symp.*, Z.G. Seydim, Z.Y. Ekinci, and A. Seydim, Eds, p. 68, Isparta, Turkey, May 24–28, 2004.
20. Schultz, M. and Sartor, R.B., Probiotics and inflammatory bowel diseases, *Am. J. Gastroenterol.*, 95, 19S–21S, 2000.
21. Guandalini, S., et al., *Lactobacillus* GG administered in oral rehydration solution to children with acute diarrhoea: A multicenter European trail, *J. Pediatr. Gastroenterol. Nutr.*, 30, 54, 2000.
22. He, T., The role of colonic metabolism in lactose intolerance, *Eur. J. Clin. Invest.*, 38, 541, 2008.

23. Savaiano, D.A., ElAnovar, A.A., Smith, J., and Levitt, M.D., Lactose malabsorption from yogurt, pasteurized yogurt, sweet acidophilus milk, and cultured milk in lactose-deficient individuals, *Am. J. Clin. Nutr.*, 40, 1219, 1984.
24. Gilliland, S.E., Acidophilus milk products: A review of potential benefits to consumers. *J. Dairy Sci.*, 72, 10, 2483, 1989.
25. Özbaş, Z.Y., *Bifidobakterler* ve *Lactobacillus acidophilus*: özellikleri, diyetetik amaçlar için kullanımları, yararlı etkileri ve ürün uygulamaları, *Gıda Dergisi*, 4, 247, 1993.
26. Shah, N.P., Fedorak, R.N., and Jelen, P., Food consistency effects of quarg in lactose adsorption by lactose intolerant individuals, *Int. Dairy J.*, 2, 257, 1992.
27. Yoon, H., Benamouzig, R., Little, J, Francois-Collange, M., and Tome, D., Systematic review of epidemiological studies on meat, dairy products, and egg consumption and risk of colorectal adenomas, *Eur. J. Cancer Prev.*, 9, 151, 2000.
28. Singh, J., et al., *Bifidobacterium longum* and *Lactobacillus acidophilus* producing intestinal bacteria inhibits colon cancer and modulates the intermediate biomarkers of colon carcinogenesis, *Carcinogenesis*, 18, 833, 1997.
29. Wollowski, I., Ji, S.T., Bakalinsky, A.T., Neudecker, C., and Pool-Zobel, B.L., Bacteria used for the production of yogurt inactivate carcinogens and prevent DNA-damage in the colon cells, *J. Nutr.*, 129, 77, 2001.
30. Goldin, B.R. and Gorbach, S.L., The effect of milk and *Lactobacillus* feeding on human intestinal bacterial enzyme activity, *Am. J. Clin. Nutr.*, 39, 756, 1984.
31. Cenci, G., Rossi, J., Throtta, F., and Caldini, G., Lactic acid bacteria isolated from dairy products inhibit genotoxic effect of 4-nitroquinoline-1-oxide in SOS-chromotest, *Syst. Appl. Microbiol.*, 25, 483, 2002.
32. Salminen, S., Playne, M., and Lee, Y.K., Successful probiotic lactobacilli: Human studies on probiotic efficacy, in *Handbook of Functional Dairy Products*, C. Shortt and J. O'Brien, Eds, p. 13, CRC Press, Boca Raton, 2004.
33. Liong, M.T. and Shah, N.P., Effect of *Lactobacillus casei* synbiotic on serum lipoprotein, intestinal microflora, and organic acids in rats, *J. Dairy Sci.*, 89, 1390, 2006.
34. Klaver, F.A.M and Meer, R.V.D., The assumed assimilation of cholesterol by lactobacilli and *Bifidobacterium bifidum* is due to their bile salt deconjugating activity, *Appl. Environ. Microbiol.*, 59, 1120, 1993.
35. Taranto, M.P., et al., Evidence for hypocholesterolemic effect of *Lactobacillus reuteri* in hypercholesterolemic mice, *J. Dairy Sci.*, 81, 2336, 1998.
36. Xiao, J.Z., et al., Effects of milk products fermented by *Bifidobacterium longum* on blood lipids in rats and healthy adult male volunteers, *J. Dairy Sci.*, 86, 2452, 2003.
37. Marin, M.L., et al., Differential cytokine production in clonal macrophage and T-cell lines cultured with bifidobacteria, *J. Dairy Sci.*, 80, 2713, 1997.
38. Marin, M.L., et al., Stimulation of cytokine production in clonal macrophage and T cell models by *Streptococcus thermophilus*: Comparison with *Bifidobacterium* spp. and *Lactobacillus bulgaricus*, *J. Food Protect.*, 61, 859, 1998.
39. Tejeda-Simon, M.V., Lee, J.H., Ustunol, Z., and Pestka, J.J., Ingestion of yogurt containing *Lactobacillus acidophilus* and *Bifidobacterium* to potentiate immunoglobulin A responses to chlora toxin in mice, *J. Dairy Sci.*, 82, 649, 1999.
40. Navra, M., Nevala, R., Poussa, T., and Korpela, R., The effect of *Lactobacillus helveticus* fermented milk on acute changes in calcium metabolism in postmenopausal women, *Eur. J. Nutr.*, 43, 61, 2004.

11 Immunity and Functional Dairy Foods in the Human Life Cycle

Bilkay Baştürk

CONTENTS

11.1   INTRODUCTION

Immunity is a way of protection from diseases. And as a part of the immune system, the cells and molecules are responsible for constituting the immune system. Immune responses are coordinated with complex responses which are made of against harmless agents.

Our environment contains a great variety of infectious microbes that can cause diseases. Because of the immune system combats, harmless agents such as microorganisms are short-lived and they leave little permanent damage. Any immune response involves, firstly, recognition of the pathogen and, secondly, a reaction to eliminate it. Innate and adaptive immune systems work together for this combat, and the innate and the adaptive immune system include lots of factors. The first line of defense against pathogens is a physical barrier including mucosa. Adaptive immune system protects us against specific pathogens. T and B lymphocytes and antibodies are composed of adaptive immune response. Colostrum is a premilk substance that is produced after birth, and human milk contains highly beneficial nutrition for the newborn. Colostum and human milk include several immune factors, for example, T cells B cells, immunoglobulins, complement components, antimicrobials peptides, lactoferrin, lysozymes, macrophages, neutrophils, cytokines, vitamins, prebiotics, and probiotics. Probiotics are live microorganisms and they are beneficial to health. The best examples of probiotics are *Bifidobacterium* and *Lactobacillus*. Breastfeeding provides both defense against pathogens and development in intestinal mucosa. Studies showed the relationship between several diseases (such as allergies, infectious diseases, and cancer), breastfeeding, and probiotics.

In this chapter we focus on human milk, probiotics, and their immune properties.

11.2   GENERAL FEATURES OF THE IMMUNE SYSTEM

The immune system protects us against potential pathogens. It must be able to distinguish foreign non-self-antigens from self-antigens. The same immune system should respond with immunological tolerance against our own tissues, and other antigens as well as foods. It starts to develop during embryogenesis, when the first hematopoietic cells develop outside the embryo, in the yolk sac. In week six of gestation, hematopoietic stem cells are developed. In week seven, cells seed the developing thymus.[1] There are two types of organs in the immune system: primary organs and secondary organs. Bone marrow, where T and B cells are produced and B cells are developed, and the thymus, where T cells are developed, are primary organs. T and B cells are activated in secondary organs like spleen, lymph nodes, and mucosa-associated lymphoid tissue (MALT). Activated T and B cells result in the clonal expansion of lymphocytes. The immune system is constituted by cells and molecules that are responsible for immunity. Defense against infectious and noninfectious foreign substances is the physiological function of the immune system. The immune system consists of two parts: the innate (natural or native) immune system and the adaptive immune system. Innate immune response to antigens stimulates the adaptive immune response and adaptive immune response uses the many of the effector mechanisms of innate immunity.

11.2.1 INNATE IMMUNE SYSTEM

The first line of defense against infections is the innate immune system, which is acting within minutes of exposure to pathogenic microorganisms. Innate immunity components include barriers and these barriers are provided by epithelial and mucosal surfaces. Also these barriers allow microbial entry. The other components, such as phagocytes and the complement system, are normally inactive but are also poised to respond quickly. The innate immune system also involves various substances to prevent entry or colonization of infectious agents such as enzymes, proteins, peptides, low pH, and fatty acids.

The skin, gastrointestinal and respiratory tracts, and mucosal surface are the main interfaces between the host and the environment. Physical barriers are formed by intact epithelial surfaces and loss of integrity predisposes the organism to infections.[2] Peptides that have a natural antibiotic function are produced by epithelia. Defensins are also produced by epithelia. Defensins have a natural antibiotic function, which kills a variety of bacteria and fungi. Collectins are surfactant proteins and act on the epithelial surface of lung alveoli to bind microbes, leading to aggregation, opsonization, and increased clearance of organisms by alveolar macrophage.[3] Phagocytes are ingesting and destroying microbes. Neutrophils, which generally migrate more rapidly than macrophages, are effective in the earliest phase of infection, and the second are macrophages and monocytes are effector cells for elimination of infectious and noninfectious foreign substances. In the innate immune system, these cells' functions are fundamentally similar. At the site of initial infection the innate immune system is active primarily.

Natural killer (NK) cells are derived from bone marrow precursors. NK cells are a subset of lymphocytes that kill virus-infected cells and tumor cells. They can mediate antibody-dependent cellular cytotoxicity (ADCC), and also secrete cytokines, mainly interferon-γ (IFN-γ).

The complement system is a cascade of enzymatically activated proteins yielding molecules that function immunologically. There are several plasma proteins which consist of the complement system. The principal functions of the complement system include opsonization of the organism and immune complexes for phagocytosis. Another function cell lysis, which is mediated by the membrane attack complex. Classical and alternate pathways function to activate complement. Both pathways induce the formation of C3b. C3b is an opsonin and acts to cleave C5 into C5a that functions as a chemoattractant and C5b that is a part of the membrane attack complex of the classical pathway. In the alternate pathway, complement components are direct binding microorganisms.

Cytokines are proteins that mediate many of the responses of innate and adaptive immunity. Cytokines are synthesized in response to inflammatory or antigenic stimuli. Secretion of cytokines mediates many of the effector functions of innate immunity.[2,4]

11.2.2   ADAPTIVE IMMUNE SYSTEM

Adaptive immunity develops as a response to infection and adapts to infection, so it is called adaptive immunity or acquired immunity or specific immunity. The lymphocytes (T and B) and their products are the components of adaptive immunity. The adaptive immune response is activated along with the innate defense system. Phagocytes play an important role in both innate and adaptive immune response. In the thymus T lymphocytes develop in a process that involves rearrangement of the T cell receptors (TCRs) followed by selection against self-antigens. NK cells and dendritic cells (DC) take place in the thymus. Thymus development commences during early fetal life and it reaches its maximum size in relation to total body weight soon after birth. Thymus plays a central role in the development of T cells. TCR rearrangement and thymocyte differentiation into mature T cells occur in the thymus. Cell-mediated immunity, cellular immunity, is mediated by T lymphocytes.

These effector cells originate from a common stem cell in the bone marrow, attack the specific pathogen and generate memory cells that can prevent reinfection on exposure to the same organism. T lymphocytes function in the regulation of antigen-specific immune response, both helping and suppressing specific activities. T cells can be subdivided into T helper cells and T cytotoxic cells. Helper T (Th) lymphocytes, which express CD4 molecules on the cell surface, secrete cytokines, whereas cytotoxic T lymphocytes (CTL), which express CD8 molecules on the cell surface, act by killing cells that express foreign antigens. T cells cannot recognize the antigen by themselves. Antigenic determinant must be presented by an appropriate major histocompatibility complex (MHC) molecule. They recognize their antigens through their TCR in the form of an MHC peptide complex. MHC class I molecules are expressed at the surface of all nucleated cells, but MHC class II molecules are expressed only by professional antigen presenting cells like DC. CTL and NK cells kill infected cells via proteins named perforin and enzymes named granzymes. Perforin creates pores in the cell membrane and the granzymes enter through these pores to induce apoptosis of target cells.[4,5] Humoral immunity and cell-mediated immunity, which are mediated by different components of the immune system, are types of adaptive immune response.

The principal defense mechanism against extracellular microbes and their toxins is humoral immunity. It is mediated by molecules in the blood called antibodies. Antibodies are produced by B cells and on the bone marrow they developed. Antibodies function either alone through neutralization or with complement and phagocytes to inactivate infectious organisms. Different types of antibodies may activate different effector mechanisms. The development of lymphoid cells requires growth factors. At birth, the lymphoid system is not yet mature and all T and B cells are naïve.

Active immunity is induced by exposure to a foreign antigen. Immunity can also be conferred by transferring serum or lymphocytes, which is called passive immunity. The infant's immune system is supported by passive immunity transferred from mother to child. Maternal immunoglobulins and breast milk are composed of passive immunity and both of them are the best examples of passive immunity. Transplacental transfer of IgG from the mother to the infant is a selective process. Only IgG and IgG subclasses are across the placenta. The majority of the transfer of IgG occurs in the third trimester. These antibodies enable newborns to combat infections.

Specificity, diversity, memory, specialization, self-limitation, and nonreactivity to self are cardinal features of adaptive immune responses.

11.2.3 DIFFERENCES BETWEEN ADULTS' AND NEONATES' IMMUNE SYSTEM

Human infants are born immature and to reach the level of adult function human infants need a period of maturation. In innate immunity neutrophils play an important role and in neonates the number of circulating neutrophils is higher[6] but production of hydroxyl radicals for killing pathogens may be lower than in adults.[7] Neutrophil cytotoxicity in normal neonates seems similar to that in adults.[8] NK cells of infants have decreased cytotoxic activity and decreased ADCC. This situation continues through 6 months of life.[9] In complement system, C8 and C9 components levels are low at all gestational ages.[10] Except C5 and C7, most of the complement protein concentrations are lower than in adults until 18 months of age.[11,12] Neonatal T lymphocytes produce less IFN-γ, interleukin-2 (IL-2), IL-4, IL-10, and tumor necrosis factor-β than adult T lymphocytes produced after stimulation.[13,14] The decreased cytokine production is certainly a function of the limited numbers of memory T-lymphocytes. There is also decreased cytotoxic activity of CD8+ lymphocytes in the newborns.[15] There are increased numbers of T lymphocytes in cord blood or adults. The number of T lymphocytes decreases after the neonatal period.[16] B lymphocytes contribute the pathogen-specific immunity. Neonatal B cells produce primarily immunoglobulin M (IgM) and limited amounts of IgA and IgG. IgM production can occur in the fetus in response to an intrauterine infection. After birth one of the major defense mechanisms is passive immunity, which is provided by maternal antibodies. Maternal IgG is transported across the placenta and ingested IgG antibodies are also transported across the gut epithelium into the circulation of the newborn. The majority of the transfer of IgG occurs in the third trimester.[2] The infant begins to actively produce IgG antibody on exposure to antigens. Premature infants have very low levels of IgG antibody, but mean concentration increases with increasing gestational age.

11.2.4 IMMUNITY AT OLD AGE

Old age is accompanied by variety of health problems, which are mainly due to a gradual decline in the function of the various organ systems. Changes in the aging immune system are of particular importance, as they result in the decrease in the capacity of an organism to defend itself against pathogens. Aging is related to impairment of immunity, mostly cell-mediated immunity. Thymus is a primary lymphoid organ where the T cells are maturated. Thymus involution begins at 10 years, and it is completely replaced by adipose tissue at 50 years, and the thymic hormones disappear at about 60 years.[17] Age-related T cell-mediated immunity dysfunction has been implicated in the ethiology of many of the chronic degenerative diseases of the elderly. Age-associated thymic involution decreases the ability of the elderly to generate naïve T cells,[18] resulting in the accumulation of memory cells and reduction in naïve T cell repertoire.[19] The level of cholesterol, which increases in the old age period, affects lipid rafts in T cell membrane. A major factor influencing the assembly of the signaling apparatus is cell membrane fluidity. And due to this, signaling in T cell membrane decreases. As a result of this, decrease in T cell functions may occur.[20] The majority of changes seen in humoral immunity in the elderly are likely to be due to altered T cell help. The antigen presenting cell function of DC is generally well retained in the elderly[21] but their numbers are reduced with age.[22] In the elderly, production and proliferation rates of NK cells are lower than in the young.[23]

11.2.5 MUCOSAL IMMUNE SYSTEM

The mucosal epithelia of the gastrointestinal, respiratory, and reproductive systems consist of the mucosal immune system. It has several functions including gas exchange, food absorption, and protection against microorganisms and foreign proteins, and it is composed of innate mechanism of protection. Some of the innate mechanisms acting at the mucosal surfaces include pH or acidity, enzymes, chemicals, immunoglobulins, and mucus. IgA is the major class of antibody that is produced in the mucosal immune system. Defense against microbes is provided by antibody, largely IgA. Antibody responses to antigens encountered by ingestion or inhalation are typically dominated by IgA. In mucosal secretions IgA binds to microbes and toxins present in the lumen and neutralizes them by blocking their entry into the host.[2,4] Mucus production is another innate mechanism of defense, blocking adherence of pathogens to epithelial cells. Intestinal epithelium and mucus function as a barrier, limiting the entry of microorganisms from the lumen into the interior of the host.

The MALT is located adjacent to the mucosal surfaces: tonsils and adenoids of Waldeyer's ring at the back of the mouth, Peyer's patches in the small intestine and appendix, and isolated B-cell follicles in the distal large intestine. In MALT tissue, some of the epithelial cells overlying Peyer's patches are specialized M (membranous) cells. M cells lack microvilli, are actively pinocytic, and transport macromolecules from the intestinal lumen into subepithelial tissues. They are thought to play an important role in delivering antigens to Peyer's patches. MALT is activated by the postnatal exposure of the mucosal surfaces to numerous antigens. The lactating mammary glands in the mother are an integral part of MALT. It is important that mucosal immunity also undergoes a period of postnatal development.[2,4]

11.3 HUMAN MILK

11.3.1 PROPERTIES OF COLOSTRUM

Colostrum is a premilk substance that is produced after birth and this is a gift for the newborn. Colostrum includes proteins, different types of sugar, fats, and micronutrients in the form of vitamins and minerals. Colostrum consists of several immune factors; for example, secretory IgA (SIgA) component is a cardinal feature of colostrums. IgA binds to microbes and toxins and then neutralizes them by blocking their entry into the host. IgG, IgE, IgM, IgA, and IgD are subgroups of immunoglobulins and they play an important role in defense both in the treatment and prevention of viral and bacterial infections and allergies. Vital growth factors stimulate growth and help in the regeneration and repair of muscle, skin, collagen, and nerve tissue.

Colostrum lasts 2–4 days after birth, but on the other hand, breast milk provides a number of bioactive factors as well as colostrums.

11.3.2 IMMUNOLOGICAL CONTENTS OF HUMAN MILK

The neonatal immune system functions are different from that of adult. After birth, neonates are exposed to a large number of microorganisms and foreign proteins, and resistance to infection relies both on the protective factors in milk and on the infant developing his or her own innate and adaptive immunity. The relationship between breastfeeding and healthy babies has been noted over the past years. In infants, human milk provide a development of elements in acquired and innate immune system. The innate immune system is the first defense mechanism. Human milk includes several components that are effective in the innate immune system.

11.3.2.1 Properties of the Innate Immune System in Human Milk

11.3.2.1.1 Fatty Acids and Monoglycerides

They have antiviral, antiprotozoal and antibacterial activity and this activity may augment the ability of the stomach to act as a barrier against ingested pathogens. Oleic acid and linoleic acid have very high activity at killing of enveloped viruses. Oleic acid is released from milk in the highest concentration so it is the primary source of protection to the breastfed infant.[24]

11.3.2.1.2 Antimicrobial Peptides

Antimicrobial peptides are abundant in human milk. Many peptides must be secreted in their inactive forms to become active only in particular locations and specific conditions. Peptides at different local concentrations may have different functions. Without inflammation some peptides may be optimized to inhibit pathogens but others inhibit best in an inflamed environment.

11.3.2.1.3 Lactoferrin

Lactoferrin is the major protein in human milk. It has anti-inflammatory, antiviral, and antibacterial properties. It is a ferric iron-binding glycoprotein that inhibits the growth of pathogens by competing with bacteria for ferric ion. It can prevent reproduction of bacteria. Lactoferrin and its fragments are bactericidal for many Gram-positive and Gram-negative bacteria. Lactoferrin has the capacity to enter the nuclei of leukocytes and block the transcription factor NF-κB and this effect suppresses proinflammatory cytokine synthesis.

11.3.2.1.4 Lysozymes

Lysozymes are an antimicrobial peptide that cleaves peptidoglycans in cell walls of bacteria and it contains proteolytic enzymes that degrade proteins capable of destroying infectious agent on contact.

11.3.2.1.5   Leukocyte

Prevent infection and stimulate cytokine secretion, especially IFN.

11.3.2.1.6   Lactalbumins

Active agent against several cancer and viral infections.

11.3.2.1.7   Proline-Rich Peptides

They can stimulate the thymus to regulate the immune system.

11.3.2.1.8   Oligopolysaccharides

They bind the bacteria and prevent their entry into the mucosal surface. Breast milk contains 80 different oligosaccharides. Many of these function as a receptor analogue that inhibits the binding of bacterial or viral pathogens, or toxins to gut epithelial cells.

11.3.2.1.9   Glycans

Glycoproteins, glycolipids, mucins, and glycosaminoglycans are composed of glycans. Human milk glycans are protecting nursing infants from enteric pathogens.

11.3.2.1.10   Vitamins and Minerals

They are essential for the normal metabolism, growth, and development. Vitamins A, C, E, and the others make colostrums serve as antioxidant in the body.

11.3.2.1.11   Macrophages

Macrophages play important roles in innate and adaptive immune responses and they are activated by microbial products such as endotoxin and by T cell cytokine such as IFN-γ. Activated macrophages phagocytose and kill microorganisms, secrete proinflammatory cytokines and present antigens to helper T cell. Milk macrophages contain engulfed SIgA, which can be released on contact with bacteria in the gut, and breast milk-derived macrophages express CD14, whose function is to bind the complex of lipopolysaccharides (LPS) required for LPS-induced macrophage activation, and CD11c, whose function is phagocytosis and likely act on infant T and B cells, demonstrate phagocytic activity and secrete immunoregulatory factors.[25,26]

11.3.2.1.12   Neutrophils

The number of neutrophils is higher in neonates than in adults. Neutrophils are recruited to inflammatory sites and they are capable of phagocytosing and enzymatically digesting microbes. Human milk neutrophils show decreased adherence and motility and express high levels of CD11b, whose function is phagocytosis of C3b-coated particles, and adhesion to endothelium, and low levels of L-selectin (CD62L), whose function is homing of naïve T cells to peripheral lymph nodes, these molecules show prior activation.[27]

11.3.2.1.13   Cytokines

Cytokines are principal mediators of the communication between the immune system's cells. Cytokines are proteins that are produced by many different cell types that mediate inflammatory and immune reactions. Human milk contains an array of cytokines and chemokines. The primary source of these cytokines is the mammary gland and leukocytes recovered from expressed human milk have been shown to be capable of producing a number of cytokines.[28] Human milk contains both proinflammatory cytokines (TNF-α, IL-6, IL-8) and anti-inflammatory cytokines (IL-10, TGF-β).

11.3.2.1.14 Polyamines

Human breast milk is the main source of polyamines for the newborns. The synthesis of polyamines gradually increases in the mammary gland during pregnancy and lactation. Polyamines are involved in the differentiation of immune cells and the regulation of the inflammatory response.

11.3.2.2 Properties of the Acquired Immune System in Human Milk

There are two types of immune response in the acquired immune system: cell-mediated immune response and humoral immune response. T and B cells are the main effector cells in cell-mediated immune response. The majority of lymphocytes in milk are T cells. CD4+ T cells are present in an activated state and CD4+ cells express activation markers and immunological memory-associated protein. In human milk, the CD4+/CD8+ cells ratio is decreased and the NK cells ratio is increased, so there is a negative correlation between CD4+/CD8+ cells and NK cells. CD8+ T cells have selectively homed from the maternal mucosal immune system to the mammary gland.[29] IgA plays an important role in the humoral immune response in human milk. Breast milk contains 0.4–1.0 g/L SIgA. SIgA is directed specifically against enteric and respiratory pathogens. Ingested IgA can neutralize pathogenic organisms that attempt to colonize the infant's gut.

11.4 BREASTFEEDING AND MUCOSAL IMMUNITY

11.4.1 Functions of Mucosal Immunity

The mucosal surfaces of the body play a vital role in the interaction between the external and internal environments. Lots of microorganisms infecting humans use the mucosa as portals of entry. Microbial colonization of intestinal flora begins at birth. The maternal microflora can be a source of bacteria that colonize the newborn's intestine. Colonization can also be affected by environmental factors and also by infant-feeding patterns. Colonization with bacteria is critical for the normal structural and functional development and optimal function of the mucosal immune system.[30]

Mucosal epithelia cover an area at least 200 times that of the skin. Gut-associated lymphoid tissues (GALT) is the largest collection of lymphoid tissues in the body. Mucins are secreted by goblet cells. Mucin-rich glycocalyx is the major physical barrier of the gut.[31] The compositions of intestinal glycocalyx and mucins differ between neonates and adults; this is the primary determinant of the distinct differences in microbial composition of the intestine of neonates and adults.[32] Other barriers are antimicrobial peptides, which are produced by paneth cells.[33] Paneth cells are found at the bottom of each transcript and secrete also lysozymes. DC, which are present in luminal antigens to T lymphocytes, are important factors for GALT.[34] Peyer's patches are dome-like follicle-associated epithelial structures and contain M cells. M cells take the antigens with the apical (luminal) side and present these antigens with the basal side to mucosal lymphoid elements.[35] Human milk triglyceride is digested by infants' lingual and gastric lipases into free fatty acid and monoglyceride. Free fatty acid and monoglyceride are toxic to many pathogens and high concentrations of these are found in the infant's stomach.

Lactating mammary glands are part of the integrated mucosal immune system and milk antibodies reflect antigenic stimulation of MALT both in the gut and airways.

11.4.2 How Breastfeeding Affects the Mucosal Immunity?

A relationship between breastfeeding and infant health has been reported for thousands of years. Breastfeeding protects the infant against wide range of infectious and other disease.

Some immunomodulatory molecules such as soluble TNF-α receptors, IL-1 receptor antagonist (IL-1RA), and cytokines such as transforming growth factor β (TGF-β), IL-6, and IL-10 are found in breast milk. TNF-α receptors and IL-1RA suppress proinflammatory TNF-α and IL-1 activity.[36] TGF-β and IL-10 are anti-inflammatory cytokines and both of them are locally released from milk macrophages and they are stimulated in the neonatal gut and thereby enhance the development of mucosal immunity.

At birth, mucosal IgA- and IgM-producing cells are very rare in intestinal tissue. The numbers of intestinal IgM- and IgA-producing cells increase rapidly after 2–4 weeks.[37] TGF-β, IL-6, and IL-10 play an important role in developing and differentiation of IgA-producing cells.[38,39] Differentiated B cells produce dimmers or larger polymers of IgA (pIgA). Like SIgA, pIgA are transported externally by an epithelial glycoprotein called membrane secretory component (SC) or the polymeric Ig receptor (pIgR).[40] SIgA is protected against proteolytic degradation by SC and SIgA inhibits colonization and invasion by pathogens. pIgA, which is transported by pIgR and IgM antibodies, may inactivate viruses such as rotavirus and influenza virus, and SIgA antibodies may block microbial invasion.[40] In addition SIgA can interfere with growth factors and enzymes that are necessary for pathogenic bacteria and parasites.

Breast milk includes free SC. Free SC blocks its own epithelial adhesion and so limit infection by enterotoxigenic *Escherichia coli*[41] and inhibit the effect of bacterial toxins such as *Clostridium difficile* toxin A.[42]

Human milk also contains both complement components and anti-inflammatory factors, which are capable of inhibiting complement activation.[43] C3, C4, and C1q are found in early colostrums and continue at low levels up to 18 months of lactation. Human milk macrophages are able to synthesize all the components of the complement system. The presence of cytokines in human milk is the effect of local synthesis of the complement by human milk macrophages. Bacteria coated with C3 fragments can be ingested by phagocytic cells in the absence of antibodies. C3 fragments are also known to enhance the opsonizing effects of IgG.[44,45]

Human milk accelerates maturation of the gut barrier function, and breastfed infants had a predominance of *Lactobacillus bifidus*, thought to acidify the gut and inhibit enteric pathogens from infecting breastfed.

11.5   PREBIOTICS AND PROBIOTICS AND THE IMMUNE SYSTEM

11.5.1   PREBIOTICS

Prebiotics, which can occur naturally (breast milk), are nondigestible oligosaccharides that enter the colon and fermented to change the colonic environment to stimulate the increased proliferation of certain commensal bacteria, namely bifidobacteria and *Lactobacillus*. Prebiotics undergoes fermentation in the colon producing a lower pH.[46] Prebiotics present in human milk are primarily oligosaccharides. Oligosaccharides are one of the four main components (lactose, lipids, oligosaccharides, and protein) of human breast milk. The quantity of them is highest in colostrum and low in mature milk.

11.5.2   PROBIOTICS

Human milk consists of commensal bacteria for the infant's gut. Among the bacteria found in human milk, those belonging to the species *Staphylococcus*, *Lactococcus*, *Enterococcus*, and *Lactobacillus* are the most frequent.[47] Probiotics are live microorganisms that are beneficial to health. The best examples of probiotics are *Bifidobacterium* and *Lactobacillus*. Lactobacilli and bifidobacteria inhibit the growth of pathogen microorganisms such as *Staphylococcus aureus*, *Salmonella typhimurium*, *Yersinia enterocolitica*, and *Clostridium perfringens*.[48] *B. lactis* transiently trigger innate signal transduction and pro-inflammatory gene expression in the intestinal epithelium[49] and a study show that individuals who consumed *B. lactis*-supplemented milk or milk alone showed enhanced phagocyte-mediated bactericidal activity.[50] *L. casei* reduces the number of activated T lymphocytes and reduces the expression of the antiapoptotic protein Bcl-2 in the lamina propria of Crohn's disease mucosa.[51] Dietary consumption of probiotic lactic acid bacteria in a milk-based diet may offer benefit to elderly consumers to combat some of the deleterious effects of immunosenescence on cellular immunity.[52] Administration of fermented milk containing the probiotic *L. johnsonii* La1 may contribute to suppressing infections by improving nutritional and immunological status in the elderly.[53] *L. salivarius* strain isolated from breast milk and it may be responsible for its antimicrobial activity.[54] *Lactobacillus* are able to activate mucosal B-cell responses and generate divergent immune responses.[55] The different lactobacillus strains have different effects on immune system. The effect of *Lact. fermentum* CECT5716 is immunostimulatory in contrast to the antiinflammatory effect of *Lact. salivarius* CECT5713.[56] A study showed that *Lactobacillus rhamnosus* GG has immunostimulating effects on oral mucosa seen as increased allergen specific IgA levels in saliva.[57] Oral administration of the strain *L. fermentum* CECT5716 potentates the immunologic response of an anti-influenza vaccine and may provide enhanced systemic protection from infection by increasing the T-helper type 1 response and virus-neutralizing antibodies.[58] Daily intake of *Lactobacillus casei* strain Shirota has a positive effect on NK-cell activity.[59,60] Probiotic bacteria possess a heat-stable antiproliferative component(s) and may be used to generate microbiologically nonviable yet immunologically active probiotic food products.[61] Probiotic supplementation may prevent and treat antibiotic-associated diarrhea. Specific probiotics may modulate the intestinal mucosa by antagonizing pathogens through the production of antimicrobial compounds and chemicals.[62]

Bacterial cells enhance the proliferation of immune cells and bacterial cells induce the production of proinflammatory cytokines, but probiotic bacteria mediate the suppression of lymphocyte proliferation and cytokine production by T cells.[63] Probiotics stimulate the production of IL-10, which is produced by DC, monocytes, B cells, and regulatory T cells. IL-10 has anti-inflammatory effects and primarily IL-10 acts both to inhibit the proinflammatory response and to maintain tolerance to commensal intestinal bacteria.[64] Probiotics can induce an anti-inflammatory action on the intestinal mucosal immune system by suppressing T cell proliferation and probiotics can reduce T cell activation. Oral induction of lactobacilli can enhance nonspecific host resistance to microbial pathogens. Oral intake of *L. acidophilus* enhances phagocytosis in humans. Phagocytic activity results in the further recruitment of immunocompetent cells and the generation of inflammatory response. Probiotic bacteria modulate phagocytosis differentially in healthy and allergic subjects. In healthy people, probiotics have immunostimulatory effects, but in allergic people, it down-regulates the inflammatory response.[65] Probiotics determine the proinflammatory/anti-inflammatory balance but some of them influence both subsets.

11.6 IMMUNOLOGICAL TOLERANCE

Immunological tolerance is defined as the unresponsiveness to an antigen and this is induced by prior exposure to that antigen. All of the following determine the development of the T cell response: the type of antigen, the route of antigen entry, and the dose of antigen. Upon antigen exposure, immune cells respond with the release of a host of cytokines that then direct the subsequent immune responses. Th1- and Th2-type cells produce different types of cytokines. IL-4 is a Th2-type cytokine and it leads to enhanced IgE production. Another important cytokine is TGF-β. TGF-β participates both in oral immunization by production of IgA in mucosal tissue and in systemic tolerance. Inadequate production of TGF-β predisposes a person to sensitization by a low dose of antigens.[66] The oral administration of a protein antigen often leads to marked suppression of systemic humoral and cell-mediated immune response. This is called oral tolerance. In the context of inflammation, the altered rate, route, and mode of antigen presentation may lead to abrogation of oral tolerance. The intestinal immune system plays an important role in tolerance. It must encounter all antigens in order to determine which ones require an immune response and which ones can be safely tolerated. The mucosal immune system normally maintains itself to a state that favors tolerance and IgA production.

11.7 ALLERGIES AND NUTRITION

Allergy is a form of atopy and it often refers to type of antigen. Allergic diseases are common but some patients have an occasional mild allergic reaction, some suffer life-long debilitating disease, while more rarely, some react with severe or fatal anaphylactic shock. T lymphocyte-mediated response to common environmental allergens is biased toward anti-inflammatory (Th2) activity. Th2-type lymphocytes release cytokines such as IL-4, IL-5, and IL-13. IL-4 promotes differentiation of B cells specific for that antigen into IgE-producing cells.

Primary sensitization to allergen at pregnancy is via the fetal gut during the second trimester; there is also an exposure to allergen via the fetal circulation in the third trimester. This is predominantly a consequence of active transport of IgG antibody across the placenta complexed with antigens and allergens.[67]

In early childhood the greatest possible impact of primary dietary allergy is food allergy, particularly cow's milk allergy and atopic dermatitis (eczema). Later in childhood, allergies to inhalant allergens typically occur and asthma and rhinoconjuctivitis develop.[68]

11.7.1 ALLERGIES AND HUMAN MILK

Breastfeeding provides a prolonged benefit for infants in terms of protection against allergic disease. Some elements of breast milk are protective against the development of allergies, whereas others sensitize the individual. Cytokine concentrations can play a role in the immunogenicity of breast milk. IL-4, IL-5, and IL-13 are responsible for IgE production and induction of the eosinophilic response. These cytokines are present at higher concentration in the breast milk of atopic mothers.[69] Breast milk contains bioactive components such as functional proteins like growth factors and polyunsaturated fatty acids (PUFA).[70] PUFA are cellular membrane phospholipids that contribute to membrane fluidity and they support gut maturation, thus providing protection against infectious disease and development of allergies.

IgA production against β-lactoglobulin, casein, ovalbumin, and gliadin is essential for gut protection. TGF-β, which is the predominant cytokine in breast milk, stimulates the IgA production.

The presence of cytokines in human milk would tend to favor local synthesis of the complement by breast milk macrophages.[71] Human breast milk has a relative contribution of the complement which is transported from the serum, as well as the role and the control of the local synthesis. The rate of secretion of C2 and factor B, which activates C3, by milk macrophages has been found to be 8- and 2.5-fold, respectively, that of blood monocytes.[44] C3 is also a potent immunosuppressor, which may modulate the production of IgE antibodies directed against food and other allergens.[72] C3 may also be involved in the observed induction of a memory suppressor subset of lymphocytes, which regulates the production of IgE antibodies.[73]

Human breast milk contains another important cytokine, which is called TGF-β. TGF-β maintains oral tolerance, and infants with food allergy have been reported to display a defect in TGF-β as it has direct suppressive effects on both Th1 and Th2 responses[74] and it is a stimulation for the production of IgA antibodies.[75]

CD14 is a molecule that is known as a receptor for LPS and is required for LPS-induced macrophage activation. Breast milk contains very high levels of soluble CD14, which has been postulated to have a sentinel role enabling LPS-induced activation of membrane CD14$^-$ cells, such as intestinal epithelial cells, in the neonatal gut.[76] sCD14 in breast milk plays an important role in the induction of the T-helper lymphocyte response to bacteria and can also protect against development of allergies.

There is a significant association between reduced breast milk sCD14 levels and a diagnosis of eczema by 6 months of age.

Evidence suggests that exclusive breastfeeding for at least the first 6 months of life can decrease the incidence of atopic allergies.

11.7.2 ALLERGIES AND PROBIOTICS IN COMMERCIAL DAIRY PRODUCTS

Differences in the composition of intestinal microbiota influence the incidence of certain pathologies with an important immunological component, such as the allergic or inflammatory process. The antiallergic effect of probiotics could be explained on the Th1/Th2 balance. Th2-type cytokines are responsible for allergic response. Probiotics induce a Th1-type response and downregulate the production of Th2-type response. Breast milk probiotic *L. gasseri* CECT5714 and *L. coryniformis* CECT5711 together reduces the incidence and severity of allergic response in an animal model.[77] Several studies suggest that probiotics can be useful in the treatment and prevention of allergies when administered in infancy, but are less useful for adults.[78–80]

11.8 INFECTIOUS DISEASE AND BREAST MILK

Breastfeeding is important for infant and child health to protect them from infectious diseases. Breastfeeding is considered to decrease the incidence and severity of infection and malnutrition by several mechanisms. Human milk is nutritionally ideal for infants and contains factors that both passively prevent infection and actively promote the infant's own immune function. Breastfeeding protects against infectious and immunological diseases such as asthma and allergy, autoimmune diseases, and also tumors. One simple example for the benefits of breastfeeding during infection is the improved outcome for infants with diarrhea.

11.8.1 DIARRHEA AND BREASTFEEDING

Diarrhea is a common cause of death at infancy and is a major factor for infant mortality and it is obviously important to determine the protective capacity of breastfeeding. Breastfeeding is associated with a marked reduction in morbidity and mortality.[81,82]

Breastfeeding protects against gastroenteritis during the first year of life, and exclusive breastfeeding for 6 months results in fewer cases of gastroenteritis than exclusive breastfeeding for 3 months.[83,84]

Soluble IgA is an important factor for the protection against diarrhogenic bacteria and their toxins. Enterotoxigenic *E. coli*, *Shigella*, *Salmonella*, *Vibrio cholerae*, *G. lamblia*, and virus are responsible for diarrheal disease.[85,86] Breastfeeding is associated with a fivefold lower risk of the diarrhea caused by *G. lamblia* when compared with no breastfeeding.[87]

Multiple mechanisms of protection against gastrointestinal illness are provided by human milk. The presence of SIgA prevents the attachment of enteropathogens and prevents microbes from reaching the mucosal membranes, so that they cannot cause infections. The specificity of SIgA antibodies in milk is based on the incorporation of the microbes into the numerous aggregates of lymphoid cells in the mother's gut.

These antibodies are primarily directed against the microflora in the mother's gut. SIgA specific to many pathogens has been found in human milk such as *Salmonella*, *Shigella*, *H. influenza*, *E. coli*, poliovirus, influenza virus, and others.[88] The human peptide antisecretory and anti-inflammatory factor, which can be induced in human milk, is produced in response to bacterial enterotoxins. It gives protection against acute diarrhea.[89] Lactoferrin has antimicrobial activities. It also affects the bacterial outer membrane, it inhibits the growth of pathogens and it can prevent reproduction of bacteria.

Human milk contains substantial amounts of oligosaccharides, which play an important role in diarrhea. For the infections to occur, the microbes must attach themselves to mucosal cells, and different microbes bind different carbohydrate structures on the cell surface.[90] The carbohydrates function as receptor analogues so they prevent microbes from binding to the mucosal epithelium.

Worldwide, breastfeeding is a major protective factor against diarrheal diseases.

11.8.2 OTHER INFECTIONS AND BREASTFEEDING

Respiratory tract infections are a major source of morbidity and mortality in infancy. Breastfeeding has been shown to protect against a variety of respiratory pathogens and it may protect against upper respiratory infections especially pneumonia.[91,92] On the other hand, a study shows that there are no significant differences in risk of respiratory infections when comparing infants exclusively breastfed for 3 and 6 months.[84]

Ear infections are not only less common in breastfed infants, but also are less likely to become chronic.[93] The Eustachian tube closes in breastfed infants while they are nursing, thereby preventing reflux of milk into the middle ear, which can lead to inflammation and subsequent blockage of tube.

SIgA or oligosaccharides may interfere with bacterial adhesion to urinary epithelium. The increased excretion in urine of lactoferrin may also contribute to a decreased frequency of urinary tract infections in breastfed infants.

11.8.2.1 Breastfeeding and Transmission of HIV-1

Maternal viral infections may be a different case. There is evidence that several viruses including HIV,[94] hepatitis C,[95] and cytomegalovirus[96] can be transmitted by breastfeeding. Prolonged breastfeeding is estimated to cause one third to half of new infant HIV-1 infections worldwide.[97] During breastfeeding, HIV can be introduced into the gastrointestinal tract submucosa of the infant by a breach in the integrity of the epithelial cell layer. Since gastric acid production in the neonate is reduced, more virus, either cell-free or cell-associated, may reach the monostratified intestinal mucosa.[98] Breast milk viral load is highest immediately after birth.[99] Colostrum is richer in lymphocytes when compared with mature breast milk, and cell-associated virus may be seen at higher concentrations in colostrums than in mature milk. HIV has been detected in both the liquid phase of breast milk and breast milk cells.[100,101] But at the same time, many innate mechanisms may contribute to prevention of HIV-1 transmission. Breast milk is a complex fluid that contains factors with diverse antimicrobial and immunomodulatory properties. The effects of these soluble factors on HIV infection are diverse. The secretory leukocyte protease inhibitor (SLPI) is found in breast milk. It is secreted polymorphonuclear and epithelial cells and SLPI plays an important role in reducing HIV-1 transmission through breast milk.[102] Another mechanism for protection against HIV is antibodies. Colostrum as well as mature breast milk of HIV-infected women contains SIgA, IgM, and IgG against HIV antigens. IgG is the predominant isotype of HIV-specific antibodies in breast milk.[103]

11.9   CANCER AND HUMAN MILK

Cancer is a major health problem worldwide and it arises from the uncontrolled proliferation and spread of clones of transformed cells. Malignant tumors are able to evade or overcome the mechanisms of host defense. Cancers can be eradicated by specific immune responses and the physiological function of the immune system is to recognize and destroy clones of transformed cells before they grow into tumors and kill tumors after they are formed.

Breastfeeding protects against tumors in childhood such as acute lymphoblastic leukemia, Hodgin's disease, and neuroblastoma.[104] Human milk contains α-lactalbumin, which is the form of "human α-lactalbumin made lethal to tumor cells" (HAMLET). The HAMLET complex consists of α-lactalbumin and oleic acid, and is formed under acidic conditions in the presence of free oleic acid of which large amounts are released from milk into the stomach and transported to the nucleus and leading to apoptosis in malignant cells.[105] Tumors in adulthood such as prostate, colorectal, and gastric cancers are not reduced by breastfeeding but there is reduction in premenopausal breast cancer.[106]

11.10   COMMERCIAL MILK PRODUCTS AND IMMUNITY

Yogurt is a coagulated milk product that results from fermentation of lactic acid in milk.[107] Although yogurt and milk have similar vitamin and mineral compositions they have a few differences. During fermentation, vitamins B-6, B-12, and C are decreased and folic acid is produced. When milk is converted into yogurt, some compositional changes occur; for example, calcium is more bioavailable from yogurt than from milk. It is believed that yogurt has a stimulatory effect on the immune system and this effect is due to yogurt's bacterial components. Yogurt includes lactic acid bacteria. Lactic acid bacteria are Gram-positive bacteria and their cell wall is composed of techoic acid, peptidoglycan, and polysaccharide. All of the components have immunostimulatory properties.[108] Teichoic acids stimulate the production of IL-1, TNF-α, and IL-6 by monocytes *in vitro*.[109] Regular intake of lactic acid bacteria is able to enhance the function of the immune system and reduce the incidence of infectious diarrhea, acute gastroenteritis, allergic symptoms, and lactose intolerance. The inhibitory effects of lactic acid bacteria against gastrointestinal disorders are due to organic acid and bacteriocin, which are metabolites of lactic acid fermentation.[110-112]

REFERENCES

1. Plum, J., De Smedt, M., Verhasselt, B., Kerre, T., Vanhecke, D., Vandekerckhove, B., and Leclercq, G., Human T lymphopoiesis. *In vitro* and *in vivo* study models, *Ann. NY Acad. Sci.*, 917, 724–731, 2000.

2. Abul, K. Abbas, and Andrew, H., *Lichtman, Cellular and Molecular Immunology*, 5th edition, Elsevier Saunders, Philadelphia, Pennsylvania, 2005.
3. Whitsett, J.A., Surfactant proteins in innate host defense of the lung, *Biol. Neonate.*, 135, 1308–1312, 2005.
4. Ivan Roitt, Jonathan Brostoff, and David Male, *Immunology*, 6th edition, Mosby, London, 2001.
5. Phillips, H.J., Hori, T., Nagler, A., Bhat, N., Spits, H., and Lanier. L.L., Ontogeny of human natural killer (NK) cells: Fetal NK cells mediate cytolytic function and express cytoplasmic CD3 epsilon, delta proteins, *J. Exp. Med.*, 175, 1055–1066, 1992.
6. Christensen, R.D., MacFarlane, J.L., Taylor, N.L., Hill, H.R., and Rothstein, G., Blood and marrow neutrophils during experimental group B streptococcal infection: Quantification of the stem cell, proliferative, storage and circulating pools, *Pediatr. Res.*, 16, 549–553, 1982.
7. Strauss, R.G. and Synder, E.L., Activation and activity of the superoxide-generating system of neutrophils from human infants, *Pediatr. Res.*, 17, 662–664, 1983.
8. McCracken, G.H. Jr. and Eichenwald, H.F., Leucocyte function and the development of opsonic and complement activity in the neonate, *Am. J. Dis. Child.*, 121, 120, 1971.
9. Nair, M.P., Schwartz, S.A., and Menon, M., Association of decreased natural and antibody-dependent cellular cytotoxicity and production of natural killer cytotoxic factor and interferon in neonates, *Cell Immunol.*, 94, 159–171, 1985.
10. Wolach, B., Dolphin, T., Regev, R., Gilboa, S., and Schlesinger, M., The development of the complement system after 28 weeks gestation, *Acta Pediartr.*, 86, 523–527, 1978.
11. Anderson, D.C., Hughes, B.J., Edwards, M.S., Buffone, G.J., and Baker, C.J., Impaired chemotaxigenesis by type III group B streptococci in neonatal sera: Relationship to diminished concentration of specific anticapsular antibody and abnormalities of serum complement, *Pediatr. Res.*, 17, 496–502, 1983.
12. Edwards, M.S., Buffone, G.J., Fuselier, P.A., Weeks, J.L., and Baker, C.J., Deficient classical complement pathway activity in newborn sera, *Pediatr. Res.*, 17, 685–688, 1983.
13. Kilpinen, S. and Hurme, M., Low CD3 + CD28-induced interleukin-2 production correlates with decreased reactive oxygen intermediate formation in neonatal T cells, *Immunology*, 94, 167–172, 1998.
14. Lewis, D.B., Yu, C.C., Meyer, J., English, B.K., Kahn, S.J., and Wilson, C.B., Cellular and molecular mechanisms for reduced interleukin 4 and interferon-gamma production by neonatal T cells, *J. Clin. Invest.*, 87, 194–202, 1991.
15. Palacios, R. and Andersson, U., Autologous mixes lymphocyte reaction in human cord blood lymphocytes: Decreased generation of helper and cytotoxic T cell functions and increased proliferative response and induction of suppressor t cells, *Cell Immunol.*, 66, 88–98, 1982.
16. Hannet, I., Erkeller-Yuksel, F., Lydyard, P., Deneys, V., and De-Bruyere, M., Developmental and maturational changes in human blood lymphocyte subpopulations, *Immunol. Today*, 13, 215–218, 1992.
17. Lewis, V.M., Twomwrt, J.J., Bealmear, P., Goldstein, G., and Good, R.A., Age thymic involution and circulating thymic hormoneactivity, *J. Clin. Endocrinol. Metabolism*, 47, 145–150, 1978.
18. Lesourd, B.M. and Meaume, S., Cell mediated immunity changes in ageing, relative importance of cell subpopulation switches and of nutritional factors, *Immunol. Lett.*, 40, 235–242, 1994.
19. Goronzy, J.J., Lee, W.W., and Weyand, C.M., Aging and T cell diversity, *Exp. Gerontol.*, 42, 400–406, 2007.
20. Larbi, A., Dupuis, G., Khalil, A., Douziech, N., Fortin, C., and Fulop, T., Jr, Differential role of lipid rafts in the functions of CD4+ and CD8+ human T lymphocytes with aging, *Cell Signal.*, 18, 1017–1030, 2006.

21. Agrawal, A., Agrawal, S., and Gupta, S., Dentritic cells in human aging, *Exp. Gerontol.*, 42, 421–426, 2007.
22. Della-Bella, S., Bierti, L., Presicce, P., Arienti, R., Valenti, M., Saresella, M., Vergani, C., and Villa, M.L., Peripheral blood dentritic cells and monocytes are differently regulated in the elderly, *Clin. Immunol.*, 122, 220–228, 2007.
23. Zhang, Y., Wallace, D.L., de Lara, C.M., Ghattas, H., Asquith, B., Worth, A., Griffin, G.E., Taylor, G.P., Tough, D.F., Beverley, P.C., and Macallan, D.C., *In vivo* kinetics of human natural killer cells: The effects of ageing and acute and chronic viral infection, *Immunology*, 121, 258–265, 2007.
24. Thapa, B.R., Health factors in colostrums, *Indian J. Pediatr.*, 7, 579–581, 2005.
25. Newburg, S.D., Innate immunity and human milk, *J. Nutr.*, 5,1308–1312, 2005.
26. Brandtzaeg, P., Mucosal immunity: Integration between mother and the breast-fed infant, *Vaccine*, 24, 3382–3388, 2003.
27. Rivas, R.A., el Mohandes, A.A., and Katona, I.M., Mononuclear phagocytic cells in human milk: HLA-DR and Fc gamma R ligand expression, *Biol. Neonate.*, 66, 195–204, 1994.
28. Kim, S.K., Keeney, S.E., Alpard, S.K., and Schmalstieg, F.C., Comparison of L-selectin and CD11b on neutrophils of adults and neonates during the first month of life, *Pediatr. Res.*, 53, 132–136, 2003.
29. Hawkes, J.S., Brya, D.L., and Gibson, R.A., Cytokine production by human milk cells and peripheral blood mononuclear cells from same mothers, *J. Clin. Immunol.*, 22, 338–344, 2002.
30. Forchielli, M.L. and Walker, W.A., The role of gut-associated lymphoid tissues and mucosal defence, *Br. J. Nutr.*, 93 (Suppl. 1), 41–48, 2005.
31. Gork, A.S., Usui, N., Ceriati, E., Drongowski, R.A., Epstain, M.D., Coran, A.G., and Harmon, C.M., The effect of mucin on bacterial translocation in I-407 fetal and Caco-2 adult enterocyte cultured cell lines, *Pediatr. Surg. Int.*, 15, 155–159, 1999.
32. Nathakumar, N.N., Dai, D., Newburg, D.S., and Walker, A.W., The role of indigenous microflora in the development of murine intestinal fucosyl- and sialyltransferases, *FASEB*, 17, 44–46, 2003.
33. Ouelette, A.J., Paneth cell alpha-defensins: Peptide mediators of innate immunity in the small intestine, *Springer Semin. Immunopatol.*, 27, 133–146, 2005.
34. Escigno, M. and Barrow, P., The host pathogen interaction: New themes from dentritic cell biology, *Cell*, 106, 267–270, 2001.
35. Nagler-Anderson, C., Man the barrier! Strategic defenses in the intestinal mucosa, *Nat. Rev. Immunol.*, 1, 59–67, 2001.
36. Buescher, E.S. and Malinowska, I., Soluble receptors and cytokines antagonists in human milk, *Pediatr. Res.*, 40, 839–844, 1996.
37. Conley, M.E. and Delacroix, D.L., Intravascular and mucosal immunoglobulin A: Two separate but related systems of immune defence? *Ann. Intern. Med.*, 106, 892–899, 1987.
38. Buescher, E.S., Antiinflammatory characteristics of human milk: How, where, why, *Adv. Exp. Med. Bio.*, 501, 207–222, 2001.
39. Brandtzaeg, P., Farstad, I.N., Johansen, F.-E., Morton, H.C., Norderhaug, I.N., and Yamanaka, T., The B cell system of human mucosea and exocrine glands, *Immunol. Rev.*, 171, 45–87, 1999.
40. Norderhaug, I.N., Johansen, F.E., Schjerven, H., and Brandtzaeg, P., Regulation of the formation and external transport of secretory immunoglobulins, *Crit. Rev. Immunol.*, 19, 481–508, 1999.
41. de Olivera, I.R., de Araujo, An, Bao, S.N., and Giugliano, L.G., Binding of lactoferrin and free secretory component to enterotoxigenic *Escherichia coli*, *FEMS Microbiol. Lett.*, 203, 29–33, 2001.
42. Dallas, S.D. and Rofle, R.D., Binding of *Clostridium difficile* toxin A to human milk secretory component, *J. Med. Microbiol.*, 47, 879–888, 1998.

43. Ogundele, M.O., Inhibitors of complement activity in human breast milk: A proposed hypothesis of their physiological significance, *Mediators Inflamm.*, 8, 69–75, 1999.
44. Cole, F.S., Schneeberg, E.E., Lichtenberg, N.A., and Colten, H.R., Complement biosynthesis in human milk macrophages and blood monocytes, *Immunology*, 46, 429–441, 1982.
45. Ogundele, M.O., Role and significance of the complement system in mucosal immunity: Particular reference to the human breast milk complement, *Immunol. Cell Biol.*, 79, 1–10, 2001.
46. Moro, G., Minoli, I., Mosca, M., Fanaro, S., Jelinek, J., Stahl, B., and Boehm, G., Doseage related bifidogenic effects of galacto- and fructooligosaccharides in formula-fed term infants, *J. Pediatr. Gasrtoenterol. Nutr.*, 34, 291–295, 2002.
47. Martin, R., Langa, S., Reviriego, C., Jiminez, E., Marin, M.L., Xaus, J., Fernandez, L., and Rodrigues, J.M., Human milk is a source of lactic acid bacteria for the infant gut, *J. Pediatr.*, 143, 754–758, 2003.
48. Gilliland, S.E. and Speck, M.L., Antagonistic action of lactobacillus acidophilus toward intestinal and food borne pathogens in associative cultures, *J. Food Prot.*, 40, 820–823, 1977.
49. Ruiz, P.A., Hofmann, M., Szcesny, S., Blaut, M., and Haller, D., Innate mechanisms for *Bifidobacterium lactis* to activate transient pro-inflammatory host responses in intestinal epithelial cells after the colonization of germ-free rats, *Immunology*, 115, 441–450, 2005.
50. Arunchalam, K., Gil, H.S., and Chandra, R.K., Enhancement of natural immune function by dietary consumption of *Bifidobacterium lactis* (HN019), *Eur. J. Clin. Nutr.*, 54, 263–267, 2000.
51. Carol, M., Borruel, N., Antolin, M., Lipois, M., Casellas, F., Guarner, F., and Malagelada, J.R., Modulation of apoptosis in intestinal lymphocytes by a probiotic bacteria in Chron's disease, *J. Leukoc. Biol.*, 79, 917–922, 2006.
52. Gill, H.S., Rutherfurd, K.J., and Cross, M.L., Dietary probiotic supplementation enhances natural killer cell activity in the elderly: An investigation of age-related immunological changes, *J. Clin. Immunol.*, 21, 264–271, 2001.
53. Fukushima, Y., Miyaguchi, S., Yamano, T., Kaburagi, T., Iino, H., Ushida, K., and Sato K., Improvement of nutritional status and incidence of infection in hospitalised, enterally fed elderly by feeding of fermented milk containing probiotic *Lactobacillus johnsonii* La1 (NCC533)., *Br. J. Nutr.* 5, 969–977, 2007.
54. Martín, R., Jiménez, E., Olivares, M., Marín, M.L., Fernández, L., Xaus, J., and Rodríguez, J.M., *Lactobacillus salivarus* CECT5713, a potential probiotic strain isolated from infant feces and breast milk of a mother-child pair, *Int. J. Microbiol.*, 112, 35–43, 2006.
55. Ibnou-Zekri, N., Blum, S., Schiffrin, E.J., and von der Weid, T., Divergent patterns of colonization and immune response elicited from two intestinal *Lactobacillus* strains that display similar properties in-vitro, *Infect. Immunol.*, 71, 428–436, 2003.
56. Diaz Ropero, M.P., Martin, R., Sierra, S., Lara-Villoslada, F., Rodriguez, J.M., Xanus, J., and Olivares, M., Two *Lactobacillus* strains, isolated from breast milk differently modulate the immune response, *J. Appl. Microbiol.*, 102, 337–343, 2006.
57. Piirainen, L., Haahtela, S., Helin, T., Korpela, R., Haahtela, T., and Vaarala, O., Effect of *Lactobacillus rhamnosus* GG on rBet v1 and rMal d1 specific IgA in the saliva of patients with birch pollen allergy., *Ann. Allergy Asthma Immunol.*, 4, 338–342, 2008.
58. Olivares, M., Diaz, Ropero, M.P., Sierra, S., Lara-Villoslada, F., Fonolla, J., Navas, M., Rodriguez, J.M., and Xanus, J., Oral intake of *Lactobacillus fermentum* CECT5716 enhance the effect of influenza vaccination, *Nutrition*, 23, 254–260, 2007.
59. Takeda, K., and Okumura, K., Effects of a fermented milk drink containing *Lactobacillus casei* strain Shirota on the human NK cell-activity, *J. Nutr.*, 3 (suppl 2), 791S–793S, 2007.
60. Ogawa, T., Asai, Y., Tamai, R., Makimura, Y., Sakamoto, H., Hashikawa, S., and Yasuda, K., Natural killer cell activities of symbiotic *Lactobacillus casei* ssp. *casei* in conjunction with dextran, *Clin. Exp. Immunol.*, 143, 103–109, 2006.

61. Pessi, T., Sutas, Y., Salexin, M., Kallininen, H., and Isolauri, E., Antiproliferative effects of homogenates derived from five strains of candidate probiotic bacteria, *Appl. Environ. Microbiol.*, 65, 4725–4728, 1999.
62. Rohde, C.L., Bartolini, V., and Jones, N., The use of probiotics in the prevention and treatment of antibiotic-associated diarrhea with special interest in Clostridium difficile-associated diarrhea, *Nutr. Clin. Pract.*, 1, 33–40, 2009.
63. Kuhn, R., Lohler, J., Rennick, D., Rajewsky, K., and Muller, W., Interleukin-10 deficient mice develop chronic enterocolitis, *Cell*, 75, 263–276, 1993.
64. Sutas, Y., Soppi, E., Korhonen, H., et al., Supression of lymphocyte proliferation *in vitro* by bovine caseins hydrolyzed with *Lactobacillus casei* GG-derived enzymes, *J. Allergy Clin. Immunol.*, 98, 216–224, 1996.
65. Pelto, L., Isolauri, E., Lilius, E.M., Nuutila, J., and Salminen, S., Probiotic bacteria down-regulate the milk-induced inflammatory response in milk-hypersensitive subjects but have an immunostimulatory effect in healthy subjects, *Clin. Exp. Allergy*, 28, 1474–1479, 1998.
66. Strober, W., Kelsall, B., and Marth, T., Oral tolerance, *J. Clin. Immunol.*,18, 1–30, 1998.
67. Warner, J.O., Early life nutrition and allergy, *Early Human Dev.*, 83, 777–783, 2007.
68. Høst, A., Halken, S., Muraro, A., et al., Dietary prevention of allergic diseases in infants and small children, *Pediatr. Allergy Immunol.*, 19, 1–4, 2008.
69. Schneider, A.P., Stein, R.T., and Fritscher, C.C., The role of breastfeeding, diet and nutritional status in the development of asthma and atopy, *J. Bras. Pneumol.*, 33, 454–462, 2007.
70. Hosea, Blewett, H.J., Cicalo, M.C., Holland, C.D., and Field, C.J., The immunological components of human milk, *Adv. Food Nutr. Res.*, 54, 45–80, 2008.
71. Goldman, A.S., Chheda, S., Garofalo, R., and Schmalstieg, F.C., Cytokines in human milk: Properties and potential effects upon the mammary gland and the neonate, *J. Mammary Gland Biol. Neoplasia.*, 1, 251–158, 1996.
72. Weigle, W.O., Goodman, M.G., Morgan, E.L., and Hugli, T.E., Regulation of immune response by components of the complement cascade and their activated fragments, *Springer. Semin. Immunopathol.*, 6, 173–194, 1983.
73. Ogundale, M., Role and significance of the complement system in mucosal immunity: Particular reference to the human breast milk complement, *Immunol. Cell Biol.*, 79, 1–10, 2001.
74. Perez-Machado, M.A., Ashwood, P., Thomson, M.A., et al., Reduced transforming growth factor-beta 1-producing T cells in the duedonal mucosa of children with food allergy, *Eur. J. Immunol.*, 33, 2307–2315, 2003.
75. Stavnezer, J., Regulation of antibody production and class switching by TGF-beta, *J. Immunol.*, 155, 1647–1651, 1995.
76. Labeta, M.O., Vidal, K., Nores, J.E., et al., Innate recognition of bacteria in human milk is mediated by a milk-derived highly expressed pattern recognition receptor soluble CD14, *J. Exp. Med.*, 191, 1807–1812, 2000.
77. Olivares, M., Diaz–Ropero, M.P., Gomez, N., Lara-Villoslada, F., Sierra, S., Maldonada, J.M., Martin, R., Rodriguez, J.M., and Xanus, J., The consumption of two new probiotic strains, *Lactobacillus gasseri* CECT5714 and *Lactobacillus coryniformis* CECT5711, boost the immune system of health adults, *Int. Microbiol.*, 9, 47–52, 2006.
78. Kalliomaki, M., Salminen, S., Arvilommi, H., Kero, P., Koskinen, P., and Isolauri, E., Probiotics in primary prevention of atopic disease: A randomised placebo-controlled trial, *Lancet*, 357, 1076–1079, 2003.
79. Taylor, A.L., Dunstan, J.A., and Prescott, S.L., Probiotics supplementation for the first 6 months of life fails to reduce the risk of atopic dermatitis and increases the risk of allergen sensitization in high-risk children: A randomized controlled trial, *J. Alllergy Clin. Immunol.*, 119, 184–191, 2007.

80. Kukonnen, K., Savilahti, E., Haahtela, T., Juntunen-Backman, K., Korpela, R., Poussa, T., Tuure, T., and Kuitunen, M., Probiotics and prebiotic galactooligosaccharides in the prevention of allergic disease; a randomized double-blind, placebo-controlled trial, *J. Allergy Clin. Immunol.*, 119, 192–198, 2007.

81. Howie, P.W., Forsyth, J.S., Ogston, S.A., Clark, A., and Florey, C.V., Protective effect of breast feeding against infection, *Br. Med. J.*, 300, 11–16, 1990.

82. Victoria, C.G., Smith, P.G., Vaughan, J.P., Nobre, L.C., Lombardi, C., Teixeria, A.M., Fuchs, S.M., Moreira, L.B., Gigante, L.P., and Barros, F.C., Evidence for protection by breast feeding against infant deaths from infectious disease in Brazil, *Lancet*, 2, 319–322, 1987.

83. Kramer, M.S., Chalmers, B., Hodnett, E.D., et al., Promotion of breastfeeding intervention trial (PROBIT): A randomized trial in the Republic of Belerus, *J. Am. Med. Assoc.*, 285, 413–420, 2001.

84. Kramer, M.S., Guo, T., Platt, R.W., Sevkovskaya, Z., Dzikovich, I., Collet, J.P., et al., Infant growth and health outcomes associated with 3 compared with 6 mo of exclusive breastfeeding, *Am. J. Clin. Nutr.*, 78, 291–295, 2003.

85. Hayani, K.C., Guerrero, M.L., Morrow, A.L., Gomez, H.F., Winsor, D.K., Ruiz-Palacios, G.M., and Cleary, T.G., Concentration of milk secretory immunoglobulin A against Shigelle virulence plasmid-associated antigens as a predictor of symptom status in Shigella-infected breast-fed infants, *J. Pediatr.*, 121, 852–856, 1992.

86. Glass, R.I., Svennerholm, A,M., Stoll, B.J., Khan, S.R., Hassain, K.M.B., Huq, M.I., and Holmgren, J., Protection against cholera in breast-fed children by antibodies in breast-milk, *New Engl. J. Med.*, 308, 1389–1392, 1983.

87. Goldman, A.S., The immune system of human milk: Antimicrobial, anti-inflammatory and immunomodulating properties, *Pediatr. Infect. Dis. J.*, 12, 664–671, 1993.

88. Marrow, A.L., Reves, R.R., West, M., Guerrero, M.L., Ruiz-Palacios, G.M., and Pickering, L.K., Protection against infection with *Giardia lamblia* by breast-feeding in cohort of Mexican infants, *J. Pediatr.*, 121, 363–370, 1992.

89. Zaman, S., Mannan, J., Lange, S., Lönnrot, I., and Hanson, L.A., B 221, a medical food containing antisecretory factor reduces child diarrhoea: A placebo controlled trial, *Acta Pediatr.*, 96, 1655–1659, 2007.

90. Newburg, D.S., Ruiz-Palacios, G.M., and Morrow, A.L., Human milk glycans protect infants against enteric pathogens, *Ann. Rev. Nutr.*, 25, 37–58, 2005.

91. Cesar, J.A., Victora, C.G., Barros, F.C., Santos, I.S., and Flores, J.A., Impact of breast feeding on admission for pneumonia during postneonatal period in Brazil: Nested case-control study, *BMJ*, 318, 1316–1320, 1999.

92. Oddy, W.H., Sly, P.D., de Klerk, N.H., Landau, L.I., Kendall, G.E., Holt, P.G., and Stanley, F.J., Breast feeding and respiratory morbidity in infancy: A birth cohort study, *Arch. Dis. Childhood*, 88, 224–228, 2003.

93. Beaudry, M., Dufour, R., and Marcoux, S., Relation between infant feeding and infectious during the first six months of life, *J. Pediart.*, 126: 191–197, 1995.

94. Leroy, V., Newel.-L., Dabis, F., Peckham, C., Van de Perre, P., Bulterys, M., Kind, C., Simonds, R.J., Wiktor, S., and Msellati, P., International multicentre pooled analysis of late postnatal mother-to-child transmission of HIV-1 infection, *Lancet*, 352, 597–600, 1998.

95. Kumar, R.M. and Shahul, S., Role of breast-feeding in transmission of hepatitis C virus to infants of HCV-infected mothers, *J. Hepatol.*, 29, 191–197, 1998.

96. Vochem, M., Hamprecht, K., Jahn, G., and Speer, C.P., Transmission of cytomegalovirus to preterm infants through breast milk, *Pediatr. Infect. Dis. J.*, 17, 53–58, 1998.

97. Fowler, M.G. and Newel, M.L., Breast-feeding and HIV-1 transmission in resource-limited settings, *J. AIDS*, 30, 230–239, 2002.

98. Meng, G., Wei, X., Wu, X., et al., Primary intestinal epithelial cells selectively transfer R5 HIV-1 to CCR5+ cells, *Nat. Med.*, 8, 150–156, 2002.

99. Rousseau, C.M., Nduati, R.W., Richardson, B.A., et al., Longitudinal analysis of HIV-1 RNA in breast milk and its relationship to infant infection and maternal disease, *J. Infect. Dis.*, 187, 741–747, 2003.

100. Lewis, P., Nduati, R., Kreiss, J.K., et al., Cell free human immunodeficiency virus type 1 in breastmilk, *J. Infect. Dis.*, 177, 134–149, 1998.

101. Willumsen, J., Filteau, S.M., Coutsoudis, A., et al., Breastmilk RNA viral load in HIV-1 infected South African women: Effects of subclinical mastitis and infant feeding, *AIDS*, 17, 407–14, 2003.

102. Farquhar, C., VanCott, T.C., Mbori-Ngacha, D.A., Horani, L., Bosire, R.K., Kreiss, J.K., Richardson, B.A., and John-Stewart, G.C., Salivary secretory leukocyte protease inhibitor is associated with reduced transmission of human immunodeficiency virus type 1 through breast milk. *J. Infect. Dis.*, 15, 1173–1176, 2002.

103. Becquart, P., Hocini, H., Garin, B., et al., Compartmentalization of the IgG immune response to HIV-1 in breast milk, *AIDS*, 13, 1323–1331, 1999.

104. Martin, R.M., Gunnel, D., Owen, C.G., and Smith, G.D., Breastfeeding and childhood cancer: A systematic review with metaanalysis, *Int. J. Cancer*, 117, 1020–1031, 2005.

105. Gustafsson, L., Boiers, C., Hallgren, O., Mossberg, A.K., Pettersson, J., Fischer, A.W., Aronsson, A., and Svanborg, C., HAMLET kills tumor cells by apoptosis: Structure, cellular mechanisms, and therapy, *J. Nutr.*, 135, 1299–1303, 2005.

106. Martin, R.M., Middleton, N., Gunnell, D., Owen, C.G., and Smith, G.D., Breast-feeding and cancer: The Boyd Orr cohort and a systematic review with meta-analysis, *J. Nat. Cancer Inst.*, 97, 1446–1457.

107. Bourlioux, P. and Pochart, P., Nutritional and health properties of yogurt, *World Rev. Nutr. Diet.*, 56, 217–58, 1988.

108. Takahashi, T., Oka, T., Iwana, H., Kuwata, T., and Yamamoto, Y., Immune response of mice to orally administered lactic acid bacteria, *Biosci. Biotechnol. Biochem.*, 57, 1557–1560, 1993.

109. Heumann, D., Barras, C., Severin, A., Glauser, M.P., and Tomasz, A., Gram-positive cell walls stimulate synthesis of tumor necrosis factor-alpha and interleukin-6 by human monocytes, *Infect. Immun.*, 62, 2715–2721, 1994.

110. Kim, H.S. characterization of lactobacilli and bifidobacteria as applied to dietary adjuvants, *J. Cult. Dairy Prod.*, 23, 6–9, 1988.

111. Gorbach, S.L., Chang, T.W., and Goldin, B.R., Successful treatment of relapsing *Clostridium difficile* colitis with *Lactobacillus* GG, *Lancet*, 2, 43, 1987.

112. Meydani, S.N. and Woel-Kyu, H. Immunologic effects of yogurt[1–4], *Am. J. Clin, Nutr.*, 71, 861–872, 2000.

12 Functional Dairy Foods and Flora Modulation

Theodoras H. Varzakas, Ioannas S. Arvanitoyannis, and Eugenia Bezirtzoglou

CONTENTS

12.1 INTRODUCTION

Functional foods are foods going beyond providing simple nutrition and also having some beneficial effects on their host. Fermented products have been known for thousands of years, as already in the Bible, the term "acid milk" was first used. Knowledge of the health benefits of fermented dairy foods goes back to the 1900s, when Metchnikoff [1], in his Thesis entitled "The prolongation of life," correlated the intake of large quantities of Bulgarian fermented milk with the longetivity of the Caucasian people. Moreover, Metchnikoff stated that the variety in the different microflora profile is a determinant for the well-being of the host and stressed the importance of interactions between the host and bacteria [1,2]. Escherich claimed that a global assessment of the intestinal microflora was essential for solid knowledge of the host digestion mechanisms, but also for understanding the pathology and therapy of microbial intestinal diseases [3].

Since then, multiple strategies and approaches were created for the development of effective functional foods. Many functional foods now exist in various countries. However, internationally they are grouped into three main classes: probiotics, prebiotics, and synbiotics. Regulatory authorities and legislative frameworks in different countries divulged the features of functional foods. Japan seems to be the country strongly cognizant and supportive of the public health benefits of functional foods, as more than 200 functional foods are proposed to be marketed under the FOSHU (Foods for Specialised Health Use) legislation. Accordingly, the Food and Drug

339

Administration (FDA) in the United States imposed legislation allowing more than 15 food categories grouping different functional foods.

Through centuries, fermented cultures were developed from empirical cultures with beneficial action to artificial cultures with particular beneficial action and finally to artificial probiotic cultures with choosen enterical bacteria. One of the most promising areas for the development of functional foods lies in modification of the activity of the gastrointestinal (GI) tract by use of probiotics, prebiotics, and synbiotics [4]. Since 2000, genetically selected probiotic therapeutic cultures with reinforced properties stimulated the researcher's interest. A plethora of healthful effects have been attributed to the probiotic lactic acid bacteria (LAB).

The contribution of biotechnology has been very important by selection of new strains, improvement of specific functional properties, nutritional improvement of foods and, finally, improvement of the sensory and textural qualities of the final product. However, a major role of functional foods is the stimulation of the host immune system and preservation of the microbial intestinal balance via the "barrier effect." Specifically, dairy functional foods showed important health benefits [5,6], which included (a) increased nutritional value, (b) promotion of intestinal lactose digestion, (c) positive influence on intestinal and urogenital flora and, finally, (d) prevention and reduction of intestinal tract infections by inhibiting colonization by enteric pathogens.

Dairy products have so far been in the front line in the development of functional foods. Fermented dairy products have traditionally been considered to have health benefits, and thus broadening the product range to other types of health-promoting products is quite natural for the dairy industry. Probiotic dairy products, which contain health-promoting LAB and/or bifidobacteria in addition to traditionally used starter LAB, are a good example of a successful functional dairy product. Others include products supplemented with prebiotics, fibers, calcium, Omega-3, plant stanols, and bioactive peptides produced by LAB. Functional dairy products are increasingly available in the daily-dose product format, which has gained increasing popularity in the past few years. Consumers' concerns about personal health are key drivers in creating markets for functional food products [7].

Dairy products and milk components with bioactive functions are consumed daily for our nutrition. Dairy products form the major part of functional products. To understand their successful involvement as functional foods, it is important to understand that milk is a natural and highly nutritive part of a balanced daily diet. Moreover, milk offers an ideal substratum. The composition and properties of human milk, such as high lactose, low casein and calcium phosphate, and low buffering capacity, seem to favor the development of *Bifidobacterium* [8,9]. By modifying or enriching the base dairy product, a powerful functional food is obtained. Milk and some other dairy products have been known to be important foods since 8000 BC. In the Bible, fermented dairy foods were called "acid milk" [10]. The Roman historian Plinio observed that the use of some fermented milk preparations was able to alleviate or treat GI disease.

In the 1900s, the French pediatrician Tissier observed the "bifid microflora" in breastfed infants and understood their role in preventing intestinal infections in infants. This was confirmed by Metchnikoff [1,2,10], who concluded that fermented milk could inhibit the putrefactive intestinal microflora. Thus, multiple fermented dairy products reinforced with selected probiotic bacteria have developed into specific functional foods by the aid of the food industry. These functional foods include dairy products, such as yogurt and other fermented dairy foods, milk, colostrum, cheese, whey protein concentrates, or isolates and milk protein concentrates.

Dairy products contain proteins, peptides, lipids, minor carbohydrates, minerals, and vitamins. It is believed that almost all the above milk components may contribute to health benefits. A relationship between bioactive function and milk components is established. Normal intestinal flora has an important role in the digestion and metabolism of nutrients. Additionally, the flora has the capacity to transform precarcinogenic compounds in carcinogenics by the aid of bacterial enzymes including glycosidase, β-glucuronidase, nitroreductase, and azoreductase [11,12]. Several milk bioactive substances seem to offer protection against some cancers [13–15], such as whey protein concentrates, bovine serum albumin, lactoferrin, α-lactalbumin, different peptides, sphingolipids, conjugated linoleic acids (CLA), butyric acid, and calcium.

Anti-inflammatory and antimicrobial effects are associated with peptides, colostrums, and immune whey protein concentrates lactoferrin and lactoperoxidase. Finally, promotion of bifidobacterial growth seems to be associated with casein glycomacropeptide, amino sugars, and oligosaccharides. Almost all components of milk have a multifunctional physiological role in nutrition with the aim to protect basically intestinal health and enhance the immune system functions.

Dairy foods can be included in the functional food category, not only for their potential to be the electic carrier for probiotic cultures, but because of their calcium content, which can help to reduce the risk of osteoporosis [16] and hypertension [17]. Nevertheless, the future for dairy functional foods appears extremely promising [18]; it is ultimately associated with the strain, bioactive substance, or substrate specificity, which provides evidence of their efficacy, safety, and organoleptic quality.

Recently, intensive scientific research and efforts to develop innovative dairy products have focused particular attention on the many promising health effects of both functional and medicinal dairy products. It is obvious that cooperative research in different parts of the world need to widen our knowledge about the global ecology of the intestinal ecosystem [19–21] and particularly of factors modulating its integrity and its ecological stability [22].

LAB have received much attention in the past few decades for their use as probiotic microorganisms traditionally used in food fermentation [23]. Probiotics are defined as live microbial feed supplements that beneficially affect the host animal by improving its intestinal microbial balance [24]. FAO/WHO (2001) proposed a new definition for probiotics: "live microorganisms that, when being administered in appropriate dose, confer a benefit of health to the receiver." There are many reports showing that such beneficial effects may be mediated, at least partly, by the immunomodulatory capacity of certain probiotic strains [25].

Probiotics play a key role as functional dairy foods, as they are destined to protect the integrity of the intestinal system. Different ways of action are associated with their presence in the intestinal system [5], such as (i) competition for space (spatial arrangement), (ii) competition for nutrients found in limited quantities, (iii) maintenance of an acid pH on the epithelium, (iv) production of H_2O_2, (v) production of antimicrobial substances, organic acids, or bacteriocins, (vi) synthesis of nutrients reported as the source of energy for epithelial cells or bacteria, and (vii) immune system stimulation. The theoretical basis for selection of probiotic microorganisms includes (i) safety, (ii) functional behavior (survival, adherence, colonization, antimicrobial production, immune stimulation, antigenotoxic activity, and prevention of pathogens such as *Helicobacter pylori*, *Salmonella*, *Listeria*, and *Clostridium*), and (iii) technological aspects (growth in milk, sensory properties, stability, phage resistance, and viability in processes). In general, strains for pilot testing should be selected based on established *in vitro* scientific data. Naturally, the safety of probiotic strains has been of prime importance and new guidelines have been developed [26–30]. Current safety criteria and functional properties for successful probiotics have been defined in recent reviews [31–33]. These include the following specifications: (i) strains for human use are preferably of human origin, (ii) they are isolated from the GI tract of a healthy human, (iii) they have a history of being nonpathogenic even in immunocompromised hosts, and (iv) they have no history of association with diseases such as infective endocarditis or GI disorders.

Probiotic dairy foods and cultures have a long history and large consumption in the Nordic diet. Industrial products, including cultured dairy products, and their probiotic properties have been studied for many decades. The objective of the Nordic program (from 1994 to the end of 1997) was to validate industrial probiotic strains with regard to *in vitro* functionality. Strains were provided by project participants Arla (Sweden), Christian Hansen (Denmark), Norwegian Dairies (Norway), and Valio Ltd (Finland). Strains studied included the following: *Lactobacillus paracasei* subsp. *paracasei* strains E-94506 and E-94510, *Lactobacillus rhamnosus* strains E-94509 and E-94522, *Lactobacillus acidophilus* E-94507, *Lactobacillus plantarum* E-79098, *Lactococcus lactis* subsp. *lactis* E-90414, *Lactobacillus lactis* subsp. *cremoris* E-94523, *Bifidobacterium animalis* (*lactis*) E-94508, and *Bifidobacterium longum* E-94505 [34]. Microorganisms applied in probiotic products are given in Table 12.1.

Certain bacterial species are able to stimulate the mucus secretion [35]. Recently, a direct probiotic effect was observed through the induction of intestinal mucin gene expression in epithelial cells [36]. Thus, probiotic dairy products preserve the integrity of the intestinal immunological status by stimulating the inflammatory response, particularly through production of intestinal immunoglobulin A (IgA) [37]. Probiotics have recently been shown to provide benefits to subjects with particular needs, as well as to combat lifestyle-related disorders and degenerative diseases. Among these are stress, lactose intolerance, type 2 diabetes, obesity, aging, kidney failure, and oral and skin health [38]. Albeit the fact that for a long time probiotics have been known for their production of specific antimicrobial substances [11,39–41], recent studies confirmed their ability to reduce the activity of procarcinogenic enzymes [13,14].

Additionally probiotic species seem to decrease mutagens and secondary bile salts that are potentially involved in colon carcinogenesis [14,15]. Probiotics can reduce the luminal pH leading to a reduction in colonic pH and thus inhibit the growth of anaerobic bacteria [42]. It is believed that increased production of short-chain fatty acids, such as acetate, propionate, and butyrate, following gut fermentation has been associated with the decrease of the colonic pH [42], which carry out stimulation of cell proliferation in normal cells, while restraining proliferation in

TABLE 12.1

Microorganisms Applied in Probiotic Products

Yeasts	LAB	*Bifidobacterium* sp.	*Lactobacillus* sp.
Saccharomyces cerevisiae	*Enterococcus faecalis*	*B. adolescenentis*	*L. rhamnosus*
Saccharomyces boulardii	*Enterococcus faecium*	*B. animalis*	*L. kefir*
	Lactococcus lactis subsp. *lactis*	*B. bifidum*	*L. delbrueckii* subsp. *bulgaricus*
	Lactococcus lactis subsp. *cremaris*	*B. breve*	*L. helveticus*
	Leuconostoc mesenteroides subsp. *dexiranicus*	*B. infantis*	*L. GG*
	Pediococcus acidilacticus	*B. lactis*	*L. curvatus*
	Sporolactobacillus inulinus		*L. brevis*
	Propionibacterium freundenreichii		*L. acidophilus*
	Streptococcus thermophilus		*L. casei*
			L. crispatus
			L. gallinarum
			L. gasseri
			L. johnsonni
			L. paracasei subsp. *paracasei*
			L. plantarum
			L. reuteri
			L.cellobiosus

altered or carcinogenic cells [13–15], making us expect promising therapeutics for the treatment of chronic bowel diseases or colon cancer. Another aspect focuses on the principle of a bioactivity associated with the production of secondary metabolites such as short-chain fatty acids mentioned above or short bioactive peptides following cleavage from milk or other proteins in the intestine [13–15].

Adhesion of probiotic strains to human intestinal cells and the subsequent colonization of the human GI tract have been suggested as an important prerequisite for probiotic action. Adhesion verifies the potential of the strain to inhabit the intestinal tract and to grow in intestinal conditions. Adhesion also provides an interaction with the mucosal surface, facilitating contact with gut-associated lymphoid tissue, mediating local and systemic immune effects. Thus, only adherent probiotics have been thought to induce immune effects and to stabilize the intestinal mucosal barrier [43]. The Nordic program project results of *in vitro* adhesion assays gave a clear indication of differences and variation between assays and different strains [44,45].

Prebiotics have the following properties [46,47]: (i) they are nonhydrolyzed or absorbable in the intestine, (ii) they are metabolized selectively by the beneficial microflora, (iii) they promote the growth and metabolic capacity of the beneficial microflora, (iv) they show resistance to acids, bile, and pancreatic secretions, and (v) they promote the well-being of the host. They belongi to the class of carbohydrates known as dietetic fibers nondigestible. The results of their action include (i) increase in bacterial mass and volume in the stools, (ii) modification of pH, and (iii) reduction of volatile fatty acids and gas. Finally, a mixture of probiotics and prebiotics gave us the synbiotics (from the Greek word meaning "to live together"), which combine both effects.

This last aspect links the probiotic flora to the prebiotic substrate and may explain mechanisms resulting in health benefits. The word *prebiotic* originates from the Greek words *pre* (support and substrate) and *bios* (life) and this explains the capacity of the prebiotics to alter the bacterial composition of the intestinal lumen by being a substrate to stimulate the growth or activity of one or a limited number of probiotic bacteria in the colon [48–52]. Prebiotics are characterized as carbohydrates nondigestible bioactive substances, which are acting in a beneficial way on the intestinal microflora of the host. The results of their action are grouped into the following: (i) increasing bacterial mass and volume in the stools, (ii) modification of pH, and (iii) production of volatile fatty acids and gas. Prebiotic substances are food in different foods, such as inulin, soya-oligosaccharides, fructo-oligosaccharides (FOS), galacto-oligosaccharides (GOS), lactosucrose, isomalto-oligosaccharides (IMO), and xylo-oligosaccharides (XOS).

The last generation of functional foods is based on the addition of specifically targeted substances (i.e., CLA or polyunsaturated fatty acids, etc.). Nowdays, much interest is focused on the role of dairy functional foods as mild therapeutical agents. The role of functional foods in the maintenance of a healthy intestinal system is well known [53–55].

Some additional roles are associated with them, such as regulation of the gut motility, decreased incidence and duration of diarrhea, maintenance of mucosal integrity, improvement of the immune system, and reduction of catabolic products eliminated by kidney and liver. In previous years, some studies reported their role in the prevention of colon cancer as they have anticarcinogenic and antimutagenic action and some other studies reported their antiallergic activities [13].

It is evident that their anticancer activity remains the most controversial. Experimentation is based on the profile of specific biomarkers for colon cancer risk in dietary intervention studies. These include colonic mucosal markers, fecal water markers, and immunological markers. It is clear, however, that there are no direct experimental data on cancer regression in human as a result of consumption of dairy lactic cultures [11].

Diets based on meat consumption seem to cause changes to the intestinal microflora. The microflora changes are associated with cancer disease. It is also known that the occurrence of intestinal cancer shows an increasing incidence in developed countries due to the high consumption of meat [56]. Moreover, it is clear that there are components in a plant-based diet other than traditional nutrients that can reduce cancer risk [11].

Their role in prevention of osteoporosis seems to be real, as they stimulate and support the production of calcium. They are known to exercise a hypocholestemic action and, constructively, they compensate us with a sense of well-being. Another type of functional dairy foods embeds prebiotics that are nondigestible bioactive substances acting in a beneficial way on the intestinal microflora of the host [39,40,57].

Since antiquity, various LAB are implemented in fermentation of milk to produce a variety of dairy products. This is very well documented in the scientific literature by many researchers who studied the microbiota of various "ethnic" products [58–60]. The fermentations occur either "spontaneously" by raw milk's microbiota or after inoculation of a starter culture. In Greece and particularly in Epirus, the "pytia" (rennet) serves for centuries as a starter. To the best of our knowledge, this is the first study investigating thoroughly the LAB originating from "pytia" with respect to their physiological and biochemical technological properties as well as their probiotic potential [61].

12.2 MICROFLORA OF FUNCTIONAL FOODS

Different foods, such as milk and milk solids, yoghurt and kefir, contain probiotics that have the ability to exercise a beneficial effect on the intestinal microflora composition through various mechanisms as described above. The human GI tract harbors a large variety of microorganisms.

Nevertheless, it is known that the human newborn is devoid of bacteria before birth. Bacteria start appearing from the first days of life [62]. Within a few hours the newborn develops its normal bacterial flora, which originates principally from the immediate environment [63], the hospital staff [64–67], and the effect of feeding [8,68,69]. The composition of the newborn bowel flora depends on age, race, and basically on the diet of the person [70–75].

In the newborn intestine, probiotic bacteria and especially *Bifidobacterium* sp., either alone or through the changes they bring to the intestinal flora, have been shown to have positive effects on the intestinal flora, as well as resistance to disease [62,68]. Their ability to do so is potentially governed mainly by inhibiting or eventually interrelationships with other intestinal bacteria. Although the *Bifidobacterium* sp. are important regulators, when involved in dietary means as feeding, they are large in number and maintain the balance of the intestinal microflora. It has been more than an axiom that in breastfed infants the intestinal flora is dominated by *Bifidobacterium* [8,68]. The effect of human milk seemed to be the result of *Bifidobacterium bifidum* proliferation, in contrast to artificial alimentation that seemed to favor *Clostridium perfringens* implantation [9]. Indeed human milk frequently contains low amounts of nonpathogenic bacteria such as *Streptococcus*, *Micrococcus*, *Lactobacillus*, *Staphylococcus*, diphteroids, and *Bifidobacterium*. Under breastfeeding, the flora is less diversified than under bottlefeeding. However, by about the end of the second year, the fecal flora of both groups of infants resembles that of adults. An antagonism between these bacteria seems to be established in the newborn intestine, via the alimentation [9,69].

The different parts of the GI ecosystem seem to carry different bacterial populations concerning as well qualitative and quantitative differences [62,71,72]. Bacterial numbers are increasing as they move down the alimentary tract, where the bacterial population can reach extremely high numbers such as more than 10 million bacteria/mL of fecal fluid.

It is also important to state that bacteria carry out a number of biochemical functions [76,77]. These biochemical functions include the deconjugation and dehydroxylation of bile acids by *Escherichia coli, Bacillus cereus, Streptococcus faecalis, Bacteroides* spp., *Eubacterium* spp., and *Clostridium* spp. [76], the conversion of bilirubin to urobilinogen by *Clostridium ramosum* [78], the metabolism of cholesterol to coprostanol by strains of the genus *Eubacterium* [79], as well as in short-chain fatty acids feature [80] and tryptic activity [81].

Bacteria belonging to the normal intestinal microflora, such as *Bacteroides, Eubacterium, Propionibacterium, Fusobacterium, Bifidobacterium, Lactobacillus, Clostridium, Enterobacterium, Veillonella, Enterococcus, Enterobacteria,* and *Streptococcus*, participate in the production of different vitamins and folic acids [82]. A trilogue seems to characterize this complex ecosystem based on gut epithelial cells, microbiota, which is a newly introduced term to describe the collective societies of bacteria assembled on the mucosal surfaces of an individual [83], and finally, the gut-associated lymphoid tissue (GALT) [41].

Members of genera *Lactobacillus* are normal residents of the complex ecosystem of the human GI tract [41,61,84]. As already discussed, much interest is focused on their beneficial effect by improving the human intestinal microflora [38,85–87] via different actions and so they are called probiotics. Moreover, probiotics produce nutrients, bacteriocins, and antimicrobial substances, they are able to eliminate toxins and protect food from putrefaction. It is then obvious that the probiotic approach will help to determine the role of the bacterial species as well as ingredients in promoting their growth in the GI tract. Clearly, the beneficial potential of the human microflora is qualified together with the deficiencies in the gut flora, as a tool having a protecting effect on the gut microbiota. *Lactobacillus*, which are facultatively anaerobic or aerobic rods, are an important part of the human microflora by inhabiting various organs without usually exercing any pathogenic effect [38,62,88].

However, specific factors determining the development of the human lactic acid microflora are not yet completely elucidated, and studies focusing on the distribution of different strains in various human organs could clarify this crucial problem. Attachment to epithelial cells explains *Lactobacillus*-selective adherence to a particular ecosystem. Enterobacterial strains that determine intestinal infections exhibit specific adhesins that mediate bacterial adhesion and subsequent colonization of intestinal mucosa. Nonpathogenic anaerobic bacteria belonging to *Lactobacillus* and *Bifidobacterium* genera could inhibit the adhesion and invasion capacity of some enteropathogenic enterobacterial strains [89].

Despite the large numbers of studies on *Lactobacillus* and their effect as probiotics, precise knowledge of their colonization potential in healthy subjects is still inadequate. The rural people still produce unpasteurized fermented milk and other dairy products with live cultures of *Lactobacillus, Bifidobacterium,* and other probiotics by using traditional methods and technology. However, it is different from having complete information on the nutritional habits of a population. Children are considered to consume more frequently milk and dairy products than adults. Various bacterial species used in fermentation of dairy products often colonize the children in high numbers: *Lactobacillus paracasei, Lactobacillus delbrueckii lactis, Lactobacillus lactis lactis,* and *Leuconostoc. Bifidobacterium* is also found in the microflora of children (10%) [8], as well as in the microflora of old persons (5%) sparsely.

Furthermore, old persons have particular dietetic habits and a key portion of their nutrition comes from traditional foods. It is then assumed to be inhabited as well by bacterial species used for traditional food preparation. Clearly, healthy subjects of all ages are colonized by a predominant lactoflora (100%). However, there are differences in the species numbers and distribution during aging. Stability in *Lactobacillus* numbers was also observed by other authors [88], together with the stable persistence of the same biotype species during aging.

Furthermore, prolonged biological isolation of healthy persons, as it is the case of space flight or special trainings, causes alterations in the intestinal microflora. Moreover, stress influence seems to provide the GI microflora with putrefactive bacteria and especially increase in *C. perfringens* numbers [89–91]. GI infections, bacterial or viral diarrhea disease, pseudomembranous colitis, and antibiotic-associated diarrhea have been treated successfully by using some pharmaceutical probiotics such as *Saccharomyces boulardii*, *Lactobacillus casei* GG, *Lactobacillus acidophilus*, and *Enterococcus faecium*.

Surprisingly, high levels of intestinal *Lactobacillus* and/or *Enterococcus* were seen in infants with rotavirus diarrhea [92], as well as in inhabitants of the Chernobyl area after the atomic explosion [93]. Although some authors report missing *Lactobacillus* in the fecal flora of elderly people, most of the scientific world agrees on the predominance of *Lactobacillus* in all ages [94]. As already mentioned, *Lactobacillus* were reported to be extremely sensitive to environmental factors, diet, antibiotics [38,87,93], and stress [89–91]. Dissemination of antibiotic resistances into dairy products and into consumers following overuse of them could make some bacterial species prevail over others [38,88].

C. perfringens strains isolated from foods showed resistances in different antibiotics ranging from 8% to 49%. Resistant *C. perfringens* strains must be predominant in the elderly intestinal flora. In Greece, multiresistance in hospitalized patients and outpatients is reported [95]. The case of outpatients is somewhat interesting; as these patients had not received systematically antibiotics, the observation of frequent multiresistance was unexpected in this group of patients. The reasons for the resistance patterns observed may be due to the feed ingested. It is of considerable interest to note that in our country, for improving the quality of animals, antibiotics are added in their food. Antibiotics could be present at high levels in animals and their products ingested by human. It is then conceivable and understandable that the presence of multiresistance observed in most of our isolates may not be underestimated.

Lactobacillus predominates as well the healthy vaginal flora [88,94]. During delivery, excessive hygienic habits as decontamination of the birth canal by some antiseptics may select species of the vaginal microflora and so then limiting the species capable of colonizing the newborn intestine. *Lactobacillus* sp. are very susceptible to antiseptics [69]. Adhesion of *Lactobacillus* to the epithelial cells is directly connected with the mucus integrity, as the species have the ability to ferment monosaccharides of mucin in order to keep their stable population level. Antibiotics are able to cause breakdown of mucins [35]. Specifically, *Lactobacillus* were reported to be inhibitory to some other microorganisms and this is the basis of their ability to improve the keeping quality and safety of many food products [96]. The production of bacteriocins by LAB has been reported. Bacteriocins are bactericidal peptides that are active against other microbial species [97,98].

C. perfringens and *Escherichia coli* were predominant mainly in adults and elderly microflora. *C. perfringens* (25%) was shown in children microflora followed by *Escherichia coli* (10%), together with lower levels of *Bacillus* sp. (2.5%) and *Staphylococcus aureus* (2.5%) [62]. In subjects of all ages, *C. perfringens* was found in vegetative and spore forms [62,70]. Frequency of *C. perfringens* spore forms was higher in children (20%) and old people (87.5%) when compared to the *C. perfringens* total numbers. The absence of *C. perfringens* vegetative forms in children and old people is shown to be real in ages where lactobacilli prevail the fecal flora [62]. *C. perfringens* vegetative forms were more frequent (70%) in healthy adults [70].

The interactions among infection and immunity in the GI tract are illustrated by current studies on the interactions among *H. pylori*, the development of gastritis, and duodenal ulceration. *H. pylori* infection is present in 40% of the adult population and is now recognized as the major cause of duodenal ulceration. This invasive infection induces inflammation within the gastric mucosa greatly increasing the release of gastrin. Eradication of *H. pylori* decreases gastrin-mediated acid secretion by 60%. Studies in a mouse model of *Helicobacter* infection using *Helicobacter felis* have indicated that the development of hypergastrinemia does not correspond to the onset of bacterial infection but with inflammatory infiltrate. It is thought that gastrin release is not directly due to the bacterium but is due to cytokines released by cells involved in the inflammatory response [99].

It is likely that many of the bacteria isolated from the stomach are allochthonous, originating in the oral cavity or are ingested with food [100]. One important exception is *H. pylori*, evolved for gastric colonization and occurring in approximately 40% of the adult population in developed countries. *H. pylori* possesses a number of unique ecological adaptations that allow it to colonize in the stomach [101].

It appears that the presence of predominant cell types and associated environment in different regions of the GI tract will facilitate certain infections and perhaps inhibit others [102]. For example, whereas *H. pylori* is predominantly a gastric infection, *Vibrio cholerae*, *Shigella*, and *Salmonella* (*Salmonella typhi* and *Salmonella paratyphi*) mainly infect the small intestine causing inflammation and malabsorption. The nontyphoidal salmonellae (*Salmonella typhimurium* and *Salmonella enteritidis*) produce gastroenteritis with a neutrophilic infiltrate that can involve the small intestine and colon [103]. Studies in the mouse on *Trichinella spiralis* infection in which mast cells in the mucosa of the distal colon are triggered to release prostaglandins and leukotrienes have shown that dietary aspirin can suppress mucosal immune response of the distal colon without affecting a similar immune response in the small intestine [104].

The small intestine is also relatively sparsely populated, with the rapid transit of digesta driven by peristalsis limiting microbial colonization. The digestive capabilities of the small intestine and biliary secretions also inhibit microbial colonization in this region of the gut. Indeed it is not until the distal ileum that microbial populations start to increase in number significantly. Here numbers of facultative lactobacilli, streptococci, and enterobacteria, as well as some anaerobic bifidobacteria, *Bacteroides* spp., and clostridia reach population levels of about 10^4–10^8 CFU/mL. The ileocecal valve, in health, effectively limits the spread of a more diverse and dense microflora moving proximally from the colon [100,102].

Lactobacillus helveticus is an industrially important thermophilic starter for the fermentation of foods. It is mostly employed for cheese manufacture [105]. This species, known for its high proteolytic activities [106], releases oligopeptides from milk proteins [107]. These oligopeptides can be hydrolyzed to bioactive peptides by GI enzymes. In their study, the high performance liquid chromatography (HPLC) elution patterns as well as the sodium dodecyl sulphate-polyacrylamide gel electrophoresis (SDS-PAGE) study of milks fermented by *Lactobacillus helveticus* R389 demonstrated the high proteolytic activity of this strain, which was enhanced when the pH was kept at 6 (optimum pH for lactic acid bacteria proteases activity during fermentation [108]).

12.3   FLORA MODULATION

Optimum (optimized) nutrition will aim at maximizing the physiological functions of each individual, in order to ensure both maximum well-being and health but, at the same time, a minimum risk of disease throughout life. In other words, it will have to aim at maximizing a healthy lifespan. At the same time, it will have to match an individual's unique biochemical needs with a tailored selection of nutrient intakes for that individual. Such a selection will be based on a better understanding of the interactions between genes and nutrition [109]. These interactions include polymorphism and interindividual variations in response to diet, dietary alteration and modulation of gene expression, and dietary effects on disease risk. These interactions play a role both in the modulation of specific physiological functions and/or pathophysiological processes by given food components, as well as in their metabolism by the body. They control the responsiveness of a particular individual to both the beneficial and deleterious effects of their diet.

"Target function" refers to genomic, biochemical, physiological, psychological, or behavioral functions that are relevant to the maintenance of a state of well-being and health or to the reduction of the risk of a disease. Modulation of these functions should be quantitatively evaluated by measuring change in serum or other body fluids of the concentration of a metabolite, a specific protein or a hormone, change in the activity of enzymes, change in physiological parameters (e.g., blood pressure, GI transit time, etc.), change in physical or intellectual performances, and so on [110].

Probiotic bacteria have been shown to promote the endogeneous host defense mechanisms. In addition to effects on the nonimmunological gut defense, characterized by stabilization of the gut microflora [111], probiotic bacteria have been shown to enhance nonspecific host resistance to microbial pathogens [112]. Several strains of LAB have been shown to induce *in vitro* the release of proinflammatory cytokines, tumor necrosis factor-α, and interleukin-6 (IL-6), reflecting stimulation of nonspecific immunity [113]. Enhanced phagocytosis has also been reported in humans by *Lactobacillus acidophilus* strain La1 [114] and *Lactobacillus rhamnosus* GG [115]. Phagocytosis is responsible for early activation of the inflammatory response before antibody production. Recently, probiotic bacteria were shown to modulate phagocytosis differently in healthy and allergic subjects: in the former, an immunostimulatory effect, and in the latter, downregulation of the inflammatory response were detected, substantiating the immunoregulatory role of the gut microflora in the gut-associated lymphoid tissue [115].

Animal models offer an opportunity to test new therapeutic agents. Although experience has shown that several agents are beneficial in the treatment of experimental inflammatory bowel disease (IBD), drugs of totally different origin, composition, and function appear to be effective in animal models with completely diverse mechanisms of inflammation. Although the enormous list of "effective" agents points to a lack of specificity of inflammatory pathways, the efficacy of each therapy can make sense depending on the model, particularly in those with a well-defined immunological mechanism. In the mouse model of trinitrobenzene sulfonic acid-induced colitis, modulation of the cytokines predicted to be important for sustaining immune reactivity is effective: administration of antibodies against IL-12 abrogates even established inflammation, as does induction of oral tolerance resulting in TGF-β-mediated resolution of colitis [116,117]. The possibility that mechanisms responsible for IBD in animals and humans are diverse is real, but whether imbalances of immunoregulatory, proinflammatory, and immunosuppressive cytokines can be manipulated in humans as effectively as in animal models remains to be proved [118].

Cross et al. [119] have suggested that dietary consumption of fermented foods, such as yogurt, can alleviate some of the symptoms of atopy and might also reduce the development of allergies, possibly via a mechanism of immune regulation. Controlled studies have indicated that consumption of fermented milk cultures containing LAB can enhance production of type I and type II interferons at the systemic level. In animal models, LAB have been shown to promote interferon expression, and to reduce allergen-stimulated production of IL-4 and IL-5 in some cases. Recent results have shown that LAB are potent inducers of prointerferon monokines (IL-12 and IL-18), and that cytokine secretion is stimulated by the interaction of Gram(+) cell wall components with surface receptors of mononuclear phagocytes, via NF-κB and signal transducers and activators of transcription (STAT) signaling pathways. However, it is clear that the extent and quality of LAB-induced immunoregulation are strain-dependent.

The probiotic effects ascribed to LAB and their fermented dairy products arise not only from whole microorganisms and cell wall components, but also from peptides and extracellular polysaccharides (exopolysaccharides) produced during the fermentation of milk. There is a lack of knowledge concerning the immune mechanisms induced by exopolysaccharides produced by LAB, which would allow a better understanding of the functional effects described. The aim of the study by Vinderola et al. [120] was to investigate the *in vivo* immunomodulating capacity of the exopolysaccharide produced by *Lactobacillus kefiranofaciens* by analyzing the profile of cytokines and immunoglobulins induced at the intestinal mucosa level, in the intestinal fluid and blood serum. BALB/c mice received the exopolysaccharide produced by *Lactobacillus kefiranofaciens* for 2, 5, or 7 consecutive days. At the end of each period of administration, control and treated mice were sacrificed and the numbers of IgA+ and IgG+ cells were determined on histological slices of the small and large intestines by immunofluorescence [121]. Cytokines (IL-4, IL-6, IL-10, IL-12, IFNc, and TNF-α) were also determined in the gut lamina propria as well as in the intestinal fluid and blood serum [122]. There was an increase of IgA+ cells in the small and large intestine lamina propria, without change in the number of IgG+ cells in the small intestine. This study reports the effects of the oral administration of the exopolysaccharide produced by *Lactobacillus kefiranofaciens* on the number of IgA+ cells in the small and large intestines, comparing simultaneously the production of cytokines by cells of the lamina propria and in the intestinal fluid and blood serum. The increase in the number of IgA+ cells was not simultaneously accompanied by an enhancement of the number of IL-4+ cells in the small intestine. This finding would be in accordance with the fact that, in general, polysaccharide antigens elicit a T-independent immune response. For IL-10+, IL-6+, and IL-12+ cells, the values found were slightly increased compared to control values, while IFNc+ and TNF-α+ cells did not change compared to control values. The effects observed in immunoglobulins and in all the cytokines assayed in the large intestine after kefiran administration were of greater magnitude than the ones observed in the small intestine lamina propria, which may be due to the saccharolytic action of the colonic microflora. In the intestinal fluid, only IL-4 and IL-12 increased compared to control values. In blood serum, all the cytokines assayed followed a pattern of production quite similar to the one found for them in the small intestine lamina propria [120].

The effect of long-term administration of commercial fermented milk containing probiotic bacteria on the mucosal immune response and peritoneal macrophages was analyzed. BALB/c mice were fed with fermented milk for 98 consecutive days. The small and large intestines were removed for histology; IgA, CD4, and CD8 cells and cytokines-producing cells were counted. The influence on the immune cells associated with bronchus and mammary glands as well as on peritoneal macrophages was also analyzed. Continuous oral administration of fermented milk increased IgA+ cells in both parts of the intestine (the small and large intestines). IL-10, a regulatory cytokine, increased in the intestinal cells in most samples. TNF-α, IFN-γ, and IL-2-producing cells were also enhanced. Values for CD4 and CD8+ cell populations in the lamina propria of the intestine were increased in relation to the control throughout the assay [123]. No modifications in the histology of intestines were observed. Long-term consumption of fermented milk enhanced intestinal mucosa immunity, mediated by IgA+ cells and by cytokine production [124]. This improvement of gut immunity was maintained and downregulated by cytokines such as IL-10, preventing gut inflammatory immune response. The effect of this fermented milk on mucosal sites distant to the gut, such as bronchus and mammary glands, showed that in both tissues the increase in IgA+ cells was only observed at the beginning of the continuous consumption and no modifications in the number of cytokine-positive cells were found. Similar observations were found when phagocytic activity of peritoneal macrophages was measured. It was demonstrated that the most evident effect of long-term consumption of fermented milk was observed in the intestine. Immunomodulatory effects and the maintenance of intestinal homeostasis without secondary effects after long-term administration of fermented milk were also observed [123].

Innate immunity that protects against pathogens in the tissues and circulation is the first line of defense in the immune reaction, where macrophages have a critical role in directing the fate of the infection. We recently demonstrated that kefir modulates the immune response in mice, increasing the number of IgA+ cells in the intestinal and bronchial mucosa and the phagocytic activity of peritoneal and pulmonary macrophages. The aim of this study was to further characterize the immunomodulating capacity of the two fractions of kefir (F1: solids including bacteria and F2: liquid supernatant), by studying the cytokines produced by cells from the innate immune system: peritoneal macrophages and the adherent cells from Peyer's patches. BALB/c mice were fed with either kefir solid fraction (F1) or kefir supernatant (F2) for 2, 5, or 7 consecutive days. The number of cytokine (IL-1α, IFN-γ, TNF-α, IL-6, and IL-10)-producing cells was determined on peritoneal macrophages and adherent cells from Peyer's patches [125]. Both kefir fractions (F1 and F2) induced similar cytokine profiles on peritoneal macrophages (only TNF-α and IL-6 were upregulated) [126]. All cytokines studied on adherent cells from Peyer's patches were enhanced after F1 and F2 feeding, except for IFN-γ after F2 administration. Moreover, the percentage of IL-10+ cells induced by fraction F2 on adherent cells from Peyer's patches was significantly higher than the one induced by fraction F1. Different components of kefir have an *in vivo* role as oral biotherapeutic substances capable of stimulating immune cells of the innate immune system, to downregulate the Th2 immune phenotype or to promote cell-mediated immune responses against tumors and also against intracellular pathogenic infections [125].

Bacterial infections in the GI tract represent a major global health problem, even in the presence of normally effective mucosal immune mechanisms. Milk fermented by *Lactobacillus helveticus* R389 (FM) or its nonbacterial fraction obtained by milk fermentation at controlled pH 6 (NBF) are able to activate the small intestine mucosal immune response according to previous studies. In a completely randomized design, BALB/c mice received FM or NBF for 2, 5, or 7 consecutive days, followed by a single oral challenge with *Salmonella typhimurium* (107 cells/mouse). The increase in the number of IgA+ cells in the lamina propria of the small intestine, after the feeding periods, was accompanied by an increase in the luminal content of total S-IgA. However, no antibodies were produced against the NBF. In mice given the FM or the NBF for 7 consecutive days, lower levels of liver colonization on day 7 postchallenge with *Salmonella typhimurium*, higher luminal contents of specific anti-*Salmonella* S-IgA, higher percentages of survival to infection, and lower numbers of macrophage inflammatory protein (MIP)-1α+ cells in the lamina propria were observed. In this work, we observed that in both the FM and the NBF, there are active principles that confer enhanced protection against *Salmonella typhimurium* infection. However, the mechanisms underlying mucosal immunomodulation and protection are different. In those mechanisms, the mucosal immune response would seem to be more involved than the competitive or exclusion mechanisms between *Lactobacillus helveticus* R389 and *Salmonella enteritidis* serovar Typhimurium [127].

LAB are probiotics widely used in functional food products, with a variety of beneficial effects reported. Recently, intense research has been carried out to provide insights into the mechanism of action of probiotic bacteria. We have used gene array technology to map the pattern of changes in the global gene expression profile of the host caused by *Lactobacillus* administration. Affymetrix microarrays were applied to comparatively characterize differences in gene transcription in the distal ileum of normal microflora (NMF) and germ-free (GF) mice evoked by oral administration of two *Lactobacillus* strains used in fermented dairy products today—*Lactobacillus paracasei* ssp. *paracasei* F19 (*Lactobacillus* F19) or *Lactobacillus acidophilus* NCFB 1748. Nerstedt et al. [128] show that feeding either of the two strains caused very similar effects on the transcriptional profile of the host. Both *Lactobacillus* F19 and *Lactobacillus acidophilus* NCFB 1748 evoked a complex response in the gut, reflected by differential regulation of a number of genes involved in essential physiological functions such as immune response, regulation of energy homeostasis, and host defense. Notably, the changes in intestinal gene expression caused by *Lactobacillus* were different in the mice raised under GF versus NMF conditions, underlying the complex and dynamic nature of the host–commensal relationship. Differential expression of an array of genes described in this report evokes a novel hypothesis of possible interactions between the probiotic bacteria and the host organism and warrants further studies to evaluate the functional significance of these transcriptional changes on the metabolic profile of the host.

Infection with the Gram(−) microaerophilic bacterium *H. pylori* is typically acquired in childhood. About 10% of patients develop symptoms of gastritis, peptic ulcer disease, or MALT lymphoma, but anemia and growth retardation are also associated with *H. pylori* colonization in children [129]. The infection is a relevant health problem since approximately half of the world population is infected with *H. pylori*. In particular, high prevalence rates exist in developing countries and in populations with low socioeconomic standard and poor hygienic conditions. *H. pylori* can be eradicated by antimicrobial therapy (typically amoxicillin plus clarithromycin or amoxicillin plus metronidazole) plus a proton pump inhibitor [129–131].

However, using the current antibiotic combinations, complete eradication rate has not been achieved and current therapy is associated with GI side effects. There is increasing evidence that probiotics do not completely eradicate *H. pylori* but maintain lower levels of this pathogen in the stomach. This reduction in bacterial load seems to increase the efficacy of standard eradication therapies. Furthermore, the use of probiotics may reduce the rate of adverse effects of current standard therapies [132]. School children from a low socioeconomic area of Santiago de Chile that received 1 month live *Lactobacillus johnsonii* La1 (but not *Lactobacillus paracasei* ST11 or heat-killed *Lactobacillus johnsonii* La1) showed moderately reduced delta over baseline (DOB) values in the (13)C-urea breath test, indicating a direct modulation in *H. pylori* colonization by living *Lactobacillus johnsonii* La1 [133].

One of the mechanisms by which probiotics may confer a health benefit on the host is the modulation of the intestinal microbiota [134]. Accordingly, food supplements such as prebiotics, probiotics, and synbiotics are generally developed to improve the population and/or the activity of lactobacilli and bifidobacteria within the gut microbiota. One of the most promising properties of dairy propionibacteria, in this context, is their bifidogenic effect. Some strains of *Propionibacterium freudenreichii* were shown to enhance the growth of bifidobacteria *in vitro* and their population in the gut. In this respect, propionibacterial metabolites would best fit to the first definition of probiotics being "growth promoting factors produced by microorganisms" [135].

Indeed, a bifidogenic effect was observed *in vitro* for cell-free extracts of *P. freudenreichii* [136] and is due to the presence of 2-amino-3-carboxy-1,4-naphthoquinone [137] and 1,4-dihydroxy-2-naphthoic acid [138]. Moreover independent studies showed that ingestion of *P. freudenreichii*, under the form of whey cultures, either heat-inactivated [139] or not [140], or of freeze-dried live bacteria [141], resulted in a higher fecal bifidobacteria concentration in humans. This was linked to an increased number of defecations in constipated female volunteers [140].

The best and first recognized effect of probiotics is the alleviation of lactose intolerance by LAB, mainly *Streptococcus thermophilus* and *Lactobacillus bulgaricus* used as yoghurt starters. The genetically programmed drop in human enterocyte lactase activity in childhood [142], as well as disorders leading to small intestinal mucosa damages or increase of the GI transit time [143], triggers lactose malabsorption responsible for GI symptoms such as bloating, flatulence, abdominal pain, and diarrhea [144].

LAB have proved useful in this context to improve lactose dairy propionibacteria as probiotics via their lactase activity [145,146]. Among the carbon sources used by dairy propionibacteria, lactose of dairy origin can be used for the production of propionic acid [147]. Utilization of lactose requires the expression of lactase, or β-galactosidase, by the bacterium, in order to convert the disaccharide lactose into the monosaccharides galactose and glucose. Indeed, the genome sequence of *P. freudenreichii* CIP103027 suggests the existence of a β-galactosidase (118 kDa, 41% identical to *Actinobacillus pleuropneumoniae* β-galactosidase) and the corresponding activity was evidenced in the species *P. freudenreichii* and *Propionibacterium acidipropionici*. *In vitro*, this activity was shown to be increased in the extracellular medium by the presence of raw bile or bile salts, probably via permeabilization of propionibacteria [148]. The impact of physicochemical parameters on this activity suggests that propionibacterial β-galactosidase may be active within the gut [149]. Accordingly, feeding mice with *P. acidipropionici*, either as pure cultures in milk or in conjunction with *Streptococcus thermophilus* and *Lactobacillus bulgaricus* in Swiss-type cheeses, resulted in a significant increase in β-galactosidase activity within the small bowel and the cecum of mice, compared to sterile milk [150].

The development of probiotics for use in children is a challenging task. Due to the flexibility of the developing microbiota in early childhood, there is a clear potential to influence and modulate the intestinal microbiota to achieve health benefits. Furthermore, there are several defined applications where probiotics have been shown to give therapeutic benefit. The therapeutic applications include relevant disorders with high incidence such as infectious enteritis, *H. pylori* infection, or allergy. Already these few applications mean that probiotics could be relevant for potentially every child [151].

However, there are several risks and questions that have not been answered yet: there is still some uncertainty about the safety of probiotics in very young children with an immature immune system as addressed earlier. In fact, there are few reports of sepsis in patients treated with *Lactobacillus rhamnosus* GG. A 6-week-old full-term baby with double outlet right ventricle and a 6-year-old child with jejunostomy and several infections are among those reported [152]. There are also reports of fungaemia by *Saccharomyces boulardii* (*Saccharomyces cerevisiae* Hansen CBS 5926) after therapeutic use as probiotic [153–155].

Dogi et al. [156] analyzed the gut immune stimulation induced by Gram(+) bacteria: nonprobiotic *Lactobacillus acidophilus* CRL 1462 and *Lactobacillus acidophilus* A9; two potentially probiotic strains: *Lactobacillus acidophilus* CRL 924 and *Lactobacillus delbrueckii* subsp. *bulgaricus* CRL 423; comparatively with a probiotic strain: *Lactobacillus casei* CRL 431. They also studied Gram(−) bacteria: *Escherichia coli* 129 and *Escherichia coli* 13-7 in BALB/c mice. All the strains increased the number of IgA+ cells. We analyzed the cytokines IFNc, TNF-α, IL-17, IL-12, IL-6, and MIP-1α. The Gram(+) strains increased the number of IL-10+ cells. Gram(−) strains did not increase IL-10+ cells, but they increased the number of IL-12+ cells. The probiotic strain increased mainly IFNc and TNF-α. In the study of the receptors TLR-2, TLR-4, and CD-206, the researchers demonstrated that only the probiotic strain increased the number of CD-206+ cells. All the Gram(+) strains increased the number of TLR-2+ cells and the Gram(−) strains of the TLR-4+ cells. The probiotic strain induced the release of IL-6 by a preparation enriched in intestinal epithelial cells (IEC). Gram(+) and Gram(−) bacteria activated different immune receptors and induced a different cytokine profile. The probiotic strain showed a great activity on the immune cells and the enriched population in IEC, activating mainly cells of the innate immune system.

A decisive pathophysiological factor for many infectious diseases such as diarrhea for example is the ability of microbial pathogens to adhere to the mucosal surface and their subsequent spreading, colonization, and invasion (e.g., for *Escherichia coli*, *Helicobacter jejuni*, *Shigella* strains, *Vibrio cholerae*, and *Salmonella* species) in the gut [157,158]. Bacterial adhesion is often a receptor-mediated interaction between structures on the bacterial surface and complementary ligands on the mucosal surface of the host [159]. The various ligand specificities, for example, of *Escherichia coli* strains could explain the different intestinal colonization of breast-fed versus formula-fed newborns [160]. Human milk, with its high amount and large variety of oligosaccharides (5–10 g/L milk, 4150 different structures), might prevent the intestinal attachment of microorganisms by acting as soluble analogues competing with epithelial receptors for bacterial binding or binding of other pathogens.

FOS such as inulin or oligofructose are well-characterized components. GOS can be produced from lactose through specific processes. They consist of a number of β1-6-linked galactosyl residues bound to a terminal glucose unit via an α1-4 linkage. A thorough review of this topic has been given by Tungland and Meyer [161]. In human milk, however, small oligosaccharides are fucosylated or sialylated, but solely galactosylated components do not occur. In addition, the linkage between monosaccharides is important for biological effects as well. Although the amount of oligosaccharides in milk of most animal species is low compared with human milk, recent data indicate significant differences among milk from farm animals [162]. Whether some of these oligosaccharides are good candidates for clinical studies needs to be further investigated. Currently, there is only a limited amount of quantitative data on the total amount of oligosaccharides and on individual components in animal milk, for example, in bovine, goat, or buffalo milk.

Regarding biological functions certain structural prerequisites are necessary for milk oligosaccharides to be effective in different *in vitro* systems. Often prebiotic oligosaccharides (PBOs) from plants are obtained by technological means and are considered to be similar or even identical to HMOs. However, there is no evidence for this speculation as PBOs are structurally quite different from HMOs. Whether

PBOs exert comparable functional effects remains to be investigated. If this were the case, then their addition to infant formula may be useful in the context of mimicking biological functions of human milk constituents [163].

The immune enhancing properties of *Lactobacillus acidophilus* LAFTI L10 and *Lactobacillus paracasei* LAFTI L26 in mice were investigated. Each mouse (BALB/c) was orally fed with cultures of either *Lactobacillus acidophilus* or *Lactobacillus paracasei* at 10^8 CFU/50 μL per day for 14 days. The effect of these strains on IgA, IL-10, and IFN-γ-producing cells in the gut immune system was determined by immunofluorescence assays. Systemic immune responses were analyzed in mice serum upon euthanizing after a 14-day feeding trial to estimate cytokines such as IL-10 and IFN-γ by enzyme-linked immunosorbent assays. *Lactobacillus acidophilus* and *Lactobacillus paracasei* strains demonstrated an increase in the number of IgA-producing cells, IL-10, and IFN-γ cytokine-producing cells in the small intestine. In the systemic immune response, mice fed with *Lactobacillus acidophilus* or *Lactobacillus paracasei* also enhanced the secretion of anti-inflammatory cytokine (IL-10) and proinflammatory cytokine (IFN-γ). The results of this study suggest that *Lactobacillus acidophilus* and *Lactobacillus paracasei* were able to enhance specific gut and systemic immune responses in mice [164].

The increased number of IgA-producing cells was significantly different ($P < 0.001$) between mice fed with *Lactobacillus acidophilus* or *Lactobacillus paracasei*. The external secretions of IgA in the GI tract play an active role in protecting the surface of the mucus membrane from pathogenic infections and carcinogens [165].

Mice fed with *Lactobacillus acidophilus* or *Lactobacillus paracasei* also demonstrated differences ($P < 0.001$) in enhancing IL-10 and IFN-γ cytokine levels in the serum. Human volunteers fed with lyophilized lactobacilli showed an increased production of IFN-γ in serum [166]. Schultz et al. [167] reported that oral administration of *Lactobacillus rhamnosus* GG to healthy human volunteers stimulated an increased secretion of anti-inflammatory cytokines (IL-10 and IL-4) and decreased secretion of proinflammatory cytokines (IFN-γ, TNF-α, and IL-6). In the present study, IL-10 was significantly increased in the systemic immune response of mice fed with *Lactobacillus acidophilus* or *Lactobacillus paracasei*. The magnitude of the increment of IL-10 was higher than that of the Th1 cytokine IFN-γ, which may be necessary to control the increase of the proinflammatory cytokine IFN-γ.

The aim of the work of Vinderola et al. [168] was to gain further knowledge of the previously observed immunomodulating capacity of milk fermented by *Lactobacillus helveticus* R389 by the study of the mucosal immunomodulation exerted by the non-bacterial fraction of the milk fermented at a constant pH 6 (NBFpH6). The effects of small intestine epithelial cells on IL-6 production; the profile of IgA+ and cytokine+ cells (IL-2, IL-6, IL-10, TNF-α, and IFN-γ) induced in the gut lamina propria; and the levels of total and specific secretory IgA in the lumen of BALB/c mice that received NBFpH6 for 2, 5, or 7 days were examined. There was an increase in the number of IgA+, IL-10+, IL-2+, and IL-6+ cells after all feeding periods. Total S-IgA in the small intestine lumen increased in mice that received NBFpH6 for 2 days. However, no specific antibodies against NBFpH6 were detected. Feeding with NBFpH6 for 7 days significantly ($P < 0.05$) enhanced

IL-6 secretion by the small intestine epithelial cells. NBFpH6 induced a nonspecific mucosal response that was downregulated for protective immunity, enhancing IL-6 production by epithelial cells and IgA production in the small intestine. These events improve the immunological defenses at the intestinal level, increasing host protection against pathologies. Because mucosal immune responses induced by certain dietary antigens play a large part in the prevention of GI diseases, the oral administration of a mucosal adjuvant such as NBFpH6 may positively affect the milieu of the intestinal lumen. The opportunity exists then to manipulate the constituents of the lumen of the intestine through dietary means, thereby enhancing the health condition of the host.

The oral administration of the nonbacterial fractions of milks fermented by *Lactobacillus helveticus* R389 modulated the gut mucosa immune response. There was an increase in the number of IgA+ cells in the lamina propria of the small intestine. That increase, which was greater in mice that received NBFpH6 than in the ones that received NBF or nonfermented 12% milk, was probably due to the greater content of bioactive peptides in NBFpH6. Feeding of 12% milk also induced an increase in the number of IgA+ cells by day 7, possibly due to the presence of endogenous preformed immunoregulatory peptides in bovine milk [169] or other factors not controlled in this study. Vinderola et al. [168] observed that the greater the amount of peptides formed in milk, the greater the effect on the number of IgA+ cells in the small intestine lamina propria. Since the greatest effects on the number of IgA+ cells were observed when mice received NBFpH6, they decided to further characterize its effects on the gut mucosa.

Studies with mice found strong immuno-enhancing effects of whey proteins, especially in combination with whey phospholipids. The serum IgM levels were more than doubled in mice fed with diets based on whey protein and fresh whey cream [170]. Inclusion of total whey protein in experimental diets has been correlated with stimulatory effect for the immune system [171], a low-density lipoprotein (LDL)-cholesterol-lowering effect and increased production of cholecystokinin involved in appetite suppression [172]. It is likely that at least some of these properties are linked to the individual protein species included in the total whey protein. Both of the two major whey proteins, α-lactalbumin and β-lactalbumin, can be considered as having physiological properties. The uniqueness of α-lactalbumin as a calcium-binding protein has been known for some time [173,174].

Rats initiated with azoxymethane (AOM) and fed with a semipurified diet supplemented with *Bifidobacterium longum* had a significantly lower incidence and multiplicity of colonic tumors than control rats. Colonic proliferation and the expression of ras-p21 oncoprotein were also decreased in rats treated with probiotics, suggesting a mechanism for the observed inhibition of colon carcinogenesis [175]. Although this report suggests a protective effect of probiotics, other studies have shown that this effect is not completely consistent and may depend on the experimental conditions. Goldin et al. [176] demonstrated that while *Lactobacillus rhamnosus* (strain GG) reduced colon cancer when given to rats 3 weeks before carcinogen administration, it was not active if given after the ninth week of DMH treatment. Goldin and Gorbach [177] reported that the incidence of colon cancer induced by DMH in rats treated with *Lactobacillus acidophilus* was lower after 20 weeks of induction, but this protective effect was not observed after 36 weeks, thus suggesting that these bacteria may increase the latency for induction of experimental carcinogenesis.

Lactobacillus delbrueckii subsp. *bulgaricus* were tested for the ability to inhibit DMH-induced colon carcinogenesis in BD6 rats [178]. Both strains induced pro-differentiation markers and inhibited ear tumors (that are sometimes induced with DMH treatment). However, one of the strains decreased carcinogenesis in both the colon and small intestine, while the other one was inactive in the colon. Different strains of probiotic bacteria were also studied on DMH-induced colon carcinogenesis in Sprague–Dawley rats. Only *Lactobacillus acidophilus* (strain Delvo Pro LA-1) caused a significant reduction in colon tumors, whereas strains such as *Lactobacillus rhamnosus* (GG), *Bifidobacterium animalis* (CsCC1941), or *Streptococcus thermophilus* were not active [179]. These data together with those of Balansky et al. [178] suggest that different results can be obtained, depending on the probiotic strain tested.

Coconnier et al. [180] reported that *Lactobacillus acidophilus* strain LB was able to protect against *H. pylori* infection in conventional mice. Inhibition of stomach colonization by *H. felis* (closely related to *H. pylori*) was observed and no evidence of gastric histopathological lesions was found. Recently, probiotic combination containing *Lactobacillus acidophilus* R0052 and *Lactobacillus rhamnosus* R0011 reduced the effects of *H. pylori* infection in a C57BL/6 mice model through reducing *H. pylori* colonization and ameliorating *H. pylori*-induced inflammation of the stomach [181]. Also, the same probiotic preparation has proved effective in a Mongolian gerbil model of *H. pylori* infection via its attenuating effect on the *H. pylori* colonization, the mucosal inflammation, and the impairment of gastrin–somatostatin link [182]. Studies by Sgouras et al. [183,184] in a C57BL/6 mice model demonstrated that *Lactobacillus casei* strain Shirota and *Lactobacillus johnsonii* La1, both administered in drinking water, attenuated *H. pylori* infection-induced gastric mucosa inflammation. However, only *Lactobacillus casei* strain Shirota was able to downregulate the colonization of *H. pylori* to gastric mucosa.

Administration of *Lactobacillus reuteri* R2LC, but not *Lactobacillus rhamnosus* GG, significantly attenuated inflammation in acetic acid- or methotrexate-induced colitis in rats [185–187]. Conversely, *Lactobacillus rhamnosus* GG and VSL#3 demonstrated a protective effect in the iodoacetamide model of colitis [188]. *Bifidobacterium infantis* 35624 also limited inflammation, and its protective effects were evident outside the context of established inflammation and at the preinflammatory stage [189,190]. Some examples of flora modulation are shown in Table 12.2.

12.4 CONCLUSIONS

Functional foods probably first arose through the necessity to supplement the diet with vitamins. Certainly the first generation of functional foods involved the addition of trace minerals to appropriate foodstuffs. It is the case that most current thinking and product development is centered toward GI activity and microbial interactions specifically. Probiotics have a long history of use in humans, but have never realized their full potential. This is probably because of some poor science that has been associated with the concept. Often trials have been carried out in a very subjective manner [110].

TABLE 12.2
Flora Modulation

Product	Active Ingredient	Dose	Test Animal	Application Time	Results	Reference
Yoghurt	Lactobacillus, bifidobacteria	—	Mice	—	– Enhanced protection against intercellular bacterial pathogens – Control of tumor growth in mice	Cross et al. [119]
Milk	Lactobacillus kefiranofaciens	100 mg/kg body weight/day	6–8-week-old female BALB/c mice	2, 5, and 7 consecutive days	– Increase of IgA+ cells – Determination of cytokines in the gut lamina propria – Without change in the IgG+ cells in the small intestine	Vinderola et al. [120]
Fermented milk	Lactobacillus delbrueckii subsp. Bulgaricus, Streptococcus thermophilus, Lactobacillus casei	10⁸ CFU/mL, 10⁸ CFU/mL, 10⁷ CFU/mL in drinking water of rodents	6-week-old mice	98 consecutive days	– Increase of IgA+ cells in both the small and large intestines – IL-10 increased in intestinal cells – No modification in the histology of intestines	De Moreno de LeBlanc et al. [123]
Milk protein	Lactobacillus kefiranofaciens	200 µL/day	6–8-week-old female BALB/c mice	2, 5, and 7 consecutive days	– Adherent cells from Peyer's patches	Vinderola et al. [125]

continued

TABLE 12.2   (continued)

Product	Active Ingredient	Dose	Test Animal	Application Time	Results	Reference
Fermented milk	*Lactobacillus helveticus* R389	100 µg of total protein/day/mouse 200 µL in drinking water	6–8-week-old BALB/c mice	2, 5, and 7 consecutive days	– Increase of the number of IgA+ cells in the small intestine – Increase of the luminal content of total S-IgA	Vinderola et al. [127]
Fermented milk	*Lactobacillus acidophillus* CRL924	The daily dose was previously selected by determination of absence of intestinal disturbance in the NMF	6–8-week-old BALB/c mice	2, 5, and 7 consecutive days	– Increases mainly IFN-γ and TNF-α – Increase the number of CD-206+ cells	Dogi et al. [156]
Yoghurt	*Lactobacillus delbrueckii* subsp. *bulgaricus*					
Skimmed milk powder	*Lactobacillus acidophillus* LAFTI L10, *Lactobacillus paracasei* LAFTI L26	10^8 CFU/50 µL/day	6–8-week-old male BALB/c mice	14 days	– Increase the number of IgA-producing cells – Increase of IL-10 and IFN-γ cytokine-producing cells in the small intestine	Paturi et al. [164]
Fermented milk	*Lactobacillus helveticus* R389	100 µg of total protein/day 200 µL of 12% skim milk	6–8-week-old male BALB/c mice	2, 5, and 7 consecutive days	– Increase of total S-IgA in the small intestine lumen	Vinderola et al. [168]
High-temperature processed milk	*Lactobacillus acidophillus* NCFB1748, *Lactobacillus paracasei* F19	10^9 CFU/mL	6–8-week-old GF and NMF male mice	10 days	– Both strains evoked a complex response in the gut	Nerstedt et al. [128]

Features of a functional food are defined as

a. Conventional or everyday food consumed as part of the normal diet
b. Composed of naturally occurring components, sometimes in increased concentration or present in foods that would not normally supply them
c. Scientifically demonstrated positive effects on target functions beyond basic nutrition
d. Provide enhancement of the state of well-being and health to improve the quality of life and/or reduce the risk of disease
e. Supported by claims authorized by a relevant authority [191–193]

Functional dairy products clearly possess the potential to improve intestinal health. Milk as such is a healthy food. Certain lactobacilli strains already have established evidence for their shortening effect on the duration of acute diarrhea, especially in rotavirus infections. However, vaccination against rotavirus is starting to be developed and the need for improved treatment may be reduced. There are still only a few studies on the successful treatment of invasive acute diarrhea with native lactobacilli, but a promising experimental trial to bind cholera toxin with a genetically modified probiotic strain has recently been published [194].

Physiological functions and the dairy products and components associated with these functions include the following:

1. Immunomodulation (modified whey protein concentrate, colostrums, probiotics, lactoferrin, lactoperoxidase, κ-casein glycomacropeptide, CLA, and calcium)
2. Antimicrobial/antiviral activity (lactoferrin/lactoferricin, lactoperoxidase, lactalbumin, and casein glycomacropeptide)
3. Microbial toxin binding (whey protein concentrate, β-lactoglobulin, α-lactalbumin, and casein glycomacropeptide)
4. Protection from some cancers (whey protein concentrate, lactoferrin, α-lactalbumin, peptides, sphingolipids, CLA, and butyric acid)
5. Anti-inflammatory activity (peptides, colostrums, and immune milk)
6. Antithrombotic activity (lactoferrin and peptides)
7. Reduction in cholesterol levels (whey protein concentrates, whey protein isolates, and stearic acid)
8. Opioid-like activity (peptides)
9. Prebiotic effects such as stimulation of growth of bifidobacteria (casein glycomacropeptide, oligosaccharides, and amino sugars)
10. Maintaining a healthy gut (dairy products containing probiotic microorganisms)
11. Antioxidative effects (whey protein concentrates/isolates, lactoferrin, bovine serum albumin, and vitamin C)
12. Protection from hypertension (immune whey protein concentrate, whey protein isolates, and minerals such as Ca, Mg, and K), especially the role of fermented dairy products in improving cardiovascular health by regulating blood pressure, has been emphasized tremendously during the past few years [195–203]

Probiotics are not selected among pathogens and, by definition, have a high safety profile, and the tolerance is usually excellent. Many of the commercial probiotic products have been officially designated as "generally regarded as safe," and the deliberate ingestion of lactobacilli or bifidobacteria does not pose a greater risk of infection than that associated with the commensal strains [204].

To be recognized as functional food components, they should demonstrate the following properties: acid and bile stability, adhesion to intestine surface, resistance to digestive enzymes, antagonistic activity against human pathogens, anticarcinogenic and antimutagenic activity, cholesterol-lowering effects, stimulation of the immune system without inflammatory effects, enhancement of bowel motility, maintenance of mucosal integrity, improvement of bioavailability of food compounds, and production of vitamins and enzymes [205].

Understanding the mechanisms by which bifidobacteria affect the host is essential to support their possible role in functional foods. This requires more than the insight we have accumulated so far on the diversity, survival, and general activity of bifidobacteria. At least three complementary lines of research need to be further developed. These include the development of (i) functional genomics to determine the global activity of bifidobacteria, (ii) genetic tools to allow for testing hypotheses of the bifidobacterial function, and (iii) models and real-life studies that show the impact of bifidobacteria on the host and its intestinal microbiota [206].

Engineered probiotics may eventually be developed for specific food applications, although the pharmaceutical industry will likely capitalize first on genetically modified organisms for medical applications. The bottom line is that explorations of whole bacterial systems at the genomic level will ultimately advance the fields of functional foods and probiotics at a rapid pace unimaginable before the advent of functional genomics [207].

Today, the concept of gut flora modulation is enjoying new popularity and it is imperative that well-conducted human studies are used to test and validate probiotics, prebiotics, and synbiotics. These should have rigorous control and include appropriate placebo. New advances in molecular biology allow a highly sophisticated tracking of the microbiota changes in response to dietary intervention. Similarly, this chapter has reviewed the use of certain animal models for probiotic use. Here, many hypotheses have arisen on immunological status. Again, these need to be confirmed in humans. It is implicit that any effects seen through the use of functional foods identify a plausible mechanism of effect. It is important that diet fulfills all the nutritional requirements of humans; however, an added bonus may be the health-enhancing effects. While the population ages and pharmaceutical expenses increase, the route of using diet for the prophylactic management of disorder is an attractive concept—especially when the human gut is considered [110].

The initial step in the characterization of the mechanism of action for functional food products is the identification of a specific interaction between the active component of this food and an effect on the host organism that is potentially beneficial for health. One approach to investigate these interactions is to map the changes in the transcription profile of the host organism caused by nutrient intake. The recent development of expression profiling by the use of microarray technology has made it possible to monitor the expression of thousands of genes simultaneously, allowing systematic analysis of complex biological processes and offering the advantage of reducing bias in data collection, compared with the candidate gene-based approaches [208].

The rapid expansion of genetic tools and genomic sequencing of LAB have yielded vast amounts of molecular information in a short time span of several years. Commercial applications of LAB and other beneficial bacteria in functional foods including dairy products will continue to evolve rapidly with the proliferation of knowledge of bacterial biological systems. Functional genomics will immediately impact the science of natural strain selection in the food industry. By comparing gene content and gene expression profiles in various environmental conditions including animal models, natural LAB strains may be evaluated for specific beneficial or metabolic functions and high-throughput screening may be feasible. Rational selection based on particular biological features will be possible using highly parallel investigations of gene content and gene expression of entire bacterial chromosomes [207].

Mucosal T cells—in particular allergen-specific Th2 CD4 T cells, eosinophils, and mast cells—appear to play central roles in the development of allergic reactions in the GI mucosa [209]. In "classic" food allergy, the immediate allergic reactions are initiated by the cross-linking of mast-cell-bound IgE by the cognate antigen (type-I hypersensitivity reaction). The relevance of this threesome of effector immune cells (Th2 T cells, eosinophils, and mast cells) in combination with allergen-specific IgE for the development of eosinophil-associated GI allergies was formally demonstrated in a mouse model of eosinophil-associated GI allergy. Intraperitoneal priming with a model antigen (ovalbumin), followed by oral challenge with encapsulated antigen, resulted in blood eosinophilia and increased levels of circulating antigen-specific IgE and IgG1 (i.e., Th2-dependent immunoglobulins). These changes were associated with an increase of eosinophils in the intestinal lamina propria of challenged mice. Upon antigen-specific challenge of the sensitized mice, eosinophils appeared not only in the small intestine and stomach, but also in the esophagus that in healthy mice normally lacks eosinophils [210].

Oligonucleotide microarrays were applied to compare global transcriptional profiles in the distal ileum of mice receiving *Lactobacillus paracasei* ssp. *paracasei* F19 (*Lactobacillus* F19) or *Lactobacillus acidophilus* NCFB 1748 with the control group of mice receiving a placebo product. The effects of the two *Lactobacillus* strains were evaluated both in GF and NMF mice. *Lactobacillus* F19 and *Lactobacillus acidophilus* NCFB 1748, in combination with *Bifidobacterium lactis* Bb12, have been shown to efficiently restore the intestinal microflora during antibiotic treatment [207].

The mucosal mast cells exert important functions in the recruitment of leukocyte subsets due to their rapid secretion of chemokines and inflammatory cytokines upon activation. Together with leukotrienes and histamine, which are also released by activated mast cells, these mediators may substantially affect the tissue microenvironment for the subsequent local differentiation of effector cells of hypersensitivity reactions [211]. Through the potent production of IL-4, IL-5, and IL-13, antigen-specific Th2 CD4 T cells are key to the differentiation of B cells into IgE-producing plasma cells and to the activation of eosinophils, and thus to the induction of type-I hypersensitivity reactions [212].

REFERENCES

1. Metchnikoff, E., Études sur la flore intestinale, *Ann. Inst. Pasteur Paris*, 22, 929–955, 1908.
2. Metchnikoff, E., Études sur la flore intestinale, Deuxième mémoire, *Ann. Inst. Pasteur Paris*, 24, 755–770, 1910.
3. Escherich, T., The intestinal bacteria of the neonate and breast-fed infant, *Forschritte der Medizin* (3) *Rev. Infect. Dis.*, 10 (3),1220–1225, 1885.
4. Dairy Council Digest, available at www.nationaldairycouncil.org, 70 (6), November–December 1999.
5. Bezirtzoglou, E., Probiotics and the intestinal flora overtime and space, in *Current Topics on Bioprocesses in Food Industry*, A. Koutinas, A. Pandey, and C. Larroche, Eds, Vol. II, Chapter 18, pp. 281–288, API Asia Tech Publishers, Inc., New Delhi, 2006.
6. Bishop-MacDonald, H., Dairy food consumption and health: State of the science on current topics, *J. Am. College Nutr.*, 24 (6), 525–535, 2005.
7. Saarela, M. (Ed.), *Functional Dairy Products*, Vol. 2, preface: xvii, CRC Press, Cambridge, England, 2007.
8. Bezirtzoglou, E. and Romond, C., Occurrence of *Bifidobacterium* in the faeces of newborns delivered by cesarian section, *Biol. Neonate*, 58 (5), 175–180, 1990.
9. Bezirtzoglou, E., Romond, M.B., and Romond, C., Modulation of *C. perfringens* intestinal colonization in infants delivered by caesarean section, *Infection*, 17, 232–236, 1989.
10. Kurmann, J.A., Une nouvelle generation de cultures en industrie laitiere, *Lett. Appl. Microbiol.*, 42 (6), 12–18, 1993.
11. Mata, L.J., Mejicanos, M.L., and Jimenez, F., Studies on the indigenous flora of Guatemalan children, *Am. J. Clin. Nutr.*, 25, 1380–1390, 1972.
12. Mullie, C., Romond, M.B., Yazourh, A., Bezirtzoglou, E., and Romond, C., Modification to intestinal glycosidase activities following *Bifidobacterium breve* C50 oral challenge in C3H mice, *Anaerobe*, 3, 9–12, 1999.
13. Rafter, J.J., Scientific basis of biomarkers and benefits of functional foods for reduction of disease risk: Cancer, *Br. J. Nutr.*, 88 (2), S219–S224, 2002.
14. Cruise, J.P., Lewin, M.R., Ferulano, G.P., and Clark, C.G., Experimental evidence against the bile salt theory of colon carcinogenesis, *Eur. Surg. J.*, 13 (2), 117–124, 1981.
15. Thomas, W.E.G., Gastric morphological and functional changes produced by bile in the canine stomach, *Eur. Surg. Res.*, 13, 125–133, 1981.
16. Bonjour, J.P., Dietary protein: An essential nutrient for bone health, dairy food consumption and health, *State J. Am. College Nutr.*, 24 (6), 525S–535S, 2005.
17. Parvez, S., Malik, K.A., Ah-Kang, A., and Kim, H.Y., Probiotics and their fermented food products are beneficial for health, *J. Appl. Microbiol.*, 100, 1171–1185, 2006.
18. McFarland, L.V. and Elmer, G.W., Biotherapeutical agents: Past, present and future, *Microecol. Ther.*, 23, 46–73, 1995.
19. Van der Kaaij, N.P., The patient with decreased resistance to infections, *Microecol. Ther.*, 22, 1–4, 1996.
20. Levi, F., La Vecchia, C., Lucchini, F., and Negri, E., Cancer mortality in Europe, 1990–92, *Eur. J. Cancer Prev.*, 4, 389–417, 1995.
21. Mostratos, Z., Domeyer, P.R., and Michalis, D., Cancer mortality in Greece: Where are we heading? A 20-year comparative study in four Greek counties, *Cent. Eur. J. Public Health*, 14, 113–116, 2006.
22. Mullie, C., Romond, M.B., Yazourh, A., Libersa, C., Bezirtzoglou, E., and Romond, C., Influence of stress on faecal carriage of *C. perfringens*, *Micr. Ecol. Health Dis.*, 14, 118–121, 2002.

23. de Roos, N.M. and Katan, M.B., Effects of probiotic bacteria on diarrhea, lipid metabolism, and carcinogenesis: A review of papers published between 1988 and 1998, *Am. J. Clin. Nutr.*, 71, 405–411, 2000.

24. Fuller, R., History and development of probiotics, in *Probiotics*, R. Fuller, Ed., pp. 1–8, Chapman & Hall, New York, 1992.

25. FAO/WHO, Evaluation of health and nutritional properties of powder milk and live lactic acid bacteria, Food and Agriculture Organization of the United Nations and World Health Organization Expert Consultation Report, 2001, available at http://www.fao.org/es/ESN/probio/probio.htm.

26. Aguirre, M. and Collins, M.D., Lactic acid bacteria and human clinical infection, *J. Appl. Bacteriol.*, 75, 95–107, 1993.

27. Donohue, D.C. and Salminen, S.J., Safety of probiotic bacteria, *Asia Pacific J. Clin. Nutr.*, 5, 25–28, 1996.

28. Saxelin, M., Rautelin, H., Salminen, S., and Makela, H., The safety of commercial product with viable *Lactobacillus* strains, *Inf. Dis. Clin. Practice*, 5, 331–335, 1996.

29. Adams, M.R. and Marteau, P., On safety of lactic acid bacteria from food, *Int. J. Food Microbiol.*, 27, 263–264, 1995.

30. Salminen, S., Ouwqhand, A.C., and Isolauri, E., Clinical applications of probiotic bacteria, *Int. Dairy J.*, 8, 563–572, 1998.

31. Lee, Y.K. and Salminen, S., The coming of age of probiotics, *Trend Food Sci. Technol.*, 6, 241–245, 1995.

32. Salminen, S., Von Wright, A., Laine, M., Vuopio-Varkila, J., Korhonen, T., and Mattila-Sandholm, T., Development of selection criteria for probiotic strains to assess their potential in functional foods: A Nordic and European approach, *Biosci. Microbiol.*, 15(2), 61–67, 1996.

33. Salminen, S., Von Wright, A., Morelli, L., Marteau, P., Brassart, D., De Vos, W., Fonden, R., Saxelin, M., Collins, K., Mogenden, G., Birkeland, S.E., and Mattila-Sandholm, T., Demonstration of safety of probiotics: A review, *Int. J. Food Microbiol.*, 44 (1–2), 93–106, 1998.

34. Mattila-Sandholm, T. and Saarela, M., in *Functional Foods—Concept to Product*, G.R. Gibson and C.M. Williams, Eds, Chapter 12, pp. 292–294, CRC Press, Cambridge, England, 2000.

35. Midtvedt, T., Carlstedt-Duke, B., Höverstad, T., Midtvedt, A.C., Norin, K.E., and Saxerholt, H., Establishment of a biochemically active intestinal ecosystem in ex-germfree rats, *Appl. Environ. Microbiol.*, 53, 2866–2871, 1987.

36. Buisine, M.P., Desreumaux, P., Leteurtre, E., Copin, M.C., Colombel, J.F., Porchet, N., and Aubert, J.P., Mucin gene expression in intestinal epithelial cells in Crohn's disease, *Gut*, 49, 544–551, 2001.

37. Fukushima, Y., Kawata, Y., Hara, H., Terada, A., and Mitsuoka, T., Effect of a probiotic formula on intestinal immunoglobulin A production in healthy children, *Int. J. Food Microbiol.*, 42 (1), 39–44, 1998.

38. Ljungh, A. and Wadstrom, T., Lactic acid bacteria as probiotics, *Curr. Issues Intest. Microbiol.*, 7, 73–89, 2006.

39. Grajek, W., Olejnik, A., and Sip, A., Probiotics, prebiotics and antioxidants as functional foods, *Acta Biochim. Polon.*, 52 (3), 665–671, 2005.

40. Fuller R., Probiotics in man and animals, *J. Appl. Bacteriol.*, 66, 5365–378, 1989.

41. Falk, P.G., http://mmbr.asm.org/cgi/content/full/62/4/1157—FN151. Hooper, L.V., Midtvedt, T., and Gordon J.I., Creating and maintaining the gastrointestinal ecosystem: What we know and need to know from gnotobiology, *Microbiol. Mol. Biol. Rev.*, 62 (4), 1157–1170, 1998.

42. Saikali, J., Picard, C., Freitas, M., and Holt, P., Fermented milks, probiotic cultures and colon cancer, *Nutr. Cancer*, 49 (1), 14–24, 2004.

43. Crittenden, R.G. and Playne, M.J., Production, properties and applications of food-grade oligosaccharides, *Trend Food Sci. Technol.*, 7, 353–360, 1998.
44. Salminen, S., Isolauri, E., and Salminen, E., Probiotics and stabilisation of the gut mucosal barrier, *Asia Pacific J. Clin. Nutr.*, 5, 53–56, 1996.
45. Toba, T., Virkola, R., Westerlund, B., Bjorkman, Y., Sillanpaa, J., Vartio, T., Kalkkinen, N., and Korhonen, T.K., A collagen binding S-layer protein in *Lactobacillus crispatus*, *Appl. Environ. Microbiol.*, 61, 2467–2471, 1995.
46. Westerlund, B. and Korhonen, T., Bacterial proteins binding to the mammalian extracellular matrix, *Mol. Microbiol.*, 9, 687–694, 1993.
47. Roberfroid, M.B., Prebiotics and probiotics: Are they functional foods? *Am. J. Clin. Nutr.*, 71, 1682S–1687S, 2000.
48. Gibson, G.R. and Rastall, B., in *Prebiotics: Development and Application,* G.R. Gibson and B. Rastall, Eds, Wiley & Sons, Oxford, UK, 2006.
49. Dimerc, C. and Gibson, G.R., An overview of probiotics, prebiotics and synbiotics in the functional food concept: Perspectives and future strategies, *Int. Dairy J.*, 8 (5–6), 473–479, 1998.
50. Manning, T.S. and Gibson, G.R., Prebiotics, *Best Pract. Res. Clin. Gastrenterol*, 18, 287–298, 2004.
51. Savage, D.C., Microbial ecology of the gastrointestinal tract, *Ann. Rev. Microbiol.*, 31, 107–133, 1977.
52. Asp, N.G., Mollby, R., Norin, L., and Wadstrm, T., Probiotics in gastric and intestinal disorders as functional food and medicine, *Scand. J. Nutr.*, 48 (1), 15–25, 2004.
53. Libbey, J., *Functional Dairy Products, Eurotext, Nutrition and Health Collection*, John Libbey & Company Ltd, CIC Edizione Internazionali, Roma, Italia, available at http://www.john-libbey-eurotext.fr, 2002.
54. Jones, P.J., Clinical nutrition: Functional foods—more than just nutrition, *CMAJ*, 11(12), 166–169, 2002.
55. Toma, M.M. and Pokrotnieks, J., Probiotica and medical aspects, *Acta Univ. Latviens., Biol.*, 710, 117–129, 2006.
56. Rabiu, B.A. and Gibson, G.R., Carbohydrates: A limit on bacterial diversity within the colon, *Biol. Rev. Camb. Philos. Soc.*, 77 (3), 443–453, 2002.
57. Sanz, Y., Probiotics: Nature's own functional agents, Scientific Report, Ministeri de Education y Ciencia, CSIC, FFnet.
58. Hossain, M.A., Ralman, M.S., Chowdhury, S., and Rashid, M.A., Bioactivities of Sesbania sesban extractives, *Dhaka Univ. J. Pharm. Sci.*, 6, 47–50, 2007.
59. Kebede, A., Viljoen, B.C., Gadga, T.H., Narvhus, J.A., and Lourens-Hattingh, A., The effect of container type on the growth of yeast and lactic acid bacteria during production of Sethemi, South African spontaneously fermented milk, *Food Res. Int.*, 40 (1), 33–38, 2007.
60. Psoni, L., Tzannetakis, N., and Litopoulou-Tzannetaki, E., Characteristics of Batzos cheese made from raw pasteurized and/or pasteurized standardized goat milk and a native culture, *Food Control*, 17 (7), 533–539, 2003.
61. Vassos, D., Voidarou, C., Alexopoulos, A., Rozos, G., Maipa, V., and Bezirtzoglou, E., Isolation, identification and properties of lactic acid bacteria isolated from "pytia" (rennet), a traditional starter culture used in the region of Epirus in Greece, *Appl. Environ. Microbiol.*, 2008 (in press).
62. Bezirtzoglou, E., Contribution a l' etude de l' implantation de la flore fecale anaerobie du nouveau-ne mis au monde par cesarienne, Doctorat no. 13, Paris-Sud, 1985.
63. Bezirtzoglou, E., Romond, M.B., and Romond, C., Modulation of *C. perfringens* intestinal colonization in infants delivered by cesarian section, *Infection*, 17 (4), 232–236, 1989.
64. Bezirtzoglou, E. and Romond, C., Comportement du *C. perfringens* dans l' intestin du nourisson par cesarienne, *Ann. Pediatr.*, 1, 5–9, 1991.

65. Bezirtzoglou, E., Chavatte, P., and Romond, C., A quantitative study of faecal and other bacteria floras of newborns delivered by cesarian section, *G. I. Pat. Clin. IV*, 2, 39–43, 1989.

66. Bezirtzoglou, E. and Romond, C., Effect of the feeding practices on the establishment of bacterial interactions in the intestine of the newborn delivered by cesarian section, *J. Perinat. Med.*, 17, 139–143, 1989.

67. Midtvedt, T., Bjerneklett, A., Carlstedt-Duke, B., Gustafsson B.E., Hoverstad, T., Lingaas, E., Norin K.E., Saxerholt, H., and Steinbakk, M., The influence of antibiotics upon microflora associated characteristics in man and mammals, *Microecol. Ther.*, 14, 297–298, 1984.

68. Shooter, R.A., Asheshov, E.H., Bullimore, J.F., Morgan, G.M., Parker, M.T., Walker, K.A., and Williams, V.R., Faecal carriage of *Ps. aeruginosa* in hospital patients, *Lancet*, 2, 1331–1334, 1966.

69. Lundequist, B., Nord C.E., and Winberg, J., The composition of the fecal microflora in breast-fed and bottle-fed infants from birth to eight weeks, *Acta Paediatr. Scand.*, 74, 45–51, 1985.

70. Ellis-Pegler, R.B., Crabtree, C., and Lambert, H.P., The fecal flora of children in U.K., *J. Hyg.*, 75, 135–142, 1975.

71. Mitsuoka, T. and Kimura, T.N., Die Fakalflora bei Menschen. Zentralbl. Bakteriol. Parasit, *Infekt. Hyg.*, 1 A 226, 469–478, 1973.

72. Gorbach, S.L., Nahas, L., Lerner, P.I., and Weinstein, L., Studies of intestinal microflora, *Gastroenterology*, 53, 845–855, 1967.

73. Drasar, B.S. and Hill, M.J., *Human Intestinal Flora*, Academic Press, New York, 1974.

74. Finegold, S., Sutter, V., and Mathisen, G., Human intestinal microflora in health and disease. Academic Press, London, 1983.

75. Bennet, R. and Nord, C.E., The regulatory and protective role of the normal flora, Stockton Press, Stockholm, 1988.

76. Midtvedt, T., Microbial bile acid transformation, *Am. J. Clin. Nutr.*, 27, 1341–1347, 1974.

77. Midtvedt, T., Intestinal microflora-associated characteristics, *Microecol. Ther.*, 16, 121–130, 1986.

78. Midtvedt, T. and Gustafsson, B.E., Microbial conversion of bilirubin to urobilins *in vitro* and *in vivo*, *Acta Pathol. Microbiol. Scand. Sect. B*, 89, 57–60, 1981.

79. Sadzikowski, M.R., Sperry, J.F., and Wilkins, T.D., Cholesterol reducing bacterium from human feces, *Appl. Environ. Microbiol.*, 34, 355–362, 1977.

80. Bezirtzoglou, E., Norin, E., Chen, J., and Midtvedt, T., Influence of roxithromycin on the fecal excretion of short-chain fatty acids, *Microecol. Ther.*, 23, 106–109, 1995.

81. Bezirtzoglou, E., Norin, E., and Midtvedt, T. Influence of roxithromycin on the fecal tryptic activity, *Microecol. Ther.*, 23, 102–106, 1995.

82. Gustafsson, B.E., Vitamin K deficiency in germfree rats, *Ann. NY Acad. Sci.*, 78, 166–173, 1959.

83. Savage, D.C., Microbial ecology of the gastrointestinal tract, *Ann. Rev. Microbiol.*, 31, 107–133, 1977.

84. Fuller, R., Probiotics in human medicine, *Gut*, 1, 439–449, 1991.

85. McFarland, L.V. and Elmer, G.W., Pharmaceutical probiotics for the treatment of anaerobic and other infections, *Anaerobe*, 3, 73–78, 1997.

86. Tannock, G.W., Molecular assessment of intestinal microflora, *Am. J. Clin. Nutr.*, 73 (2), 410S–414S, 2001.

87. Mahida, Y.R. and Rolfe, V.E., Host bacterial interactions in inflammatory bowel disease, *Clin. Sci.*, 107, 331–341, 2004.

88. Mikelsaar, M., Mandar, R., and Sepp, E., Lactic acid microflora in the human microbial ecosystem, in *Lactic Acid Bacteria*, S. Salminen and A. Von Wright, Eds, Marcel Dekker, New York and Basel, 1988.

89. Lazar, V., Bezirtzoglou, E., Vezyraki, P., Voidarou, C., Tsiotsias, A., Bulai, D., Gernat, R., and Herlea, V., Influence of *L. casei* strains on the adhesion and invasion capacity of some opportunistic bacteria's rain to HeLa cell line, *Microecol. Ther.*, 30, 121–127, 2001.

90. Tsiotsias, A., Voidarou, C., Skoufos, J., Simopoulos, C., Konstadi, M., and Kostakis, D., Stress-induced alterations in intestinal microflora, *Micr. Ecol. Health Dis.*, 16, 28–31, 2004.

91. Konstadi, M., Voidarou, C., Papadaki, E., Tsiotsias, A., Kostovolou, O., and Envangelou, E., Stress modifies the vaginal flora in cyclic female rats, *Micr. Ecol. Health Dis.*, 18, 161–169, 2006.

92. Gaon, D., Garcia, H., Winter, L., Rodriguez, N., Quintas, R., Gonzalez, S., and Oliver, G., Effect of *Lactobacillus* strains and *Saccharomyces boulardii* on persistent diarrhea in children, *Medicina*, 63 (4), 1–10, 2003.

93. Tokai, Y., Effects on caecum content in rats, *Chiba Hyg. Coll. Bull. (Jpn)*, 5, 2–15, 1987.

94. Bezirtzoglou, E. and Romond C., Occurrence of *Lactobacillus* sp. in newborns delivered by caesarean section, *Rev. Med. Microbiol.*, 8, 101–103, 1997.

95. Bezirtzoglou, E., Alexopoulos, A., and Voidarou, C., Apparent antibiotic misuse in environmental ecosystems and food, *Micr. Ecol. Health Dis.*, 20 (4), 197–198, 2008.

96. Ingrassia, I., Leplingard, A., and Darfeuille-Michaud, A., *L. casei* DN-114001 inhibits the ability of adherenr—invasive *E. coli* isolated from Crohn's disease patients to adhere to and to invade intestinal epithelial cells, *Appl. Environ. Microbiol.*, 71 (6), 2880–2887, 2005.

97. Eijsink, V.G., Brurberg, M.B., Middelhoven, P.H., and Nes, I.F., Induction of bacteriocins production in *L. sake* by a secreted peptide, *J. Bacteriol.*, 178 (8), 2232–2237, 1996.

98. Maldonado, A., Jimenez-Diaz, R., and Ruiz-Barba, J.L. Induction of plantaricin production NC8 after coculture with specific G(+) bacteria is mediated by an autoinduction mechanism, *J. Bacteriol.*, 186, 1556–1564, 2004.

99. Williams, C., MacDonald, K., and Mowat, A., Stomach lymphocytes in experimental *Helicobacter* infection, *Adv. Exp. Med. Biol.*, 371B, 927, 1995.

100. Gorbach, S.L., Perturbation of intestinal microflora, *Vet. Hum. Toxicol.*, 35, S15–S23, 1993.

101. Sachs, G., Moo Shin, J., Vagin, O., Munson, K., Weeks, D., Scott, D.R., and Voland, P., Current trends in the treatment of upper gastrointestinal disease, *Baillieres Best Pract. Res. Clin. Gastroenterol.*, 16 (6), 835–849, 2002.

102. Conway, P.L., Microbial ecology of the human large intestine, in *Human Colonic Bacteria: Role in Nutrition, Physiology and Pathology*, G.R. Gibson and G.T. MacFarlane, Eds, pp 1–24, CRC Press, Boca Raton, 1995.

103. Cunningham-Rundles, S. and Ho Lin, D., Nutrition and the immune system of the gut, *Nutrition*, 14 (7/8), 573–579, 1998.

104. Broaddus, R.R. and Castro, G.A., Mast cell-mediated colonic immune function and its inhibition by dietary aspirin in mice infected with *Trichinella spiralis*, *Int. Arch. Allergy Immunol.*, 105, 135, 1994.

105. Fortina, M.G., Nicastro, G., Carminati, D., Neviani, E., and Manachini, P.L., *Lactobacillus helveticus* heterogeneity in natural cheese starters: The diversity in phenotypic characteristics, *J. Appl. Microbiol.*, 84, 72–80, 1998.

106. Luoma, S., Peltoniemi, K., and Joutsjoki, V., Expression of six peptidases from *Lactobacillus helveticus* in *Lactococcus lactis*, *Appl. Environ. Microbiol.*, 67, 1232–1238, 2001.

107. Foucaud, C. and Juillard, V., Accumulation of casein-derived peptides during growth of proteinase-positive strains of *Lactococcus lactis* in milk: Their contribution to subsequent bacterial growth is impaired by their internal transport, *J. Dairy Res.*, 67, 233–240, 2000.

108. Frey, J.P., Marth, E.H., Johnson, M.E., and Olson, N.F., Peptidases and proteases of lactobacilli associated with cheese, *Milchwissenschaft*, 41, 622–627, 1986.
109. Fuller, P., in *Probiotics* 2: *Applications and Practical Aspects*, R. Fuller, Ed., Chapman & Hall, London, 1997.
110. Rastall, R.A., Fuller, R., Gaskins H.R., and Gibson, G.R., Colonic functional foods, in *Functional Foods—Concept to Product*, G.R. Gibson and C.M. Williams, Eds, pp 77, 95, CRC Press, Cambridge, England, 2000.
111. Isolauri, E., Kaila, M., Mukkanen, H., Ling W.H., and Salminen, S., Oral bacteriotherapy for viral gastroenteritis, *Dig. Dis. Sci.*, 39, 2595–2600, 1994.
112. Ouwehand, A., Sutas, Y., Salminen, S., and Isolauri, E., Probiotic therapies: Present and future, *Int. Semin. Paediatr. Gastroenterol. Nutr.*, 7, 7–15, 1998.
113. Mittinen, M., Vuopio-Varkila, J., and Varkila, J., Production of human tumor necrosis factor alpha, interleukin-6 and interleukin-10 is induced by lactic and bacteria, *Infect. Immun.*, 64, 5403–5405, 1996.
114. Schiffrin, E.J., Rochat, F., Link-Amster, H., Aeschlimann J.M., and Donnet-Hughes, A., Immunomodulation of human blood cells following the ingestion of lactic acid bacteria, *J. Dairy Sci.*, 78, 491–497, 1994.
115. Pelto, L., Salminen, S., Lilius E.M., and Isolauri, E., Milk hypersensitivity—key to poorly defined gastrointestinal symptoms in adults, *Allergy*, 53, 307–310, 1998.
116. Neurath, M.F., Fuss, I., Kelsall, B.L., Presky, D.H., Waegell, W., and Strober, W., Experimental granulomatous colitis in mice is abrogated by induction of TGF-β-mediated oral tolerance, *J. Exp. Med.*, 183, 1–12, 1996.
117. Neurath, M.F., Fuss, I., Kelsall, B.L., Stuber, E., and Strober, W., Antibodies to interleukin 12 agrogate established experimental experimental colitis in mice, *J. Exp. Med.*, 182, 1281–1290, 1995.
118. Fiocchi, C., Inflammatory bowel disease: Etiology and pathogenesis, *Gastroenterology*, 115, 182–205, 1998.
119. Cross, M.L., Stevenson M.L., and Gill, H.S., Anti-allergy properties of fermented foods: An important immunoregulatory mechanism of lactic acid bacteria? *Int. Immunopharmacol.*, 1, 891–901, 2001.
120. Vinderola, G., Perdigan, G., Duarte, J., Farnworth, E., and Matar, C., Effects of the oral administration of the exopolysaccharide produced by *Lactobacillus kefiranofaciens* on the gut mucosal immunity, *Cytokine*, 36, 254–260, 2006.
121. Brandtzaeg, P., Bjerke, K., Kett, K., Kvale, D., Rognum T.O., and Scott, H., Production and secretion of immunoglobulins in gastrointestinal tract, *Ann. Allergy*, 59, 21–39, 1987.
122. Husband, A.J., Beagly, K.W., and McGhee, J.R., Mucosal cytokines, in *Mocusal Immunology*, P.L. Ogra, M.E. Lamm, J. Brenenstock, and J.R. McGhee, Eds, pp. 541–557, Academic Press, New York, 1999.
123. De Moreno de LeBlanc, A., Chaves, S., Carmuega, E., Weill, R., Antoine, J., and Perdigon, G., Effect of long-term continuous consumption of fermented milk containing probiotic bacteria on mucosal immunity and the activity of peritoneal macrophages, *Immunobiology*, 213, 97–108, 2008.
124. De Moreno de LeBlanc, A., Matar, C., LeBlanc, N., and Pedrigon, G., Effects of milk fermented by *Lactobacillus helveticus* R389 on a murine breast cancer model, *Breast Cancer Res.*, 7, 477–486, 2005.
125. Vinderola, G., Perdigon, G., Duarte, J., Thangavel, D., Farnworth, E., and Matar, C., Effects of kefir fractions on innate immunity, *Immunobiology*, 211, 149–156, 2006.
126. Roit, I.M. and Delves, P.J., Immunologia. Fundamentos. Editoral Medica Panamericana, Buenos Aires, 2003.
127. Vinderola, G., Matar, C., and Perdigon, G., Milk fermented by *Lactobacillus helveticus* R389 and its non-bacterial fraction confer enhanced protection against *Salmonella enteritidis* serovar Typhimurium infection in mice, *Immunobiology*, 212, 107–118, 2007.

128. Nerstedt, A., Nilsson E.C., Ohlson, K., Hakansson, J., Thomas Svensson, L., Lowendler, B., Sversson U.K., and Mahlapuu, M., Administration of *Lactobacillus* evokes coordinated changes in the intestinal expression profile of genes regulating energy homeostasis and immune phenotype in mice, *Br. J. Nutr.*, 97, 1117–1127, 2007.
129. Czinn, S.J., *Helicobacter pyroli* infection: Detection, investigation and management, *J. Pediatr.*, 146, S21–S26, 2005.
130. Bourke, B., Ceponis, P., Chiba, N., Czinn, S., Ferraro, R., Fischbach, L., Gold, B. et al., Canadian *Helicobacter* Study Group Consensus Conference: Update on the approach to *Helicobacter pyroli* infection in children and adolescents—an evidence-based evaluation, *Can. J. Gastroenterol.*, 19, 399–408, 2005.
131. Elitsur, Y. and Yahar, J., *Helicobacter pyroli* infection in pediatrics, *Helicobacter*, 10 (1), 47–53, 2005.
132. Gotteland, M., Brunser, O., and Cruchet, S., Systematic review: Are probiotics useful in controlling gastric colonization by *Helicobacter pyroli*? *Aliment. Pharmacol. Ther.*, 23, 1077–1086, 2006.
133. Cruchet, S., Obregon, M.C., Salazar, G., Diaz, E., and Gotteland, M., Effect of the ingestion of a dietary product containing *Lactobacillus johnsonii* La1 on *Helicobacter pyroli* colonization in children, *Nutrition*, 19, 716–721, 2003.
134. Ouwehand, A.C., Salminen, S., and Isolauri, E., Probiotics: An overview of beneficial effects, *Anton. Leeuw. Int. J.G.*, 82, 279–289, 2002.
135. Lilly, P.M. and Stillwell, R.H., Probiotics: Growth-promoting factors produced by microorganisms, *Science*, 147, 747–748, 1965.
136. Kaneko, T., Mori, H., Iwata, M., and Meguro, S., Growth stimulation for bifidobacteria produced by *Propionibacterium freudenreichii* and several intestinal bacteria, *J. Dairy Sci.*, 77, 393–404, 1994.
137. Mori, H., Sato, Y., Taketomo, N., Kamiyama, T., Yoshiyama, Y., Meguro, S., Sato, H., and Kaneko, T., Isolation and structural identification of bifidogenic growth stimulator produced by *Propionibacterium freudenreichii*, *J. Dairy Sci.*, 80, 1959–1964, 1997.
138. Isawa, K., Hojo, K., Yoda, N., Kamiyama, T., Makino, S., Saito, M., Sugan, H., et al., Isolation and identification of a new bifidogenic growth stimulator produced by *Propionibacterium freudenreichii* ET-3, *Biosci. Biotechnol. Biochem.*, 66, 679–681, 2002.
139. Satomi, K., Kurihara, H., Isawa, K., Mori, H., and Kaneko, T., Effects of culture-powder of *Propionibacterium freudenreichii* ET-3 on fecal microflora of normal adults, *Biosci. Microfl.*, 18, 27–30, 1999.
140. Hojo, K., Yoda, N., Tsuchita, H., Ohtsu, T., Sehi, K., Taketomo, N., Murayama, T., and Lino, H., Effect on ingested culture of *Propiobacterium freudenreichii* ET-3 on fecal microflora and stool frequency in healthy females, *Biosci. Microfl.*, 21, 115–120, 2002.
141. Bougle, D., Vaghefi-Vaezzadeh, N., Roland, N., Bouvard, G., Arhan, P., Bureau, F., Neuville, D., and Maubois, J.L., Influence of short-chain fatty acids on iron absorption by proximal colon, *Scand. J. Gastroenterol.*, 37, 1008–1011, 2002.
142. Wang, Y., Harrey, C.B., Holloc, E.J., Phillips, A.P., Poulter, M., Clay, P., Walker-Smith, J.A., and Swallow, D.M., The genetically programmed down-regulation of lactase in children, *Gastroenterology*, 114, 1230–1236, 1998.
143. Labayen, I., Forga, L., Gonzalez, A., Lenoir-Wijnkoop, I., Nutr, R., and Martinez, J.A., Relationship between lactose digestion, gastrointestinal transit time and symptoms in lactose malabsorebers after dairy consumption, *Aliment. Pharmacol. Ther.*, 15, 543–549, 2001.
144. Swan, A.D. and Davies, G.J., Lactose in tolerance: Problems in diagnosis and treatment, *J. Clin. Gastroenterol.*, 28, 208–216, 1999.

145. De Vrese, M., Stegelmann, A., Richter, B., Fenselau, S., Laue, C., and Schrezenmeir, J., Probiotics compensation for lactase in sufficiency, *Am. J. Clin. Nutr.*, 73, 421S–429S, 2001.

146. Montalto, M., Curigliano, V., Santoro, L., Vastola, M., Cammarota, G., Manna, R., Gasbarrini, A., and Gasbarrini, G., Management and treatment of lactose malabsorption, *World J. Gastroenterol.*, 12, 187–191, 2006.

147. Jin, Z. and Yang, S.T., Extractive fermentation for enhanced propionic acid production from lactose by *Propionibacterium acidipropionici*, *Biotechnol. Prog.*, 14, 457–465, 1998.

148. Zarate, G., Gonzalez, S., Perez Chaia, A.P., and Gonzalez, S.N., Adhesion of dairy propionibacteria to intestinal epithelial tissue *in vitro* and *in vivo*, *J. Food Protect.*, 65, 534–539, 2002.

149. Zarate, G., Chaia, A.P., Gonzalez, S., and Oliver, G., Viability and beta-galactosidase activity of dairy propionibacteria subjected to digestion by artificial gastric and intestinal fluids, *J. Food Protect.*, 63, 1214–1221, 2000.

150. Perez Chaia, A. and Zarate, G., Dairy propionibacteria from milk or cheese diets remain viable and enhance propionic acid production in the mouse cecum, *Lait*, 85, 85–98, 2005.

151. Lukewille, U. and Uhlig, H.H., Dairy products, probiotics and the health of infants and children, in *Functional Dairy Products*, M. Saarela, Ed., Vol. 2, p. 74, CRC Press, Cambridge, England, 2007.

152. Land, M.H., Rouster-Stevens, K., Woods, C.R., Cannon, M.L., Cnota, J., and Shetty, A.K., *Lactobacillus sepsis* associated with probiotic therapy, *Pediatrics*, 115, 178–181, 2005.

153. Hennequin, C., Kauffmann-Lacroix, C., Jobert, A., Viard J.P., Ricour, C., Jacquemin J.L., and Berche, P., Possible role of catheters in *Saccharomyces boulardii fungemia*, *Eur. J. Clin. Microbiol. Infect. Dis.*, 19, 16–20, 2000.

154. Herbrecht, R. and Nivoix, Y., *Saccharomyces cerevisiae fungemia*: An adverse effect of *Saccharomyces boulardii* probiotic administration, *Clin. Infect. Dis.*, 40, 1635–1637, 2005.

155. Rijnders, B.J., Van Wijngaarden, E., Verwaest, C., and Peetemans, W.E., *Saccharomyces fugemia* complicating *Saccharomyces boulardii* treatment in a non-immunocompromised host, *Intensive Care Med.*, 26, 825, 2000.

156. Dogi, C.A., Maldonado Galdeana, C., and Perdigon, G., Gut immune stimulation by non pathogenic Gram(+) and Gram(–) bacteria. Comparison with a probiotic strain, *Cytokine*, 41, 223–231, 2008.

157. Beachy, E.H., Bacterial adherence: Adhesin-receptor interactions mediating the attachment of bacteria to mucosal surfaces, *J. Infect. Dis.*, 143, 325–345, 1981.

158. Ofek, I. and Sharon, N., Adhesins as lectins: Specificity and role in infection, *Curr. Topics Microbiol. Immunol.*, 151, 91–114, 1990.

159. Karlsson, K.A., Microbial recognition of target-cell glycocojugates, *Curr. Opin. Struct. Biol.*, 5, 622–635, 1995.

160. Kunz, C., Rudloff, S., Baier, W., Klein, N., and Strobel, S., Oligosaccharides in human milk. Structural, functional and metabolic aspects, *Ann. Rev. Nutr.*, 20, 699–722, 2000.

161. Tungland, B.C. and Meyer, P.D., Dietary fiber and human health, *Comp. Rev.Food Sci. Food Saf.*, 2, 73–77, 2002.

162. Martinez-Ferez, A., Rudloff, S., Guadix, A., Henkel C.A., Pahlentz, G., Boza J.J., Guadix E.M., and Kunz, C., Goats' milk as a natural source of lactose-derived oligosaccharides: Isolation by membrane technology, *Int. Dairy J.*, 16, 173–181, 2006.

163. Kunz, C. and Rudloff, S., Review: Health promoting aspects of milk oligosaccharides, *Int. Dairy J.*, 16, 1341–1346, 2006.

164. Paturi, G., Phillips, M., Jones, M., and Kailasapathy, K., Immune enhancing effects of *Lactobacillus acidophilus* LAFTI L10 and *Lactobacillus paracasei* LAFTI L26 in mice, *Int. J. Food Microbiol.*, 115, 115–118, 2007.

165. Mestecky, J. and McGhee, J.R., Immunoglobulin A (IgA): Molecular and cellular interactions involved in IgA biosynthesis and immune response, *Adv. Immunol.*, 40, 153–245, 1987.

166. De Simone, C., Vesely, R., Bianchi-Salvadori, D., and Jirillo, E., The role of probiotics in modulation of the immune system, *Immunotherapy*, 9, 23–28, 1993.

167. Schultz, M., Linde H.J., Lehn, N., Zimmermann, K., Grossmann, J., Falk, W., and Scholmerich, J., Immunomodulatory consequences of oral administration of *Lactobacillus rhamnosus* strain GG in healthy volunteers, *J. Dairy Res.*, 70, 165–173, 2003.

168. Vinderola, G., Matar, C., Palacios, J., and Perdigon, G., Immunomodulation by the nonbacterial fraction of milk fermented by *Lactobacillus helveticus* R389, *Int. J. Food Microbiol.*, 115, 180–186, 2007.

169. Gill, H.S., Doull, F., Rutherfurd, K.J., and Cross, M.L., Immunoregulatory peptides in bovine milk, *Br. J. Nutr.*, 84, S111–S117, 2000.

170. Chinniah, T.B., Pedersen, M., and Jimenez-Flores, R., Effect of whey diets on serum immunoglobulin M levels in mice, *J. Dairy Sci.*, 81 (1), 134, 1997.

171. Bounous, G., Kongshavn, P.A.L., and Gold, P., The immunoenhancing property of dietary whey protein concentrate, *Clin. Invest. Med.*, 12, 343–349, 1988.

172. Zhang, X. and Beynen, A., Lowering effect of dietary milk-whey protein v. casein on plasma and liver cholesterol concentrations in rats, *Br. J. Nutr.*, 70, 139–146, 1993.

173. Hiraoka, Y., Segawa, T., Kuwajima, K., Sugai, S., and Murai, N., α-Lactalbumin: A calcium metalloprotein, *Biochem. Biophys. Res. Commun.*, 95, 1098–1106, 1980.

174. Bernal, V. and Jelen, P., Effect of calcium binding on thermal denaturation of bovine α-lactalbumin, *J. Dairy Sci.*, 67, 2452–2454, 1984.

175. Singh, J., Rivernson, A., Tomita, M., Shimamura, S., Ishibashi, N., and Reddy, B.S., *Bifidobacterium longum*, a lactic acid producing intestinal bacterium inhibits colon cancer and modulates the intermediate biomarkers of colon carcinogenesis, *Carcinogenesis*, 18, 833–841, 1997.

176. Goldin, B.R., Gualtieri, L.J., and Moore, R.P., The effect of *Lactobacillus* GG on the initiation and promotion of DMH-induced intestinal tumours in the rat, *Nutr. Cancer*, 25, 197–204, 1996.

177. Goldin, B.R. and Gorbach, S.L., Effect of *Lactobacillus acidophilus* dietary supplementation on 1,2-dimethylhydrazine-dihydrochloride-induced intestinal cancer in rats, *J. Natl. Cancer Inst.*, 64, 263–265, 1980.

178. Balansky, R., Gyosheva, B., Ganchev, G., Mircheva, Z., Minkova, S., and Georgiev, G., Inhibitory effects of freeze-dried milk fermented by selected *Lactobacillus bulgaricus* strains on carcinogenesis induced by 1,2-dimethylhydrazine in rats and by diethylnitrosamine in hamsters, *Cancer Lett.*, 147, 125–137, 1999.

179. McIntosh, G.H., Royle, P.J., and Playne, M.J., A probiotic strain of *L. acidophilus* reduces DMH induced large intestinal tumors in male Sprague–Dawley rats, *Nutr. Cancer*, 35 (2), 153–159, 1999.

180. Coconnier, M.H., Lievin, V., Hemery, E., and Servin, A.L., Antagonistic activity against *Helicobacter* infection *in vitro* and *in vivo* by the human *Lactobacillus acidophilus* strain LB, *Appl. Environ. Microbiol.*, 64 (11), 4573–4580, 1998.

181. Johnson-Henry, K.C., Mitchell, D.J., Avitzur, Y., Galindo-Mata, E., Jones, N.L., and Sherman, P.M., Probiotics reduce bacterial colonization and gastric inflammation in *H. Pylori* infected mice, *Dig. Dis. Sci.*, 49 (7), 1095–1102, 2004.

182. Brzozowski, T., Konturek, P.C., Mierzwa, M., Drozdowicz, D., Bielanski, W., Kwiecien, S., Konturek, S.J., Pawlik, W.W., and Hahn, E.G., Effect of probiotics and triple eradication therapy on the cyclooxygenase (COX)-2 expression, apoptosis, and functional gastric mucosal impairment in *Helicobacter pylori* infected Mongolian gerbils, *Helicobacter*, 11, 10–20, 2006.

183. Sgouras, D., Maragkoudakis, P., Petraki, K., Martinez-Gonzalez, B., Eriotou, E., Michopoulos, S., Kalantzopoulos, G., Tsakalidou, E., and Mentis, A., *In vitro* and *in vivo* inhibition of *Helicobacter pylori* by *Lactobacillus casei* strain shirota, *Appl. Environ. Microbiol.*, 70, 518–526, 2004.

184. Sgouras, D.N., Panayotopoulou, E.G., Martinez-Gonzalaz, B., Petraki, K., Michopoulos, S., and Mentis, A., *Lactobacillus johnsonii* La1 attenuates *Helicobacter pylori*-associated gastritis and reduces levels of proinflammatory chemokines in C57BL/6 mice, *Clin. Diag. Lab. Immunol.*, 12 (12), 1378–1386, 2005.

185. Fabia, R., Ar'Rajab, A., Johansson, M.L., Willen, R., Andersson, R., Molin, G., and Bengmark, S., The effect of exogenous administration of *Lactobacillus reuteri* R2LC and oat fiber on acetic acid-induced colitis in the rat, *Scand. J. Gastroenterol.*, 28, 155–162, 1993.

186. Holma, R., Salmenpera, P., Lohi, J., Vapaatalo, H., and Korpela, R., Effects of *Lactobacillus rhamnosus* GG and *Lactobacillus reuteri* R2LC on acetic acid-induced colitis in rats, *Scand. J. Gastroenterol.*, 36, 630–635, 2001.

187. Mao, Y., Nobaek, S., Kasravi, B., Adawi, D., Stenram, U., Molin, G., and Jeppsson, B., The effects of *Lactobacillus* strains and oat fiber on methotrexate-induced enterocolitis in rats, *Gastroenterology*, 111, 334–344, 1996.

188. Shibolet, O., Karmeli, F., Eliakim, R., Swennen, E., Brigidi, P., Gionchetti, P., Campieri, M., Morgenstern, S., and Rachmilewitz, D., Variable response to probiotics in two models of experimental colitis in rats, *Inflamm. Bowel Dis.*, 8, 399–406, 2002.

189. McCarthy, J., O'Mahony, L., O'Callaghan, L., Sheil, B., Vaughan, E.E., Fitzsimos, N., Fitsgibbon, J., O'sullivan, G.C., Kiely, B., Collins, J.K., and Shanajan, F., Double blind, placebo controlled trial of two probiotic strains in interleukin 10 knockout mice and mechanistic link with cytokine balance, *Gut*, 52, 975–980, 2003.

190. Sheil, B., MacSharry, J., O'Callaghan, L., O'Riordan, A., Waters, A., Morgan, J., Collins, J.K., O'Mahony, L., and Shanahan, F., Role of interleukin (IL-10) in probiotic-mediated immune modulation: An assessment in wild-type and IL-10 knock-out mice, *Clin. Exp. Immunol.*, 144, 273–280, 2006.

191. Clydesdale, F., A proposal for the establishment of scientific criteria for health claims for functional foods, *Nutr. Rev.*, 55, 413–422, 1997.

192. Bellisle, F., Diplock A.T., and Hornstra, G., Functional food science in Europe, *Br. J. Nutr.*, 80, S3–S4, 1998.

193. Roberfroid, M.B., Concepts and strategy of functional food science: The European perspective, *Am. J. Clin. Nutr.*, 71, 1660S–1664S, 2000.

194. Focareta, A., Paton, J.C., Morona, R., Cook, J., and Paton, A.W., A recombinant probiotic for treatment and prevention of cholera, *Gastroenterol*, 130 (6), 1688–1695, 2006.

195. Agerholm-Larsen, L., Raben, A., Haulrik, N., Hansen, A.S., Manders, M., and Astrup, A., Effect of 8 week intake of probiotic milk products on risk factors for cardiovascular diseases, *Eur. J. Clin. Nutr.*, 54 (4), 288–297, 2000.

196. Hata, Y., Yamamoto, M., Ohni, M., Nakajimi, K., Nakamura, Y., and Takano, T., A placebo controlled study of the effect of sour milk on blood pressure in anti-hypertensive subjects, *Am. J. Clin. Nutr.*, 64, 767–771, 1996.

197. Hayakawa, K., Kimura, M., Kasaha, K., Matsumoto, K., Sansawa, H., and Yamori, Y., Effect of a gamma-aminobutyric acid-enriched dairy product on the blood pressure of spontaneously hypertensive and normotensive Wistar–Kyoto rats, *Br. J. Nutr.*, S92 (3), 411–417, 2004.

198. Mizuno, S., Matsuura, K., Gotou, T., Nishimura, S., Kajimoto, O., Yabune, M., Kajimoto, Y., and Yamamoto, N., Antihypertensive effect of casein hydrolysate in a placebo-controlled study in subjects with high-normal blood pressure and mild hypertension, *Br. J. Nutr.*, 94 (1), 84–91, 2005.

199. Seppo, L., Jauhiainen, T., Poussa, T., and Korpela, R., A fermented milk high in bioactive peptides has a blood pressure-lowering effect in hypertensive subjects, *Am. J. Clin. Nutr.*, 77, 326–330, 2003.
200. Sipola, M., Finckenberg, P., Korpela, R., Vapaatalo, H., and Nurminen, M.L., Effect of longterm intake of milk products on blood pressure in hypertensive rats, *J. Dairy Res.*, 69 (1), 103–111, 2002.
201. Takano, T., Anti-hypertensive activity of fermented dairy products containing biogenic peptides, *Antonie Van Leeuwenhoek*, 82 (1–4), 333–340, 2002.
202. Tuomilehto, J., Lindstrom, J., Hyyrynen, J., Korpela, R., Karhunen, M.L., Mikkola, L., Jauhiainen, T., and Seppo, L., Effect of ingesting sour milk fermented using *Lactobacillus helveticus* bacteria producing tripeptides on blood pressure in subjects with mild hypertension, *J. Hum. Hypertens.*, 18, 795–802, 2004.
203. Flambard, B. and Johansen, E., Developing a functional dairy product: From research on *Lactobacillus helveticus* to industrial application of Cordi-04™ in novel antihypertensive drinking yoghurts, in *Functional Dairy Products*, M. Saarela, Ed., Vol. 2, Chapter 23, pp. 507–508, CRC Press, Cambridge, England, 2007.
204. Ouwehand, A., Kirjavainen, P., Shortt, C., and Salminen, S., Probiotics: Mechanisms and established effects, *Int. Dairy J.*, 9 (1), 43–45, 1999.
205. Borriello, S.P., Hammes, W.P., Holzapfel, W., Marteau, P., Schrezenmeir, J., Vaara, M., and Valtonen, V., Safety of probiotics that contain lactobacilli or bifidobacteria, *Clin. Infect. Dis.*, 36, 775–780, 2003.
206. Klaassens, E.S., de Vos, W.M., and Vaugham, E.E., Molecular approaches to assess the activity and functionality of commensal and ingested bifidobacteria in the human intestinal tract, in *Functional Dairy Products*, M. Saarela, Ed., Vol. 2, Chapter 15, p. 326, CRC Press, Cambridge, England, 2007.
207. Jones, S.E. and Versalovic, J., Genetics and functional genomics of probiotic bacteria: Translation to application, in *Functional Dairy Products*, M. Saarela, Ed., Vol. 2, Chapter 16, p. 353, CRC Press, Cambridge, England, 2007.
208. Sallivan, A., Barkholt, L., and Nord, C.E., *Lactobacillus acidophilus*, *Bifidobacterium lactis* and *Lactobacillus* F19 prevent antibiotic-associated ecological disturbances of *Bacteroides fragilis* in the intestine, *J. Antimicrob. Chemother.*, 52, 308–311, 2003.
209. Dombrowicz, D. and Capron, M., Eosinophils, allergy and parasites, *Curr. Opin. Immunol.*, 13 (6), 716–720, 2001.
210. Hogan, S.P., Mishra, A., Bradt, E.B., Foster, P.S., and Rothernberg, M.E., A critical role for eotaxin in experimental oral antigen-induced eosinophilic gastrointestinal allergy, *Proc. Natl. Acad. Sci. USA*, 97 (12), 6681–6686, 2000.
211. Gordon, C. and Wofsy, D., Effects of recombinant murine tumor necrosis factor-alpha on immune function, *J. Immunol.*, 144 (5), 1753–1758, 1990.
212. Kweon, M.N., Yamamoto, M., Kajiki, M., Takahashi, I., and Kiyono, H., Systemically derived large intestinal CD4(+) Th2 cells play a central role in STAT6-mediated allergic diarrhea, *J. Clin. Invest.*, 106 (2), 199–206, 2000.

13 Application of Functional Dairy Products from IBS to IBD

Tarkan Karakan

CONTENTS

13.1 INTRODUCTION

Probiotics are organisms that provide health benefits as opposed to the pathogens invading gut mucosa. Probiotics have been derived from a wide range of sources including the commensal microbiota of a particular soldier in the World War I trenches, who proved resistant to dysentery (*Escherichia coli* Nissle 1917), neonatal stool (*Bifidobacterium infantis*), and starter cultures for yoghurt (*Bifidobacterium longum*). Typically, 1×10^{10} organisms are given daily with the idea of significantly changing the gut microbiota. An important safety feature is that all probiotics have a short lifespan within the gut and need recurrent dosing to achieve a constant level. Studies measuring fecal probiotics indicated that fecal probiotic microorganisms disappear from the feces after 1 week of cessation of oral intake [1,2]. Prebiotics are an alternative strategy for altering the gut microbiota by providing regular doses of a specific substrate engineered to be readily metabolized by specific desirable bacteria, thereby encouraging their growth. Combinations of prebiotics and probiotics are called "synbiotics."

In order to realize the mechanism of beneficial effects of probiotics, we should first be familiar with the normal microbiota of the gut. The primary defense mechanisms against bacteria are bacteriocidal salivary lysozyme and gastric acid followed by bile salts and Paneth cell-derived defensins that kill most of the bacteria [3]. Therefore, the bacterial density is high in the mouth, up to 10^6 colony-forming units (CFU), and then rapidly falls to nearly zero in the stomach, and gradually increases to 10^1–10^2 CFU in the jejunum and finally reaches back to 10^6 in the distal ileum [4]. In the colon, bacterial density is extremely high, reaching 10^{13}–10^{15}; however, the tight junctions between cells and thick mucous layer prevents bacterial translocation. Furthermore, macrophages and immunocytes in the subepithelium protect bacterial penetration.

Although more than 400 classes of commensal gut bacteria are present, demonstration of each species is extremely difficult due to the different culture medium requirements of each bacterium. Recent advances enabled the documentation of whole microbiota using the culture-independent approach. Extracted DNAs from the feces are used for amplifying DNA sequences coding for 16S ribosomal RNA via polymerase chain reaction (PCR) followed by denaturing gradient gel electrophoresis (DGGE) [5,6]. This has opened new frontiers in the understanding of gut microbiota and related disorders [7].

13.2   IRRITABLE BOWEL SYNDROME AND PROBIOTICS

Irritable bowel syndrome (IBS) is a chronic condition that severely impacts the quality of life of affected individuals [8,9]. The prevalence of IBS in the general population ranges from 3% to 25% [10]. IBS is characterized by intermittent abdominal pain, altered bowel habits (diarrhea and/or constipation), and other gastrointestinal symptoms such as bloating and flatulence in the absence of structural abnormalities in the intestine. The pathophysiology of IBS is multifactorial and may include motor and sensory dysfunction, immune responses, food sensitivities, and genetic predisposition [10,11]. Risk factors include female gender (2–3 times more common), acute gastrointestinal infections (e.g., *Campylobacter* or *Salmonella*), and psychological factors [10,12,13]. As no curative treatments are available, therapy for IBS is palliative and supportive, targeting specific symptoms, but is notoriously unsatisfactory [14,15]. Although 30% of patients report resolution of symptoms within 1 year, nearly 70% report that symptoms recur within 5 years [10].

Probiotics are recently claimed to improve the symptoms of IBS. However, the question of what IBS mechanisms might be influenced by treatment with probiotics should be answered. The mechanisms influenced by probiotics that are of potential relevance to the development of IBS include immune function, motility, and intraluminal milieu.

13.2.1   Immune Function

IBS follows an acute, presumably infectious diarrhea in ~15% of IBS patients. These patients may have a persistent, mild inflammatory state, which may result in changes in mucosal function such as increased mucosal permeability, change in mucosal structure, or increases in serotonin-containing enteroendocrine cells, or infiltration with inflammatory cells in bowel mucosa biopsies [16]. One study showed proximity of mast cells to nerve cells in the lamina propria [17]. The latter cells seem to produce substances that activate receptors involved in visceral sensation such as proteinase-activated receptors (PAR-2) [18,19].

13.2.2 CHANGES IN COLONIC BACTERIAL FLORA

Genomic DNAs examined in 1 g fecal samples of patients with different bowel functions [20] showed lower numbers of *Lactobacillus* species in the samples of patients with the diarrhea-predominant irritable bowel syndrome (IBS-D), whereas increased numbers of *Veillonella* species were detected in those with the constipation-predominant irritable bowel syndrome (IBS-C). In contrast, counts of bifidobacterial species were unaltered. These are intriguing observations given the fact that a therapeutic trial suggests that a particular bfidobacterial species rather than a *Lactobacillus* species was efficacious in the treatment of IBS symptoms.

Colonic bacteria normally metabolize nutrient substrates, reaching the colon with the formation of gas and production of short-chain fatty acids. The latter may induce propulsive contraction [21] and accelerate transit, or enhance fluid and sodium absorption in the colon [22].

Some patients with functional diarrhea show evidence of bile acid malabsorption [23]; di-α-hydroxyl bile acids (chenodeoxycholic and deoxycholic acids) induce colonic secretion [24] or propulsive contractions in the colon [25]. Lactobacilli and bifidobacteria subspecies are able to deconjugate and absorb bile acids [26,27]. This may reduce the bile acid load in the colon and potentially reduce the colonic mucosal secretion of mucin and fluids or the induction of propulsive colonic contractions that may be contributing to the symptoms of patients with functional diarrhea or IBS-D.

13.2.3 EFFECT OF COLONIC TRANSIT ON COLONIC MICROBIOTA

Under physiological circumstances, microbial fermentation is maximal in the right colon and gradually decreases toward the left or distal colon. Diminished available substrate for fermentation at the distal colon or decreased water content of feces may contribute to these metabolic changes. However, stimulation of colonic transit via pharmacological agents such as cisapride causes an increased production of short-chain fatty acids, particularly propionic acid and butyric acid, and an enhancement of the rate of fermentation of a nonstarch polysaccharide fiber [28]. Supplementation of wheat bran or senna further accelerates proximal colonic transit and leads to greater capability of fermentation of resistance starch in the distal colon, generating higher levels of short-chain fatty acids [29,30]. Psychological stress is believed to worsen symptoms of IBS, which is mediated via corticotrophin-releasing peptide and altered autonomic outflow through the brain stem. The resulting acceleration of colonic transit alters microbiota in patients with IBS-D.

13.2.4 IS THERE A PREEXISTING ABNORMAL MICROBIOTA IN IBS?

As mentioned above, colonic transit time and diet-induced changes in the fiber content are related to abnormal microbiota in IBS. Other factors are also described such as episodes of bacterial gastroenteritis or antibiotic-associated microbial changes (depletion of normal anaerobic organisms such as *Bacteroides* spp., *Bifidobacterium* spp., lactobacilli spp., and others). Some patients may benefit from dietary exclusion of poorly absorbed nonstarch polysaccharide together with poorly absorbed di- and/or monosaccharides (e.g., lactulose and fructose) and polyhydric alcohols (sorbitol) [31–33]. Although many patients express a beneficial effect of exclusion-specific foods from diet, no placebo-controlled trial is available. Indirect evidence comes from alteration of breath hydrogen response after such exclusion diets [34].

Conventional techniques (culture-based techniques) were used in many earlier studies in patients with IBS. IBS patients had fewer *Lactobacillus* spp., coliforms, and bifidobacteria spp. [35] and a greater instability of the microbiota [36]. Recent studies using DNA-based techniques also evaluated the temporal changes in microbiota in specific IBS subgroups. Matto et al. compared fecal composition of 21 IBS and 17 controls [37]. Although the proportion of *Bacteroides* spp., *Bifidobacterium* spp., lactobacilli spp., and coliforms were similar, there was a slight increase in total aerobes. More strikingly, there was a greater temporal instability in the bacterial microbiota in IBS patients with 9 out of 21 IBS patients showing PCR-DGGE profiles that were clearly different on different occasions during the 6 month follow-up study, something that was true in only 5 out of 17 controls. Part of this instability was explained by the greater consumption of antibiotics. IBS patients have many nongastrointestinal complaints, which increase the number of doctor visits and antibiotic consumption [38,39]. Antibiotic consumption is a risk factor for developing IBS [40].

Another study investigated IBS subgroups, namely IBS-D and IBS-C. Patients with IBS-D had lower numbers of lactobacilli spp., whereas those with IBS-C had increased amounts of *Veillonella* spp. [41]. However, studies are limited to small groups of patients and new technologies of fecal microbiota measurements are not widely available. Given the heterogeneity of IBS patients, larger studies are needed to determine profiles of microbiota in specific subgroups of IBS patients [42].

13.3 LUMINAL VERSUS MUCOSAL MICROBIOTA

Gastrointestinal microbiota is divided into two distinct subgroups: intraluminal microbiota (bound to foods or liquid feces) and mucosa-associated microbiota (attached to the mucus layer adjacent to the intestinal epithelium). These two ecosystems have their own microenvironment. Luminal microbiota is largely responsible for intraluminal fermentation and related products such as intestinal gas and short-chain fatty acids. However, mucosal microbiota is in close contact with the epithelial immune system and is responsible for many immune-mediated consequences in IBS. Luminal microbiota represents most of the microbiota, and mucosal microbiota is relatively scarce in amount [43].

Mucosa-associated microbiota requires endoscopic and microscopic examination of the gastrointestinal tract. They are bound to the mucus layer containing glycosylated polysaccharides and glycocalyx. The mucus layer contains binding sites for both commensal and pathogenic bacteria, which minimize the adherence of these bacteria to the epithelium below [44]. Studies in healthy volunteers showed that the apical colonic epithelium has scattered contact with bacteria [45]. Only bacteria, which have suitable adhesion proteins, can directly interface with the apical surface [46]. Luminal interaction takes place via pattern-recognition receptors (PRRs) such as toll-like receptors (TLRs). TLRs are expressed on the apical and basolateral surfaces of entero-cytes and on the processes of dendritic cells. Dendritic cells can pass through the tight junctions of enterocytes into the lumen from the lamina propria. Each TLR has a specific ligand, such as lipopolysaccharide (LPS), the epitope for TLR4 [47]. Bacteria can also pass through epithelial layer via M cells, and once they reach the lamina propria, they are presented to dendritic cells and macrophages directly.

The pathogenicity of the bacteria depends on the cytokine response that they generate. For instance, commensal bacteria stimulate dendritic cell IL-10 and transforming growth factor β (TGF-β), which induce tolerance. However, pathogenic bacteria stimulate proinflammatory cytokines and evoke an aggressive response. The disruption of mucosa-associated microbiota might result in upregulation of the immune system [48].

One study examined mucosal microbiota using fluorescent *in situ* hybridization (FISH) [49]. Although the examined IBS patients were the healthy controls of inflammatory bowel disease (IBD) patients, the results were interesting. In comparison with 20 controls, there was a nonsignificant trend toward higher numbers of adherent bacteria ($8.9 \log_{10}$ CFU versus $8.3 \log_{10}$ CFU). The predominant mucosal bacterium in IBS was clostridia and there was less diversity than that of controls.

In conclusion, IBS patients have some differences in colonic microbiota from healthy volunteers and patients with IBD. However, the role of mucosa-associated microbiota is still unclear and further studies are needed to determine the exact role of this microbiota.

13.3.1 CLINICAL TRIALS OF PROBIOTICS IN IBS

Although probiotics are used in antibiotic-associated diarrhea and traveler's diarrhea since the 1990s, studies on IBS are lacking until the last decade [50–52]. The main reason for this discrepancy is the lack of a clear therapeutic target in IBS patients. Although, as mentioned above, there are many changes in microbiota in IBS, which organism is responsible for the harmful effect and which mechanism (inflammation, hypersensitivity, increased fermentation, or colonic transit) is the therapeutic target are still unanswered questions. Disturbed commensal microbiota shows substantial interindividual variability (probiotics might reverse abnormal colonic microbiota; however, many studies lack any confirmation of post-therapy changes in microbiota). Furthermore, IBS patients are a heterogeneous group, which include somatization and anxiety disorders. These differences in patient groups affect the evaluation of symptom-based scores.

Nobaek et al. used *Lactobacillus plantarum*, a bacterium that is commonly found on healthy gut mucosa through the jejunum to the rectum [52] (Table 13.1). *L. plantarum* decreases the number of sulfite-producing clostridia spp. within a week after

TABLE 13.1

Summary of Recent RCTs of Probiotics in IBS

Reference	Probiotic	N	Design	CFU	Weeks	Outcome
Nobaek et al. [52]	L. plantarum 299 V	60	RCT	5×10^7	4	Improved flatulence
Kajander et al. [54]	L. rhamnosus LC705, Bifidobacterium breve Bb99, P. freudenreichii spp. shermanii JS	81	RCT	$8–9 \times 10^9$	24	Reduction in GSS
Guyonnet et al. [55]	Bifidobacterium animalis DN 173 010	274	RCT	1.2×10^{10}	6	Stool frequency increased (IBS-C)
Whorwell et al. [56]	Bifidobacterium infantis 35624 in 3 doses	362	RCT	1×10^6 1×10^8 1×10^{10}	4	Reduction in abdominal pain and GSS
Gawronska et al. [57]	L. rhamnosus GG	37	RCT	1×10^9	4	Reduction in GSS
Kajander et al. [58]	L. rhamnosus LC705, Bifidobacterium breve Bb99, P. freudenreichii spp. shermanii JS	103	RCT	$8–9 \times 10^9$	24	Reduction in GSS
Kim et al. [59]	VSL#3	48	RCT	1×10^{10}	4	Reduction in flatulence
Bausserman and Michail [60]	Lactobacillus GG	50	RCT	1×10^{10}	6	No benefit over placebo
Niv et al. [61]	L. reuteri ATCC 55730	54	RCT	1×10^8	26	No benefit over placebo

O'Mahony et al. [62]	L. salivarius UCC4331, Bifidobacterium infantis 35624	67	RCT	1×10^{10}	8	Bifidobacterium infantis showed significant improvement in GSS over placebo, L. salivarius failed to show benefit
Tsuchiya et al. [63]	L. helveticus, L. acidophilus, Bifidobacterium	68	SB, RCT	1×10^{9}	12	Global assessment 80% versus 10%
Sen et al. [64]	L. plantarum 299 V	12	RCT	1×10^{7}	4	No benefit over placebo
Niedzielin et al. [65]	L. plantarum 299 V	40	OL, RCT	1×10^{7}	4	Pain score reduction in all patients
Drouault-Holowacz et al. [66]	Four strains of lactic acid bacteria	116	DB, RCT	1×10^{10}	4	IBS symptoms were unchanged, abdominal pain decreased
Kim et al. [67]	Bacillus subtilis, Streptococcus faecium (Medilac DS)	40	DB, RCT	?	4	No significant difference in bloating, frequency of gas expulsion, frequency of defecation, and hardness of stool. Abdominal pain decreased
Bittner et al. [68]	29 soil-based microorganisms	25	First period DB-RCT, second period OL	2.4×10^{8}	52	Improvement in subsyndromes

RCT: Randomized controlled trial, SB: single blind, DB: double blind, GSS: global symptom score, OL: open label, IBS-C: constipation-predominant irritable bowel syndrome.

starting intake [53]. The study period was 4 weeks and *L. plantarum* 299 V (10^{10}) was given to 60 patients. The authors reported that improvement was significant in only flatulence, as expected.

Kajander et al. [54] used a combination of probiotics: *Lactobacillus rhamnosus* LC705, *Bifidobacterium breve* Bb99, and *Propionibacterium freudenreichii* spp. *shermanii* JS. Treatment duration was 20 weeks on 86 patients. There was a significant reduction in the global symptom score (GSS).

Guynonnet et al. investigated the effects of *Bifidobacterium animalis* DN 173 010 (fermented milk) on 274 IBS-C patients in a randomized-controlled trial (RCT) [55]. The treatment duration was 6 weeks. They observed significant improvement over the baseline but no benefit over the placebo group.

Whorwell et al. investigated the effects of *Bifidobacterium infantis* 35624 (10^8) on 362 IBS patients in an RCT [56]. The duration of treatment was 4 weeks. They reported reductions in the pain score and the GSS over the placebo.

Gawronska et al. studied a large cohort of patients (children) with functional abdominal pain syndromes [57]. Subgroup analysis of 37 IBS patients treated with *Lactobacillus* GG (10^9) for 4 weeks revealed a GSS of 33% versus 5.1% ($p < 0.04$).

Kajander et al. [58], unlike in their previous study, enrolled a larger cohort (103 patients) and longer treatment period (26 weeks). They used the combination of probiotics, *L. rhamnosus* LC705, *Bifidobacterium breve* Bb99, and *P. freudenreichii* spp. *shermanii* JS. They reported significant reduction in GSS ($p < 0.015$).

Kim et al. [59] investigated the effects of VSL#3 (10^{10}) on 48 patients in an RCT. The duration of treatment was 4 weeks. There was a reduction in flatulence scores; however, they failed to show improvement in bloating scores.

Bausserman and Michail used *Lactobacillus* GG (10^{10}) in 50 IBS patients for 6 weeks. There was no difference in GSS over the placebo (children) [60]. Niv et al. randomized 54 patients to *Lactobacillus reuteri* ATCC 55730 (10^8) for 26 weeks [61]. They failed to show benefit in GSS over the placebo.

O'Mahony et al. investigated the effects of *Bifidobacterium infantis* 35624 (10^{10}), *Lactobacillus salivarius* UCC4331 on 67 patients for 8 weeks [62]. *Bifidobacterium infantis* improved GSS over placebo; however *L. salivarius* had no effect.

Tsuchiya et al. used *Lactobacillus helveticus*, *Lactobacillus acidophilus*, and *Bifidobacterium* (10^9) in 68 patients for a period of 12 weeks [63]. The global assessment score was 80% versus 10% in the treatment and placebo arms, respectively. This was a single-blind, RCT. Sen et al. and Niedzelin et al. used *L. plantarum* 299 V in the amount of 10^7. No effect was detected on GSS. Flatulance was improved only in the second study; however, the placebo response was also augmented in this study (100% versus 55%) [64,65].

In a recent study (double-blind, RCT), 116 patients with IBS were randomized to placebo or a combination of probiotics (10^{10}). One hundred subjects completed the study (48 probiotic combinations and 52 placebos). The probiotic combination was not superior to the placebo in relieving the symptoms of IBS (42.6% versus 42.3% improvement). However, the decrease of abdominal pain between the first and the fourth week of treatment was significantly higher in probiotic-treated patients (−41.9% versus −24.2%, $p = 0.048$). Interesting findings from the IBS subgroups were also observed, such as a lower pain score at end point in patients with alternating bowel habits ($p = 0.023$) and an increase of stool frequency in the constipated subgroup from the first week of probiotic treatment ($p = 0.043$). The probiotic combination was not significantly superior to the placebo in relieving the symptoms of IBS. Despite the apparent high placebo response, interesting findings from IBS subgroups were observed in the field of abdominal pain and stool frequency [66].

Regardless of medical requirements, public consumption of probiotics is progressively increasing. Probiotics are commonly integrated in diary foods. Although there is strong evidence of benefit in probiotic usage for antibiotic-associated diarrhea and traveler's diarrhea, there is relatively weaker evidence on the benefits of probiotic prescription in IBS. The most commonly encountered benefit is improvement of flatulence in IBS patients.

Safety of probiotics is never questioned or suspected until 2008. A Dutch trial, PROPATRIA, showed unexpectedly high mortality in patients with severe acute pancreatitis who had enteral nutrition with multispecies probiotics [69]. Although the study is performed on patients with severe inflammatory response, prolonged administration of probiotics on populations without severe inflammation (such as IBS) should also be carefully observed.

13.4 PROBIOTICS IN IBD

IBDs, which include Crohn's disease (CD) and ulcerative colitis (UC), are chronic relapsing disorders of unknown cause characterized by inflammation of the gastrointestinal tract. The two main conditions are CD and UC, while 10–15% of cases are difficult to distinguish and are given the term "indeterminate colitis" [70,71]. A variety of etiological factors have been linked to CD and UC, including socioeconomic determinants such as smoking, and use of the oral contraceptive pill, but the actual pathogenesis is still not completely understood [72–76]. Whereas UC is mostly limited to the colon, CD can spread from the mouth to the anus. Both conditions may require extensive surgery, for either life-threatening or neoplastic complications. The pathogenesis of IBD involves an interaction between genetically determined host susceptibility, dysregulated immune response, and the enteric microbiota. Host susceptibility is related to genetic polymorphisms in intestinal defense mechanisms (e.g., defensins) or in altered recognition of microbial signals in enterocytes, immune cells, or Paneth cells (e.g., NOD2-CARD15 and TLR4 polymorphisms) [77].

Enteric microbiota is thoroughly studied in IBD patients. It was shown that *Lactobacillus* and bifidobacteria counts are significantly reduced in feces of patients with IBD compared to controls, suggesting that normalization of gut flora is a logical means of treatment [78,79]. Experiments in rodents have demonstrated the potential of this approach, and preliminary studies in humans have been reported [80]. Historical evidence comes from the observations of two very important drugs used for the treatment of IBD: sulfasalazine and its derivative 5-aminosalicylate (5-ASA) had some antibacterial activity. Some of the beneficial effects of these drugs are attributed to their antibacterial activity. It was postulated that the flare of UC and CD might have some connection with intestinal microflora [80].

The chronic inflammation of the gut in patients with IBD seems to be the result of an altered response to endogenous microbiota [81]. Thus, modification of intestinal microflora might have a therapeutic potential in IBD. The human large intestine contains a diverse microbiota composed of several hundred different species and strains of bacteria [82]. The intestinal microbiota plays an important role in host physiology and metabolism [83]. Although the major components of intestinal bacteria are similar in different people, interindividual differences exist at the bacterial species level [84]. The microbiota established after birth is considered essential in priming the immune system during ontogeny, to limit dysfunctional responses. Recent evidence clearly demonstrated that commensal bacteria regulate intestinal development and function, and interruption of these interactions results in pathological features [81]. Gut microflora has several beneficial effects on the health of the intestine. Commensal bacteria maintain a physical barrier against colonization of pathogen bacteria, facilitate digestion of nutrients, and provide immunological surveillance signals at the gut–mucosa lumen interface.

13.4.1 Pathogenesis of Probiotic-Induced Benefit in IBD

Probiotics exert their beneficial effects through different pathways. We can classify these pathogenetic mechanisms into four groups [85]:

- *Inhibition of pathogenic enteric bacterial growth*: Probiotics diminish bacterial adherence to the intestinal epithelium, decrease luminal pH, produce local antibiotic-like substances (bacteriocins), and decrease colonization of pathogenic bacteria.
- *Improvement in epithelial and mucosal barrier function*: Probiotics produce short-chain fatty acids (e.g., butyrate) that are nutrients for enterocytes, enhance mucus production, and increase barrier integrity.
- *Alteration of immunoregulation*: Probiotics favor Th2 cytokine response. They decrease the production of proinflammatory cytokines (IFN-γ, TNF-α, and IL-12) and increase IL-10 and TGF-β.
- *Downregulation of proinflammatory cytokines*: Probiotics inhibit NF-κB activation, modulate PepT1 activity, decrease number of intraepithelial lymphocytes, and modulate TLR9, TLR2 signaling, and alter PPARγ activity.

13.4.2 Clinical Trials of Probiotics in Ulcerative Colitis

Rembacken et al. investigated the effects of *E. coli* Nissle 1917 in patients with UC. The duration of study was 1 year. Induction and maintaining of remission were similar to 5-ASA [86]. Kruis et al. also investigated the effects of *E. coli* Nissle 1917 on 120 patients for a shorter duration of time (12 weeks). Relapse rate of UC was similar to 5-ASA [87]. Venturi et al. and recently Bibiloni et al. investigated VSL#3 in patients with UC in open label trials [88,89]. Both studies indicated a 75–77% remission rate. Kruis et al., using *E. coli* Nissle 1917, found that after 1 year of treatment on 327 patients, 5-ASA is superior to probiotic treatment in maintaining remission in UC [90]. Ishikawa et al. used milk with bifidobacteria for 1 year in UC. Patients on probiotic treatment achieved higher rates of remission over the control group (27%

versus 9%) [91]. Guslandi et al. investigated the role of *Saccharomyces boulardii* for 4 weeks on patients with UC and on treatment with 5-ASA. This was an open trial and 71% of patients have maintained remission [92]. Kato et al. conducted an RCT of bifidobacteria-fermented milk (BFM) supplementation as a dietary adjunct in treating active UC [93]. Twenty patients with mild to moderate, active, UC randomly received 100 mL/day of BFM or placebo for 12 weeks with conventional treatment. The post-treatment endoscopic activity index and histological score were significantly reduced in BFM, but not in the placebo group. Increases in fecal butyrate, propionate, and short-chain fatty acid concentrations were significant in BFM, but not the placebo group.

Probiotics may inhibit potentially pathogenic bacteria such as *Bacteroides vulgatus* in the intestinal flora; however, alternative mechanisms might play a role in the beneficial effects of probiotics, such as modulation of host signaling events that drive the intestinal inflammatory response. In IBD, IL-10 is a cytokine of particular therapeutic interest since it has been shown in animal models that IL-10-deficient mice spontaneously develop intestinal inflammation. IL-10 plays a central role in the control of inflammatory responses to enteric organisms [94–97]. A recent study investigated the anti-inflammatory activity of probiotic bifidobacteria in BFM, which is effective against active UC and exacerbations of UC, and underlying immunoregulatory mechanisms [98]. Peripheral blood mononuclear cells (PBMNC) from UC patients or HT-29 cells were cocultured with heat-killed probiotic bacteria or culture supernatant of *Bifidobacterium breve* strain Yakult (BbrY) or *Bifidobacterium bifidum* strain Yakult (BbiY) to estimate the amount of IL-10 or IL-8 secreted. Both strains of probiotic bifidobacteria contained in the BFM induced IL-10 production in PBMNC from UC patients, although BbrY was more effective than BbiY. Conditioned medium (CM) and DNA of both strains inhibited IL-8 secretion in HT-29 cells stimulated with TNF-α, whereas no such effect was observed with heat-killed bacteria. The inhibitory effect of CM derived from BbiY was greater than that of CM derived from BbrY. DNAs of the two strains had a comparable inhibitory activity against the secretion of IL-8. CM of BbiY induced a repression of IL-8 gene expression with a higher expression of IκB-ζ mRNA 4 h after culture of HT-29 cells compared to that in the absence of CM. The authors concluded that probiotic *Bifidobacterium* strains in BFM enhance IL-10 production in PBMNC and inhibit IL-8 secretion in intestinal epithelial cells, suggesting that BFM has anti-inflammatory effects against UC.

Several studies investigated the role of probiotics in induction of remission in patients with active UC. Mitsuyama et al. studied the efficacy of germinated barley foodstuff (30 g) for 4 weeks in 10 patients in an open label trial. This study found no effect on induction of remission [99]. Tursi et al. compared VSL#3 plus balsalazide (2.25 g) versus balsalazide (4.25 g) plus mesalazine (2.4 g) for 8 weeks on 90 patients in a randomized open label trial. In the study and control groups, 80% and 77% of patients achieved remission, respectively ($p < 0.02$) [100].

In patients with UC, probiotics might provide little benefit in the induction of remission and debate over a matter of safety issues. However, for maintaining remission in patients with UC, data are more solid than the former and larger studies are needed to reach a conclusion. Current algorithms do not mention routine application of probiotics in UC.

13.4.3 Studies Investigating the Role of Probiotics in CD

CD is characterized by transmural inflammation and skip lesions that can spread all along the gastrointestinal tract. Typical features are granuloma, strictures, and fistula. Medical treatment includes 5-ASA, antibiotics (mainly ciprofloxacin and metranidazol), corticosteroids, anti-TNF agents (infliximab and adalimumab), and immunomodulatory agents (azathioprine, 6-mercaptopurine, etc.). Unlike in UC, surgery is not a curative treatment in CD. However, it may be considered in patients with severe complications.

The studies on probiotic usage in CD can be divided into three categories [101]:

1. Probiotic versus placebo
   a. *Outcome defined by Crohn's disease activity index (CDAI)*: There are three studies in this category: *E. coli* Nissle compared to placebo ($p = 0.11$) [102], patients with surgically induced remission receiving *Lactobacillus* GG compared to placebo ($p = 0.59$) [103], and patients with medically induced remission with *Lactobacillus* GG ($p = 0.77$) [104]. None of these studies were able to show the benefit of probiotics over placebo.
   b. *Outcome defined endoscopically*: Only one study investigated whether the probiotic *Lactobacillus* GG alters endoscopical findings [103]. There was no significant change over placebo in terms of endoscopical scores.
2. Probiotic versus maintenance treatment
   a. *Outcome defined by CDAI*: Zocco et al. compared *Lactobacillus* GG versus mesalazine for maintenance treatment of CD [105]. This was a small study and, after 1 year of treatment, *Lactobacillus* GG supplementation was not superior to mesalazine (relative risk: 0.50, 95% CI: 0.18–1.40).
   b. *Outcome defined endoscopically*: Campieri et al. compared VSL#3 over mesalazine for maintaining remission in CD. There was no statistically significant difference between VSL#3 and mesalazine [106].
3. Probiotic plus maintenance therapy versus maintenance treatment alone: This small study (Guslandi et al.) showed that *Lactobacillus* GG has no benefit over standard therapy for the prevention of recurrence in CD [107].

Very few studies focused on the efficacy of probiotics and/or prebiotics in induction of remission in patients with active CD. Malchow et al. studied the effect of *E. coli* Nissle (100 mg) versus placebo on 28 patients for 12 weeks. *E. coli* Nissen had no effect on the induction of remission [108]. Gupta et al. investigated the efficacy of *L. rhamnosus* GG ($>10^{10}$ CFU) for 24 weeks on only four patients. Remission rate was 100% [109]. Finally, Lindsay et al. studied the effect of fructo-oligosaccharide (prebiotic) 15 g/day for 3 weeks on 10 patients. The remission rate was 40% [110].

One of the most popular indications of probiotics in IBD is pouchitis. Pouchitis is the inflammation of the ileoanal pouch (frequently for UC). The etiopathogenesis of pouchitis includes altered microbial flora in the pouch (which is a small intestine ileum) and decreased levels of butyrate (essential nutrient for small intestinal epithelial cells). The most compelling evidence for the use of probiotics in IBD comes from randomized double-blind placebo-controlled trials of VSL#3 (a mixture of four species of lactobacilli, three species of bifidobacteria and *Streptococcus thermophilus*; Vsl Pharmaceuticals Inc., Gaithersburg, MD, USA) in patients with pouchitis. Gionchetti et al. have assessed the efficacy of VSL#3 as a maintenance treatment in 40 patients with chronic relapsing pouchitis after antibiotic-induced remission. After 4 months, fewer relapses were found to occur in the intervention group than in the control group. Moreover, all patients were subsequently found to relapse 3 months after cessation of VSL#3 [111]. The same groups have assessed VSL#3 in the primary prevention of pouchitis in 40 patients following surgery. The incidence of pouchitis was found to be reduced and the quality of life improved in the VSL#3-treated group compared with the placebo group at the end of the intervention period; these beneficial effects were associated with fecal colonization with the probiotics [112]. Finally, a further study (Mimura et al.) has confirmed the effectiveness of VSL#3 as maintenance therapy in patients with recurrent or chronic pouchitis [113]. Importantly, these studies demonstrate high relapse rates of pouchitis in the placebo group, perhaps reflecting intensive patient follow-up, resulting in the detection of relapse that may have otherwise remained subclinical.

In conclusion, probiotics are promising agents in the treatment of patients with UC or CD. The role of probiotics is nearly established in patients with pouchitis. Further studies, including strict patient follow-up, are needed to assess the individual role of certain probiotics in patients with IBD.

REFERENCES

1. Goossens, D., Jonkers, D., Russel, M., Stobberingh, E., Van Den, B.A., and Stockbrugger, R., The effect of *Lactobacillus plantarum* 299v on the bacterial composition and metabolic activity in faeces of healthy volunteers: A placebo-controlled study on the onset and duration of effects, *Aliment. Pharmacol. Ther.*, 18, 495–505, 2003.
2. Alander, M., Satokari, R., Korpela, R., Saxelin, M., Vilpponen-Salmela, T., Mattila-Sandholm, T., and von, W.A., Persistence of colonization of human colonic mucosa by a probiotic strain, *Lactobacillus rhamnosus* GG, after oral consumption, *Appl. Environ. Microbiol.*, 65, 351–354, 1999.
3. Spiller, R., Review article: Probiotics and prebiotics in irritable bowel syndrome, *Aliment. Pharmacol. Ther.*, 28, 385–396, 2008.
4. Posserud, I., Stotzer, P.O., Bjornsson, E., Abrahamsson, H., and Simren, M., Small intestinal bacterial overgrowth in patients with irritable bowel syndrome, *Gut*, 56, 802–808, 2007.
5. Satokari, R.M., Vaughan, E.E., Akkermans, A.D., Saarela, M., and De Vos, W.M., Polymerase chain reaction and denaturing gradient gel electrophoresis monitoring of fecal bifidobacterium populations in a prebiotic and probiotic feeding trial, *Syst. Appl. Microbiol.*, 24, 227–231, 2001.
6. Zoetendal, E.G., Akkermans, A.D., and De Vos, W.M., Temperature gradient gel electrophoresis analysis of 16S rRNA from human fecal samples reveals stable and host-specific communities of active bacteria, *Appl. Environ. Microbiol.*, 64, 3854–3859, 1998.
7. Backhed, F., Ley, R.E., Sonnenburg, J.L., Peterson, D.A., and Gordon, J.I., Host-bacterial mutualism in the human intestine, *Science*, 307, 1915–1920, 2005.
8. Cain, K.C., Headstrom, P., Jarrett, M.E., Motzer, S.A., Park, H., Burr, R.L., Surawicz, C.M., and Heitkemper, M.M., Abdominal pain impacts quality of life in women with irritable bowel syndrome, *Am. J. Gastroenterol.*, 101, 124–132, 2006.

9. Ford, A.C., Forman, D., Bailey, A.G., Axon, A.T., and Moayyedi, P., Initial poor quality of life and new onset of dyspepsia: Results from a longitudinal 10-year follow-up study, *Gut*, 56, 321–327, 2007.

10. Cremonini, F. and Talley, N.J., Irritable bowel syndrome: Epidemiology, natural history, health care seeking and emerging risk factors, *Gastroenterol. Clin. North Am.*, 34, 189–204, 2005.

11. Saito, Y.A., Cremonini, F., and Talley, N.J., Association of the 1438G/A and 102T/C polymorphism of the 5-HT2A receptor gene with irritable bowel syndrome 5-HT2A gene polymorphism in irritable bowel syndrome, *J. Clin. Gastroenterol.*, 39, 835, author reply, 835–836, 2005.

12. Spiller, R., Aziz, Q., Creed, F., Emmanuel, A., Houghton, L., Hungin, P., Jones, R., Kumar, D., Rubin, G., Trudgill, N., and Whorwell, P., Guidelines on the irritable bowel syndrome: Mechanisms and practical management, *Gut*, 56, 1770–1798, 2007.

13. Ruigomez, A., Garcia Rodriguez, L.A., and Panes, J., Risk of irritable bowel syndrome after an episode of bacterial gastroenteritis in general practice: Influence of comorbidities, *Clin. Gastroenterol. Hepatol.*, 5, 465–469, 2007.

14. Agrawal, A. and Whorwell, P.J., Irritable bowel syndrome: Diagnosis and management, *BMJ*, 332, 280–283, 2006.

15. Cremonini, F. and Talley, N.J., Treatments targeting putative mechanisms in irritable bowel syndrome, *Nat. Clin. Pract. Gastroenterol. Hepatol.*, 2, 82–88, 2005.

16. Spiller, R.C., Infection, immune function, and functional gut disorders, *Clin. Gastroenterol. Hepatol.*, 2, 445–455, 2004.

17. Barbara, G., Stanghellini, V., De Giorgio, R., et al., Activated mast cells in proximity to colonic nerves correlate with abdominal pain in irritable bowel syndrome, *Gastroenterology*, 126, 693–702, 2004.

18. Barbara, G., Cremon, C., Vicini, R., et al., Colonic mucosal mast cell mediators from patients with irritable bowel syndrome excite enteric cholinergic motor neurons, *Gastroenterology*, 128, A-58, 2005.

19. Cenac, N., Chapman, K., Andrade-Gordon, P., et al., Role for proteases and protease-activated receptor-2 (par2) in pain associated with irritable bowel syndrome (IBS), *Gastroenterology*, 128, A-14, 2005.

20. Malinen, E., Rinttila, T., Kajander, K., et al., Analysis of the fecal microbiota of irritable bowel syndrome patients and healthy controls with real-time PCR, *Am. J. Gastroenterol.*, 100, 373–382, 2005.

21. Kamath, P.S., Phillips, S.F., O'Connor, M.K., et al., Colonic capacitance and transit in man: Modulation by luminal contents and drugs, *Gut*, 31, 443–449, 1990.

22. Binder, H.J. and Mehta, P., Short-chain fatty acids stimulate active sodium and chloride absorption *in vitro* in the rat distal colon, *Gastroenterology*, 96, 989–996, 1989.

23. Luman, W., Williams, A.J., Merrick, M.V., et al., Idiopathic bile acid malabsorption: Long-term outcome, *Eur. J. Gastroenterol. Hepatol.*, 7, 641–645, 1995.

24. Chadwick, V.S., Gaginella, T.S., Carlson, G.L., et al., Effect of molecular structure on bile acid-induced alterations in absorptive function, permeability, and morphology in the perfused rabbit colon, *J. Lab. Clin. Med.*, 94, 661–674, 1979.

25. Bampton, P.A., Dinning, P.G., Kennedy, M.L., et al., The proximal colonic motor response to rectal mechanical and chemical stimulation, *Am. J. Physiol.*, 282, G443–G449, 2002.

26. Tannock, G., Dashkevicz, M.P., and Feighner, S.D., Lactobacilli and bile salt hydrolase in the murine intestinal tract, *Appl. Environ. Microbiol.*, 55, 1848–1851, 1989.

27. Kurdi, P., Tanaka, H., van Veen, H.W., et al., Cholic acid accumulation and its diminution by short-chain fatty acids in bifidobacteria, *Microbiology*, 149, 2031–2037, 2003.

28. Oufir, L.E., Barry, J.L., Flourie, B., Cherbut, C., Cloarec, D., Bornet, F., and Galmiche, J.P., Relationships between transit time in man and *in vitro* fermentation of dietary fiber by fecal bacteria, *Eur. J. Clin. Nutr.*, 54, 603–609, 2000.

29. Lewis, S.J. and Heaton, K.W., Increasing butyrate concentration in the distal colon by accelerating intestinal transit, *Gut*, 41, 245–251, 1997.

30. Govers, M.J., Gannon, N.J., Dunshea, F.R., Gibson, P.R., and Muir, J.G., Wheat bran affects the site of fermentation of resistant starch and luminal indexes related to colon cancer risk: A study in pigs, *Gut*, 45, 840–847, 1999.

31. Nanda, R., James, R., Smith, H., Dudley, C.R., and Jewell, D.P., Food intolerance and the irritable bowel syndrome, *Gut*, 30, 1099–1104, 1989.

32. Parker, T.J., Naylor, S.J., Riordan, A.M., and Hunter, J.O., Management of patients with food intolerance in irritable bowel syndrome: The development and use of an exclusion diet, *J. Human Nutr. Diet.*, 8, 159–166, 1995.

33. Atkinson, W., Sheldon, T.A., Shaath, N., and Whorwell, P.J., Food elimination based on IgG antibodies in irritable bowel syndrome: A randomised controlled trial, *Gut*, 53, 1459–1464, 2004.

34. King, T.S., Elia, M., and Hunter, J.O., Abnormal colonic fermentation in irritable bowel syndrome, *Lancet*, 352, 1187–1189, 1998.

35. Balsari, A., Ceccarelli, A., and Dubini, F., The fecal microbial population in the irritable bowel syndrome, *Microbiologica*, 5, 185–194, 1982.

36. Bradley, H.K., Wyatt, G.M., Bayliss, C.E., and Hunter, J.O., Instability in the faecal flora of a patient suffering from food-related irritable bowel syndrome, *J. Med. Microbiol.*, 23, 29–32, 1987.

37. Matto, J., Maunuksela, L., Kajander, K., Palva, A., Korpela, R., Kassinen, A., and Saarela, M., Composition and temporal stability of gastrointestinal microbiota in irritable bowel syndrome—a longitudinal study in IBS and control subjects, *FEMS Immunol. Med. Microbiol.*, 43, 213–222, 2005.

38. Thompson, W.G., Heaton, K.W., Smyth, G.T., and Smyth, C., Irritable bowel syndrome in general practice: Prevalence, characteristics, and referral, *Gut*, 46, 78–82, 2000.

39. Mendall, M.A. and Kumar, D., Antibiotic use, childhood affluence and irritable bowel syndrome (IBS), *Eur. J. Gastroenterol. Hepatol.*, 10, 59–62, 1998.

40. Maxwell, P.R., Rink, E., Kumar, D., and Mendall, M.A., Antibiotics increase functional abdominal symptoms, *Am. J. Gastroenterol.*, 97, 104–108, 2002.

41. Malinen, E., Rinttila, T., Kajander, K., Matto, J., Kassinen, A., Krogius, L., Saarela, M., Korpela, R., and Palva, A., Analysis of the fecal microbiota of irritable bowel syndrome patients and healthy controls with real-time PCR, *Am. J. Gastroenterol.*, 100, 373–382, 2005.

42. Kassinen, A., Krogius-Kurikka, L., Makivuokko, H., Rinttila, T., Paulin, L., Corander, J., Malinen, E., Apajalahti, J., and Palva, A., The fecal microbiota of irritable bowel syndrome patients differs significantly from that of healthy subjects, *Gastroenterology*, 133, 24–33, 2007.

43. Macfarlane, S., Hopkins, M.J., and Macfarlane, G.T., Bacterial growth and metabolism on surfaces in the large intestine, *Microbiol. Ecol. Health Dis.*, 12 (Suppl. 2), 64–72, 2000.

44. Magalhaes, J.G., Tattoli, I., and Girardin, S.E., The intestinal epithelial barrier: How to distinguish between the microbial flora and pathogens, *Semin. Immunol.*, 19, 106–115, 2007.

45. Swidsinski, A., Loening-Baucke, V., Theissig, F., et al., Comparative study of the intestinal mucus barrier in normal and inflamed colon, *Gut*, 56, 343–350, 2007.

46. Swidsinski, A., Sydora, B.C., Doerffel, Y., et al., Viscosity gradient within the mucus layer determines the mucosal barrier function and the spatial organization of the intestinal microbiota, *Inflamm. Bowel Dis.*, 13, 963–970, 2007.

47. Furrie, E., Macfarlane, S., Thomson, G., et al., Toll-like receptors-2, -3 and -4 expression patterns on human colon and their regulation by mucosal-associated bacteria, *Immunology*, 115, 565–574, 2005.

48. Hart, A.L., Lammers, K., Brigidi, P., et al., Modulation of human dendritic cell phenotype and function by probiotic bacteria, *Gut*, 53, 1602–1609, 2004.

49. Swidsinski, A., Weber, J., Loening-Baucke, V., et al., Spatial organization and composition of the mucosal flora in patients with inflammatory bowel disease, *J. Clin. Microbiol.*, 43, 3380–3389, 2005.

50. Siitonen, S., Vapaatalo, H., Salminen, S., Gordin, A., Saxelin, M., Wikberg, R., and Kirkkola, A.L., Effect of *Lactobacillus* GG yoghurt in prevention of antibiotic associated diarrhoea, *Ann. Med.*, 22, 57–59, 1990.

51. Oksanen, P.J., Salminen, S., Saxelin, M., Hamalainen, P., Ihantola-Vormisto, A., Muurasniemi-Isoviita, L., Nikkari, S., Oksanen, T., Porsti, I., and Salminen, E., Prevention of travellers' diarrhoea by *Lactobacillus* GG, *Ann. Med.*, 22, 53–56, 1990.

52. Nobaek, S., Johansson, M.L., Molin, G., Ahrne, S., and Jeppsson, B., Alteration of intestinal microflora is associated with reduction in abdominal bloating and pain in patients with irritable bowel syndrome, *Am. J. Gastroenterol.*, 95, 1231–1238, 2000.

53. Johansson, M.L., Nobaek, S., Berggren, A., Nyman, M., Bjorck, I., Ahrne, S., Jeppsson, B., and Molin, G., Survival of *Lactobacillus plantarum* DSM 9843 (299v), and effect on the short-chain fatty acid content of faeces after ingestion of a rose-hip drink with fermented oats, *Int. J. Food Microbiol.*, 42, 29–38, 1998.

54. Kajander, K., Myllyluoma, E., Rajilic-Stojanovic, M., et al., Clinical trial: Multispecies probiotic supplementation alleviates the symptoms of irritable bowel syndrome and stabilizes intestinal microbiota, *Aliment. Pharmacol. Ther.*, 27, 48–57, 2008.

55. Guyonnet, D., Chassany, O., Ducrotte, P., et al., Effect of a fermented milk containing Bifidobacterium animalis DN-173010 on the health-related quality of life and symptoms in irritable bowel syndrome in adults in primary care: A multicentre, randomized, double-blind, controlled trial, *Aliment. Pharmacol. Ther.*, 26, 475–486, 2007.

56. Whorwell, P.J., Altringer, L., Morel, J., et al., Efficacy of an encapsulated probiotic *Bifidobacterium infantis* 35624 in women with irritable bowel syndrome, *Am. J. Gastroenterol.*, 101, 1581–1590, 2006.

57. Gawronska, A., Dziechciarz, P., Horvath, A., et al., A randomized double-blind placebo-controlled trial of *Lactobacillus* GG for abdominal pain disorders in children, *Aliment. Pharmacol. Ther.*, 25, 177–184, 2007.

58. Kajander, K., Hatakka, K., Poussa, T., et al., A probiotic mixture alleviates symptoms in irritable bowel syndrome patients: A controlled 6-month intervention, *Aliment. Pharmacol. Ther.*, 22, 387–394, 2005.

59. Kim, H.J., Vazquez Roque, M.I., Camilleri, M., et al., A randomized controlled trial of a probiotic combination VSL#3 and placebo in irritable bowel syndrome with bloating, *Neurogastroenterol Motil.*, 17, 687–696, 2005.

60. Bausserman, M., and Michail, S., The use of *Lactobacillus* GG in irritable bowel syndrome in children: A double-blind randomized control trial, *J. Pediatr.*, 147, 197–201, 2005.

61. Niv, E., Naftali, T., Hallak, R., et al., The efficacy of *Lactobacillus reuteri* ATCC 55730 in the treatment of patients with irritable bowel syndrome—a double blind, placebo controlled, randomized study, *Clin. Nutr.*, 24, 925–931, 2005.

62. O'Mahony, L., McCarthy, J., Kelly, P., et al., *Lactobacillus* and *Bifidobacterium* in irritable bowel syndrome: Symptom responses and relationship to cytokine profiles, *Gastroenterology*, 128, 541–551, 2005.

63. Tsuchiya, J., Barreto, R., Okura, R., et al., Single-blind follow up study on the effectiveness of a symbiotic preparation in irritable bowel syndrome, *Chin. J. Dig. Dis.*, 5, 169–174, 2004.

64. Sen, S., Mullan, M.M., Parker, T.J., et al., Effect of *Lactobacillus plantarum* 299v on colonic fermentation and symptoms of irritable bowel syndrome, *Dig. Dis. Sci.*, 47, 2615–2620, 2002.

65. Niedzielin, K., Kordecki, H., and Birkenfeld, B., A controlled, double-blind, randomized study on the efficacy of *Lactobacillus plantarum* 299 V in patients with irritable bowel syndrome, *Eur. J. Gastroenterol. Hepatol.*, 13, 1143–1147, 2001.

66. Drouault-Holowacz, S., Bieuvelet, S., Burckel, A., Cazaubiel, M., Dray, X., and Marteau, P., A double blind randomized controlled trial of a probiotic combination in 100 patients with irritable bowel syndrome, *Gastroenterol. Clin. Biol.*, 32, 147–152, 2008.

67. Kim, Y.G., Moon, J.T., Lee, K.M., Chon, N.R., and Park, H., The effects of probiotics on symptoms of irritable bowel syndrome, *Korean J. Gastroenterol.*, 47, 413–419, 2006.

68. Bittner, A.C., Croffut, R.M., Stranahan, M.C., and Yokelson, T.N., Prescript-assist probiotic–prebiotic treatment for irritable bowel syndrome: An open-label, partially controlled, 1-year extension of a previously published controlled clinical trial, *Clin. Ther.*, 29, 1153–1160, 2007.

69. Besselink, M.G., van Santvoort, H.C., Buskens, E., Boermeester, M.A., van Goor, H., Timmerman, H.M., Nieuwenhuijs, V.B., Bollen, T.L., van Ramshorst, B., Witteman, B.J., Rosman, C., Ploeg, R.J., Brink, M.A., Schaapherder, A.F., Dejong, C.H., Wahab, P.J., van Laarhoven, C.J., van der Harst, E., van Eijck, C.H., Cuesta, M.A., Akkermans, L.M., and Gooszen, H.G., Dutch Acute Pancreatitis Study Group. Probiotic prophylaxis in predicted severe acute pancreatitis: A randomised, double-blind, placebo-controlled trial, *Lancet*, 371, 651–659, 2008.

70. Sands, B.E., From symptom to diagnosis: Clinical distinctions among various forms of intestinal inflammation, *Gastroenterology*, 126, 1518–1532, 2004.

71. Gasche, C., Scholmerich, J., Brynskav, J., et al., A simple classification of Crohn's disease: Report of the Working Party for the World Congresses of Gastroenterology, Vienna 1998, *Inflamm. Bowel Dis.*, 6, 8–15, 2000.

72. Lewkonia, R.M., and McConnell, R.B., Progress report. Familial inflammatory bowel disease—heredity or environment? *Gut*, 17, 235–243, 1976.

73. Begleiter, M.L. and Harris, D.J., Familial incidence of Crohn's disease, *Gastroenterology*, 88, 221, 1985.

74. Orholm, M., Munkholm, P., Langholz, E., et al., Familial occurrence of inflammatory bowel disease, *N. Engl. J. Med.*, 324, 84, 1991.

75. Timmer, A., Sutherland, L.R., and Martin, F., Oral contraceptive use and smoking are risk factors for relapse in Crohn's disease. The Canadian Mesalamine for Remission of Crohn's Disease Study Group, *Gastroenterology*, 114, 1143–1150, 1998.

76. Somerville, K.W., Logan RFA, Edmond, M., and Langman MJS. Smoking and Crohn's disease, *Br. Med. J.*, 289, 954–956, 1984.

77. Wehkamp, J., and Stange, E.F., A new look at Crohn's disease: Breakdown of the mucosal antibacterial defense, *Ann. NY Acad. Sci.*, 1072, 321–331, 2006.

78. Bai, A.P. and Ouyang, Q., Probiotics and inflammatory bowel diseases, *Postgrad. Med. J.*, 82, 376–382, 2006.

79. Chermesh, I. and Eliakim, R., Probiotics and the gastrointestinal tract: Where are we in 2005? *World J. Gastroenterol.*, 12, 853–857, 2006.

80. Campieri, M. and Gionchetti, P., Bacteria as the cause of ulcerative colitis, *Gut*, 48, 132–135, 2001.

81. Grangette, C., Nutten, S., Palumbo, E., et al., Enhanced anti-inflammatory capacity of a Lactobacillus planetarium mutant synthesizing modified teichoic acids, *Proc. Natl. Acad. Sci. USA*, 102, 10321–10326, 2005.

82. Macfarlane, S. and Macfarlane, G.T., Bacterial diversity in the large intestine, *Adv. Appl. Microbiol.*, 54, 261–289, 2004.

83. Cummings, J.H. and Macfarlane, G.T., Colonic microflora: Nutrition and health, *Nutrition*, 13, 476–479, 1997.

84. Steed, H., Macfarlane, G.T., and Macfarlane, S., Prebiotics, synbiotics and inflammatory bowel disease, *Mol. Nutr. Food Res.*, 52, 898–905, 2008.

85. Mach, T., Clinical usefulness of probiotics in inflammatory bowel diseases, *J. Physiol. Pharmacol.*, 57 (Suppl. 9), 23–33, 2006.

86. Rembacken, B.J., Snelling, A.M., Hawkey, P.M., Chalmers, D.M., and Axon, A.T., Non-pathogenic Escherichia coli versus mesalazine for the treatment of ulcerative colitis: A randomized trial, *Lancet*, 354, 635–639, 1999.

87. Kruis, W., Schutz, E., Fric, P., Fixa, B., Judmaier, G., and Stolte, M., Double-blind comparison of an oral *Escherichia coli* preparation and mesalazine in maintaining remission of ulcerative colitis, *Aliment. Pharmacol. Ther.*, 11, 853–858, 1997.

88. Venturi, A., Gioncherti, P., Rizzelo, P., et al., Impact on the composition of the faecal flora by a new probiotic preparation: Preliminary data on maintenance treatment of patients with ulcerative colitis, *Aliment. Pharmacal. Ther.*, 13, 1103–1108, 1999.

89. Bibiloni, R., Fedorak, R.N., Tannack, G.W., et al., VSL#3 probiotic-mixture induces remission in patients with active ulcerative colitis, *Am. J. Gastroenterol.*, 100, 1539–1546, 2005.

90. Kruis, W., Fric, P., and Stolte, M., Maintenance of remission in ulcerative colitis is equally effective with *Escherichia coli* Nissle 1917 and with standard mesalamine, *Gastroenterology*, 120 (S1), 73, 2001.

91. Ishikawa, H., Akedo, I., Umesaki, Y., Tanaka, R., Imaoka, A., and Otani, T., Randomized controlled trial on the effect of bifidobacteria-fermented milk on ulcerative colitis, *J. Am. Coll. Nutr.*, 22, 56–63, 2003.

92. Guslandi, M., Giollo, P., and Testoni, P.A., A pilot trial of *Saccharomyces boulardii* in ulcerative colitis, *Eur. J. Gastroenterol. Hepatol.*, 15, 697–698, 2003.

93. Kato, K., Mizuno, S., Umesaki, Y., Ishii, Y., Sugitani, M., Imaoka, A., Otsuka, M., Hasunuma, O., Kurihara, R., Iwasaki, A., and Arakawa, Y., Randomized placebo-controlled trial assessing the effect of bifidobacteria-fermented milk on active ulcerative colitis, *Aliment. Pharmacol. Ther.*, 20, 1133–1141, 2004.

94. Rennick, D.M. and Fort, M.M., Lessons from genetically engineered animal models. XII. IL-10-deficient (IL-10(−/−) mice and intestinal inflammation, *Am. J. Physiol. Gastrointest. Liver Physiol.*, 278, G829–G833, 2000.

95. Asseman, C., Read, S., and Powrie, F., Colitogenic Th1 cells are present in the antigen-experienced T cell pool in normal mice: Control by CD4+ regulatory T cells and IL-10, *J. Immunol.*, 171, 971–978, 2003.

96. Takahashi, I., Matsuda, J., Gapin, L., DeWinter, H., Kai, Y., Tamagawa, H., Kronenberg, M., and Kiyono, H., Colitis-related public T cells are selected in the colonic lamina propria of IL-10-deficient mice, *Clin. Immunol.*, 102, 237–248, 2002.

97. Sydora, B.C., Tavernini, M.M., Wessler, A., Jewell, L.D., and Fedorak, R.N., Lack of interleukin-10 leads to intestinal inflammation, independent of the time at which luminal microbial colonization occurs, *Inflamm. Bowel Dis.*, 9, 87–97, 2003.

98. Imaoka, A., Shima, T., Kato, K., Mizuno, S., Uehara, T., Matsumoto, S., Setoyama, H., Hara, T., and Umesaki, Y., Anti-inflammatory activity of probiotic *Bifidobacterium*: Enhancement of IL-10 production in peripheral blood mononuclear cells from ulcerative colitis patients and inhibition of IL-8 secretion in HT-29 cells, *World J. Gastroenterol.*, 14, 2511–2516, 2008.

99. Mitsuyama, K., Saiki, T., Kanauchi, O., et al., Treatment of ulcerative colitis with germinated barley foodstuff feeding: A pilot study, *Aliment. Pharmacol. Ther.*, 12, 1225–1230, 1998.

100. Tursi, A., Brandimarte, G., Giorgetti, G.M., Forti, G., Modeo, M.E., and Gigliobianco, A., Low-dose balsalazide plus a high-potency probiotic preparation is more effective than balsalazide alone or mesalazine in the treatment of acute mild-to-moderate ulcerative colitis, *Med. Sci. Monit.*, 10, I126–I131, 2004.

101. Rolfe, V.E., Fortun, P.J., Hawkey, C.J., and Bath-Hextall, F., Probiotics for maintenance of remission in Crohn's disease, *Cochrane Database Syst. Rev.*, 4, CD004826, 2006.

102. Malchow, H.A., Crohn's disease and Escherichia coli. A new approach in therapy to maintain remission of colonic Crohn's disease? *J. Clin. Gastroenterol.*, 25, 653–658, 1997.

103. Prantera, C., Scribano, M.L., Falasco, G., Andreoli, A., and Luzi, C., Ineffectiveness of probiotics in preventing recurrence after curative resection for Crohn's disease: A randomised controlled trial with *Lactobacillus* GG, *Gut*, 51, 405–409, 2002.

104. Schultz, M., Timmer, A., Herfarth, H.H., Sartor, R.B., Vanderhoof, J.A., and Rath, H.C., *Lactobacillus* GG in inducing and maintaining remission of Crohn's disease, *BMC Gastroenterol.*, 4, 5, 2004.

105. Zocco, M.A., Zileri Dal Verme, L., Armuzzi, A., et al., Comparison of *Lactobacillus* GG and mesalazine in maintaining remission of ulcerative colitis and Crohn's disease, *Gastroenterology*, 124 (Suppl. 1), A201, 2003.

106. Campieri, M., Rizzello, F., Venturi, A., et al., Combination of antibiotic and probiotic treatment is efficacious in prophylaxis of post-operative recurrance of Crohn's disease: A randomized controlled study versus mezalamine, *Gastroenterology*, 118 (4, Suppl. 2), A781, 2000.

107. Guslandi, M., Mezzi, G., Sorghi, M., and Testoni, P.A., *Saccharomyces boulardii* in maintenance treatment of Crohn's disease, *Dig. Dis. Sci.*, 45, 1462–1464, 2000.

108. Malchow, H.A., Crohn's disease and *Escherichia coli.* A new approach in therapy to maintain remission of colonic Crohn's disease? *J. Clin. Gastroenterol.*, 25, 653–658, 1997.

109. Gupta, P., Andrew, H., Kirschner, B.S., and Guandalini, S., Is *Lactobacillus* GG helpful in children with Crohn's disease? Results of a preliminary, open-label study, *J. Pediatr. Gastroenterol. Nutr.*, 31, 453–457, 2000.

110. Lindsay, J.O., Whelan, K., Stagg, A.J., Gobin, P., Al-Hassi, H.O., Rayment, N., Kamm, M.A., Knight, S.C., and Forbes, A., Clinical, microbiological, and immunological effects of fructo-oligosaccharide in patients with Crohn's disease, *Gut*, 55, 348–355, 2006.

111. Gionchetti, P., Rizzello, F., Venturi, A., Brigidi, P., Matteuzzi, D., Bazzocchi, G., Piggoli, G., Miglioli, M., and Campieri, M., Oral bacteriotherapy as maintenance treatment in patients with chronic pouchitis: A double-blind, placebo-controlled trial, *Gastroenterology*, 119, 305–309, 2000.

112. Gionchetti, P., Rizzello, F., Helwig, U., Venturi, A., Lammers, K.M., Brigidi, P., Vitali, B., Piggoli, G., and Miglioli. M., Campieri M Prophylaxis of pouchitis onset with probiotic therapy: A double-blind, placebo-controlled trial, *Gastroenterology*, 124, 1202–1209, 2003.

113. Mimura, T., Rizzello, F., Helwig, U., Poggioli, G., Schreiber, S., Talbot, I.C., Nicholls, R.J., Gionchetti, P., Campieri, M., and Kamm, M.A., Once daily high dose probiotic therapy (VSL#3) for maintaining remission in recurrent or refractory pouchitis, *Gut*, 53, 108–114, 2004.

14 Functional Dairy Products and Probiotics in Infectious Diseases

Meltem Yalinay Cirak

CONTENTS

14.1 INTRODUCTION

The growing awareness of the relationship between diet and health has led to an increasing demand for food products that support health. Today, probiotic-containing foods are commonly found all over the world. By and large, functional dairy products that contain probiotics comprise fermented milk products or yogurt. The ancient Assyrian word for yogurt, "lebeny," means life. It is interesting to note that the modern word "probiotic" is derived from words meaning "for life" (Greek *pro*: for and *bios*: life).

Generally, probiotics are known as "friendly bacteria" or "good bacteria." Probiotics are defined by the World Health Organization and the Food and Agriculture Organization of the United Nations as "live microorganisms, which, when administered in adequate amounts, confer a health benefit on the host" [1].

Most probiotics are microorganisms known as lactic acid bacteria (LAB) and are normally consumed in the form of yogurt, fermented milks, or other fermented foods [2]. LAB are known to exert a wide range of effects on the immune system, and are defined as "generally recognized as safe" (GRAS). While the most common microorganisms used as probiotics are from the LAB such as lactobacilli, lactococci, and streptococci [3,4], these are not the only good bugs in our gut. *Bifidobacterium* genera [5] and other bacterial genera, including *Enterococcus*, *Streptococcus*, and *Escherichia* [6], and the yeast *Saccharomyces boulardii* [7], are also used as probiotics.

The most popular LAB have a long history of safe use [8]. Almost a century ago, the Russian microbiologist Elie Metchnikoff suggested that consuming the live microbes in fermented milk products may be responsible for the longevity of certain ethnic groups. He credited his relatively long life in part to the lactic bacilli in his diet, and hypothesized, "When people have learnt how to cultivate a suitable flora in the intestines of children as soon as they are weaned from the breast, the normal life may extend to twice my 70 years" [9].

In 1907, Metchnikoff proposed that fermented milk could be used as a source of beneficial lactobacilli and that regular consumption would improve health and prolong life [10]. He began to modify the colonic microflora through ingestion of soured milks like Bulgarian peasants, who consumed large quantities of fermented milk and had longevity [11]. He used a Gram-positive rod, which he called the Bulgarian bacillus and later *Bacillus bulgaricus* [12], which probably became known as *Lactobacillus bulgaricus* and is now called *Lactobacillus delbrueckii* ssp. *bulgaricus*, which together with *Streptococcus thermophilus*, is responsible for the traditional fermentation of milk into yogurt [11]. Up to Metchnikoff's theory of the prolongation of life by lactobacilli in yogurt, probiotic LAB have shown numerous strain-dependent beneficial roles in the protection of host organisms against a wide variety of enteropathogens [13].

These effective microorganisms in foods, especially in dairy products, present a new term "functional food" [14,15]. The term "functional foods" comprises not only some bacterial strains but also products of plant and animal origin containing physiologically active compounds beneficial for human health and reducing the risk of chronic diseases [16]. Among the best-known functional compounds and products, probiotics, prebiotics, and synbiotics should be assumed as examples.

14.1.1 DEFINITIONS

A probiotic has been defined as a live microbial food ingredient that, when ingested in sufficient amounts, exerts beneficial effects on health [17]. In order to consider organisms as probiotics [18,19], it has to be demonstrated that it should (a) be nonpathogenic and nontoxigenic, (b) have a proven beneficial effect on health, (c) protect against pathogenic microorganisms [20–23], (d) be isolated from the same species as its intended host, (e) be able to survive transit of the upper gastrointestinal tract (GIT) [24], (f) adhere to mucus or the intestinal epithelium [25], (g) temporarily colonize sites in the GIT [26,27], and (h) remain viable for a long time.

Prebiotics, on the other hand, have been defined as nonabsorbable food ingredients that promote the growth or activity of a limited number of bacterial species for the benefit of human health [28]. Prebiotics are found naturally in many foods that provide fermentable fiber, and can also be isolated from plants. The most commonly used prebiotics are carbohydrate substrates such as fructans and nonfructan prebiotics like resistant starch [29].

Synbiotics is the word used for the combined administration of probiotic bacteria with prebiotics that support their growth to provide definite health benefits by synergistic action [18].

14.2   MICROBIOTA OF GUT AND PROBIOTICS

Gram-positive cocci and Gram-positive and Gram-negative rods constitute most of the microbiota. It has been estimated that there are at least 20 genera of which 500 different microbial species exist in the GIT [18]. Not only are the vast majority of microorganisms anerobic, but many different species are present in large numbers. The predominant species are streptococci, acid-tolerant lactobacilli, diphtheroids, *Bacteroides*, *Eubacterium*, *Bifidobacterium*, *Fusobacterium*, *Peptostreptococcus*, enterococci, and members of the family *Enterobacteriaceae*. The initial residents of the colon of breast-fed infants are members of the Gram-positive *Bifidobacterium* genus, because human milk contains a disaccharide amino sugar that *Bifidobacterium* species require as a growth factor [30].

Different microbes have been studied as probiotics. Most of the currently available probiotics are LAB such as lactobacilli, lactococci (e.g., *Lactococcus lactis* and *Lactobacillus rhamnosus* GG), streptococci (e.g., *Streptococcus thermophilus*), *Bifidobacterium* species, and the yeast *Saccharomyces boulardii* [31]. Live active cultures in fermented dairy products such as kefir, yogurt, and cheeses are a source of these microorganisms [29]. In probiotic foods and supplements, the bacteria may have been present originally or added during preparation. Probiotics are available in foods and dietary supplements as capsules, tablets, and powders. Currently studies have shown the oral doses of probiotics as 1–10 billion colony-forming units (CFU) per dose, with administration frequency ranging from twice daily to intermittent weekly schedules. Intent of probiotics-like treatment or prophylaxis may have an effect on dosing as well [32].

Starter bacteria used in yogurt cultures include *Lactobacillus delbrueckii* ssp. *bulgaricus* and *Streptococcus thermophilus*; however, it is not clear whether these bacteria are capable of colonization of the human GIT and generally do not reach the GIT in very high numbers. It is believed constant replenishment by periodic ingestion of yogurt might be needed for these bacteria to persist in the GIT [33]. However, as these starter bacteria have been shown to improve lactose digestion in people lacking lactase and have demonstrated some immunity-enhancing effects, they are often considered as "probiotic" [31].

14.3 MECHANISM OF ACTION IN INFECTIOUS DISEASES

Probiotics can affect the host by multiple mechanisms but there are some essential mechanisms in infectious disease:

- Improvement of healthy intestinal microflora
- Prevention of enteric infections
- Stimulation and alteration of the immune system

Improvement of healthy intestinal microflora: Probiotics help normalization of unbalanced microflora and improve healthy gut microflora by specific strains. Fundamentally, this constitutes the rationale of probiotic therapy [18,32].

Prevention of enteric infections: Probiotic microorganisms can block epithelial attachment or invasion by a competitive mechanism and can enhance mucosal barrier function by stimulating mucus production; thus they resist colonization of pathogenic bacteria. Probiotics suppress the growth of pathogens directly by producing bacteriocins or antimicrobial substances, by decreasing luminal pH, or by stimulating defensin production by epithelial cells [11,34–36]. Defensins enhance mucosal barrier function by stimulating the phosphorylation of actinin and occludin in tight junctions or by inhibiting cytokine-induced apoptosis [37,38].

Stimulation and alteration of the immune system: One of the important mechanisms by which probiotics prevent infectious diseases is through stimulation of the immune system by inducing the expression of cytokines IL-10 (interleukin-10) and TGF-β (transforming factor-β). In a study, it was found that *Escherichia coli* and lactobacilli suppress monocyte populations and proinflammatory cytokine expression and increase the anti-inflammatory IL-10 production [39]. Probiotics stimulate secretory IgA production at the same time [36,40]. Moreover, they decrease the production of proinflammatory cytokines such as IFN-γ (interferon-γ), TNF-α (tumor necrosis factor-α), and IL-12 [41–43].

Probiotics enhance host immune mechanisms by strengthening tight junctions between enterocytes and producing metabolically active substances that act as protective nutrients (arginine, glutamine, and short-chain fatty acids) for the gut [44].

14.4 CLINICAL USES OF PROBIOTICS

To date, there have been a large number of publications on probiotics (PubMed search: 4529 papers). In these studies, experimentally or *in vivo*, different health effects of probiotics are mentioned [36,45–48]. Probiotics are basically used for the prevention or treatment of

- Infectious diseases
  - Intestinal infections (diarrheal diseases)
    - Infectious diarrhea (bacterial and viral diarrhea)
    - Antibiotic-associated diarrhea (AAD)
    - Human immunodeficiency virus (HIV) infection-related diarrhea
    - Radiation-induced diarrhea

- ○ *Helicobacter pylori* infections
- ○ Urinary tract infections (UTIs) or female genital tract infections (e.g., bacterial vaginosis)
- ○ Pancreatitis
- ○ Respiratory infections
- ○ Skin infections
- ○ Dental caries and periodontal diseases
- Irritable bowel syndrome
- Inflammatory bowel disease (e.g., ulcerative colitis and Crohn's disease)
- Lactose intolerance
- Pouchitis (a condition that can follow surgery to remove the colon)
- Cancer
- Allergic diseases
- Atopic dermatitis (eczema)

In the scope of this chapter, the importance of probiotics in infectious diseases is reviewed.

14.5 PROBIOTICS IN INFECTIOUS DISEASES

14.5.1 Diarrheal Diseases

Studies concerning the clinical uses of probiotics have been mainly focused on gastrointestinal disorders [44–54]. Probiotics have been demonstrated to be beneficial to infectious (bacterial or viral) diarrhea, AAD, HIV infection-related diarrhea, and radiation-induced diarrhea [11,36,49–55].

14.5.1.1 Infectious Diarrhea

Diarrhea is one of the most common gastrointestinal disorders all over the world. In the developing countries, children are especially affected with 6–12 episodes per year, but in the developed countries elderly and immuno-compromised patients are the targeted group [51]. Not only bacterial (e.g., enterotoxigenic, enteropathogenic, enterohemorrhagic, enteroinvasive, enteroadherent *Escherichia coli*, *Shigella*, *Campylobacter*, and *Clostridium difficile*) but also viral agents (e.g., *rotavirus*) cause infectious diarrhea. Studies about the effects of probiotics on infectious diarrhea are frequently focused on traveler's diarrhea as one of the most common encountered bacterial diarrhea and rotavirus diarrhea as an example of acute viral diarrhea.

Traveler's diarrhea: Traveler's diarrhea is a disease occurring in healthy ones who travel to subtropical and tropical countries. Its incidence is about 20–50% depending on the origin and the destination of the traveler [52]. The most common causative agent is enterotoxigenic *Escherichia coli*. There are multiple studies about the beneficial effects of various probiotics (e.g., *Lactobacillus*, *Bifidobacterium*, *Streptococcus*, and *Saccharomyces*) on traveler's diarrhea [56–58]. Probiotics can prevent or ameliorate diarrhea through their effects on mucosa and the immune system. *Lactobacillus* GG is the most studied bacterial strain.

In a study by Oksanen et al. in which the efficacy of *Lactobacillus* GG strain has been evaluated in 820 persons for preventing diarrhea, no significant difference was found between the incidences of diarrhea in the placebo group (46.5%) and in the patients receiving *Lactobacillus* GG (41%) [56]. On the other hand, a placebo-controlled double-blind study showed that *Lactobacillus* GG reduced the occurrence of traveler's diarrhea by 39.5% [59]. In another similar study on 56 Danish tourists receiving lyophilized LAB, the incidence of diarrhea was 43%, whereas it was 71% in the placebo group [60].

Probiotics has also been examined to have potential to control infections. A meta-analysis based on 23 controlled studies involving 1917 patients deduces that the risk of diarrhea is reduced by 3 days (relative risk 0.66) and the mean duration of diarrhea with 30.5 h [61].

In a very recent experimental molecular study, the attachment of *Escherichia coli* O157:H7 (serotype of enterohemorrhagic *Escherichia coli*) to intestinal epithelial cells was shown to be inhibited significantly by *Lactobacillus acidophilus* A4 and its cell extracts [62].

Saccharomyces cerevisiae is a nonpathogenic yeast used as probiotics other than LAB. Kollaritsch et al. demonstrated the dose-dependent role of *Saccharomyces cerevisiae* in a study group with 1231 people. In this study, infection rates in the groups receiving 250 or 500 mg of *Saccharomyces cerevisiae* were 33.6% and 31.8%, respectively, compared with 42.6% in the placebo group [63].

Rotavirus diarrhea: Acute viral diarrhea is one of the prevalent conditions treated by probiotics. The use of probiotics in the treatment of acute viral diarrhea has been extensively studied by several groups in placebo-controlled studies in both Europe and the United States.

Rotavirus is the leading cause of viral diarrheal illness in infants and children worldwide. Probiotic administration has been decreasing the duration of infectious diarrheal episodes (by an average of 0.7 day) in pediatric inpatients, childcare attendees, and children with rotaviral infections [64–66]. In clinical trials, the probiotics that have been shown to shorten the duration of acute rotavirus diarrhea are *Lactobacillus rhamnosus* GG, *Lactobacillus reuteri*, *Lactobacillus casei*, *Bifidobacterium lactis*, and *Saccharomyces boulardii* [67,68].

Shornikova et al. showed that *Lactobacillus reuteri* can shorten the course of acute diarrhea in infants from 2.5 to 1.5 days [69]. Isolauri et al. demonstrated the effectiveness of *Lactobacillus casei* GG in the treatment of 74 children (aged 4–45 months) with acute diarrhea as well [70]. In a study by Kaila et al., *Lactobacillus casei* ssp. *casei* strain GG (LGG) is found to be most effective on acute rotavirus gastroenteritis duration and shown to be produced the highest titers of IgA antibodies [71].

In a meta-analysis concerning 18 studies by Huang et al. pointed out the coadministration of bacterial probiotic therapy with standard rehydration therapy reduced the duration of diarrhea by approximately 1 day [72].

Rosenfeldt et al. defined the effect of a mixture of two *Lactobacillus* strains, *Lactobacillus rhamnosus* and *Lactobacillus reuteri*; administered twice daily for 5 days to children with acute diarrhea in local daycare centers. The mean duration of diarrhea was reduced by 40 h ($P = 0.05$) in the group treated with *Lactobacillus* strains [73].

The use of *Saccharomyces boulardii* in acute diarrhea was studied in a double-blind placebo-controlled study with 130 pediatric patients (aged 3 months to 3 years). In this study 65 patients were treated with 200 mg of *Saccharomyces boulardii* in group I and the other 65 patients were treated with placebo in group II. After 24 h stool frequency was reduced in group I and after 96 h, the percentage of clinically recovered patients was significantly higher ($P < 0.001$) in *Saccharomyces boulardii*-treated group, 85% compared with 40% in the placebo group [74].

14.5.1.2   Antibiotic-Associated Diarrhea

The administration of antibiotics frequently leads to a mild-to-moderate diarrhea, termed AAD. Approximately 25% cases of AAD episodes involve *Clostridium difficile*.

Probiotics have been evaluated in the treatment and prevention of diarrhea in multiple clinical trials [75–77]. *Lactobacillus* GG produces antimicrobial substances that have a broad spectrum of activity against bacteria, including *C. difficile* [11]. A study by Siitonen et al. showed the efficacy of *Lactobacillus* GG yogurt in preventing AAD. Healthy human volunteers receiving *Lactobacillus* GG yogurt with erythromycin had less diarrhea than those receiving pasteurized yogurt. The subjects receiving *Lactobacillus* GG yogurt were colonized with these bacteria even during erythromycin treatment [78]. *Lactobacillus* GG has been shown to significantly reduce stool frequency and increase stool consistency in children treated with oral antibiotics for common childhood infections [79]. A similar result has been obtained from *Lactobacillus* GG in prevention of nosocomial diarrhea in infants [80] and another study in children reported the success of *Lactobacillus* GG in the treatment of recurrent *C. difficile* diarrhea [81]. In a large randomized controlled trial with *C. difficile*-associated colitis demonstrated that *Saccharomyces boulardii* was able to prevent disease recurrence in elderly patients who had more than one *C. difficile* sequential infection [82]. On the contrary, a systematic review pointed out the fact that the data are inadequate to justify probiotics as treatment for *C. difficile* diarrhea in adults [83].

Furthermore, total flora replacement (TFR) or fecal bacteriotherapy has been reported as an alternative treatment in severe *C. difficile* infections. It is based on transfer of fecal flora from a healthy individual, often a close relative, to a severely sick patient [18]. TFR has been used in 84 patients: 36 with *C. difficile*-associated diarrhea, 22 with *C. difficile* colitis, and 26 with pseudomembranous colitis [51,84]. 72/84 patients (86%) showed immediate resolution of the problems. Long-term cure is reported to have been achieved with a single-shot treatment in 33/36 patients (92%).

Besides the use of probiotics in treatment due to AAD, there are several studies concerning their effect in prevention of diarrhea. In two meta-analyses by Cremonini et al. and D'souza et al., probiotics treatment in prevention of AAD has been demonstrated with an odds ratio of 0.39 and 0.37, respectively [76,77]. A placebo-controlled randomized study evaluating the efficacy of *Lactobacillus* GG therapy in preventing AAD in hospitalized infants and children receiving intravenous antibiotic therapy by Shane demonstrated a benefit in reduction of diarrhea incidence [48]. In another controlled clinical trial with 740 patients undergoing cataract surgery showed that

13% of patients had diarrhea receiving antibiotics alone where the incidence of diarrhea was 0% in the patients receiving antibiotics plus *Lactobacillus* [85]. *Saccharomyces boulardii* is used in prevention of AAD as well. In a study by McFarland et al. with 193 patients receiving a broad spectrum β-lactam antibiotic, the incidence of developing diarrhea was 14.6% in the placebo group while 7.2% of those patients receiving *Saccharomyces boulardii* had no diarrheal symptoms at all [86].

Mixture of probiotics has been shown to be beneficial reducing the incidence of diarrhea in AAD. Seventy-nine hospitalized patients on treatment with ampicillin were given a mixture of *Lactobacillus acidophilus* and *Lactobacillus bulgaricus* or a placebo and 14% of patients in the control group developed diarrhea while no patients treated with lactobacilli had diarrhea [87]. In another study using a mixture of probiotics *Lactobacillus acidophilus* and *Bifidobacterium bifidum* (1.8×10^9 cfu/day) in 19 infants treated with ampicillin, the number of lactobacilli was observed to be increased significantly following the normalization of the microflora [88].

Although some authors have opposed to use of *Enterococcus faecium* as a probiotic from the point of view of safety as *Enterococcus faecium* is an important cause of dangerous infections and can contain genetic material for multiple antibiotic resistance, there are studies related to effect of this bacteria in prevention of AAD. In one of these studies, *Enterococcus faecium* SF 68 was given to 45 patients receiving a 7-day course of prophylactic antibiotics, in this group 8.7% developed diarrhea compared with 27.2% in the placebo group [89]. In another study in pediatric patients, one group of patients with diarrhea was given *Enterococcus faecium* (3×10^7 cfu) and the other group a mixture of *Lactobacillus acidophilus* (5×10^8 cfu), *Lactobacillus bulgaricus* (4×10^9 cfu), and *Streptococcus lactis* (4×10^9 cfu). Among all these study groups, the results demonstrated that the duration of diarrhea was shorter in the group treated with *Enterococcus faecium* [90].

Sullivan et al. studied the mechanism of probiotic effect in AAD and probiotics have been shown to prevent antibiotic-induced changes in *Bacteriodes fragilis* microflora cultured from human feces [91].

For further clinical studies related to AAD, Szajewska et al. [92] underlined the importance of [55]

- The identification of populations at high risk of AAD who would benefit most from probiotic therapy
- The evaluation of the efficacy of probiotics in preventing AAD caused by *C. difficile*
- The determination of the most effective dosing schedule
- Addressing the cost effectiveness of using probiotics to prevent AAD in children

The effectiveness of probiotics for the treatment and prevention of infectious and AAD is best documented and these studies show that patients would benefit from prophylactic probiotic therapy. However, all the criteria mentioned by Szajewska et al. must be taken into consideration for future clinical trials.

14.5.1.3 HIV Infection-Related Diarrhea

In HIV infection, diarrhea with unknown etiology can accompany and there are no effective treatment modalities [52]. In studies, *Saccharomyces boulardii* is the probiotic used for treatment of HIV-related diarrhea. In double-blind studies by Born et al. and Saint-Marc et al., *Saccharomyces boulardii* was used to treat 33 HIV patients with chronic diarrhea [93,94]. Fifty-six percent of patients receiving *Saccharomyces boulardii* had resolution of diarrhea compared with 9% of patients receiving placebo. In another study by Elmer et al., high doses of *Saccharomyces boulardii* reported to be effective in some patients with HIV-related chronic diarrhea [95]; however, further studies are required before firm conclusions can be drawn.

14.5.1.4 Radiation-Induced Diarrhea

Radiotherapy to abdominal, pelvic, lumbar, or para-aortic fields for pelvic malignancies causes chronic radiation damage to the gut in approximately 5% of patients. The clinical presentation varies from mild disease to debilitating rectal bleeding, diarrhea, obstruction, and fistula formation. Acute diarrhea is a common complication in cancer patients treated with radiotherapy [96].

A probiotic preparation, VSL#3 (VSL Pharmaceuticals, Fort Lauderdale, MD, USA) containing eight different probiotics (*Lactobacillus casei*, *Lactobacillus plantarum*, *Lactobacillus acidophilus*, *Lactobacillus delbruekii* ssp. *bulgaricus*, *Bifidobacterium longum*, *Bifidobacterium breve*, *Bifidobacterium infantis*, and *Streptococcus salivarius* ssp. *thermophilus*) has been evaluated for the prevention of radiation-induced diarrhea effect in patients undergoing pelvic radiation. Fifty-five percent of the patients developed more severe radiation-induced diarrhea in the placebo group compared with 38% of patients receiving VSL#3 [97].

In another study, the efficacy of *Lactobacillus rhamnosus* (*Antibiophilus*) in patients suffering from mild-to-moderate diarrhea induced by radiation therapy was evaluated. Statistical analysis of the patients' self-ratings with regard to diarrhea grade and feces consistency showed a statistically highly significant treatment-by-time interaction ($P < 0.001$) compared with the group receiving the active probiotic and placebo [98].

14.5.2 *H. pylori* Infections

H. pylori infection is a worldwide chronic bacterial infection and is associated with gastritis, gastroduodenal ulcers, gastric adenocarcinoma, lymphoma, and a number of nongastrointestinal disorders.

The internationally recommended eradication therapy for *H. pylori* infection is a bismuth-based quadruple drug regimen consisting of a proton pump inhibitor (PPI), bismuth salt, metronidazole, and tetracycline for a minimum of 7 days [99,100]. Major causes of bismuth-based quadruple therapy failure are antibiotic resistance and noncompliance [101].

The role of probiotics in the treatment of *H. pylori* infection is increasingly documented as a complement or alternative to antibiotics, and thus having the potential to decrease the use of antibiotics [102]. In clinical studies and experimental models, several probiotics have been studied, for example, *Lactobacillus acidophilus, Lactobacillus gasseri, Lactobacillus johnsonii, Lactobacillus rhamnosus, Lactobacillus casei, Lactobacillus reuteri, Saccharomyces boulardii*, and *Bifidobacterium lactis* [76,102–112]. These probiotics either improve the eradication rate by suppressing the growth of *H. pylori* and reducing gastric inflammation or alleviate the adverse effects of the anti-*Helicobacter* treatment. Some of these lactobacillus strains have the ability to tolerate low pH and survive and grow in the hostile environment of the stomach; by this way they could prevent overgrowth of *H. pylori* [113].

Clarithromycin resistance is an important obstacle in the treatment of *H. pylori* infection. Ushiyama et al. demonstrated the complementary effect of probiotics in clarithromycin-resistant *H. pylori* strains as well [114]. This study suggests that *Lactobacillus gasseri* inhibited not only the *in vitro* growth of clarithromycin-resistant *H. pylori* and the release of IL-8 from epithelial cells, but also *H. pylori* colonization in an *in vivo* mouse model.

In studies, generally probiotics have been used as a complement to antibiotics. A study by Canducci et al. showed the role of *Lactobacillus acidophilus* LB in improving the eradication rate in *Helicobacter* treatment [105]. Kim et al. evaluated the addition of probiotics to PPI-based triple therapy in the eradication rate of *H. pylori* [115]. In 347 *H. pylori*-infected patients, 168 were given yogurt with triple therapy where 179 received only triple therapy. The eradication rate in the yogurt group, 87.5% (133 of 152) was higher than that in the control group, 78.7% (129 of 164) ($P = 0.037$), but there was no reduction in the side effects. In the studies using different probiotics other than *Lactobacillus rhamnosus* GG such as *Saccharomyces boulardii, Lactobacillus reuteri*, and a combination of *Lactobacillus acidophilus* and *Bifidobacterium lactis*, adverse effects were reported to be decreased as well.

In another study, Sheu et al. pointed out the role of *Lactobacillus acidophilus* La5 and *Bifidobacterium lactis* Bb12 containing yogurt not only in increasing the eradication rate but also decreasing several side effects of the triple therapy [111].

Furthermore, Myllyluoma et al. suggested that the regular intake of probiotics does not eradicate *H. pylori*, but could be considered as an adjuvant to the conventional antibiotic therapy and the effects of probiotics are explained due to their indirect immunomodulating properties and ability to survive in the GIT despite the intensive antimicrobial therapy [116].

In their latest *in vitro* study, Myllyluoma et al. demonstrated the difference in the mechanism of probiotics alone and in combination; four probiotics (*Lactobacillus rhamnosus* GG, *Lactobacillus rhamnosus* Lc705, *Propionibacterium freudenreichii* subsp. *shermanii* Js, and *Bifidobacterium breve* Bb99) and their combination in terms of pathogen adhesion, barrier function, cell death, and inflammatory response in *H. pylori*-infected epithelial cells were tested. The anti-inflammatory effects of probiotics are found to be not persistent when they are used in combination and they suggest that the therapeutic response can be optimized if probiotic strains are characterized before using in combination [117].

In some other clinical trials, probiotics have been tested as an alternative to antimicrobials. In different studies, the regular intake of fermented milk or yogurt-containing strains of *Lactobacillus acidophilus* (*johnsonii*) La1, *Lactobacillus acidophilus* La5, or *Bifidobacterium lactis* Bb12 has been shown to cause a decrease in *H. pylori* infection-associated inflammation; however, they did not eradicate *H. pylori* in any of these studies [118–123].

Taken together, these studies suggest that consumption of probiotics may be beneficial in combating *H. pylori* infection as a complement to the first-line or the second-line eradication therapy. Probiotics have been committed to increase the efficacy of eradication therapy and prevent antibiotic-associated gastrointestinal side effects. Without antimicrobials, using probiotics as an alternative seems to be unsuccessful though probiotics have some potential in the suppression of *H. pylori* infection.

14.5.3 NECROTIZING ENTEROCOLITIS

Breast-feeding is important for the protection of infants from infectious disease and has an effect in modulating the composition of the intestinal flora. The GIT of healthy infants is colonized by nonpathologic bacteria such as lactobacilli and bifidobacteria. On the other hand, preterm infants develop a different bowel colonization pattern and this may contribute to the development of necrotizing enterocolitis (NEC), which is one of the devastating intestinal disorders. NEC occurs in 10–25% of premature infants and very-low-birth-weight babies and has a high mortality of 20–30% [18,124].

The proactive colonization of preterm infants using probiotic supplements such as *Lactobacillus acidophilus* and *Bifidobacterium infantis* is hypothesized to help decrease the incidence of NEC.

Although clinical trials have been shown to reduce the incidence and severity of NEC in premature infants given supplements of probiotics, further studies are needed before firm conclusions can be drawn [125,126].

14.5.4 URINARY TRACT INFECTIONS OR FEMALE GENITAL TRACT INFECTIONS

Recurrent UTIs, bacterial vaginosis, and yeast vaginitis are common urogenital problems. Lactobacilli dominate in normal vaginal flora of premenopausal women and unstable vaginal flora may cause vaginal infections. There are several studies concerning the beneficial effects of *Lactobacillus* species in the prevention and treatment of recurrent UTIs and resolution of bacterial vaginosis in women. The production of lactic acid and H_2O_2 is an important characteristic of bacteria that are beneficial for urogenital health [127,128].

Different randomized controlled studies by Reid et al. suggest that once weekly vaginal capsules of freeze-dried *Lactobacillus* strains GR-1 and B-54 [129] prepared with the addition of skim milk, and once daily oral capsule use of *Lactobacillus* strains GR-1 and RC-14 [130] can restore and maintain a normal urogenital flora and lower risk of UTI. Falagas et al. also mentioned the role of lactobacilli for the prevention of recurrent UTIs [131].

The effectiveness of lactobacilli in the treatment of bacterial vaginosis accompanying sexually transmitted disease, especially HIV infection, is demonstrated as well. The treatment and prevention of bacterial vaginosis by means of vaginal lactobacilli have been shown to reduce the risk of acquiring HIV-1, gonorrhea, and trichomoniasis [132–134].

14.5.5 PANCREATITIS

Severe acute pancreatitis is a very important cause of morbidity and mortality inside the context of gastrointestinal diseases. Microbial infection of the pancreatic tissue in patients with severe acute pancreatitis aggravates the disease. Colonization of the lower GIT and oropharynx with Gram-negative and Gram-positive bacteria precedes contamination of the pancreas [135]. In acute pancreatitis, there are some clinical trials with probiotics.

In a randomized double-masked study by Oláh et al., LAB was shown to be effective in reducing pancreatic sepsis by using *Lactobacillus plantarum* 299. Live and heat-killed *Lactobacillus plantarum* 299 were compared in 45 patients and significantly lower rates of infection were detected in the groups treated with the live probiotic ($P = 0.023$) [135]. Additionally, there was a trend toward a shorter mean length of stay in the live (13.7 days) versus the killed *Lactobacillus* group (21.4 days). Similar results were obtained by Pezzilli and Fantini and in animal models of acute pancreatitis in which intestinal microbial translocation was reduced as well [136,137]. On the contrary, Besselink et al. demonstrated that supplemental probiotics did not reduce the risk of infectious complications and was associated with an increased risk of mortality in a total of 296 patients with predicted severe acute pancreatitis [138]. However, the combination of probiotic strains administered is a very important component and in the latest study it was different from the other studies.

Finally, the evaluation of the effect of probiotics in acute pancreatitis has been obtained by a meta-analysis [139]. Sun et al. did a meta-analysis of randomized controlled trials with totally 428 patients including four studies by Oláh et al. [135], Oláh et al. [140], Li et al. [141], and Besselink et al. [138]. The results obtained from these studies showed that using probiotics could not reduce the risk of infection pancreatic necrosis [odds ratio (OR) = 0.56, 95% confidence intervals (CI) [0.13, 2.35]]. There is no significant difference between the two groups in mortality (OR = 0.83, 95% CI [0.14, 4.83]), the mean duration of hospital [weighted mean difference (WMD) = −1.20, 95% CI [−13.13, 10.92]], and the required operation (OR = 0.59, 95% CI [0.11, 3.07]). According to the results of the meta-analysis, enteral feeding with probiotic has been evaluated as not to reduce the infected necrosis and mortality. It seems that further large-scale, high-quality, placebo-controlled double-blind trials will better clarify the results.

14.5.6 OTHER INFECTIONS

The prophylactic use of probiotic bacteria has also been encountered in infections such as respiratory infections, dental carries, and to a lesser extent skin infections.

In common childhood infections, concerning the antibiotic resistance, there is an increased interest in alternative approaches for controlling infections [142]. A number of relevant preliminary trials suggest that in the upper respiratory tract the rate of recurrence of otitis media or streptococcal pharyngotonsillitis appears to decrease using selected bacteria with inhibitory ability against common pathogens of the upper respiratory tract in combination with appropriate antibiotic treatment [143,144]. In these studies, the results demonstrate that a regular, long-term intake of various synbiotics may improve health by reducing the incidence and severity of respiratory diseases during the cold season.

A study by de Vrese et al. investigated the effect of long-term consumption of the probiotic bacteria lactobacilli and bifidobacteria on viral respiratory tract infections (common cold and influenza) [145]. This randomized, double-blind, controlled intervention study including 479 healthy adults was performed during two winter/spring periods. The intake of the probiotic has been found to have no effect on the incidence of common cold infections, but to significantly shorten the duration of episodes by almost 2 days ($P = 0.045$), reduce the severity of symptoms, and lead to larger increases in cytotoxic T and T-suppressor cell counts and in T-helper cell counts.

On the other hand, Hatakka et al. showed that probiotics did not prevent the occurrence of acute otitis media or the nasopharyngeal carriage of otitis pathogens in otitis-prone children [146]. These accumulating data point out the need for further studies to confirm the tendency of showing a reduction in recurrent respiratory infections.

Dental caries is one of the most prevalent diseases in humans. The changes in the homeostasis of the oral cavity with an overgrowth of *Streptococcus mutans* is recognized as the primary cause of the disease [147]. The probiotic concept has also promising results in the prevention of dental caries. The probiotic properties of oral lactobacilli to combat oral diseases are conspicuous. In a number of studies, it has been suggested that lactobacilli-derived probiotics in dairy products may affect oral ecology. Being able to become a part of the supragingival dental biofilm and to compete with cariogenic microorganisms are the most mentioned properties [148–154]. Among these bacteria not only lactobacilli such as *Lactobacillus plantarum*, *Lactobacillus paracasei*, *Lactobacillus salivarius*, and *Lactobacillus rhamnosus* but also *Bifidobacterium lactis* have been shown to have the potential to be used as probiotics for oral health [148,149,153,154]. The majority of these strains suppress the growth of oral pathogenic bacteria such as mainly *Streptococcus mutans*, *Aggregatibacter actinomycetemcomitans*, *Porphyromonas gingivalis*, and *Prevotella intermedia* [148–150,153].

Dairy products supplemented with probiotics may be beneficial especially in childhood and young adults. For instance, in a study with daily consumption of ice cream containing probiotic bifidobacteria [149] and another study with milk containing *Lactobacillus rhamnosus* GG, the salivary levels of mutans streptococci have been found to decrease in young adults and children, respectively [155].

Bacteriotherapy in the form of probiotic bacteria with an inhibitory effect on oral pathogens is a promising concept, especially in childhood, but further placebo-controlled trials that assess carefully selected and defined probiotic strains using standardized outcomes are needed before any clinical recommendations can be made [151].

Finally, there are some clinical trials related to skin infections such as wound treatment and atopic dermatitis [156,157]. Inhibition of the pathogenic activity of *Pseudomonas aeruginosa* using *Lactobacillus plantarum* was demonstrated *in vitro* and *in vivo* by using a burned-mouse model in which burns infected with *Pseudomonas aeruginosa* were treated with *Lactobacillus plantarum* at 3, 4, 5, 7, and 9 days postinfection [156]. The improvement in tissue repair, enhancement of phagocytosis of *Pseudomonas aeruginosa* by tissue phagocytes, and a decrease in apoptosis at 10 days indicated the potential therapeutic role of *Lactobacillus plantarum* in the local treatment of *Pseudomonas aeruginosa* burn infections. There are also individual benefits in the prevention and treatment of atopic dermatitis in children with supplementary probiotics [157]. These are attractive studies, but the role of probiotics in skin infections needs to be validated in large cohort studies.

14.6   SAFETY

The oral consumption of viable bacteria is relatively safe but probiotics are potentially pathogenic. As a matter of fact, probiotics might cause unhealthy metabolic activities, too much stimulation of the immune system, or gene transfer (insertion of genetic material into a cell).

However, cases of infection caused by *Lactobacillus* and *Bifidobacterium* organisms are extremely rare and are estimated to occur at a rate of ~0.05–0.4% of all cases of infective endocarditis and bacteraemia [44,158].

Saccharomyces infections have been reported as fungemiae in four immunosuppressed patients who had indwelling catheters [159–161] and exacerbation of diarrhea in two patients with ulcerative colitis [162] who consumed *Saccharomyces boulardii.*

Lactobacillus bacteraemia and *Saccharomyces fungemia* are considered to be of clinical significance and the predisposing factors can be defined as immunosuppressive, prior prolonged hospitalization and surgical interventions [163]. Therefore, probiotics are not recommended to be given to those patients who are at increased risk of translocation-related problems (e.g., central venous catheters and artificial heart valves), those at high risk of developing sepsis (e.g., immunosuppressed patients having low white blood cell count), premature neonates, or those with bowel immortility problems (e.g., using D-lactic acid-producing probiotics) [55].

No serious adverse effects have been reported with the products containing lactobacilli and bifidobacteria in infants and children [158]. Nevertheless, safety assessment should be performed in clinical trials for firm results.

14.7   CONCLUSION

Probiotic microorganisms are found in large quantities in various functional dairy products. Proper use of probiotics represents a potentially beneficial adjunct to other proven therapies. Clinical trials related to the use of probiotics in infectious disease have promising results mainly in gastrointestinal diseases. Studies for understanding the mechanisms and functionality of probiotics will highlight the future of these friendly bacteria. Hereafter designating the most effective probiotic in certain clinical situations will be important. Gene technology will certainly play a role in not only clarifying the pharmacokinetic and the pharmacodynamic properties but also developing new strains. Well-designed, double-blind, placebo-controlled clinical trials are still needed to define further the role of probiotics as preventive and therapeutic agents.

REFERENCES

1. Food and Agriculture Organization of the United Nations and World Health Organization. Health and nutritional properties of probiotics in food, including powder milk with live lactic acid bacteria. World Health Organization Web site. http://www.who.int/foodsafety/publications/fs_management/en/probiotics.pdf

2. Parvez, S., Malik, K.A., Ah Kang, S., and Kim, H.Y., Probiotics and their fermented food products are beneficial for health, *J. Appl. Microbiol.*, 100 (6), 1171–1185, 2006.

3. Isolauri, E., Kirjavainen, P.V., and Salminen, S., Probiotics: A role in the treatment of intestinal infection and inflammation?, *Gut*, 50 (Suppl III), 54–59, 2002.

4. Madsen, K.L., The use of probiotics in gastrointestinal disease, *Can. J. Gastroenterol.*, 15, 817–822, 2001.

5. Reuter, G., The *Lactobacillus* and *Bifidobacterium* microflora of the human intestine: Composition and succession, *Curr. Issues Intest. Microbiol.*, 2, 43–53, 2001.

6. Katz, J.A. and Fiocchi, C., Probiotic therapy of IBD, *Inflamm. Bowel Dis.*, 2, 106–111, 2001.

7. Guslandi, M., Mezzi, G., Sorghi, M., and Testoni, P.A., *Saccharomyces boulardii* in maintenance treatment of Crohn's disease, *Dig. Dis. Sci.*, 45, 1462–1464, 2000.

8. Salminen, S. et al., Demonstration of safety of probiotics, *Int. J. Food Microbiol.*, 44, 93–106, 1998.

9. Van de Water, J., Keen, C.L., and Gershwin, M.E., The influence of chronic yogurt consumption on immunity, *J. Nutr.*, 129 (7 Suppl), 1492S-1495S, 1999.

10. Johnson, I.T., New food components and gastrointestinal health, *Proc. Nutr. Soc.*, 60 (4), 481–488, 2001.

11. Reyed, M.R., Probiotics: A new strategies for prevention and therapy of diarrhea disease, *J. Appl. Sci. Res.*, 3 (4): 291–299, 2007.

12. Metchnikoff, E., Sur la flore du corps humain, *Manchester Lit Philos Soc.*, 45, 1–38, 1901.

13. Leblanc, J., Fliss, I., and Matar, C., Induction of a humoral immune response following an *Escherichia coli* O157:H7 infection with an immunomodulatory peptidic fraction derived from *Lactobacillus helveticus*-fermented milk, *Clin. Diagn. Lab. Immunol.*, 11 (6), 1171–1181, 2004.

14. Berner, L.A. and O'Donnell, J.A., Functional foods and health claims legislation: Applications to dairy foods, *Int. Dairy J.*, 8, 355–362, 1998.

15. Dimer, C. and Gibson, G.R., An overview of probiotics, prebiotics and synbiotics in the functional food concept: Perspectives and future strategies, *Int. Dairy J.*, 8, 473–479, 1998.

16. Grajek, W., Olejnik, A., and Sip, A., Probiotics, prebiotics and antioxidants as functional foods, *Acta Biochim. Pol.*, 52, 665–71, 2005.

17. Salminen, S., Bouley, C., Boutron-Ruault, M.C., Cummings, J.H., Franck, A., Gibson, G.R., Isolauri, E., Moreau, M.C., Roberfroid, M., and Rowland, I., Functional food science and gastrointestinal physiology and function. *Br. J. Nutr.*, 80, S147–S171, 1998.

18. Harish, K., and Varghese, T., Probiotics in humans–evidence based review, *Calicut Medical Journal*, 4 (4), e3, 2006, http://www.calicutmedicaljournal.org/

19. Macfarlane, G.T. and Cummings, J.H., Probiotics, infection and immunity, *Curr. Opin. Infect. Dis.*, 15, 501–506, 2002.

20. Fujiwara, S., Seto, Y., Kimura, A., and Hashiba, H., Establishment of orally-administered *Lactobacillus gasseri* SBT2055SR in the gastrointestinal tract of humans and its influence on intestinal microflora and metabolism, *J. Appl. Microbiol.*, 90, 343–352, 2001.

21. van der Wielen, P.W., Lipman, L.J., van Knapen, F., and Biesterveld, S., Competitive exclusion of *Salmonella enterica* serovar *enteritidis* by *Lactobacillus crispatus* and

Clostridium lactatifermentans in a sequencing fed-batch culture, *Appl. Environ. Microbiol.*, 68, 555–559, 2002.

22. Asahara, T., Nomoto, K., Shimizu, K., Watanuki, M., and Tanaka, R., Increased resistance of mice to *Salmonella enterica* serovar *typhimurium* infection by synbiotic administration of bifidobacteria and transgalactosylated oligosaccharides, *J. Appl. Microbiol.*, 91, 985–996, 2001.

23. Mukai, T., Asasaka, T., Sato, E., Mori, K., Matsumoto, M., and Ohori, H., Inhibition of binding *of Helicobacter pylori* to glycolipid receptors by probiotic *Lactobacillus reuteri, FEMS Immunol. Med. Microbiol.*, 32, 105–110, 2002.

24. Bezkorovainy, A., Probiotics: Determinants of survival and growth in the gut, *Am. J. Clin. Nutr.*, 73, 399S–405S, 2001.

25. Jonsson, H., Strom, E., and Roos, S., Addition of mucin to the growth medium triggers mucus-binding activity in different strains of *Lactobacillus reuteri* in vitro, *FEMS Microbiol. Lett.*, 204, 19–22, 2001.

26. Dunne, C. et al., In vitro selection criteria for probiotic bacteria of human origin: Correlation with in vivo findings, *Am. J. Clin. Nutr.*, 73, 386S–392S, 2001.

27. Matsumoto, M., Tani, H., Ono, H., Ohishi, H., and Benno, Y., Adhesive property of *Bifidobacterium lactis* LKM512 and predominant bacteria of intestinal microflora to human intestinal mucin, *Curr. Microbiol.*, 44, 212–215, 2002.

28. Gibson, G. R. and Roberfroid, M. B., Dietary modulation of the human colonic microbiotia: Introducing the concept of prebiotics, *J. Nutr.*, 125, 1401–1412, 1995.

29. Douglas, L. C. and Sanders, M. E., Probiotics and prebiotics in dietetics practice, *J. Am. Diet Assoc.*, 108 (3), 510–521, 2008.

30. Prescott, L.M., Harley, J.P., and Klein, D.A., Symbiotic associations: Commensalism, mutualism, and the normal microbiota of the human body, *Microbiology* 4th ed., 577, McGraw-Hill Inc., USA, 1999.

31. Kaini, L., Bugs in our guts–not all bacteria are bad: How probiotics keep us healthy, 2006, http://www.csa.com/discoveryguides/discoveryguides-main.php.

32. Cabana, M.D., Shane, A.L., Chao, C., and Oliva-Hemker, M., Probiotics in primary care pediatrics, *Clin. Pediatr.*, 45, 405–410, 2006.

33. Fuller, R., Probiotics in human medicine, *Gut*, 32, 439–442, 1991.

34. Silva, M., Jacobus, N.V., Deneke, C., and Gorbach, S.L., Antimicrobial substance from a human Lactobacillus strain, *Antimicrob. Agents Chemother.*, 31, 1221–1233, 1987.

35. Sartor R.B., Probiotic therapy of intestinal inflammation and infections, *Curr. Opin. Gastroenterol.*, 21, 44–50, 2005.

36. Chermesh, I. and Eliakim, R., Probiotics and the gastrointestinal tract: Where are we in 2005?, *World J. Gastroenterol.*, 12 (6), 853–857, 2006.

37. Meier, R. and Steuerwald, M., Place of probiotics, *Curr. Opin. Crit. Care*, 11, 318–325, 2005.

38. Resta-Lenert, S. and Barrett, K. E., Live probiotics protect intestinal epithelial cells from the effects of infection with enteroinvasive *Escherichia coli* (EIEC), *Gut*, 52, 988–997, 2003.

39. Haller, D., Serrant, P., Peruisseau, G., Bode, C., Hammes, W.P., Schiffrin, E., and Blum, S., IL-10 producing CD14 low monocytes inhibit lymphocyte-dependent activation of intestinal epithelial cells by commensal bacteria, *Microbiol. Immunol.*, 46, 195–205, 2002.

40. Kaila, M., Isolauri, E., Soppi, E., Virtanen, E., Laine, S., and Arvilommi, H., Enhancement of the circulating antibody secreting cell response in human diarrhea by a human Lactobacillus strain, *Pediatr. Res.*, 32, 141–144, 1992.

41. Dotan, I. and Rachmilewitz, D., Probiotics in inflammatory bowel disease: Possible mechanisms of action, *Curr. Opin. Gastroenterol.*, 21, 426–430, 2005.

42. Yan, F. and Polk, D.B., Probiotic bacterium prevents cytokine-induced apoptosis in intestinal epithelial cells, *J. Biol. Chem.*, 277, 50959–50965, 2002.

43. Di Caro, S., Tao, H., Grillo, A., Elia, C., Gasbarrini, G., Sepulveda, A.R., and Gasbarrini, A., Effects of *Lactobacillus* GG on genes expression pattern in small bowel mucosa, *Dig. Liver Dis.*, 37, 320–329, 2005.

44. Fedorak, R.N. and Madsen, K.L., Probiotics and prebiotics in gastrointestinal disorders, *Curr. Opin. Gastroenterol.*, 20, 146–155, 2004.

45. Reid, G., Jass, J., Sebulsky, M.T., and McCormick, J.K., Potential uses of probiotics in clinical practice, *Clin. Microbiol. Rev.*, 16 (4), 658–672, 2003.

46. Guandalini, S., Probiotics for children: Use in diarrhea, *J. Clin. Gastroenterol.*, 40, 244–248, 2006.

47. Kim, M.N., The effects of probiotics on PPI-triple therapy for *Helicobacter pylori* eradication, *Helicobacter*, 13, 261–268, 2008.

48. Shane, A.L., Applications of probiotics for neonatal enteric diseases, *J. Perinat. Neonat. Nurs.*, 22 (3), 238–243, 2008.

49. Gadewar, S. and Fasano, A., Current concepts in the evaluation, diagnosis and management of acute infectious diarrhea, *Curr. Opin. Pharmacol.*, 5, 559–565, 2005.

50. Dinkçi, N., Ünal, G., Akalın, S., and Gönç, S., The importance of probiotics in pediatrics, *Pakistan J. Nutr.*, 5 (6), 608–611, 2006.

51. Bengmark, S. and Gil, A., Bioecological and nutritional control of disease: Prebiotics, probiotics and synbiotics, *Nutr. Hosp.*, 21 (Supl. 2), 72–84, 2006.

52. Rolfe, R.D., The role of probiotic cultures in the control of gastrointestinal health, *J. Nutr.*, 130, 396S–402S, 2000.

53. Sullivan, A. and. Nord, C.E, Probiotics in human infections, *J. Antimicrob. Chemother.*, 50, 625–627, 2002.

54. Alvarez-Olmos, M.I. and Oberhelman R.A., Probiotic agents and infectious diseases: A modern perspective on a traditional therapy, *Clin. Infect. Dis.*, 32, 1567–1576, 2001.

55. Heczko, P.B., Strus, M., and Kochan, P., Critical evaluation of probiotic activity of lactic acid bacteria and their effects, *J. Physiol. Pharmacol.*, 57 (Suppl 9), 5–12, 2006.

56. Oksanen, P.J., Salminen, S., Saxelin, M., Hämäläinen, P., Ihantola-Vormisto, A., Muurasniemi-Isoviita, L., Nikkari, S., Oksanen, T., Pörsti, I., and Salminen, E., Prevention of travellers' diarrhoea by *Lactobacillus* GG, *Ann. Med.*, 22, 53–56, 1990.

57. Scarpignato, C. and Rampal, P., Prevention and treatment of traveler's diarrhea: A clinical pharmacological approach, *Chemotherapy*, 41 (suppl. 1), 48–81, 1995.

58. Hilton, E., Kolakowski, P., Singer, C., and Smith, M. Efficacy of *Lactobacillus* GG as a diarrheal preventive in travelers, *J. Travel Med.*, 4, 41–43, 1997.

59. Salminen, A. and Deighton, M., Lactic acid bacteria in the gut in normal and disorders states, *Dig. Dis.*, 10, 227–238, 1992.

60. Black, F.T., Anderson, P.L., Orskov, J., Orskov, F., Gaarslev, K., and Laulund, S. Prophylactic efficacy of Lactobacilli on traveller's diarrhea, *Travel Med.*, 8, 333–335, 1989.

61. Allen, S.J, Okoko, B., Martinez, E., Gregorio, G., and Dans, L.F., Probiotics for treating infectious diarrhoea, *Cochrane Database Syst. Rev.*, 2, CD003048, 2004.

62. Younghoon, K., Inhibition of *Escherichia coli* O157:H7 attachment by interactions between Lactic Acid Bacteria and intestinal epithelial cells, *J. Microbiol. Biotechnol.*, 18 (7), 1278–1285, 2008.

63. Kollaritsch, H. and Wiedermann, G., Compliance of Austrian tourists with prophylactic measures, *Eur. J. Epidemiol.*, 8 (2), 243–51, 1992.

64. Van Niel, C.W., Feudtner, C., Garrison, M.M., and Christakis, D.A., *Lactobacillus* therapy for acute infectious diarrhea in children: A meta-analysis, *Pediatrics*, 109 (4), 678–684, 2002.

65. Rosenfeldt, V., Michaelsen, K.F., Jakobsen, M., Larsen, C.N., Møller, P.L., Tvede, M., Weyrehter, H., Valerius, N.H., and Paerregaard, A., Effect of probiotic *Lactobacillus* strains on acute diarrhea in a cohort of nonhospitalized children attending day-care centers, *Pediatr. Infect. Dis. J.*, 21 (5), 417–419, 2002.

66. Teitelbaum, J.E., Probiotics and the treatment of infectious diarrhea, *Pediatr. Infect. Dis. J.*, 24, 267–268, 2005.

67. Guandalini, S. et al., *Lactobacillus* GG administered in oral rehydration solution to children with acute diarrhea: A multicenter European trial, *J. Pediatr. Gastroenterol. Nutr.*, 30, 54–60, 2000.

68. Szajewska, H. and Mrukowicz, J.Z., Probiotics in the treatment and prevention of acute infectious diarrhea in infants and children: A systematic review of published randomized, double-blind, placebo-controlled trials, *J. Pediatr. Gastroenterol. Nutr.*, 33 (suppl 2), S17–S25, 2001.

69. Shornikova, A.V., Casas, I.A., Mykkänen, H., Salo, E., and Vesikari, T., Bacteriotherapy with *Lactobacillus reuteri* in rotavirus gastroenteritis, *Pediatr. Infect. Dis. J.*, 16, 1103–1107, 1997.

70. Isolauri, E., Juntunen, M., Rautanen, T., Sillanaukee, P., and Koivula, T., A human Lactobacillus strain (*Lactobacillus casei* sp strain GG) promotes recovery from acute diarrhea in children, *Pediatrics*, 88, 90–97, 1991.

71. Kaila, M., Isolauri, E., Saxelin, M., Arvilommi, H., and Vesikari, T., Viable versus inactivated lactobacillus strain GG in acute rotavirus diarrhoea, *Arch. Dis. Child*, 72, 51–53, 1995.

72. Huang, J.S., Bousvaros, A., Lee, J.W., Diaz, A., and Davidson, E.J., Efficacy of probiotic use in acute diarrhea in children: A meta-analysis, *Dig. Dis. Sci.*, 47, 2625–2634, 2002.

73. Rosenfeldt, V., Michaelsen, K.F., Jakobsen, M., Larsen, C.N., Møller, P.L., Pedersen, P., Tvede, M., Weyrehter, H., Valerius, N.H., and Paerregaard, A., Effect of probiotic Lactobacillus strains in young children hospitalized with acute diarrhea, *Pediatr. Infect. Dis. J.*, 21, 411–416, 2002.

74. Hotcher, D.U., Chase, W., and Hagenhoff, G., *Saccharomyces boulardii* in acute adult diarrhoea. Efficacy and tolerability of treatment, *Munch. Med. Wschr.*, 132, 188–192, 1990.

75. Wullt, M., Hagslatt, M.L., and Odenholt, I., *Lactobacillus plantarum* 299v for the treatment of recurrent *Clostridium difficile*-associated diarrhoea: A double-blind, placebo-controlled trial, *Scand. J. Infect. Dis.*, 35, 365–367, 2003.

76. Cremonini, F, Di Caro, S., Nista, E.C., Bartolozzi, F., Capelli, G., Gasbarrini, G., and Gasbarrini, A., Meta-analysis: The effect of probiotic administration on antibiotic-associated diarrhoea. *Aliment Pharmacol. Ther.*, 16, 1461–1467, 2002.

77. D'Souza, A.L, Rajkumar, C., Cooke, J., and Bulpitt, C.J., Probiotics in prevention of antibiotic associated diarrhoea: Meta-analysis, *BMJ*, 324, 1361, 2002, http://bmj.com/cgi/content/full/324/7350/1361

78. Siitonen, S., Vapaatalo, H., Salminen, S., Gordin, A., Saxelin, M., Wikberg, R., and Kirkkola, A.L., Effect of *Lactobacillus* GG yoghurt in prevention of antibiotic associated diarrhoea, *Ann. Med.*, 22, 57–59, 1990.

79. Vanderhoof, J.A., Whitney, D.B., Antonson, D.L., Hanner, T.L., Lupo, J.V., and Young, R.J., *Lactobacillus* GG in the prevention of antibiotic associated diarrhea in children. *J. Pediat.*, 135, 564–568, 1999.

80. Szajewska, H., Kotowska, M., Mrukowicz, J.Z., Armańska, M., and Mikołajczyk, W., Efficacy of *Lactobacillus* GG in prevention of nosocominal diarrhea in infants, *J. Pediat.*, 138, 361–365, 2001.

81. Biller, J.A., Katz, A.J., Flores, A F., Buie, T.M., and Gorbach, S.L., Treatment of recurrent *Clostridium difficile* colitis with *Lactobacillus* GG, *J. Pediatr. Gastroenterol. Nutr.*, 21, 224–226, 1995.

82. Lewis, S.J., Potts, L.F., and Barry, R.E., The lack of therapeutic effect of *Saccharomyces boulardii* in the prevention of antibiotic related diarrhoea in elderly patients, *J. Infect.*, 36, 171–174, 1998.

83. Dendukuri, N., Costa, V., McGregor, M., and Brophy, J.M., Probiotic therapy for the prevention and treatment of *Clostridium difficile*-associated diarrhea: A systematic review. *CMAJ*, 173, 167–170, 2005.

84. Borody, T.J., Warren, E.F., Leis, S.M., Surace, R., Ashman, O., and Siarakas, S., Bacteriotherapy using fecal microbiota. Toying with human motions, *J. Clin. Gastroenterol.*, 38, 475–483, 2004.

85. Ahuja, M.C. and Khamar, B., Antibiotic associated diarrhoea: A controlled study comparing plain antibiotic with those containing protected lactobacilli, *J. Indian Med. Assoc.*, 100, 334–335, 2002.

86. McFarland, L.V., Surawicz, C.M., Greenberg, R.N., Elmer, G.W., Moyer, K.A., Melcher, S.A., Bowen, K.E., and Cox, J.L., Prevention of β-lactam associated diarrhoea by *Saccharomyces boulardii* compared to placebo, *Am. J. Gastroenterol.*, 90, 439–444, 1995.

87. Gotz, V., Romankiewicz, J.A., Moss, J., and Murray, H.W., Prophylaxis against ampicillin associated diarrhoea with *Lactobacillus* preparation, *Am. J. Hosp. Pharm.*, 36, 754–757, 1979.

88. Zoppi, G., Deganello, A., Benoni, G., and Saccomani, F., Oral bacteriotherapy in clinical practice. I. The use of different preparations in infants treated with antibiotics. *Eur. J. Pediatr.*, 139, 18–21, 1982.

89. Wunderlich, P.F., Braun, L., Fumagalli, I., D'Apuzzo, V., Heim, F., Karly, M., Lodi, R., Politta, G., Vonbank, F., and Zeltner, L., Double bind report on the efficacy of lactic acid producing *Enterococcus* SF 68 in the prevention of antibiotic associated diarrhoea and in the treatment of acute diarrhoea, *J. Int. Med., Res.*, 17, 333–338, 1989.

90. Bellomo, G., Mangiagle, A., Nicastro, L., and Frigerio, G., A controlled double blind study of SF 68 strain as a new biological preparation for the treatment of diarrhoea in pediatrics, *Curr. Ther. Res. Clin. Exp.*, 28, 927–936, 1980.

91. Sullivan, A., Barkholt, L., and Nord, C.E., *Lactobacillus acidophilus, Bifidobacterium lactis* and *Lactobacillus* F19 prevent antibiotic-associated ecological disturbances of *Bacteroides fragilis* in the intestine, *J. Antimicrob. Chemother.*, 52, 308–311, 2003.

92. Szajewska, H., Ruszczynski, M., and Radzikowski, A., Probiotics in the prevention of antibiotic associated diarrhea in children: A meta-analysis of randomized controlled trials, *J. Pediatr.*, 149, 367–372, 2006.

93. Born, P., Lersch, C., Zimmerhackl, B., and Classen, M. The *Saccharomyces boulardii* therapy of HIV-associated diarrhea (letter), *Dtsch. Med. Wochenschr.* 118, 765, 1993.

94. Saint-Marc, T., Rossello-Prats, L., and Touraine, J.L., Efficacy of *Saccharomyces boulardii* in the treatment of diarrhea in AIDS (letter), *Ann. Med. Intern.*, 142, 64–65, 1991.

95. Elmer, G.W., Moyer, K.A., Vega, R., Surawicz, C.M., Collier, A.C., Hooton, T.M., and McFarland, L.V., Evaluation of *Saccharomyces boulardii* for patients with HIV-related chronic diarrhoea and healthy volunteers receiving antifungals, *Microecol. Ther.*, 25, 23–31, 1995.

96. Donner, C.S., Pathophysiology and therapy of chronic radiation-induced injury to the colon, *Dig. Dis.*, 16, 253–261, 1998.

97. Delia, P., Sansotta, G., Donato, V., Messina, G., Frosina, P., Pergolizzi, S., De Renzis, C., and Famularo, G., Prevention of radiation-induced diarrhea with the use of VSL#3, a new high-potency probiotic preparation, *Am. J. Gastroenterol.*, 97, 2150–2152, 2002.

98. Urbancsek, H., Kazar, T., Mezes, I., Neumann, K., Results of a double-blind, randomized study to evaluate the efficacy and safety of *Antibiophilus* in patients with radiation-induced diarrhoea, *Eur. J. Gastroenterol. Hepatol.*, 13, 391–396, 2001.

99. Malfertheiner, P., Mégraud, F., O'Morain, C., Hungin, A.P., Jones, R., Axon, A., Graham, D.Y., and Tytgat, G., European Helicobacter Pylori Study Group (EHPSG), Current

concepts in the management of *Helicobacter pylori* infection—the Maastricht 2–2000 Consensus Report, *Aliment. Pharmacol. Ther.*, 16, 167–180, 2002.

100. Malfertheiner, P., Megraud, F., O'Morain, C., Bazzoli, F., El-Omar, E., Graham, D., Hunt, R., Rokkas, T., Vakil, N., and Kuipers, E.J., Current concepts in the management of *Helicobacter pylori* infection–The Maastricht III Consensus Report, *Gut*, 56, 772–781, 2007.

101. Houben, M.H., van de Beek, D., Hensen, E.F., Craen, A.J., Rauws, E.A., and Tytgat, G.N., A systematic review of *Helicobacter pylori* eradication therapy—the impact of antimicrobial resistance on eradication rates, *Aliment. Pharmacol. Ther.*, 13, 1047–1055, 1999.

102. Myllyluoma, E., The role of probiotics in Helicobacter pylori infection, Foundation for Food Research of the Finnish Food and Drink. Industries' Federation, Helsinki, Finland, 2007, https://oa.doria.fi/bitstream/handle/10024/5622/theroleo.pdf?sequence = 1

103. Felley, C.P. et al., Favourable effect of an acidified milk (LC-1) on *Helicobacter pylori* gastritis in man, *Eur. J. Gastroenterol. Hepatol.*, 13, 25–29, 2001.

104. Armuzzi, A. et al., The effect of oral administration of *Lactobacillus* GG on antibiotic-associated gastrointestinal side effects during *Helicobacter pylori* eradication therapy. *Aliment. Pharmacol. Ther.*, 15, 163–169, 2001.

105. Canducci, F., Armuzzi, A., Cremonini, F., Cammarota, G., Bartolozzi, F., Pola, P., Gasbarrini, G., and Gasbarrini, A., A lyophilized and inactivated culture of *Lactobacillus acidophilus* increases *Helicobacter pylori* eradication rates. *Aliment. Pharmacol. Ther.*, 14, 1625–1629, 2000.

106. Gotteland, M., Brunser, O., and Cruchet, S., Systematic review: are probiotics useful in controlling gastric colonization by *Helicobacter pylori*?, *Aliment. Pharmacol. Ther.*, 23, 1077–1086, 2006.

107. Lionetti, E, Miniello, V.L., Castellaneta, S.P., Magistá, A.M., de Canio, A., Maurogiovanni, G., Ierardi, E., Cavallo, L., and Francavilla, R., *Lactobacillus reuteri* therapy to reduce side-effects during anti-*Helicobacter pylori* treatment in children: A randomized placebo controlled trial, *Aliment. Pharmacol. Ther.*, 24, 1461–1468, 2006.

108. Madden, J.A.J., Plummer, S.F., Tang, J., Garaiova, I., Plummer, N.T., Herbison, M., Hunter, J.O., Shimada, T., Cheng, L., and Shirakawa, T., Effect of probiotics on preventing disruption of the intestinal microflora following antibiotic therapy: A double-blind, placebo-controlled pilot study, *Int. Immunopharmacol.*, 5, 1091–1097, 2005.

109. Plummer, S.F., Garaiova, I., Sarvotham, T., Cottrell, S.L., Le Scouiller, S., Weaver, M.A., Tang, J., Dee, P., and Hunter, J., Effects of probiotics on the composition of the intestinal microbiota following antibiotic therapy, *Int. J. Antimicrob. Agents*, 26, 69–74, 2005.

110. Sakamoto, I., Igarashi, M., Kimura, K., Takagi, A., Miwa, T., and Koga, Y. Suppressive effect of *Lactobacillus gasseri OLL* 2716 (LG21) on *Helicobacter pylori* infection in humans, *J. Antimicrob. Chemother.*, 47, 709–710, 2001.

111. Sheu, B.S., Cheng, H.C., Kao, A.W., Wang, S.T., Yang, Y.J., Yang, H.B., and Wu, J.J., Pretreatment with *Lactobacillus*- and *Bifidobacterium*-containing yogurt can improve the efficacy of quadruple therapy in eradicating residual *Helicobacter pylori* infection after failed triple therapy, *Am. J. Clin. Nutr.*, 83, 864–869, 2006.

112. Tursi, A., Brandimarte, G., Giorgetti, G.M., and Modeo, M.E., Effect of *Lactobacillus casei* supplementation on the effectiveness and tolerability of a new second-line 10-day quadruple therapy after failure of a first attempt to cure *Helicobacter pylori* infection, *Med. Sci. Monit.*, 10, 662–666, 2004.

113. Marteau, P., Minekus, M., Havenaar, R., and Huis in't Veld, J.H., Survival of lactic acid bacteria in a dynamic model of the stomach and small intestine: Validation and the effects of bile, *J. Dairy Sci.*, 80, 1031–1037, 1997.

114. Ushiyama, A., Tanaka, K., Aiba, Y., Shiba, T., Takagi, A., Mine, T., and Koga, Y., *Lactobacillus gasseri* OLL2716 as a probiotic in clarithromycin-resistant *Helicobacter pylori* infection, *J. Gastroenterol. Hepatol.*, 18, 986–991, 2003.

115. Kim, M.N. et al., The effects of probiotics on PPI-triple therapy for *Helicobacter pylori* eradication, *Helicobacter*, 13 (4), 261–268, 2008.

116. Myllyluoma, E., Veijola, L., Ahlroos, T., Tynkkynen, S., Kankuri, E., Vapaatalo, H., Rautelin, H., and Korpela, R., Probiotic supplementation improves tolerance to *Helicobacter pylori* eradication therapy—a placebo-controlled, double-blind randomized pilot study, *Aliment. Pharmacol. Ther.*, 21 (10), 1263–1272, 2005.

117. Myllyluoma, E., Effects of multispecies probiotic combination on *Helicobacter pylori* infection in vitro, *Clin. Vaccine Immunol.*, 15 (9), 1472–1482, 2008.

118. Felley, C.P. et al., Favourable effect of an acidified milk (LC-1) on *Helicobacter pylori* gastritis in man, *Eur. J. Gastroenterol. Hepatol.*, 13, 25–29, 2001.

119. Cruchet, S., Obregon, M.C., Salazar, G., Diaz, E., and Gotteland, M.., Effect of the ingestion of a dietary product containing *Lactobacillus johnsonii* La1 on *Helicobacter pylori*-colonization in children, *Nutrition*, 19, 716–721, 2003.

120. Cats, A., Kuipers, E.J., Bosschaert, M.A., Pot, R.G., Vandenbroucke-Grauls, C.M., and Kusters, J.G., Effect of frequent consumption of a *Lactobacillus casei*-containing milk drink in *Helicobacter pylori*-colonized subjects, *Aliment. Pharmacol. Ther.*, 17, 429–435, 2003.

121. Pantoflickova, D., Corthésy-Theulaz, I., Dorta, G., Stolte, M., Isler, P., Rochat, F., Enslen, M., and Blum, A.L., Favourable effect of regular intake of fermented milk containing *Lactobacillus johnsonii* on *Helicobacter pylori* associated gastritis, *Aliment. Pharmacol. Ther.*, 18, 805–813, 2003.

122. Wang, K.Y., Li, S.N., Liu, C.S., Perng, D.S., Su, Y.C., Wu, D.C., Jan, C.M., Lai, C.H., Wang, T.N., and Wang, W.M., Effects of ingesting *Lactobacillus*- and *Bifidobacterium*-containing yogurt in subjects with colonized *Helicobacter pylori*, *Am. J. Clin. Nutr.*, 80, 737–741, 2004.

123. Wendakoon, C.N., Thomson, A.B., and Ozimek, L., Lack of therapeutic effect of a specially designed yogurt for the eradication of *Helicobacter pylori* infection, *Digestion*, 65, 16–20, 2002.

124. Yoshita, M., Fujita, K., and Sakata, H., Development of the normal intestinal flora and its clinical significance in infants and children, *Bifido. Microflora*, 10, 11–27, 1991.

125. Hoyos, A.B., Reduced incidence of necrotizing enterocolitis associated with enteral administration of *Lactobacillus acidophilus* and *Bifidobacterium infantis* to neonates in an intensive care unit, *Int. J. Infect. Dis.*, 3, 197–202, 1999.

126. Stricker, T. and Braegger, C.P., Oral probiotics prevent necrotizing enterocolitis, *J. Pediatr. Gastroenterol. Nutr.*, 42, 446–447, 2006.

127. Reid, G., Probiotic agents to protect the urogenital tract against infection, *Am. J. Clin. Nutr.*, 73 Suppl., 437–43, 2001.

128. Famularo, G., Perluigi, M., Coccia, R., Mastroiacovo, P., and De Simone, C., Microecology, bacterial vaginosis and probiotics: Perspectives for bacteriotherapy, *Medical Hypotheses*, 56, 421–30, 2001.

129. Reid, G. and Bruce, A.W., Low vaginal pH and urinary-tract infection, Lancet, Dec 23–30, 346 (8991–8992), 1704, 1995.

130. Reid, G., Beuerman, D., Heinemann, C., and Bruce, A.W., Probiotic *Lactobacillus* dose required to restore and maintain a normal vaginal flora, *FEMS Immunol. Med. Microbiol.*, 32 (1), 37–41, 2001.

131. Falagas, M.E., Betsi, G.I., Tokas, T., and Athanasiou, S., Probiotics for prevention of recurrent urinary tract infections in women: A review of the evidence from microbiological and clinical studies, *Drugs*, 66, 1253–1261, 2006.

132. Sewankambo, N. et al., *HIV-1* infection associated with abnormal vaginal flora morphology and bacterial vaginosis, *Lancet*, 350, 546–550, 1997.

133. Cohen, C.R., Duerr, A., Pruithithada, N., Rugpao, S., Hillier, S., Garcia, P., Nelson, K., Bacterial vaginosis and *HIV* seroprevalence among female commercial sex workers in Chiang Mai, Thailand, *AIDS*, 9,1093–1097, 1995.

134. Liu, J.J., Reid, G., Jiang, Y., Turner, M.S., and Tsai, C.C., Activity of *HIV* entry and fusion inhibitors expressed by the human vaginal colonizing probiotic *Lactobacillus reuteri* RC-14, *Cell Microbiol.*, 9 (1), 120–130, 2007.

135. Oláh, A., Belágyi, T., Issekutz, A., Gamal, M.E., and Bengmark, S., Randomized clinical trial of specific lactobacillus and fibre supplement to early enteral nutrition in patients with acute pancreatitis, *Br. J. Surg.*, 89, 1103–1107, 2002.

136. Pezzilli, R. and Fantini, L., Probiotics and severe acute pancreatitis, *JOP*, 7, 92–93, 2006.

137. Akyol, S. et al., The effect of antibiotic and probiotic combination therapy on secondary pancreatic infections and oxidative stress parameters in experimental acute necrotizing pancreatitis. *Pancreas*, 26, 363–367, 2003.

138. Besselink, M.G.H. et al., Dutch Acute Pancreatitis Study Group., Probiotic prophylaxis in predicted severe acute pancreatitis: A randomised, double-blind, placebo-controlled trial, Dutch Acute Pancreatitis Study Group, *Lancet*, 371, 651–659, 2008.

139. Sun, S., Yang, K., He, X., Tian, J., Ma, B., and Jiang, L., Probiotics in patients with severe acute pancreatitis: A meta-analysis. *Langenbecks Arch. Surg.*, 394, 171–177, 2009.

140. Oláh, A., Belágyi, T., Pótó, L., Romics, L. Jr., and Bengmark, S., Synbiotic control of inflammation and infection in severe acute pancreatitis: A prospective, randomized, double blind study, *Hepatogastroenterology*, 54, 590–594, 2007.

141. Li, Y.M., Adjuvant therapy for probiotics in patients with severe acute pancreatitis: An analysis of 14 cases, *World Chinese J. Digest.*, 15, 302–304, 2007.

142. Wanke, C.A., Do probiotics prevent childhood illnesses?, *BMJ*, 322, 1318–1319, 2001.

143. Falagas, M.E., Rafailidis, P.I., and Makris, G.C., Bacterial interference for the prevention and treatment of infections, *Int. J. Antimicrob. Agents.*, 31 (6), 518–522, 2008.

144. Pregliasco, F., Anselmi, G., Fonte, L., Giussani, F., Schieppati, S., and Soletti, L., A new chance of preventing winter diseases by the administration of synbiotic formulations, *J. Clin. Gastroenterol.*, 42 Suppl 3, Pt 2, S224-S233, 2008.

145. de Vrese, M. et al., Probiotic bacteria reduced duration and severity but not the incidence of common cold episodes in a double blind, randomized, controlled trial, *Vaccine*, 10, 24 (44–46), 6670–6674, 2006.

146. Hatakka, K., Blomgren, K., Pohjavuori, S., Kaijalainen, T., Poussa, T., Leinonen, M., Korpela, R., and Pitkäranta, A., Treatment of acute otitis media with probiotics in otitis-prone children-a double-blind, placebo-controlled randomised study, *Clin. Nutr.*, 26 (3), 314–321, 2007.

147. Islam, B., Khan, S.N., and Khan, A.U., Dental caries: from infection to prevention, *Med. Sci. Monit.*, 13 (11), RA196–RA203, 2007.

148. Kõll, P., Mändar, R., Marcotte, H., Leibur, E., Mikelsaar, M., and Hammarström, L., Characterization of oral lactobacilli as potential probiotics for oral health, *Oral Microbiol. Immunol.*, 23 (2), 139–147, 2008.

149. Caglar, E., Kuscu, O.O., Selvi Kuvvetli, S., Kavaloglu Cildir, S., Sandalli, N., and Twetman, S., Short-term effect of ice-cream containing *Bifidobacterium lactis* Bb-12 on the number of salivary mutans streptococci and lactobacilli, *Acta Odontol. Scand.*, 66 (3), 154–158, 2008.

150. Caglar E, Kuscu, O.O., Cildir, S.K., Kuvvetli, S.S., and Sandalli, N., A probiotic lozenge administered medical device and its effect on salivary mutans streptococci and lactobacilli. *Int. J. Paediatr. Dent.*, 18 (1), 5–9, 2008.

151. Twetman, S. and Stecksén-Blicks, C., Probiotics and oral health effects in children, Int. *J. Paediatr. Dent.*, 18 (1), 3–10, 2008.
152. Meurman, J.H. and Stamatova, I., Probiotics: Contributions to oral health, *Oral Dis.*, 13 (5), 443–451, 2007.
153. Simark-Mattsson, C., Emilson, C.G., Håkansson, E.G., Jacobsson, C., Roos, K., and Holm, S., *Lactobacillus*-mediated interference of mutans streptococci in caries-free vs. caries-active subjects, *Eur. J. Oral Sci.*, 115 (4), 308–314, 2007.
154. Caglar, E., Sandalli, N., Twetman, S., Kavaloglu, S., Ergeneli, S., and Selvi, S., Effect of yogurt with *Bifidobacterium* DN-173 010 on salivary mutans streptococci and lactobacilli in young adults, *Acta Odontol. Scand.*, 63 (6), 317–320, 2005.
155. Näse, L., Hatakka, K., Savilahti, E., Saxelin, M., Pönkä, A., Poussa, T., Korpela, R., and Meurman, J.H., Effect of long-term consumption of a probiotic bacterium, *Lactobacillus rhamnosus* GG, in milk on dental caries and caries risk in children, *Caries Res.*, 35 (6), 412–420, 2001.
156. Valdéz, J.C., Peral, M.C., Rachid, M., Santana, M., and Perdigón, G., Interference of Lactobacillus plantarum with *Pseudomonas aeruginosa* in vitro and in infected burns: The potential use of probiotics in wound treatment, *Clin. Microbiol. Infect.*, 11 (6), 472–479, 2005.
157. Plantin, P., What is the value of non-immunosuppressor therapy in the treatment of atopic dermatitis?, *Ann. Dermatol. Venereol.*, 132 Spec No 1, 1S73-1S78, 2005.
158. Borriello, S.P., Hammes, W.P., Holzapfel, W., Marteau, P., Schrezenmeir, J., Vara, M., and Valtonen, V., Safety of probiotics that contain lactobacilli or bifidobacteria, *Clin. Infect. Dis.*, 36, 775–780, 2003.
159. Thompson Healthcare. Probiotics. http://www.pdrhealth.com/drug_info/nmdrugprofiles/nutsupdrugs/pro_0034.shtml
160. Munoz, P., Bouza, E., Cuenca-Estrella, M., Eiros, J.M., Pérez, M.J., Sánchez-Somolinos, M., Rincón, C., Hortal, J., and Peláez, T., *Saccharomyces cerevisiae* fungemia: An emerging infectious disease, *Clin. Infect. Dis.*, 40, 1625–1634, 2005.
161. Riquelme, A.J., Calvo, M.A., Guzmán, A.M., Depix, M.S., García, P., Pérez, C., Arrese, M., and Labarca, J.A., *Saccharomyces cerevisiae* fungemia after *Saccharomyces boulardii* treatment in immunocompromised patients, *J. Clin. Gastroenterol.*, 36, 41–43, 2003.
162. Candelli, M., Nista, E.C., Nestola, M., Armuzzi, A., Silveri, N.G., Gasbarrini, G., and Gasbarrini, A., *Saccharomyces cerevisiae* associated diarrhea in an immunocompetent patient with ulcerative colitis, *J. Clin. Gastroenterol.*, 36, 39–40, 2003.
163. Salminen, M.K., Rautelin, H., Tynkkynen, S., Poussa, T., Saxelin, M., Valtonen, V., and Järvinen, A., Lactobacillus bacteremia, clinical significance, and patient outcome, with special focus on probiotic *L. rhamnosus* GG, *Clin. Infect. Dis.*, 38, 62–69, 2004.

Index

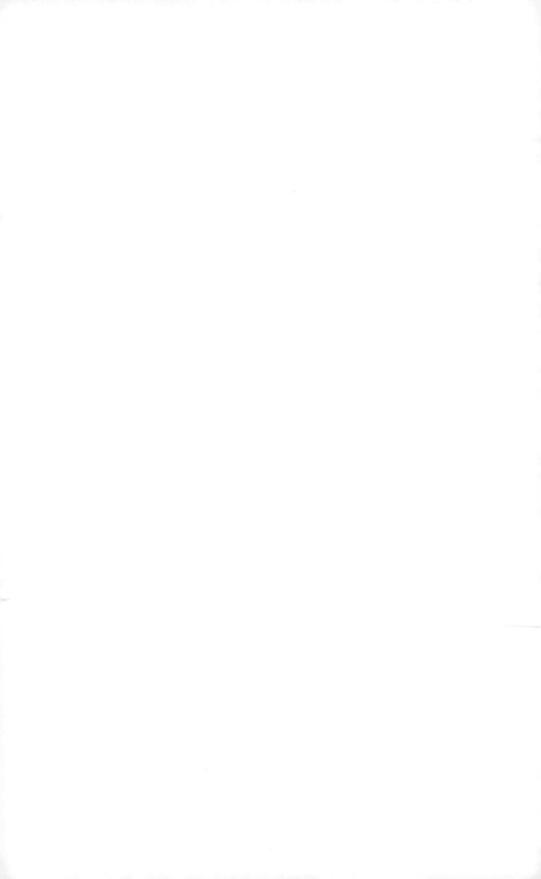

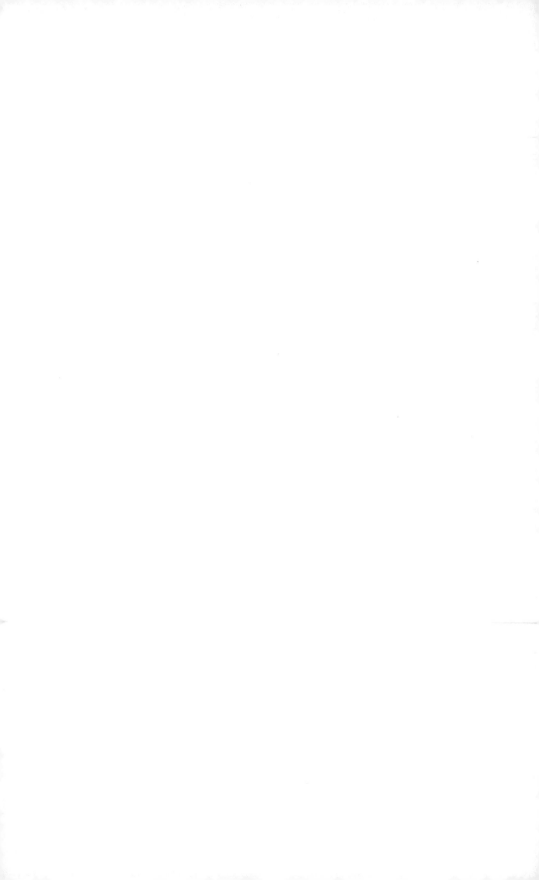

T - #0335 - 071024 - C4 - 234/156/20 - PB - 9780367384838 - Gloss Lamination